Atlas of Emergency Medicine Procedures

Latha Ganti

Editor

Atlas of Emergency Medicine Procedures

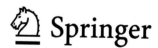

Editor
Latha Ganti
Professor of Emergency Medicine
University of Central Florida
Director, SE Specialty Care Centers of Innovation
Orlando Veterans Affairs Medical Center
Orlando, FL
USA

ISBN 978-1-4939-2506-3   ISBN 978-1-4939-2507-0   (eBook)
DOI 10.1007/978-1-4939-2507-0

Library of Congress Control Number: 2016930028

Springer New York Heidelberg Dordrecht London

Printed on acid-free paper

Springer Science+Business Media LLC New York is part of Springer Science+Business Media (www.springer.com)

To my father, my role model and career coach –
Dr. Ganti L. Rao
*Dad, I wouldn't have had the career I do were it
not for you. Your unconditional belief in me, your confidence in
my success, your never ending patience and generosity – you
lead a life of great achievements with utmost humility.
It is my privilege to be your daughter.*

Preface

The *Atlas of Emergency Medicine Procedures* is presented in the spirit of "see one, do one, teach one" and "a picture is worth a thousand words." It can be used at the bedside, both by novice practitioners and seasoned clinicians as a teaching aid. For ease of reference, the most common procedures are grouped by organ systems. Each procedure follows a standardized format, beginning with keywords, a definition if appropriate, indications, and contraindications. These are followed by materials and medications, often accompanied by a photograph of the specific equipment or setup. The procedure itself is numbered rather than bulleted, highlighting the sequence of steps. Photographs are placed where the relevant information is encountered in the text rather than at the end. Every procedure also lists complications. Finally, there is a section on pearls and pitfalls, gleaned from the collective experience of the contributors in addition to traditional teachings.

Emergency medicine, by nature, is a field best suited to a visually appealing, concise text able to deliver the information required. Much effort therefore has been dedicated to images. These are either actual photographs taken of the procedure steps or specially commissioned drawings by Springer's professional illustration team. A work of this magnitude could not have been accomplished without the expertise of my dedicated Springer team. A huge thank you to Shelly Reinhardt, Megan Ruzomberka, and Lee Klein. It is hoped that readers will find this atlas useful and practical. Feedback and suggestions for future editions are welcomed and can be sent to AtlasEMprocedures@gmail.com.

Orlando, FL, USA   Latha Ganti

Contents

Associate Editors

Lars K. Beattie, MD
Bobby K. Desai, MD
Marie-Carmelle Elie, MD
Judith K. Lucas, MD
L. Connor Nickels, MD
Department of Emergency Medicine
University of Florida
Gainesville, FL, USA

Sapna Amin, MD
Central Florida Healthcare
Mulberry, FL, USA

Ad-Hoc Reviewers

Linda Sheehan-Foster, PA-C
Jason Williams, RN
Lake City Veterans Affairs Medical Center
Lake City, Florida

Tej Geoffrey Stead
Buccholz High School
Gainesville, Florida

Models

Lars K. Beattie
Eike Flach
Tatiana Havryliuk
Katy Howard
Ben M. Mahon
Pratik S. Patel
Joseph Rabinovich
Thor Shiva Stead
Karthik Dax Stead
Clarence R. Tucker

Contributors

Michael A. Abraham, DMD United States Air Force, Dental Corps, Minot, ND, USA

Abimbola O. Adewumi, BDS, FDSR Department of Pediatric Dentistry, University of Florida College of Dentistry, Gainesville, FL, USA

Amish Aghera, MD Department of Emergency Medicine, Maimonides Medical Center, New York, NY, USA

Derek Ailes, MD Department of Emergency Medicine, Lincoln Medical and Mental Health Center, New York, NY, USA

Saadia Akhtar, MD Department of Emergency Medicine, Mount Sinai Beth Israel, New York, NY, USA

Brandon R. Allen, MD Department of Emergency Medicine, University of Florida, Gainesville, FL, USA

Hassan M. Alnuaimat, MD Department of Medicine, University of Florida, University of Florida Health Shands Hospital, Gainesville, FL, USA

Sapnalaxmi Amin, MD Department of Family Medicine/Urgent Care, Bayside Urgent Care Center, Clearwater, FL, USA

Michael Anana, MD Emergency Department, University Hospital, Rutgers New Jersey Medical School, Newark, NJ, USA

Amir Azari, DMD Department of Oral and Maxillofacial Surgery, Oregon Health and Science University, Portland, OR, USA

Lars K. Beattie, MD, MS Department of Emergency Medicine, University of Florida, Gainesville, FL, USA

Deena Bengiamin, MD Department of Emergency Medicine, University of San Francisco Fresno, Fresno, CA, USA

Justin Bennett, MD Department of Emergency Medicine, Wake Forest University School of Medicine, Winston-Salem, NC, USA

Oliver Michael Berrett, MD Department of Emergency Medicine, Lincoln Medical and Mental Health Center, New York, NY, USA

Irina Fox Brennan, MD Department of Emergency Medicine, University of Florida, Gainesville, FL, USA

Nicholas D. Caputo, MD, MSc Emergency Department Critical Care, Lincoln Medical and Mental Health Center, New York, NY, USA

Bharath Chakravarthy, MD, MPH Department of Emergency Medicine, University of California Irvine, Orange, CA, USA

Holly H. Charleton, MD Emergency Department, The Brooklyn Hospital Center, Brooklyn, NY, USA

Justin Chen, MD, MSc Department of Emergency Medicine, North Shore University Hospital, Manhasset, NY, USA

Christian Coletti, MD Department of Emergency Medicine and Internal Medicine, Christiana Care Health System, Newark, DE, USA

Ali H. Dabaja, DO Division of Critical Care, Department of Anesthesia, University of Florida, Gainesville, FL, USA

Dawood G. Dalaly, DO Department of Surgery, University of Florida, Gainesville, FL, USA

Giuliano De Portu, MD Department of Emergency Medicine, University of Florida, Gainesville, FL, USA

Bobby K. Desai, MD Department of Emergency Medicine, University of Florida, Gainesville, FL, USA

Rui Domingues, MD Department of Emergency Medicine, Lincoln Medical and Mental Health Center, New York, NY, USA

Lee Richard Donner, MD Emergency Medicine Department, Lincoln Medical and Mental Health Center, New York, NY, USA

Tina Dulani, MD Department of Emergency Medicine, New York Methodist Hospital, Brooklyn, NY, USA

Marie-Carmelle Elie, MD, RDMS Department of Emergency Medicine, University of Florida, Gainesville, FL, USA

Etan Eitches, MD Department of Emergency Medicine, Beth Israel Medical Center, New York, NY, USA

Kevin D. Ergle, MD Department of Internal Medicine, University of Florida Health Shands Hospital, Gainesville, FL, USA

Melinda W. Fernandez, MD Department of Emergency Medicine, University of Florida, Gainesville, FL, USA

Christian Fromm, MD Department of Emergency Medicine, Maimonides Medical Center, SUNY Downstate College of Medicine, New York, NY, USA

Latha Ganti, MD, MS, MBA Department of Emergency Medicine, Orlando Veterans Affairs Medical Center and University of Central Florida, Orlando, FL, USA

Diane F. Giorgi, MD Department of Emergency Medicine, Mount Sinai Queens, New York, NY, USA

Jacob J. Glaser, MD Combat Casualty Care Directorate, Naval Medical Research Unit, San Antonio, TX, USA

Jordana J. Haber, MD Department of Emergency Medicine, Maimonides Medical Center, New York, NY, USA

Jeffrey Joseph Harroch, MD Department of Emergency Medicine, University of Miami Miller School of Medicine, University of Miami Hospital, Miami, FL, USA

Tatiana Havryliuk, MD Department of Emergency Medicine, University of Colorado Denver, Denver, CO, USA

Braden Hexom, MD Department of Emergency Medicine, Mount Sinai Hospital, New York, NY, USA

Karlene Hosford, MD Department of Emergency Medicine, Lincoln Medical and Mental Health Center, New York, NY, USA

Rajnish Jaiswal, MD Department of Emergency Medicine, New York Medical College, Metropolitan Hospital Center, New York, NY, USA

Katrina John, MBBS Department of Emergency Medicine, Eisenhower Medical Center, Rancho Mirage, CA, USA

Jason Jones, MD Department of Emergency Medicine, University of Florida, Gainesville, FL, USA

Kevin M. Jones, MD Trauma and Surgical Critical Care, R Adams Cowley Shock Trauma Center, University of Maryland Medical Center, Baltimore, MD, USA

Elaine B. Josephson, MD Department of Emergency Medicine, Weill Cornell Medical College of Cornell University, Lincoln Medical and Mental Health Center, New York, NY, USA

Jeffrey Kile, MBBS, PhD, MPH Department of Emergency Medicine, Eisenhower Medical Center, Rancho Mirage, CA, USA

Bharat Kothakota, MD Department of Emergency Medicine, Lincoln Medical and Mental Health Center, New York, NY, USA

Zachary B. Kramer, MD Department of Emergency Medicine, University of Florida, Gainesville, FL, USA

Megan Kwasniak, MD Emergency Department, The Brooklyn Hospital Center, New York, NY, USA

Nathaniel Lisenbee, MD U. S. Air Force Medical Center Keesler, Biloxi, MI, USA

Judith K. Lucas, MD Department of Emergency Medicine, University of Florida, Gainesville, FL, USA

Benjamin M. Mahon, MD Ponciana Medical Center, Kissimmee, FL, USA

Clint Masterson, MD Department of Emergency Medicine, Mayo Clinic Health System in Fairmont, Fairmont, MN, USA

Lucas McArthur, MD Department of Emergency Medicine, Maimonides Medical Center, New York, NY, USA

Jay Menaker, MD Departments of Surgery and Emergency Medicine, R Adams Cowley Shock Trauma Center, University of Maryland Medical Center, Baltimore, MD, USA

Umarfarook Javed Mirza, DO Department of Emergency Medicine, Baylor University Medical Center, Dallas, TX, USA

David P. Nguyen, DO Department of Emergency Medicine, Rush-Copley Medical Center, Aurora, IL, USA

Katrina Skoog Nguyen, DO Northwest Community Hospital, Arlington Heights, IL, USA

Thomas T. Nguyen, MD Department of Emergency Medicine, Mount Sinai Beth Israel, New York, NY, USA

L. Connor Nickels, MD, RDMS Department of Emergency Medicine, University of Florida Health Shands Hospital, Gainesville, FL, USA

Marylin Otero, MD Department of Emergency Medicine, Franklin Hospital, Valley Stream, NY, USA

Eric S. Papierniak, DO Division of Pulmonary, Critical Care, and Sleep Medicine, University of Florida and Malcom Randall VA Medical Center, Gainesville, FL, USA

Ram A. Parekh, MD Department of Emergency Medicine, Icahn School of Medicine at Mount Sinai, Elmhurst Hospital Center, Elmhurst, NY, USA

Sohan Parekh, MD Department of Emergency Medicine, University of Texas at Austin Dell Medical School, Austin, TX, USA

Department of Emergency Medicine, University Medical Center Brackenridge, Austin, TX, USA

Thomas Parry, MD Department of Emergency Medicine, Lincoln Hospital and Mental Health Center, New York, NY, USA

Pratik S. Patel, MD Department of Emergency Medicine, University of Florida, Gainesville, FL, USA

Rohit Pravin Patel, MD Department of Emergency Medicine, University of Florida, Gainesville, FL, USA

Shalu S. Patel, MD Department of Emergency Medicine, Florida Hospital Tampa, Florida Hospital Carrollwood, Tampa, FL, USA

Jeffrey Pepin, MD Department of Emergency Medicine, University of Minnesota Medical Center Fairview, Minneapolis, MN, USA

Joshua Perry, DMD Department of Prosthodontics, University of Florida College of Dentistry, University of Florida Health Shands Hospital, Gainesville, FL, USA

Susana Perry, DMD Department of Pediatric Dentistry, University of Florida College of Dentistry, University of Florida Health Shands Hospital, Gainesville, FL, USA

Maritza A. Plaza-Verduin, MD Pediatric Division, Department of Emergency Medicine, Arnold Palmer Hospital for Children, Orlando, FL, USA

Joseph Rabinovich, MD Department of Emergency Medicine, Mount Sinai School of Medicine, Elmhurst Hospital Center, Elmhurst, NY, USA

Nauman W. Rashid, MD Department of Emergency Medicine, WellStar Kennestone Hospital, Marietta, GA, USA

Rosalia Rey, DDS Department of Restorative Dental Sciences, University of Florida College of Dentistry, University of Florida Health Shands Hospital, Gainesville, FL, USA

Nour Rifai, MBCHB Department of Emergency Medicine, Christiana Care Health System, Newark, DE, USA

Carlos J. Rodriguez, DO Division of Trauma Surgery, Surgical Critical Care, Walter Reed National Military Medical Center, Bethesda, MD, USA

Joseph D. Romano, MD Departments of Emergency Medicine and Internal Medicine, Christiana Care Health System, Newark, DE, USA

Mary T. Ryan, MD Department of Emergency Medicine, Lincoln Medical and Mental Health Center, New York, NY, USA

Weston Seipp, MD Department of Emergency Medicine, University of California Irvine Medical Center, Orange, CA, USA

Christopher Shields, MD Department of Emergency Medicine, Lincoln Medical and Mental Health Center, New York, NY, USA

Deylin I. Negron Smida, MD Department of Emergency Medicine, University of Pittsburgh Medical Center, Saint Margaret Hospital, Pittsburgh, PA, USA

David N. Smith, MD Department of Pediatrics, University of Alabama at Birmingham, Children's of Alabama, Birmingham, AL, USA

Christopher J. Spencer, DDS Department of Restorative Dental Sciences, University of Florida College of Dentistry, Gainesville, FL, USA

Christopher H. Stahmer, MD Department of Emergency Medicine, Lincoln Medical and Mental Health Center, New York, NY, USA

Franci Stavropoulos, DDS Department of Dental Specialties - Oral and Maxillofacial Surgery, Gundersen Health System, La Crosse, WI, USA

Kristin Stegeman, MD Department of Emergency Medicine, The Brooklyn Hospital Center, New York, NY, USA

Deborah M. Stein, MD, MPH Department of Surgery, University of Maryland School of Medicine, R Adams Cowley Shock Trauma Center, University of Maryland Medical Center, Baltimore, MD, USA

Rich Teitell, MD Department of Emergency Medicine, Waterbury Hospital, Waterbury, CT, USA

Kevin Tench, MD Department of Emergency Medicine, Banner Boswell Medical Center, Sun City, AZ, USA

Ronald Tesoriero, MD Department of Surgical Critical Care, University of Maryland School of Medicine, R Adams Cowley Shock Trauma Center, Baltimore, MD, USA

Coben Thorn, MD Department of Emergency Medicine, Bon Secours St. Francis Health System, Greenville, SC, USA

Matthew R. Tice, MD Department of Emergency Medicine, University of Florida, Gainesville, FL, USA

Tracy Timmons, MD Department of Trauma/Surgical Critical Care, R Adams Cowley Shock Trauma Center, University of Maryland Medical Center, Baltimore, MD, USA

Shannon Toohey, MD Department of Emergency Medicine, University of California Irvine Medical Center, Orange, CA, USA

Ann Tsung, MD Department of Emergency Medicine, University of Florida, Gainesville, FL, USA

Laura Tucker, DDS Department of Pediatric Dentistry, University of Florida Health Shands Hospital, Gainesville, FL, USA

Joseph A. Tyndall, MD, MPH Department of Emergency Medicine, University of Florida, Gainesville, FL, USA

Muhammad Waseem, MD Department of Emergency Medicine, Lincoln Medical and Mental Health Center, New York, NY, USA

Geraldine Weinstein, DDS Department of Restorative Dental Sciences, University of Florida College of Dentistry, Gainesville, FL, USA

Jennifer Westcott, DMD Private Practice, Palm Beach Gardens, FL, USA

Stephanie Wetmore-Nguyen, MD Department of Emergency Medicine, New York-Presbyterian Hospital/Columbia University Medical Center, New York, NY, USA

Anton A. Wray, MD Department of Emergency Medicine, The Brooklyn Hospital Center, New York, NY, USA

Henry Young II, MD Department of Emergency Medicine, University of Florida, Gainesville, FL, USA

Part I

Vascular Procedures

Arterial Cannulation (Radial and Femoral)

Jeffrey Kile, Katrina John, and Amish Aghera

Arterial cannulation is frequently performed in the care of critically ill patients for purposes of both serial arterial blood gas sampling and continuous intra-arterial blood pressure monitoring. It also provides arterial access for less common procedures, including thrombolysis, embolization, angiography, and infusion of vasoactive drugs. This chapter discusses cannulation of the radial and femoral arteries—the two most common sites for indwelling arterial catheter placement.

1.1 Indications

- Continuous monitoring of blood pressure in acute illness or major surgery
- Serial sampling of arterial blood during resuscitation
- Inability to use noninvasive blood pressure monitoring (*e.g.*, burns, morbid obesity)
- Continuous infusion of vasoactive inotropes (*e.g.*, phentolamine for reversal of local anesthesia)
- Angiography
- Embolization

1.2 Contraindications

- Absolute
  - Circulatory compromise in the extremity
  - Third-degree burns of the extremity

J. Kile, MBBS, PhD, MPH (✉) • K. John, MBBS
Department of Emergency Medicine, Eisenhower Medical Center, Rancho Mirage, CA, USA
e-mail: jeffrey.kile@gmail.com; trenjohn@me.com

A. Aghera, MD
Department of Emergency Medicine, Maimonides Medical Center, New York, NY, USA
e-mail: aaghera@maimonidesmed.org

  - Raynaud's syndrome
  - Thromboangiitis obliterans (Buerger's disease)
- Relative
  - Recent surgery in the extremity
  - Local skin infection
  - Abnormal coagulation
  - Insufficient collateral circulation
  - First- or second-degree burns of the extremity
  - Arteriosclerosis

1.3 Materials and Medications

- Radial artery cannulation: standard over-the-needle catheter assembly (Fig. 1.1)
  - Antimicrobial solution and swabs
  - Sterile gloves
  - Local anesthetic (1–2 % lidocaine without epinephrine)
  - Blunt needle
  - 25- or 27-gauge needle
  - Two 5 mL syringes
  - 4″×4″ gauze sponges
  - Standard over-the-needle catheter assembly
- Additional materials required for radial artery cannulation: over-the-needle catheter assembly with integrated guide wire
  - Over-the-needle catheter assembly with integrated guide wire
- Additional materials required for femoral artery cannulation: The Seldinger Technique
  - Introducer needle
  - Guide wire
  - Scalpel
  - Dilator
  - Arterial catheter

L. Ganti (ed.), *Atlas of Emergency Medicine Procedures*, DOI 10.1007/978-1-4939-2507-0_1

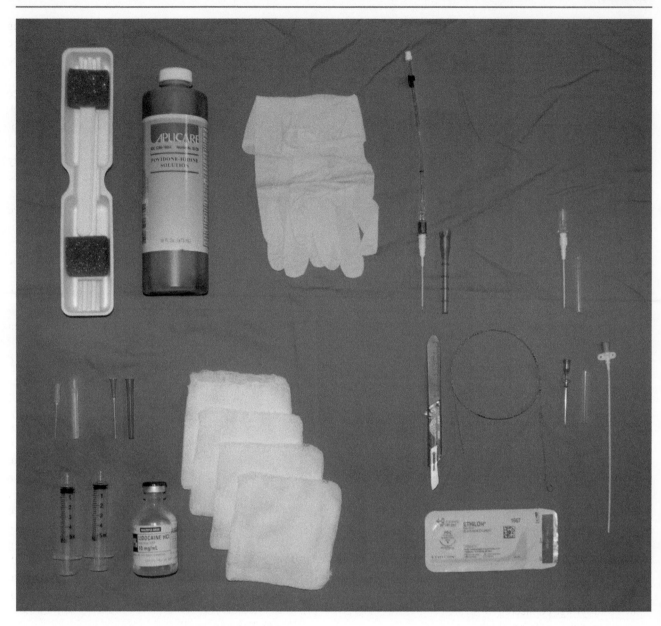

Fig. 1.1 Materials and medications

1.3.1 Procedure: Radial Artery Cannulation—Standard Over-the-Needle Catheter Assembly

1. Ensure adequate collateral flow in the selected extremity using the Allen test (see details below).
2. Immobilize the extremity by dorsiflexing the wrist to approximately 60° over a small towel roll and taping the base of the fingers to an arm board or other flat, fixed surface (Fig. 1.2).
   - Rotation of the wrist may shift the artery from its normal anatomical position, complicating cannulation.
3. Locate vessel by palpation of arterial pulse using the second and third fingers of the gloved nondominant hand.
4. Sterilize overlying skin with antimicrobial solution.
5. Inject local anesthetic to raise a small (0.5 cm) wheal using 25- or 27-gauge needle, and direct needle through wheal to infiltrate skin superficial to the artery with additional local anesthetic.
   - Infiltration of the subcutaneous tissue with local anesthetic may also reduce vessel spasm during arterial puncture.
   - Injection of local anesthetic into the vessel may precipitate arrhythmia, so draw back on the plunger prior to infiltration to ensure the tip of the needle is not inside the vessel.
   - Injection of excessive anesthetic when raising a wheal may obscure palpation of the pulse.
6. Ensure proper function of needle-cannula assembly by checking that cannula advances smoothly over needle.
7. Connect a 5 mL syringe with the plunger removed to the over-the-needle catheter assembly.
   - Attachment of syringe improves control during cannulation.
8. Hold syringe connected to needle-cannula assembly like a pen with needle bevel facing upward.
9. Directing the needle at a 30° angle to the skin, puncture the skin through the anesthetic wheal immediately overlying the palpated artery, and advance needle slowly until tip enters arterial lumen, which is confirmed by visible arterial blood flow ("flashback") into the needle hub and syringe.
   - Avoid self-puncture by maintaining adequate distance between needle tip and index finger (Fig. 1.3).

10. Reduce the angle between needle and skin (by lowering the needle) and advance an additional 2 mm to ensure catheter tip (which sits approximately 2 mm behind the needle tip) has entered the lumen.
    - Advancing the needle too far (or failing to reduce angle between needle and skin) once initial flashback is visualized may result in piercing the back side (or "double puncture") of the artery wall, in which case visible blood flow will cease; if this occurs, slowly withdraw needle several millimeters until pulsatile blood flow reappears.
11. Stabilize position of introducer needle and advance catheter alone into artery over needle until hub of catheter is in contact with the skin; blood flow from catheter hub at this point indicates successful cannulation of the artery.
    - If difficulty is encountered at this step, catheter hub may be rotated slightly to facilitate advancement.
12. Remove the needle without dislodging catheter from artery.
13. Manually apply pressure to proximal aspect of artery to occlude blood flow from the catheter.
14. Attach desired extension tubing, injection cap, and stopcock to the catheter hub.
15. Secure the catheter hub to the skin using silk (2.0) or nylon (4.0) sutures as follows. Take a 0.5 cm bite of skin under the catheter hub with the suture needle, tie several knots in the suture without pinching the skin, then tie a second set of knots around the hub of the catheter firmly. If the catheter assembly contains an integrated suture wing for fixation, take a 0.5 cm bite of skin under suture wing with the suture needle, thread suture through wing perforation, and secure wing against the skin with several knots. If suture wing has two perforations, repeat this process to secure other half of wing to skin (Fig. 1.4).
16. Cover the catheter with an appropriate self-adhesive sterile dressing.
    - A small bead of antibiotic ointment applied to the puncture site prior to dressing reduces the likelihood of cutaneous wound infection.
17. Secure the tubing connected to the catheter with gauze and adhesive tape or other sterile dressing.
18. Ensure all connections extending from catheter are tight and well secured, as accidental disconnection may result in rapid exsanguination.

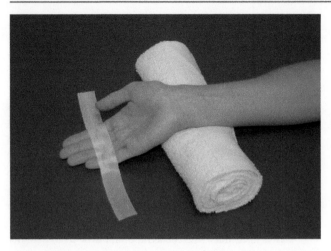

Fig. 1.2 Correct position of wrist prior to cannulation

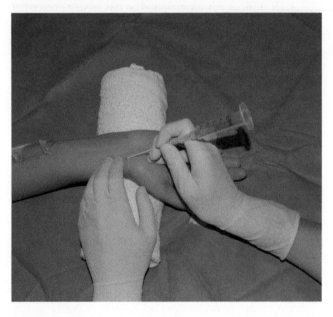

Fig. 1.3 Puncture of radial artery with standard over-the-needle catheter assembly

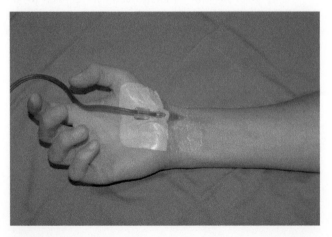

Fig. 1.4 Radial arterial catheter secured to wrist

1.3.2 Procedure: Radial Artery Cannulation—Over-the-Needle Catheter Assembly with Integrated Guide Wire (Arrow and Other Brands)

Perform steps 1–6 from the "Radial Artery Cannulation: Standard Over-the-Needle Catheter Assembly," above, and then proceed with the steps below:

1. Remove protective cap from needle-cannula assembly and ensure proper function by sliding actuation lever along extension tubing to advance and retract guide wire through needle.
2. Retract guide wire as far back as possible using actuation lever to maximize visibility arterial blood flow ("flashback") within introducer hub.

Perform steps 8–10 from the "Radial Artery Cannulation: Standard Over-the-Needle Catheter Assembly," above, and then proceed with the steps below (Fig. 1.5):

1. Hold needle stationery and slowly slide actuating lever forward to feed guide wire as far as possible into artery.
   - If resistance is met while feeding the guide wire, discontinue sliding actuating lever and withdraw entire unit from artery to prevent damage to guide wire or vessel wall
2. Advance entire assembly 1–2 mm further into vessel to ensure catheter tip (which sits approximately 2 mm behind the needle tip) has entered the lumen.
3. Stabilize clear introducer hub in position and advance catheter forward into artery over guide wire until hub of catheter is in contact with the skin.
   - If difficulty is encountered at this step, catheter hub may be rotated slightly to facilitate advancement.
4. Stabilize catheter in position and withdraw introducer needle, guide wire, and feed tube as a single unit; blood flow from catheter hub at this point indicates successful cannulation of the artery.

Perform steps 13–18 from the "Radial Artery Cannulation: Standard Over-the-Needle Catheter Assembly," above.

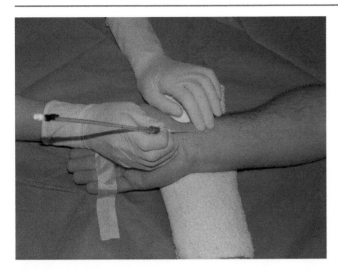

Fig. 1.5 Puncture of radial artery using over-the-needle catheter assembly with integrated guide wire

1.3.3 Procedure: Radial Artery Cannulation—The Allen Test

1. Occlude both radial and ulnar arteries of one extremity with digital pressure at wrist.
2. Instruct patient to repeatedly clench the fist tightly to exsanguinate the hand while occlusion of the arteries is maintained.
3. Without releasing digital pressure on arteries, instruct patient to extend fingers and observe palmar surface to confirm blanching of skin.
4. Release pressure on ulnar artery only and observe palmar surface for reperfusion (Fig. 1.6).
   - If reperfusion of the hand does not occur within 5–10 s, ulnar arterial blood flow may be compromised and radial artery cannulation should not be attempted. If reperfusion is brisk, repeat the test releasing pressure on radial artery only and observing palmar surface for reperfusion. If the return of rubor takes longer than 5–10 s, radial artery puncture should not be performed.

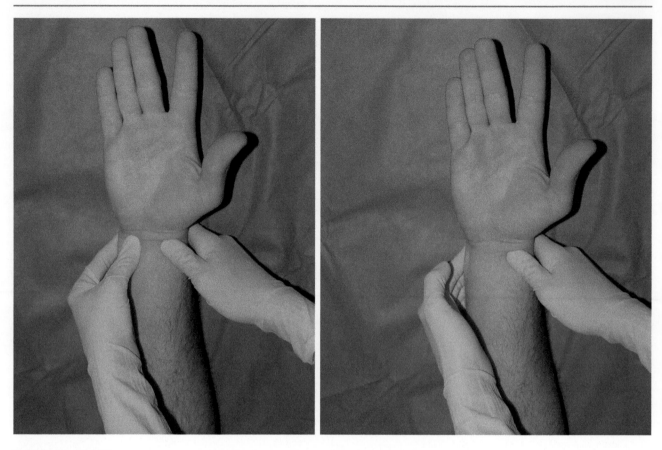

Fig. 1.6 The Allen Test

1.3.4 Procedure: Femoral Artery Cannulation—The Seldinger Technique

1. Place the patient in the supine position with the inguinal region adequately exposed.
2. Palpate the femoral pulse, located at midpoint between pubic symphysis and anterior superior iliac spine, using the second and third fingers of the gloved nondominant hand.

Perform steps 4 and 5 from the "Radial Artery Cannulation: Standard Over-the-Needle Catheter Assembly," above, and then proceed with the steps below (Fig. 1.7):

1. Attach 5 mL syringe to an introducing needle of bore sufficient to accommodate guide wire.
2. Hold syringe connected to introducing needle like a pen with needle bevel facing upward.
3. Directing the needle at a 45° angle to the skin in a cephalic direction, puncture the skin through the anesthetic wheal immediately overlying the palpated artery just distal to the inguinal ligament and advance needle slowly toward palpated artery until tip enters arterial lumen, which is confirmed by visible arterial blood flow ("flashback") into the needle hub and syringe.
   - Avoid self-puncture by maintaining adequate distance between needle tip and index finger.
   - Care must be taken to avoid trauma to the femoral nerve and vein bordering the femoral artery.
4. Hold needle stationery and remove syringe, taking care not to displace the intraluminal position of the needle tip.
   - Advancing the needle too far once initial flashback is visualized may result in piercing the back side (or "double puncture") of the artery wall, in which case visible blood flow will cease; if this occurs, slowly withdraw needle several millimeters until pulsatile blood flow reappears.
5. Occlude needle hub temporarily with gloved finger to prevent unnecessary blood loss and air embolism.
6. Thread blunt end of flexible guide wire smoothly into needle and gently into artery until at least one-quarter of guide wire is intravascular (Fig. 1.8).
   - If resistance is met while threading guide wire, remove wire from needle, reattach syringe, and aspirate blood to confirm continued intraluminal needle tip placement; if resistance is met while *removing* guide wire from needle, remove guide wire and needle from artery *as a single unit* to prevent shearing the guide wire off inside the vessel.

7. Holding the wire securely in place, remove the introducing needle.
8. Using a scalpel, make a small incision (approximately the width of the catheter to be used) through the dermis at the insertion site of the guide wire.
   - Avoid severing the guide wire by facing the sharp edge of the scalpel *away* from the guide wire.
9. While stabilizing the guide wire at its insertion site, thread the dilator over the free end of the guide wire until it is approximately one inch from the skin.
10. Grasp the free end of the guide wire protruding from the tail end of the dilator.
    - If it does not protrude from the tail end of the dilator, the guide wire must be removed sufficiently from the artery to be securely grasped; it must protrude visibly from the tail end of the dilator throughout the subsequent process of threading the dilator into the artery.
11. Holding the dilator firmly near its tip, thread the dilator over the wire into the skin with a back-and-forth twisting motion until it reaches the artery.
    - Only the skin tract should be dilated; dilation of the artery may result in excessive arterial injury and/or hemorrhage.
12. Holding the wire securely in place, remove the dilator.
13. While stabilizing the guide wire at its insertion site, thread the catheter over the free end of the guide wire until it nears the skin.
14. Grasping the guide wire where it protrudes from the tail end of the catheter, thread the catheter into the skin to its appropriate insertion length.
15. While stabilizing the catheter at its insertion site, slowly remove the guide wire.
    - If resistance is met while removing guide wire, remove guide wire and catheter from artery as a single unit to prevent shearing the guide wire off inside the vessel.
16. Secure the catheter to the skin using silk (2.0) or nylon (4.0) sutures. Take a 0.5 cm bite of skin with the suture needle. If the catheter assembly contains integrated "wings" for fixation, thread suture through the perforated wings and secure catheter against the skin with several knots. If no fixation device is included, tie several knots in the suture without pinching the skin, leaving both ends of the suture long. Using the loose ends of the suture, tie a second set of knots around the hub of the catheter, firmly, but without constricting its lumen.

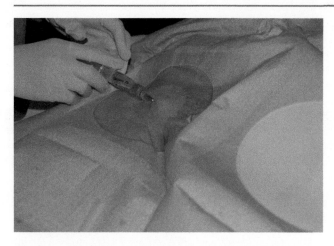

Fig. 1.7 Anesthetic injection over the femoral artery

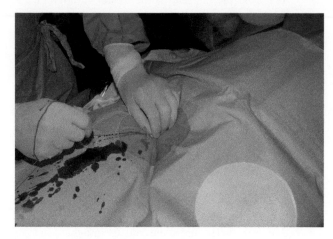

Fig. 1.8 Insertion of guide wire into femoral artery

1.4 Complications

- Hemorrhage
- Hematoma (at puncture site)
- Infection (at insertion site or systemic)
- Thrombosis
- Arteriovenous fistula
- Pseudoaneurysm formation
- Exsanguination (secondary to dislodgement of catheter)
- Cerebrovascular accident (CVA; secondary to air embolism)

1.5 Pearls and Pitfalls

- The shorter and stiffer the plastic tubing connected to the arterial cannula for blood pressure monitoring, the higher its frequency response and the accuracy of measurements.
- Use of an ultrasound probe can facilitate artery location and vessel cannulation.
- Puncture of the femoral artery proximal to the inguinal ligament, or distal to its bifurcation into superficial femoral and deep femoral arteries, may cause massive hemorrhage due to poor vessel compressibility in these regions; the artery should therefore be cannulated just distal to the inguinal ligament, where it is easily compressible against the femoral head if necessary.
- If difficulty is encountered when advancing an over-the-needle catheter into the artery, attach a 10 mL syringe containing 5 mL of sterile normal saline to the catheter hub, aspirate 1 or 2 mL of blood to confirm catheter tip placement within the vessel lumen, and then advance the catheter while gently injecting the saline-blood mixture; the jet of fluid momentarily dilates the lumen, aiding advancement of the catheter.
- An alternative approach to the over-the-needle catheter that will not fully advance is the use of a guide wire. After intraluminal placement of the cannula tip is confirmed by blood return, a guide wire is gently inserted through the catheter into the artery. The cannula is then passed along the guide wire until fully advanced. The guide wire employed must have a blunt, flexible tip to minimize the possibility of vessel wall trauma.
- Two potential consequences of arterial cannulation are vessel obstruction secondary to intravascular thrombosis and hemorrhage (the latter being the most common complication). Choice of puncture site is therefore essential. Due in part to their generous collateral blood flow, as well as ease of compressibility, the radial and femoral are the two most commonly cannulated arteries.
- Repeated puncture following unsuccessful cannulation increases the risk of arterial obstruction secondary to vessel wall damage and thrombosis.

- Double puncture of the cannulated artery by inadvertent over-insertion of the needle has not been shown to increase complications despite the additional trauma to the vessel walls.

Selected Reading

Anderson JS. Arterial cannulation: how to do it. Br J Hosp Med. 1997;57:497.

Gilchrist IC. Reducing collateral damage of the radial artery from catheterization. Catheter Cardiovasc Interv. 2010;76:677–8.

Lemaster CH, Agrawal AT, Hou P, Schuur JD. Systematic review of emergency department central venous and arterial catheter infection. Int J Emerg Med. 2010;3:409–23.

Mitchell JD, Welsby IJ. Techniques of arterial access. Surgery. 2004;22:3–4.

Wilson SR, Grunstein I, Hirvela ER, Price DD. Ultrasound-guided radial artery catheterization and the modified Allen's test. J Emerg Med. 2010;38:354–8.

Ultrasound-Guided Peripheral Intravenous Access

2

Coben Thorn and L. Connor Nickels

2.1 Indications

- Difficulty placing peripheral intravenous (PIV) using traditional methods of direct visualization and palpation
- To reduce needle sticks in a hypercoagulable patient

2.2 Contraindications

- Patient needs emergent central venous access

2.3 Materials and Medications

- Ultrasound machine
- High-frequency (5–8 MHZ) linear probe (Fig. 2.1)
- Ultrasound gel
- Minimum 1.5-in. needle length
- IV setup
- Skilled operator

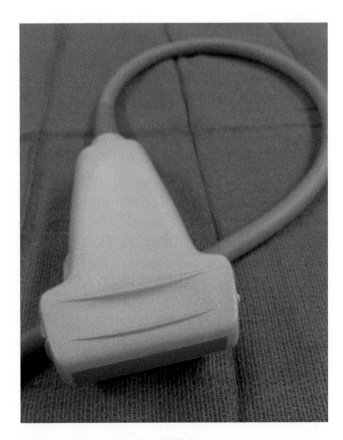

Fig. 2.1 High-frequency (5–8 MHZ) linear probe

C. Thorn, MD
Department of Emergency Medicine, Bon Secours St. Francis
Health System, Greenville, SC, USA
e-mail: cobenthorn@gmail.com

L.C. Nickels, MD, RDMS (✉)
Department of Emergency Medicine, University of Florida Health
Shands Hospital, Gainesville, FL, USA
e-mail: cnickels@ufl.edu

© Springer Science+Business Media New York 2016
L. Ganti (ed.), *Atlas of Emergency Medicine Procedures*, DOI 10.1007/978-1-4939-2507-0_2

2.4   Procedure

1. Scan the selected area to identify a target vessel for PIV cannulation.
   - Basilic (runs on the medial side of upper arm) (Fig. 2.2) and cephalic (runs on the lateral side of the upper arm) veins are good superficial veins that are generally not seen without ultrasound. The deep brachial vein is also an option; however, this is a deep vein that runs with the brachial artery, and there is higher chance for complications (Fig. 2.3).
2. Now the site should be prepared for IV insertion. It should be cleaned. An appropriate gauge long needle should be selected, and IV setup should be conveniently located for when access is obtained.
3. The ultrasound probe should be placed in the transverse plane (Fig. 2.4) to best visualize surrounding structures and vein. Alternatively, the probe can be placed longitudinally (Fig. 2.5) for better visualization of needle depth and slope.
   - Most practitioners seem to prefer the transverse approach.
4. The concept of the Pythagorean Theorem is used for accuracy. The needle should be inserted at a 45° angle to the skin and at an equal distance back from the probe as the approximate depth of the vessel vertically. The depth is given on the screen, usually at the bottom in centimeters. As soon as the needle has penetrated the skin the needle tip should be located by fanning the probe toward the needle until it is identified. The needle should then be advanced slowly always keeping the needle tip in view. Once directly on top of the vein, it should tent with pressure and then the needle should be inserted into the vein. Follow the needle in the vein as far as possible while keeping the tip of the needle in the center of the vein to make sure the catheter is securely in the vein and does not infiltrate.

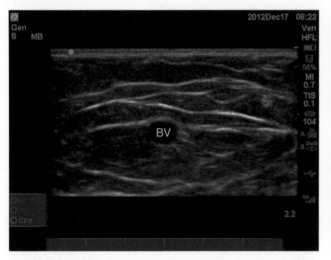

Fig. 2.2 Basilic vein (BV) located medially when scanning proximally from the antecubital fossa

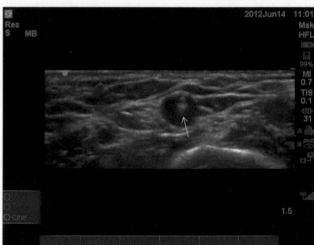

Fig. 2.4 Needle tip in vein seen in a transverse orientation

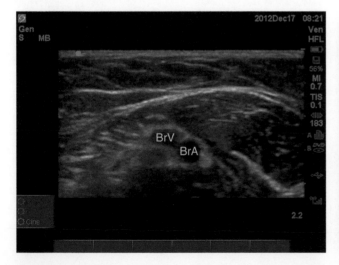

Fig. 2.3 Brachial artery (BrA) and vein (BrV). The less round, slightly compressed, anechoic structure on the left is the vein. The very circular, not compressed, anechoic structure to the right is the artery

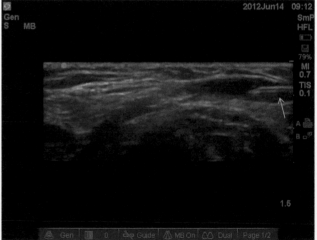

Fig. 2.5 Needle tip in vein seen in a longitudinal orientation

2.5   Complications

Inadvertent puncture of artery. Veins should be thin walled, compressible, and have no pulsations.

2.6   Pearls and Pitfalls

- Mistaking the midshaft of the needle for the needle tip. If this occurs, the needle tip is actually deeper than expected. The ultrasound machine will plot a hyperechoic "dot" on the screen for the needle tip, as long as it crosses the ultrasound beam at any point. This same "dot" will appear whether the tip is directly centered under the beam or *any* segment of the needle shaft is intersecting the beam. This can be visually deceiving and makes this procedure difficult to grasp.
- Very slow movements of the needle and the probe are important for keeping the needle tip in view. Once the needle tip is identified, the probe should be fanned forward (away from operator) just slightly and then the needle advanced until the needle tip comes into view again. This is repeated until the needle is securely moved further into the vein.

Selected Reading

Brannam L, Blaivas M, Lyon M, et al. Emergency nurses' utilization of ultrasound guidance for placement of peripheral intravenous lines in difficult-access patients. Acad Emerg Med. 2004;11:1361–3.

Constantino TG, Parikh AK, Satz WA, et al. Ultrasonography-guided peripheral intravenous access versus traditional approaches in patients with difficult intravenous access. Ann Emerg Med. 2005;46(5):456–61.

Dargin JM, Rebholz CM, Lowenstein RA, et al. Ultrasonography-guided peripheral intravenous catheter survival in ED patients with difficult access. Am J Emerg Med. 2010;28(1):1–7.

Ma JO, Mateer JR, Blaivas M. Emerg ultrasound. 2nd ed. New York: McGraw-Hill Companies, Inc.; 2008.

Saul T, Rivera M, Lewiss R. Ultrasound image quality. ACEP News. 2011;4:24–5.

Central Venous Line Placement: Internal Jugular Vein, Subclavian Vein, and Femoral Vein

3

Kevin D. Ergle, Zachary B. Kramer, Jason Jones, and Rohit Pravin Patel

3.1 Indications

- Volume replacement
- Emergent venous access
- Administration of caustic medications: vasopressors, calcium chloride, hypertonic saline, high dose of potassium
- Dialysis catheter placement (hemodialysis)
- Nutritional support (total parenteral nutrition)
- Long-term antibiotics
- Chemotherapy
- Plasmapheresis
- Frequent or persistent blood draws or intravenous therapy when unable to establish peripheral access due to edema or other causes
- Jugular and subclavian: Central venous pressure monitoring, transvenous pacing wire introduction, pulmonary artery catheterization

3.2 Contraindications

- Absolute
  - Infection at site of insertion
  - Distorted anatomy/landmarks (prior surgery, radiation, or history of thrombus in the specified vein)
  - Subclavian only: Trauma to the ipsilateral clavicle, anterior proximal rib, subclavian or superior vena cava vessels
- Relative
  - Morbid obesity
  - COPD
  - Children less than 2 years (higher complication rates)
    - Coagulopathy (although ultrasound-guided internal jugular can be done in this situation)
  - Agitated or moving patient
  - Jugular only: Trauma to the ipsilateral clavicle, anterior proximal rib, subclavian or superior vena cava vessels
  - Jugular and subclavian: Inability to tolerate potential pneumothorax of the ipsilateral thoracic cage
    - Pneumothorax or hemothorax of the contralateral thorax
    - Patients receiving ventilatory support with high-end expiratory pressures (temporarily reduce the pressures)
  - Femoral only: Intra-abdominal (or retroperitoneal) hemorrhage

3.3 Materials and Medications

- Central venous catheter tray or bundle: single/double/triple/quadruple lumen, dialysis catheter, large-bore introducer (for transvenous pacing or pulmonary artery catheter kit)
- Sterile gloves
- Sterile drapes or towels
- Sterile gown
- Hat/hair cap and mask with eye protection
- Antiseptic solution with skin swabs (e.g., chlorhexidine)
- Sterile saline flushes (one 30 mL syringe or three 10 mL syringes)
- Lidocaine 1 %

K.D. Ergle, MD
Department of Internal Medicine, University of Florida Health Shands Hospital, Gainesville, FL, USA
e-mail: kevin.ergle@medicine.ufl.edu

Z.B. Kramer, MD
Emergency Medicine Resident, University of Florida College of Medicine, University of Florida Health Shands Hospital, Gainesville, FL, USA
e-mail: zkramer@ufl.edu

J. Jones, MD • R.P. Patel, MD (✉)
Department of Emergency Medicine, University of Florida Health Shands Hospital, Gainesville, FL, USA
e-mail: jasonjones@ufl.edu; rohitpatel@ufl.edu

© Springer Science+Business Media New York 2016
L. Ganti (ed.), *Atlas of Emergency Medicine Procedures*, DOI 10.1007/978-1-4939-2507-0_3

- Sterile gauze
- No. 11 blade scalpel
- Dressing (sterile waterproof transparent dressing or sterile 4×4 gauze with tape)
- Sterile biopatch
- Suture material with needle driver if needed
- Transducing line (optional)
- Sterile probe cover (if using ultrasound guidance)

3.4   Procedures

3.4.1   Internal Jugular Vein Access Procedure

1. Obtain informed consent if not emergently indicated procedure.
2. Obtain supplies and prepare the room, ensuring that all supplies are within operator reach prior to placing gown and commencing the procedure. Include a sterile ultrasound sheath on the sterile field if ultrasound is being used.
3. Raise bed to a comfortable height for the operator.
4. Place patient with head facing away from side of central line site (if using ultrasound, other positions may be preferred). Place patient in 15–20° Trendelenburg position to help fill the upper central veins and reduce the risk of air embolism.
5. Identify the anatomy. Palpate triangle made by the clavicle and sternal and clavicular heads of the sternocleidomastoid (SCM) muscle to identify the location of the internal jugular vein (Fig. 3.1). If using ultrasound guidance, identify optimal anatomical arrangement.
6. Wash your hands and wear sterile attire using aseptic technique, including cap, mask, gown, and sterile gloves.
7. Prepare the site from the clavicle to the ear and across the trachea with antiseptic solution. Allow the antiseptic (chlorhexidine or iodine) to fully dry.
8. Drape the site and patient with sterile towels and drapes included in most CVL bundles. Make sure to cover the whole area and bed.
9. Cover the ultrasound probe with a sterile sheath. This can be done solo or by holding the sterile ultrasound sheath and having an unsterile assistant hold the probe so that the probe can be covered by the sheath.
10. Prepare the kit by checking the guide wire and flushing the tubing and lines with saline included in the kit.
11. With a 25-gauge needle, use 1 % lidocaine to anesthetize the skin at the apex of the triangle made by the SCM and clavicle. Aspirate to make sure the operator is not in a vessel and make a superficial wheel for the insertion site.
12. Preferred method is with ultrasound guidance (see steps 13–17 and Sect. 3.6 for description of ultrasound

guidance). If performing without ultrasound, palpate the carotid artery and insert needle lateral to the artery at the apex of the triangle formed by the SCM, aiming toward the ipsilateral nipple at an angle 30–45° above the horizontal plane (Fig. 3.1). Once blood returned, go to step 18.
13. Place sterile ultrasound gel over the insertion site. Use the ultrasound to identify vessel anatomy including internal jugular vein and carotid artery. Use the ultrasound probe to compress the vein, which is compressible as opposed to the carotid artery, which is not compressible (Fig. 3.2).
14. Prepare the insertion needle and syringe (if long and short needles are available, a short needle may be used to reduce posterior vein perforation) and prime the syringe by pulling back on the plunger prior to making the puncture.
15. Use the ultrasound probe to re-identify the patient's anatomy.
16. Ultrasound can be used in short axis or long axis (Fig. 3.3). Short axis is easier for novice operators due to increased ability to see the artery and vein but has a higher risk of posterior perforation if the needle tip is not visualized well. Once short axis of the vein is found, turning the probe 90° clockwise allows the operator to see the vein in long axis. The needle is better visualized in this view but technically more difficult and has less chance to penetrate the posterior wall. In patients with short necks, it may be difficult to obtain long-axis view and needle insertion in the limited space.
17. Insert the needle using the ultrasound guidance with dynamic approach preferred (see Sect. 3.6 for specifics). Make sure to aspirate while inserting the needle to identify when the venous access is obtained. The needle tip should be visualized through the whole process.
    - If using the static approach (see Sect. 3.6), insert needle lateral to carotid pulsation as this is where the vein anatomically is located. Standard method is to insert the needle as far back as the depth the vessel is visualized (e.g., if the vein is visualized 2 cm below skin surface, the needle should be inserted 2 cm behind the probe at a 45° angle).
    - If inserting the needle ~3 cm does not achieve access, gently withdraw the needle toward the surface of the skin while aspirating. Avoid withdrawing the needle completely from the skin. If needed, redirect the needle and advance until blood is aspirated. Cannulation of the vein often takes place while withdrawing the needle.
18. Hold the needle steady with your nondominant hand and remove the syringe, careful not to advance or withdraw the needle. You can place the base of your hand on the patient's chest to make your hand more stable during

this part of the procedure. Occlude the hub of the needle to prevent air embolus.

19. You may verify that you are in the vein by transducing pressure with a fluid column. The fluid should flow easily into the vein.
    - If the aspirated blood is pulsatile and moves up the column, withdraw the needle completely and apply pressure for 10–20 min while taking the patient out of Trendelenburg position (if nonemergent procedure).
20. Once it is verified that you are in the vein, insert the J-tip of the guide wire into the needle hub and advance into the vein. The J-tip can be straightened with a pinching motion (Fig. 3.4). Always keep one hand on the guide wire until it is removed from the patient. Monitor for arrhythmias as the guide wire is advanced toward the right atrium.
    - If the guide wire does not flow easily, remove the guide wire and reattach the syringe, checking for blood flow.
    - If arrhythmia occurs, slowly withdraw the guide wire until the patient's native rhythm returns.
    - Alternatively, the catheter/syringe found in most kits can be used as a bridge to guide wire placement. For the author, this has improved success when there is difficulty in wire placement. Use the same steps above with the catheter (Fig. 3.5) and when you have return of blood, advance the angiocath into the vein followed by insertion of the guide wire through the angiocath. This is especially useful in moving/agitated patients, patients who have collapsible veins due to hypovolemia, and patients who have abnormal anatomy and may have veins that take an abnormal angle shortly past the needle tip.
21. Remove the needle over the guide wire, making sure to always keep control of the guide wire.

22. Make an incision contiguous with the guide wire using a straight (No. 11) blade with the scalpel blade facing upward (away from the wire).
23. Advance the dilator over the guide wire in a twisting motion, keeping control of the guide wire.
    - The dilator only needs to go slightly beyond the anticipated depth of the patient's jugular vein. Do not advance the entire length of the dilator.
24. Withdraw the dilator and hold pressure over the wound site.
25. Advance the catheter over the guide wire while keeping control of the guide wire.
26. With the catheter inserted 10–12 in. from the skin insertion site, retract the guide wire until it comes out of the distal port. Maintain control of the guide wire and advance the catheter to the appropriate length. Usually catheters are inserted 15–16 cm from the right side and 18–20 cm from the left side (Fig. 3.6).
27. Flush each port of the catheter and check aspiration. If difficulty with aspiration or flushing, concern is raised for catheter malposition. The operator can change the depth slightly or twist the catheter and recheck.
28. At this time, an antibiotic ointment or biopatch may be applied to skin around the intersection with the lumen of the catheter. This step is based on local institutional guidelines.
29. Suture the line in place.
30. Enclose CVL site with sterile waterproof transparent dressing.
31. Confirm placement using chest X-ray (CXR). The tip of the catheter should be in the lower third of the superior vena cava (SVC) at the insertion of the SVC into the right atrium.

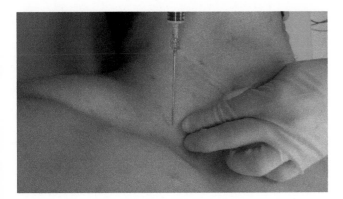

Fig. 3.1 Internal jugular blind approach; this would be the same location for probe placement if doing ultrasound guided

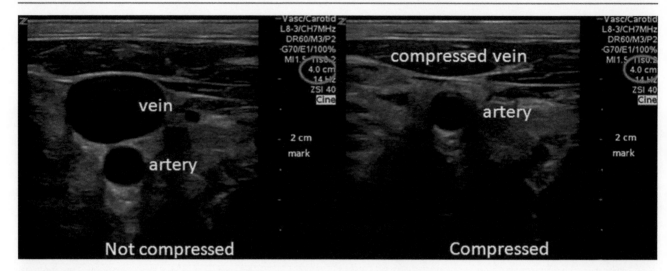

Fig. 3.2 Ultrasound showing internal jugular vein and artery with and without compression

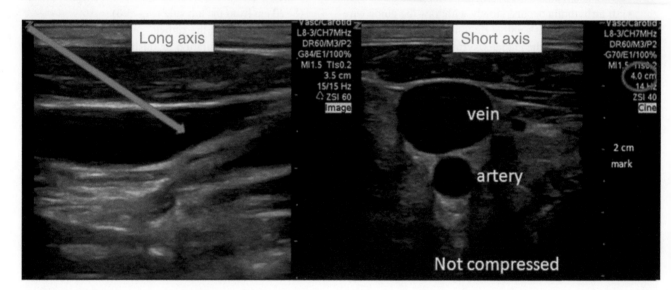

Fig. 3.3 Long- and short-axis views of the internal jugular vein

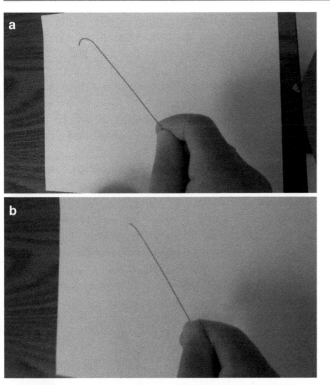

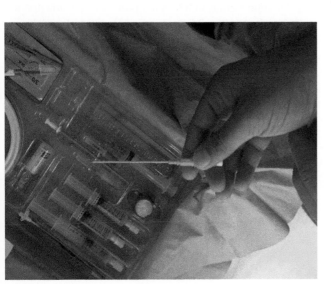

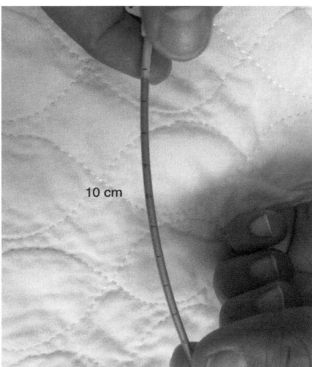

Fig. 3.4 (**a, b**) J-tip straightening using pinch/stretch method

Fig. 3.6 Length: marking seen on typical central venous catheters; number indicates distance in centimeters from distal tip

Fig. 3.5 Angiocath that can be used in difficult to cannulate/wire patients

3.4.2 Subclavian Vein Access Procedure

1. Obtain informed consent if not emergently indicated.
2. Raise bed to comfortable height for the operator.
3. Place patient in supine position and position so patient's head is at the top of the bed.
4. Place patient in 15–20° Trendelenburg position (if tolerated) to reduce risk of air embolism. Studies show this will also increase the size of the subclavian vein. Do NOT place towel between shoulder blades (arch shoulder back) as this has been shown to decrease vein diameter and affect reliability of accessibility. Keep shoulders at anatomical location (forward).
5. Prep area chosen from the anterior neck, clavicle, and upper chest (above nipple line) with chlorhexidine prep or iodine.
6. Open kit and place close to operator's dominant hand to allow for easy access. Diameter of catheter/kit used based on clinical situation:
   - Introducer or large bore if requiring large volumes of resuscitation
   - Triple lumen catheters for vasopressors
   - Introducers if anticipating pulmonary artery catheter or venous pacer
7. Operator should prepare with all aseptic techniques (e.g., hand washing) and maximal barrier precautions (e.g., sterile gowns, sterile gloves, caps, masks covering both mouth and nose, eye protection, and full-body patient drapes).
8. Once sterile and able to touch the inside of the CVL kit, the operator may want to retract the curved J-tip wire into the plastic loop sheath for easy directing into the introducer needle. The operator should also uncap all distal lumens and flush all ports with 3–5 cc of the sterile NS syringes to ensure no defects in the lumen of the catheter. Close all ports except the distal tip port (usually marked with words "distal tip") with the slide clamp.
9. Prep area chosen (right or left side) from the anterior neck, clavicle, and upper chest (above nipple line) with sterile chlorhexidine prep (this is the second cleaning).
10. Place full-body drape over patient with opening over selected side where needle will be inserted.
11. Needle insertion site options (Fig. 3.7):
    - One centimeter inferior to the junction of the middle and medial third of the clavicle
    - Just lateral to the midclavicular line, with the needle perpendicular along the inferior lateral clavicle
    - One fingerbreadth lateral to the angle of the clavicle
12. Anesthetize needle insertion site with 5–10 mL of 1 % lidocaine superficially (make sure to pull back on needle syringe to ensure operator is not in the vein or artery).
    - Never place equipment on a patient.
13. Prepare the needle and syringe by placing the long needle on the syringe. Make sure to break seal of syringe by pulling back on the plunger of the syringe prior to making incision with needle.
14. Turn patient's head to opposite of CVL placement and retract ipsilateral shoulder down to improve clavicle-vein relationship. The retraction of the arm can be done a few steps earlier and can be held in position using a person or tape/restraints.
15. Direct the insertion needle toward sternal notch in the coronal plane at an angle no greater than 10–15° while gently withdrawing the plunger of the syringe. Keep bevel of the needle facing up and in line with the numbers on the syringe until operator enters skin, then face bevel caudally to facilitate smooth progression of the guide wire down the vein toward the right atrium.
16. It helps to place nondominant hand (not holding the needle) on the sternal notch so operator can feel where sternal notch is and direct needle in that direction (Fig. 3.7).
17. NEVER increase the angle of the needle greater than 15° as pneumothorax may ensue.
18. Advance the needle under and along the inferior border of the clavicle, making sure the needle is virtually horizontal to the chest wall. Aim medially in the direction of the suprasternal notch, attempting to first aim for the clavicle then "walk" the needle below the clavicle.
19. Once under the clavicle, continue to advance the needle in a plane almost parallel to the skin approximately 2–3 cm until venous blood is freely aspirated into the syringe.
20. When venous blood is freely aspirated, disconnect the syringe from the needle, and immediately occlude the lumen to prevent air embolism and insert the guide wire. If the vein is difficult to locate, remove the introducer needle, flush it clean of clots, and try again. Change insertion sites after three unsuccessful passes with the introducer needle.
21. At this point, the hand holding the needle should be "set in stone." Use the patient's chest wall as a base to keep needle completely still as to not inadvertently advance or retract needle out of the vein.
22. Insert the guide wire through the needle into the vein with the J-tip directed caudally to improve successful placement into the subclavian vein.
    - Beware a return of red pulsatile blood. If this occurs, the wire is in an artery.
    - Beware aspirating air bubbles through the probing introducer needle. This indicates a pneumothorax.
23. Advance the wire until it is mostly in the vein or until arrythmia is seen on the cardiac monitor. Then, retract the wire 3–4 cm.
24. If the wire does not pass easily, remove the wire, reattach the syringe, and confirm that the needle is still in the

lumen of the vein before reattempting. The J-tip can be straightened with a pinching motion (Fig. 3.4).

- Alternatively, the catheter/syringe found in most kits can be used as a bridge to guide wire placement. For the author, this has improved success when there is difficulty in wire placement. Use the same steps above with the catheter (Fig. 3.5) and when you have return of blood, advance the angiocath into the vein followed by insertion of the guide wire through the angiocath. This is especially useful in moving/agitated patients, patients who have collapsible veins due to hypovolemia, and patients who have abnormal anatomy and may have veins that take an abnormal angle shortly past the needle tip.

25. Use the tip of the scalpel to make a small incision just against the needle to enlarge the catheter entry site for the dilator and catheter.
26. Holding the wire in place, withdraw the introducer needle and place in needle holder.
27. Thread the dilator over the wire and into the vein with a firm and gentle twisting motion while maintaining constant control of the wire. If a large-bore introducer is placed, the dilator/introducer goes in one step, after the introducer is inserted, hold the wire in place and remove the dilator.
28. If operator is having difficulty threading the dilator, the skin incision with the scalpel may have been too superficial or small. It may help to enlarge this incision to avoid having the dilator get caught on superficial skin or connective tissue.

29. It is helpful to have sterile gauze handy to apply pressure with the hand not holding the wire as the vein will now bleed profusely from around the wire secondary to dilation.
30. Thread the catheter until it is close to the skin insertion site. Then pull back on the guide wire until it shows outside of the distal port. Grasp the wire outside of the distal port and thread the catheter while holding onto the guide wire. Usually catheters are inserted 15–16 cm from the right side and 18–20 cm from the left side (Fig. 3.6)
31. Hold the catheter in place and remove the wire. After the wire is removed, occlude the open lumen.
32. Attach sterile saline syringe to the hub and aspirate blood. Take needed samples and then flush the line with saline and recap. Repeat this step with all lumens.
33. Place biopatch on skin around the intersection with the lumen of the catheter.
34. Suture the line in place.
35. Enclose CVL site with sterile waterproof transparent dressing.
36. Confirm placement using CXR. Tip of catheter should be in the lower third of the SVC at the insertion of SVC into right atrium (tip at right bronchiotracheal angle or up to 2.5 cm below bronchiotracheal angle).

- Alternatively, ultrasound can be used for subclavian line access but only a few limited studies have confirmed this as to date so will not describe in detail (see below for typical ultrasound technique used). See references for more information.

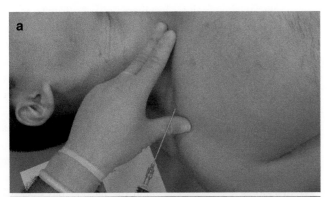

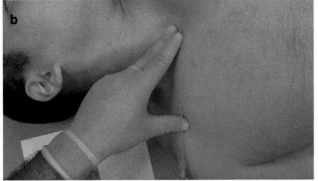

Fig. 3.7 Subclavian vein approach: wrong (**a**) and correct (**b**) angles to take when making skin puncture

3.4.2.1 Subclavian Vein Pearls and Pitfalls

- Inadequate landmark identification: operator should always palpate for landmarks and check anatomy prior to starting the procedure.
- Improper insertion position.
- Insertion of needle through periosteum.
  - Operator should NOT increase angle of needle to avoid the clavicle bone (this can cause a pneumothorax).
  - Operator should press on needle with downward pressure on chest wall to allow needle to maneuver under the clavicle without changing the angle of insertions of the needle.
- Taking too shallow a trajectory with needle.
- Aiming the needle too cephalad (aim for sternoclavicular junction).
- Failure to keep needle in place for wire passage: hand holding the needle should be planted on patient's chest for stabilization.

3.4.3   Femoral Vein Access Procedure

1. Palpate the patient's femoral artery below the inguinal ligament. This is usually found halfway between the anterior superior iliac spine (ASIS) and the midline of the symphysis pubis.
2. Trim overlying hair as necessary.
3. If ultrasound-guided approach is desired, use the linear probe (same as internal jugular) to detect the femoral vein at this location. The femoral vein will be easily compressible, while the femoral artery will be less compressible and pulsatile (Fig. 3.2).
4. Wash hands and use sterile technique to apply iodine or chlorhexidine solution (various forms available).
5. Open your femoral CVL kit and don cap, mask, sterile gown, and sterile gloves. Nonsterile assistants should wear a cap, mask, sterile gown, and sterile gloves. Flush all ports of your CVL kit with saline flushes and check for leaks or malfunction of catheter.
6. Under sterile technique, apply the drape over the area of insertion, and have an assistant extend the drape the length of the bed. Reapply sterile iodine or chlorhexidine at the site.
7. Anesthetize the skin overlying the femoral vein with lidocaine.
8. If ultrasound-guided approach is desired, have an assistant hold up the vascular ultrasound probe. Place your gloved hand through a sterile ultrasound sleeve and grasp the top of the ultrasound probe. Without breaking sterile technique, pull and invert the sterile ultrasound sleeve over the probe and cable. See Sect. 3.6 for detailed ultrasound-guided cannulation technique.

9. Insert the needle at a 45° angle, bevel down, directed superiorly, 1 cm medial to the palpable femoral artery pulse. Once the needle has broken the skin, aspirate by applying a small amount of continuous traction on the plunger of the attached syringe.
10. Advance smoothly and slowly until blood appears in the syringe. Stop once blood is aspirated. If femoral vein is not cannulated, withdraw your needle until just beneath the skin and redirect.
11. Hold the hub of the needle with thumb and forefinger to immobilize in place. Remove the syringe carefully. If blood appears arterial or pulsatile, remove the needle and hold pressure for 5–10 min.
    - Use the palm of your hand on the thigh to stabilize your hand. Not having your hand stable is a common mistake leading to needle movement out of the vein.
12. If blood appears venous (dark color, emerges as a continuous trickle, or transduced), cannulate the needle with the guide wire. Maintain a two-finger grip on the guide wire at all times. Advance the guide wire until approximately 15 cm remains.
    - Must keep handle of guide wire at ALL times and can be done through proper technique.
13. If guide wire does not advance easily, remove guide wire and reposition needle until blood aspirates easily. The J-tip can be straightened using a pinching motion if needed (Fig. 3.4)
    - Alternatively, the catheter/syringe found in most kits can be used as a bridge to guide wire placement. For the author, this has improved success when there is difficulty in wire placement. Use the same steps above with the catheter (Fig. 3.5) and when you have return of blood, advance the angiocath into the vein followed by insertion of the guide wire through the angiocath. This is especially useful in moving/agitated patients, patients who have collapsible veins due to hypovolemia, and patients who have abnormal anatomy and may have veins that take an abnormal angle shortly past the needle tip.
14. Using your scalpel, make a single 1/2 cm stab incision at the site of needle insertion to assist with dilator placement.
    - You can do the stab incision with or without the needle in place, but from experience, most novices have difficulty locating the correct stab location due to small amount of blood accumulation when the needle is taken out.
15. Remove your needle, carefully leaving guide wire in place. Apply dilator over guide wire and advance into the body with gentle pressure and a twisting motion in the same plane that you used to direct the needle.
16. Holding pressure at the insertion site with sterile gauze 4×4 pads, remove the dilator from the guide wire,

leaving the guide wire in place. Insert the central venous catheter over the guide wire until it fits snugly against the skin. Use the markings on the catheter to determine proper length placed (usually with femoral site you can "hub" the catheter) (Fig. 3.6).

17. Using a sterile saline flush, ensure that each lumen of the CVL draws blood easily and flushes easily. Carefully note any that do not and consider repositioning as needed. You can attempt moving catheter in or out a few centimeters or rotating the catheter and recheck. Apply caps to each open lumen of the CVL.

    • Remember to cover the introducer port if not using immediately. If you do not, it poses an infection and air embolism risk to the patient.

18. Suture the line in place.

19. Place an antibiotic biopatch or similar antimicrobial dressing.

20. Enclose CVL site with sterile waterproof transparent dressing.

3.4.3.1 Femoral Vein Pearls and Pitfalls

• Femoral central venous lines cannot accurately transduce central venous pressures.

• Asking the patient to perform a Valsalva maneuver has been shown to increase the width of the femoral vein by 1/3.

• The mnemonic NAVEL (Nerve Artery Vein Empty space Lymphatics) assists in remembering the order of femoral structures from lateral to medial.

• Traditionally, femoral venous lines were thought to have higher rates of infection than subclavian or internal jugular lines, but more recent analyses are challenging this belief.

    – Obesity is a more important risk factor for infection in femoral sites.

3.5   Complications

3.5.1   Jugular and Subclavian Complications

• Pneumothroax/Hemothorax
    – Prevention: Remove patient from ventilator before advancing the needle, choose the right side rather than left, and avoid multiple attempts when possible.
    – Management: Check postprocedure x-ray; if pneumothorax, arrange for thoracostomy depending on the size of the hemo-/pneumothorax.

• Catheter embolization
    – Prevention: Never withdraw a catheter past a needle bevel as this might shear off the catheter.
    – Management: X-ray the patient and contact specialist who can remove the embolized catheter.

• Arterial puncture: Hold compression if this occurs.

• Hematoma: Usually requires monitoring only.

• Thrombosis: This complication may lead to pulmonary embolism.

• Local site or systemic infection: Using maximal sterile precautions has been shown to greatly decrease rate of infection.

• Air embolism
    – May be caused by negative intrathoracic pressure when inspiration by the patient drawing air into an open line hub
    – Prevention: Be sure the line hubs are always occluded; placing the patient in the Trendelenburg position lowers the risk.
    – Management: The patient should be placed in Trendelenburg position with a left lateral decubitus tilt, which may prevent the movement of air into the right ventricle and onward into the left side of the heart. One hundred percent oxygen should be administered to speed the resorption of the air. If a catheter is located in the heart, aspiration of the air should be attempted.

• Dysrhythmias: Due to cardiac irritation by the wire or catheter tip. This can usually be terminated by simply withdrawing the line into the superior vena cava. One should always place a central venous catheter with cardiac monitoring.

• Lost guide wire: If the operator is not careful about maintaining control of the guide wire, it may be lost into the vein. This requires retrieval by interventional radiology or surgery and is an emergency.

• Catheter tip too deep: Check the postprocedure chest radiograph and pull the line back if the tip disappears into the cardiac silhouette.

• Catheter in the wrong vessel: Check the postprocedure chest radiograph for this complication; remove catheter and try again.

• Arterial puncture (subclavian only): The subclavian artery cannot be compressed; so, the subclavian approach should be avoided in anticoagulated patients.

3.5.2   Femoral Complications

• Arterial puncture: The femoral artery site can be compressed, so if punctured hold pressure.

• Hematoma: Usually requires monitoring only.

• Thrombosis: This complication may lead to pulmonary embolism.

• Catheter embolization.
    – Prevention: Never withdraw a catheter past a needle bevel which might shear off the catheter.
    – Management: X-ray the patient and contact specialist who can remove the embolized catheter.

- Lost guide wire: If the operator is not careful about maintaining control of the guide wire, it may be lost into the vein. This requires retrieval by interventional radiology or surgery and is an emergency.
- Local site or systemic infection: Using maximal sterile precautions has been shown to greatly decrease rate of infection.

3.6 Ultrasound Guided Cannulation: Tips for Each Approach

- Venous anatomy is best visualized using high-frequency (5–10 MHz) linear probe. Higher frequencies generate less penetration but better resolution.
- You can use the ultrasound to identify the location of the vessel prior to the procedure and utilize external landmarks during the procedure itself (static technique), or you can use the ultrasound to visualize cannulation of the vessel during the procedure (dynamic technique).
- Static view is advantageous in that the ultrasound transducer is not needed during the sterile portion of the procedure, but it does not allow for direct visualization of cannulation and guidance during the procedure.
- Dynamic view (preferred) allows for direct visualization during the procedure but requires more technique and requires use of transducer during the sterile portion of the procedure.
- The dynamic technique can be used in either a short-axis view, where a cross-sectional view of the vessel and needle is used, or a long-axis view, where a longitudinal view of vessel and needle is used (Fig. 3.3).
- The long-axis view allows for full visualization of the needle throughout the procedure and allows for better visualization and adjustment of needle depth. It is more difficult for lateral changes in positioning and tends to be more difficult technically.
  - Key in this view is that once a good section of vein is obtained, do not move probe to visualize the needle; move the needle into the ultrasound view by slightly adjusting trajectory.
- The short-axis view allows for lateral changes in position but is not as good at visualizing depth throughout the procedure, as visualization of the needle is in cross-sectional imaging. Perforation of the posterior wall is more common in this view.
- When using the short-axis view, remember to position the ultrasound probe such that the field of the ultrasound intersects the vessel (internal jugular, subclavian, femoral) at the anticipated site of insertion of the needle into the vein. Remember that the needle is only visualized as it intersects the plane of the ultrasound.

- When using the long-axis view, make sure to visualize the vessel with the ultrasound such that you can see the greatest diameter of the vessel along the entire length of the ultrasound probe. Keep the ultrasound steady during the procedure, and insert the needle at an angle at the lateral edge of the ultrasound probe. Using this technique, one can visualize the entire length of the needle.

3.7 Removing a Central Line

1. Place patient in supine or Trendelenburg position (for femoral removal can help decrease bleeding).
2. Remove suturing and dressing.
3. Jugular and subclavian: Have patient exhale and pull the line during the exhalation.
   - Exhalation increases intrathoracic pressure as compared to atmospheric pressure, thereby reducing the risk of air thromboembolism.
4. Hold pressure for approximately 1 min to stop bleeding.
5. Dress with a sterile dressing.
6. If central line-related infection is suspected, cut off the tip with sterile scissors and send for culture.

Selected Reading

Internal Jugular Vein Access

McGee DC, Gould MK. Preventing complications of central venous catheterization. N Engl J Med. 2003a;348(12):1123–33.

Mimoz O, et al. Chlorhexidine-based antiseptic solution vs alcohol-based providone-iodine for central venous catheter care. Arch Intern Med. 2007;167(19):2066–72.

Noble V, et al. Manual of emergency and critical care ultrasound. Cambridge: Cambridge University Press; 2007. p. 196–204.

Parry G. Trendelenburg position, head elevation and a midline position optimize right internal jugular vein diameter. Can J Anaesth. 2004;51(4):379.

Vesely T. Central venous catheter tip position: a continuing controversy. J Vasc Interv Radiol. 2003;14(5):527.

Subclavian Vein Access

Elliott TS, Faroqui MH, Armstrong RF, Hanson GC. Guidelines for good practice in central venous catheterization. Hospital Infection Society and the Research Unit of the Royal College of Physicians. J Hosp Infect. 1994;28(3):163–76.

Fortune JB, Feustel P. Effect of patient position on size and location of the subclavian vein for percutaneous puncture. Arch Surg. 2003;138(9):996–1000; discussion 1001.

Fragou M, et al. Real time ultrasound-guided subclavian vein cannulation versus the landmark method in critical care patients: a prospective randomized study. Crit Care Med. 2011;39(7):1–6.

Kilbourne MJ, Bochicchio GV, Scalea T, Xiao Y. Avoiding common technical errors in subclavian central venous catheter placement. J Am Coll Surg. 2009;208(1):104–9.

McGee DC, Gould MK. Preventing complications of central venous catheterization. N Engl J Med. 2003b;348(12):1123–33.

Femoral Vein Access

Dailey RH. Femoral vein cannulation: a review. J Emerg Med. 1985;2:367–72.

Lim T, Ryu H-G, et al. Effect of the bevel direction of puncture needle on success rate and complications during internal jugular vein catheterization. Crit Care Med. 2012;40(2):491–4.

McGee DC, Gould MK. Preventing complications of central venous catheterization. N Engl J Med. 2003c;348:1123–33.

Marik PE, Flemmer M, Harrison W. The risk of catheter-related bloodstream infection with femoral venous catheters as compared to subclavian and internal jugular venous catheters: a systemic review of the literature and meta-analysis. Crit Care Med. 2012;40:2479–85.

Swanson RS, Uhlig PN, Gross PL, et al. Emergency intravenous access through the femoral vein. Ann Emerg Med. 1984;13:244–7.

Pulmonary Artery Catheter

4

Rohit Pravin Patel and Marie-Carmelle Elie

4.1 Indications

- Prevention or treatment of multiorgan failure in high-risk patients
- Preoperative and postoperative management in high-risk patients with cardiac, pulmonary, or renal dysfunction
- Patients with anticipated large fluid shifts (sepsis, bleeding, burns, cirrhosis)
- Oliguria or hypotension not relieved by fluids
- Suspected cardiac event leading to shock
- For continuous SVO2 (central venous oxygenation) monitoring in shock
- To differentiate shock states
- For monitoring cardiac output in patients requiring high-positive end-expiratory pressure (>14 cm H20)
- Monitoring and management of complicated myocardial dysfunction or cardiogenic shock
- Congestive heart failure with poor response to afterload reduction and diuretic therapy
- Suspected tamponade or contusion from blunt chest injury
- Pulmonary hypertension with myocardial dysfunction
- Diagnosis of primary pulmonary hypertension
- Aspiration of air emboli
- Direct pulmonary artery administration of thrombolytic therapy

4.2 Contraindications

- Tricuspid or pulmonary valve mechanical prosthesis
- Right heart mass (thrombus or tumor)
- Tricuspid or pulmonary valve endocarditis

- Recurrent sepsis (catheter could serve as nidus for infection)
- Hypercoagulopathy (catheter could serve as site for thrombus formation)
- Patient known sensitivity to heparin (catheters with heparin coating)
- Electrocardiographic (ECG) monitoring encouraged in conditions of complete left bundle branch block (risk of complete heart block increased), Wolfe–Parkinson–White syndrome, and Ebstein's malformation (risk of tachyarrhythmias)

4.3 Materials

- Pulmonary artery or Swan–Ganz catheter
- Percutaneous sheath introducer and contamination shield
- Compatible cardiac output computer for measuring cardiac output by the bolus thermodilution method
- Injectate temperature sensing probe (bolus thermodilution method)
- Connecting cables
- Sterile flush system and pressure transducers
- Bedside ECG and pressure monitor system
- Appropriate ECG "slave" cables

4.3.1 Catheter Preparation

- Avoid forceful wiping or stretching of catheter to avoid injury to the thermistor wire circuitry; wiping the heparin coat may cause removal of the coating.
- In vivo calibration is required if in vitro calibration is not done; refer to the monitor operator's manual for detailed calibration instructions.
- Connect catheter's injectate and pressure-monitoring lumens to the flush system and pressure transducers; ensure all lines are free of air.
- Connect the thermistor to the monitor and confirm no fault messages appear.

R.P. Patel, MD • M.-C. Elie, MD, RDMS (✉)
Department of Emergency Medicine, University of Florida Health Shands Hospital, Gainesville, FL, USA
e-mail: rohitpatel@ufl.edu; elie@ufl.edu

© Springer Science+Business Media New York 2016
L. Ganti (ed.), *Atlas of Emergency Medicine Procedures*, DOI 10.1007/978-1-4939-2507-0_4

4.4   Procedure

1. Maintain sterile precautions including sterile cap, mask, gown, gloves.
2. Place a central venous line introducer and verify placement of introducer with chest radiograph; it is also acceptable to obtain the chest radiograph after the insertion of the pulmonary artery catheter if no complication was suspected with the central venous line introducer.
3. Cleanse the skin and introducer thoroughly with chlorhexidine.
4. Have assistant open pulmonary artery catheter kit in sterile fashion.
5. Remove pulmonary artery catheter from kit and have assistant hook up all the ports to the transducers and make sure readings are accurate as the catheter is being manipulated.
6. Gently lift the distal portion of the catheter up from the silicone gripper; do not pull the balloon through the gripper to avoid damage.
7. Have assistant check the proximal and distal ports for patency by flushing with sterile saline. Also have the assistant check the patency of the balloon with the syringe provided in the kit (Fig. 4.1). Check for major asymmetry and for leaks (optional) by submerging in sterile saline or water. Deflate balloon prior to insertion. Carefully wave the distal catheter segment up and down to confirm electrical continuity by observing a pressure tracing on monitor. Ensure proper readings, no information is sometimes better than wrong information. Make sure each port transduces appropriately *prior to* insertion.
8. Familiarize yourself with the catheter line markings. Each thin line indicates 10 cm from the tip and thick line indicates 50 cm from the tip. These are used in combination to indicate length from tip (Fig. 4.2).
9. Place the sterile plastic sleeve (lock side toward patient, Fig. 4.3) over the catheter after flushing all ports to further protect the catheter during manipulation.

10. The distal end of the catheter is inserted into the introducer hub of the central venous line and threaded to the superior vena cava. The catheter must be placed at least 30 cm into the introducer for the balloon to clear the distal end of the introducer prior to inflation. At *no point* should the catheter be withdrawn with the balloon inflated; ensure the assistant has deflated the balloon prior to withdrawal. The balloon assists in directing the catheter through the vascular system using the directional blood flow.
11. At 20 cm, the balloon should be inflated and catheter advanced through right atrium, past the tricuspid valve into the right ventricle, then past the pulmonary valve to the pulmonary artery. The waveform and pressure readings can guide you through the various locations (Fig. 4.4).
12. Once in the pulmonary artery, the catheter should be carefully and slowly advanced to wedge position. The balloon can be deflated and pulmonary artery tracings should reappear. If a wedge is obtained with less than the maximum recommended volume, the catheter should be withdrawn to a position where full inflation volume produces a wedge tracing. Avoid prolonged times when obtaining wedge pressure (2 respiratory cycles or 10–15 s), especially in patients with pulmonary hypertension.
13. General guidelines for distance necessary at various points include: right atrium 20–25 cm, right ventricle 30–35 cm, and pulmonary artery 40–45 cm; catheter usually wedges at 50–55 cm. These are dependent on the starting location you are using to advance the catheter (subclavian, internal jugular, femoral).
14. Once the catheter is in correct position, it should be locked into place with the plastic sleeve tip onto the hub of the introducer.
15. Correct placement is confirmed with chest radiograph (Fig. 4.5).

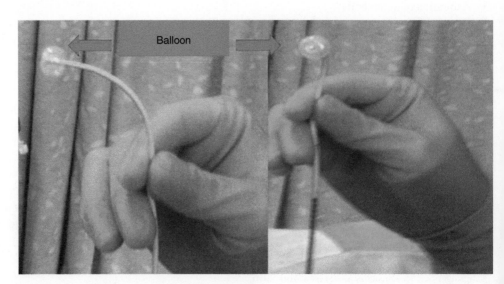

Fig. 4.1 Balloon inflation prior to insertion for evaluation of patency or leaks

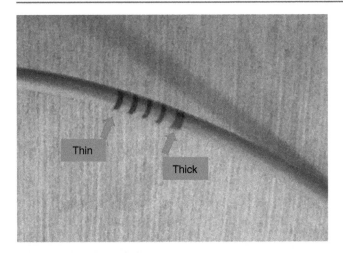

Fig. 4.2 Thick and thin markings found on the catheter representing length from distal tip

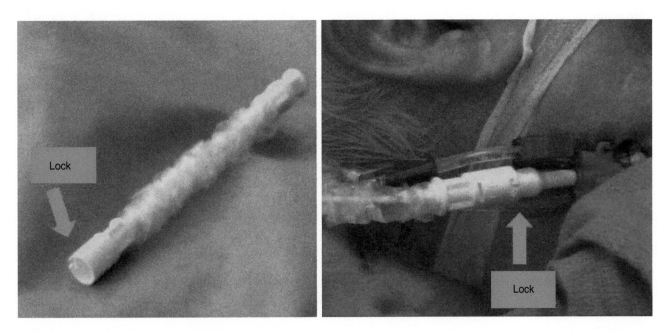

Fig. 4.3 Lock position on catheter for stabilization of catheter

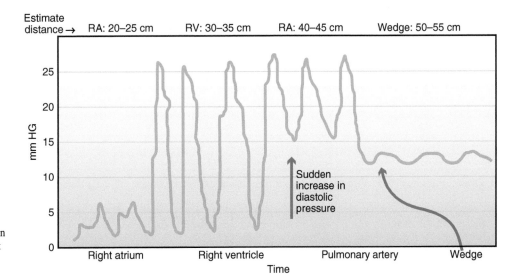

Fig. 4.4 Typical waveform seen at specific locations in the heart with associated estimated distances from catheter tip

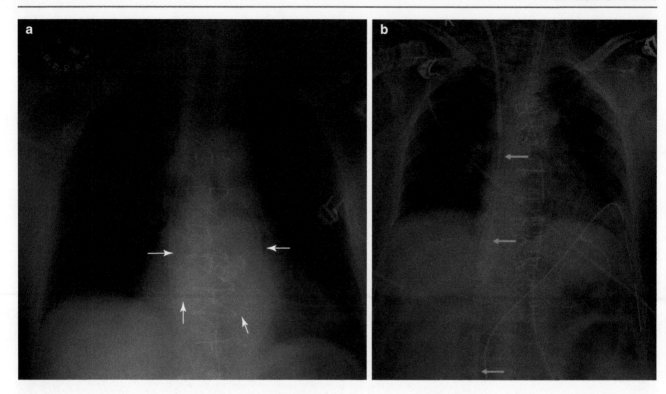

Fig. 4.5 Chest radiograph demonstrating correct (**a**) and incorrect (**b**) positioning of pulmonary artery catheter (*arrows*) (**a** Reproduced with permission from McGraw-Hill: Stead LG, et al. *First Aid for the Radiology Clerkship*. New York: McGraw-Hill; 2009; **b** Reproduced with permission from Wolters Kluwer: Jain SN. A pictorial essay: radiology of lines and tubes in the intensive care unit. *Indian J Radiol Imaging*. 2011;21(3):182–190)

4.5   Complications

- Arrhythmias: most are premature ventricular contractions that are self-limiting and resolve with advancement into pulmonary artery or withdrawal into atrium.
- Right bundle branch block: usually transient after positioning catheter into the pulmonary artery; if has already left bundle branch block may lead to complete heart block; should have temporary pacing equipment on standby.
- Knotting in the right ventricle (RV): risk increased in those with dilated cardiac chambers; a persistent RV tracing (15 cm beyond the point where initial RV tracing was observed) should alert you to this possibility.
- Pulmonary artery rupture: age >60 year, anticoagulation therapy, and presence of pulmonary hypertension increase risk of rupture; hemoptysis shortly after placement is indicative and management includes lateral decubitus positioning (bleeding side down), intubation with double lumen tube, and increasing positive end-expiratory pressure (PEEP).
- Infection.
- Pulmonary infarction: due to unintentional migration of distal tip.

4.6   Pearls and Pitfalls

- If the catheter requires stiffening during insertion, slowly perfuse the catheter with 5–10 mL of cold sterile solution as the catheter is advanced through a peripheral vessel.
- The incidence of complications increases significantly with periods of use longer than 72 h, so assess the need for the catheter on daily basis.
- Anticipate spontaneous catheter tip migration toward periphery of pulmonary bed; if a wedge tracing is observed when balloon is deflated, pull the catheter back.

Selected Reading

1. Edward Lifesciences. Pulmonary artery catheter Instruction manual. 2009. http://ht.edwards.com/resourcegallery/products/swanganz/pdfs/invasivehdmphysprincbook.pdf.
2. Edward Lifesciences. Pulmonary artery catheter Instruction manual. 2009. http://www.edwards.com/products/pacatheters/Pages/ThermodilutionCatheter.aspx.
3. Leatherman JW, Marini JJ. Clinical use of the pulmonary artery catheter. In: Hall JB, Schmidt GA, Wook LDH, editors. Principles of critical care. 3rd ed. New York: McGraw-Hill; 2005. p. 146–50.
4. Moran SE, Pei KY, Yu M. Hemodynamic monitoring: arterial and pulmonary artery catheters. In: Gabrielli A, Layon AJ, Yu M, editors. Civetta, Taylor, and Kirby's critical care. 4th ed. Philadelphia: Lippincott Williams & Wilkins; 2009.

Noninvasive Cardiac Monitoring: The Edwards Vigileo System

Dawood G. Dalaly and Rohit Pravin Patel

5.1 Indications

Cardiac output monitoring is indicated when trying to determine fluid responsiveness in patients. It assists in directing and assessing results of resuscitative efforts to ensure appropriate tissue perfusion. Although most catheters are systemically invasive, tools like the Vigileo (Edwards Lifesciences; Irvine, CA) are excellent noninvasive devices for determining values such as the stroke volume, stroke volume variation, stroke volume index, cardiac output, and cardiac index (Fig. 5.1).

D.G. Dalaly, DO
Department of Surgery,
University of Florida Health Shands Hospital,
Gainesville, FL, USA
e-mail: ddalaly@ufl.edu

R.P. Patel, MD (✉)
Department of Emergency Medicine,
University of Florida Health Shands Hospital,
Gainesville, FL, USA
e-mail: drpratik@gmail.com

© Springer Science+Business Media New York 2016
L. Ganti (ed.), *Atlas of Emergency Medicine Procedures*, DOI 10.1007/978-1-4939-2507-0_5

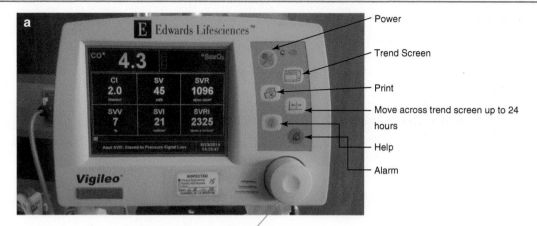

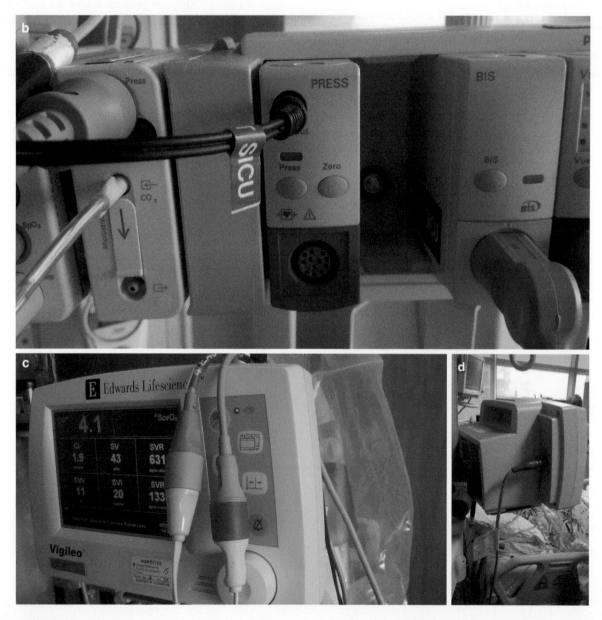

Fig. 5.1 Typical monitoring devices and connecting devices from monitor to patient: (**a**) FloTrac monitor, (**b**) FloTrac red port connects to the heart monitor, (**c**) the FloTrac system connects to the arterial line on one end and the pressure bag/monitors on the other; monitor connections are color coded, (**d**) the green port connects to the green port from the FloTrac

5.2   Contraindications

There are no contraindications to noninvasive monitoring of the heart, although most systems will need to be connected to an arterial line catheter, therefore contraindications to arterial line placement must be determined. Current literature supports the use of noninvasive monitoring to those who are 100 % supported ventilation with tidal volumes ≥8 mL/kg. There is no support for use in those with spontaneous breaths or arrhythmia. Patients with significant variation in respiratory pattern may have results that are unreliable.

5.3   Definitions and Values (Table 5.1)

Table 5.1   Cardiac output monitoring definitions

Term	Reference range	Definition
Cardiac output	4–8 L/min	Volume of blood being pumped by the heart in 1 min
Cardiac index	2.5–4 L/min/m²	Compares the amount of fluid being pumped by the heart with an individual's body surface area
Stroke volume	40–80 mL/beat	Volume of blood being pumped by the ventricle per beat
Stroke volume variation	10–15 %	Represents percentage of change between minimum and maximum stroke volumes and predictor of fluid responsiveness
Stroke volume index	33–47 mL/m²/beat	Quantity of blood ejected from the heart per beat
Mixed venous saturation (SvO_2)	60–80 %	Percentage of oxygen bound to hemoglobin in blood returning to the right side of the heart; represents oxygen delivery and consumption at the tissue level. Usually obtained from pulmonary artery catheter
Central venous oxygen saturation ($ScvO_2$)	70 %	Surrogate marker for SvO_2, usually obtained from internal jugular or subclavian catheters

5.4 Materials

- FloTrac (Edwards Lifesciences, Irvine, CA, USA)
- Vigileo monitor
- Pressure bag

5.5 Procedure

1. Connect FloTrac to arterial line and distal FloTrac port to pressure bag. Inflate bag to 300 mmHg.
2. Connect green FloTrac cord to green Vigileo cord and red FloTrac cord to arterial line port on heart monitor.
3. Turn the port on the FloTrac off to the patient and zero on your heart monitor as you would with an arterial line. At the same time, you should have pressed the "Enter" knob on the Vigileo system, scrolled it to "zero arterial pressure," and pressed the knob again for that function.
4. You should now have an arterial waveform on your heart monitor and your cardiac values on the Vigileo system.

5.6 Pearls and Pitfalls

- Some components of the values obtained are not reliable on spontaneously breathing patients and it is critical to check the ventilator waveforms for these breaths.

- Patients without adequate tidal volumes (at least 8 mL/kg) will also have unreliable values.
- Stroke volume variation usually is more reliable when greater than 13 % and indicates fluid responsiveness rather than when it is less than 13 % (similar to a low central venous pressure (CVP) being more informative than normal or high CVP levels).

Selected Reading

1. Alarcon LH, Fink MP. Chapter 13. Physiologic monitoring of the surgical patient. In: Brunicardi FC, Andersen DK, Billiar TR, et al., editors. Schwartz's principles of surgery. 9th ed. New York: McGraw-Hill; 2010.
2. Holcroft JW, Anderson JT, Sena MJ. Chapter 12. Shock and acute pulmonary failure in surgical patients. In: Doherty GM, editor. CURRENT diagnosis & treatment: surgery. 13th ed. New York: McGraw-Hill; 2009. Available at http://www.accesssurgery.com/content.aspx?aID=5212482. Accessed 22 Aug 2012.
3. Edwards Critical Care Education. Available at http://www.edwards.com/education/Pages/cceducationmap.aspx. Accessed 11 Dec 2012.

Peripheral Venous Cutdown

6

Jeffrey Kile, Katrina John, and Amish Aghera

6.1 Indications

- Distorted anatomy of peripheral venous access sites
- Unavailability of cannulable veins (e.g., in hypovolemia, burn victim, traumatic anatomy, sclerosed veins, etc.)
- Emergency venous access for infusion/transfusion
- Unavailability of central venous access or less invasive means peripherally

6.2 Contraindications

- Absolute
  - Availability of less invasive or less time-consuming means of vascular access
  - Overlying infection, traumatic tissue, burn, etc., at cutdown site
  - Traumatic injury proximal to cutdown site
- Relative
  - Coagulation disorders

6.3 Materials and Medications (Fig. 6.1)

- Sterile gloves
- Antimicrobial solution and swabs
- 4″×4″ gauze sponges
- Local anesthetic (1 % lidocaine 5 mL)
- 5-mL syringe
- Blunt needle
- 25- or 27-gauge needle
- Scalpel
- Vein dilator/lifter
- Peripheral intravenous catheter
- Curved hemostat
- 0-0 silk sutures or 4.0 nylon sutures
- Iris scissors
- Intravenous infusion tubing
- Adhesive tape

J. Kile, MBBS, PhD, MPH (✉) • K. John, MBBS
Department of Emergency Medicine, Eisenhower Medical Center,
Rancho Mirage, CA, USA
e-mail: jeffrey.kile@gmail.com; trenjohn@me.com

A. Aghera, MD
Department of Emergency Medicine, Maimonides Medical Center,
New York, NY, USA
e-mail: aaghera@maimonidesmed.org

© Springer Science+Business Media New York 2016
L. Ganti (ed.), *Atlas of Emergency Medicine Procedures*, DOI 10.1007/978-1-4939-2507-0_6

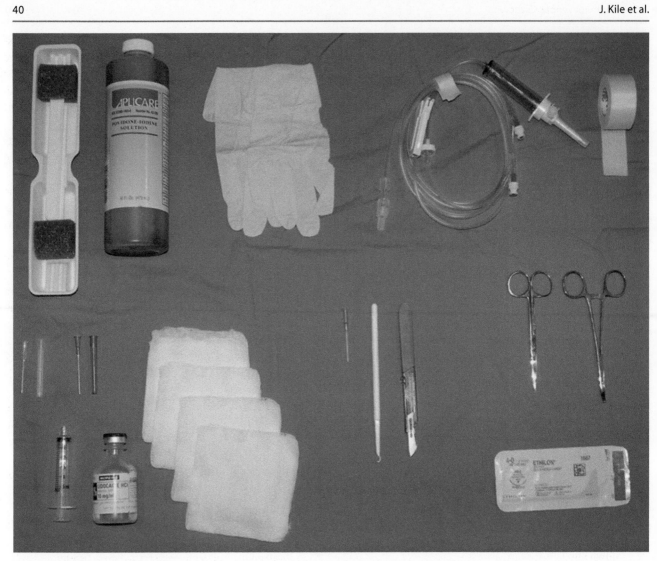

Fig. 6.1 Materials and medications

6.4   Choice of Vessel for Cutdown

- Greater saphenous vein: this vessel is the longest vein in the body, is predominantly subcutaneous, and is exposed with minimal blunt dissection just anterior to the medial malleolus at the ankle.
- Basilic vein: this vessel is reliably located 1–2 cm lateral to the medial epicondyle on the anterior aspect of the humeral region, typically catheterized just superior to the antecubital fossa approximately, and its diameter permits its localization relatively easily even in the hypotensive patient.
- Cephalic vein: this vessel runs anteromedially from the radial aspect of the wrist to the antecubital fossa, is superficial and large in diameter, and is most easily cannulated at the distal flexor crease in the antecubital fossa.

6.5   Procedure

6.5.1   Standard Venous Cutdown Technique

1. Apply antimicrobial solution liberally to the skin surrounding the incisional area.
2. Establish a sterile field by placing drapes around the incisional area.
3. Apply a tourniquet proximal to the planned cutdown site to maximize visualization of vein to be cannulated.
4. Inject local anesthetic to raise a small (0.5 cm) wheal using 25- or 27-gauge needle and then insert the tip of the needle through wheal to infiltrate skin superficial to the artery with approximately 4 mL of anesthetic.
   - Injection of local anesthetic into the vessel may precipitate arrhythmia, so draw back on the plunger prior to infiltration to ensure the tip of the needle is not inside the vessel.
5. Incise the skin with scalpel perpendicular to the course of the vein through all cutaneous layers until subcutaneous fat is visualized (Fig. 6.2).
   - Some practitioners prefer using a longitudinal incision to reduce the risk of transecting neurovascular structures, but this may not produce sufficient exposure of vein.

6. Using a curved hemostat or gloved finger, bluntly dissect the subcutaneous tissue to isolate and mobilize approximately 2–3 cm of the vein (Fig. 6.3).
   - A small self-retaining retractor or tissue spreader can be used in this step to improve visualization of vein if desired
7. Pass suture under the vein distal to the planned venous puncture site using hemostat to stabilize the vein and tie the suture over the vein (Fig. 6.4).
8. Pass a second suture under the vein proximal to the planned venous puncture site using hemostat (Fig. 6.5).
   - This step enables increased visualization, vessel control, and hemostasis during incision.
   - Leave the ends of both sutures long to facilitate maneuvering the vein.
9. Incise one-half to one-third of the diameter of the vein using a scalpel or iris scissors held at a 45° angle to the vessel (Fig. 6.6).
10. Grasping the proximal edge of the incision with a hemostat to apply counter traction (in a distal direction), insert the tip of the catheter into the venous incision (Fig. 6.7).
    - Do not force the catheter if it does not easily advance.
    - Catheter can be introduced directly through the skin incision or via skin puncture adjacent to the skin incision.
    - If the catheter lacks a tapered tip, cut the distal end of the cannula at a 45° angle to fashion a beveled tip.
11. Thread catheter into vein (Fig. 6.8).
12. Aspirate any air which may have entered the cannula during insertion.
13. Connect hub of catheter to intravenous tubing.
14. Tie the proximal suture around the vein just proximal to the venous incision, encircling both the vein and the intraluminal cannula with the suture.
15. Remove tourniquet.
16. Secure the catheter hub to the skin using nylon (4.0) sutures as follows. Take a 0.5 cm bite of skin under the catheter hub with the suture needle, tie several knots in the suture without pinching the skin, then tie a second set of knots around the hub of the catheter firmly.
17. Close the incision using nylon (4.0) sutures.
18. Dress the wound with appropriate self-adhesive sterile dressing or sterile gauze pads and adhesive tape.

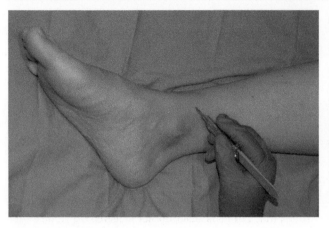

Fig. 6.2 Incision of skin

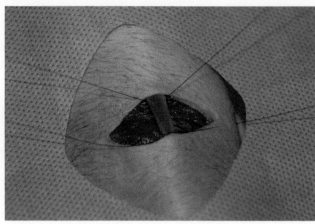

Fig. 6.5 Distal and proximal ligatures in place

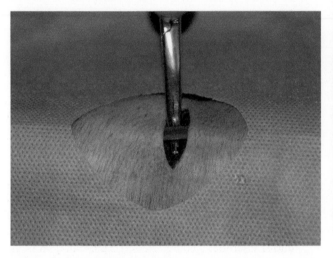

Fig. 6.3 Mobilization of vein

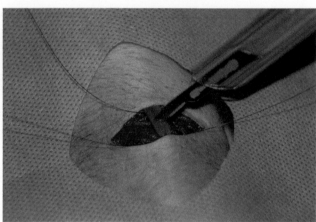

Fig. 6.6 Incision of vein

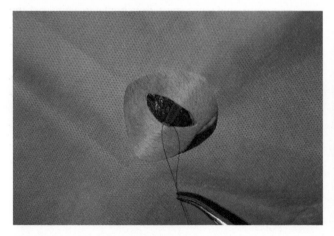

Fig. 6.4 Distal ligature tied around vein

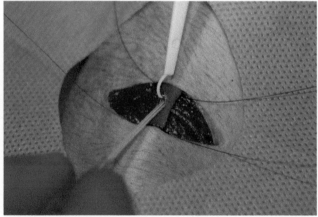

Fig. 6.7 Catheterization of vein

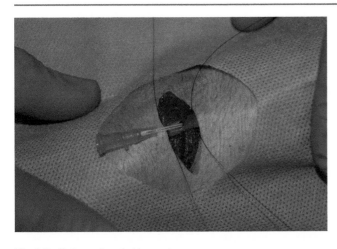

Fig. 6.8 Catheter threaded into vein

6.5.2 "Mini-Cutdown" Technique

(Perform steps 1–6 from the "Standard Venous Cutdown Technique," above, and then proceed with the steps below.)

1. Puncture the vein using a standard over-the-needle venous catheter.
   - Catheter can be introduced directly through the skin incision or via skin puncture adjacent to the skin incision.
2. Thread catheter into the vein over the needle.
3. Remove and discard the needle.
4. Aspirate any air which may have entered the catheter during insertion.
5. Connect catheter to intravenous tubing.

(Continue with steps 15–18 from the "Standard Venous Cutdown Technique," above.)

6.5.3 Modified/Guide Wire Technique

(Perform steps 1–6 from the "Standard Venous Cutdown Technique," above, and then proceed with the steps below.)

1. Insert the blunt end of the guide wire into the incised vein.
2. While stabilizing the guide wire at its insertion site, thread the dilator and sheath assembly over the free end of the guide wire until it is approximately one inch from the skin.
3. Grasp the free end of the guide wire protruding from the tail end of the assembly.
   - If it does not protrude from the tail end of the assembly, the guide wire must be removed sufficiently from the artery to be securely grasped. It must protrude visibly from the tail end of the dilator throughout the subsequent process of threading the dilator into the vein.
   - Never let go of the guide wire during this step, as insertion of the dilator and sheath assembly can otherwise push the guide wire completely into the vein.
4. Holding it firmly near its tip, thread the assembly over the wire into vessel with a gentle back-and-forth twisting motion.
5. Holding the sheath securely in the vein, remove and discard the dilator and guide wire.
6. Aspirate any air which may have entered the sheath during insertion.
7. Connect sheath to intravenous tubing.
8. Remove tourniquet.
9. Secure the sheath to the skin.
10. Close the incision using nylon (4.0) sutures.
11. Dress the wound with appropriate self-adhesive sterile dressing or sterile gauze pads and adhesive tape.

6.6 Complications

- Hematoma
- Infection
- Sepsis
- Phlebitis
- Embolization
- Wound dehiscence

6.7 Pearls and Pitfalls

- Fluids are infused most quickly via short, large-bore catheters.
- If the line is inserted for slow infusion of intravenous drugs, catheter lumen size is relatively insignificant.
- In larger children and adults, intravenous plastic tubing, small-bore pediatric feeding tubes, and Silastic catheters may be used as infusion catheters.
- Threading a 10-gauge intravenous catheter or intravenous tubing directly into the incised vein achieves excellent flow rates.
- If difficulty is encountered while threading the catheter into the incised vein, ensure an appropriately sized

catheter has been used and that the vessel lumen has been correctly identified and that no false passage has been created in the adventitia.

- As compared to the standard venous cutdown technique, the mini-cutdown technique is easier and also preserves the vein, permitting repeated catheterization if necessary.
- As compared to the standard venous cutdown technique, the modified/guide wire technique reduces procedure time and increases the likelihood of vein salvage in the event of vessel transection.

Selected Reading

1. Chappell S, Vilke GM, Chan TC, et al. Peripheral venous cutdown. J Emerg Med. 2006;31:411–6.
2. Klofas E. A quicker saphenous vein cutdown and a better way to teach it. J Trauma. 1997;43:985–7.
3. McIntosh BB, Dulchavsky SA. Peripheral vascular cutdown. Crit Care Clin. 1992;8:807–18.
4. Nocito A, Wildi S, Rufibach K, et al. Randomized clinical trial comparing venous cutdown with the Seldinger technique for placement of implantable venous access ports. Br J Surg. 2009;96:1129–34.
5. Shockley LW, Butzier DJ. A modified wire-guided technique for venous cutdown access. Ann Emerg Med. 1990;19:393–5.

Part II

Airway and Vascular Procedures

Bag-Valve-Mask Ventilation

Braden Hexom and Tatiana Havryliuk

7.1 Indications

- Hypoxia
- Hypoventilation/apnea
- Rescue maneuver if failed intubation

7.2 Contraindications

- Absolute
  - Inability to ventilate due to lack of seal (thick beard, deforming facial trauma)
  - Inability to ventilate secondary to complete upper airway obstruction
  - Active, adequate spontaneous ventilation

- Relative
  - Full stomach (aspiration risk)
  - After induction and paralysis during rapid sequence intubation (aspiration risk)

7.3 Materials (Fig. 7.1)

- Bag valve mask (BVM) with reservoir
- Oxygen connector tubing
- Nasal pharyngeal airway/oral pharyngeal airway
- Lubricant jelly

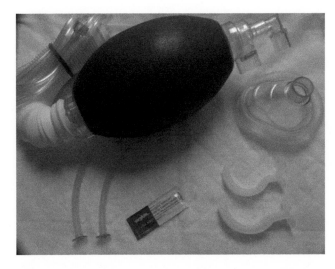

Fig. 7.1 BVM supplies: bag, mask, oral airways, nasopharyngeal airways, lubricant

B. Hexom, MD (✉)
Department of Emergency Medicine, Mount Sinai Hospital,
New York, NY, USA
e-mail: braden.hexom@mssm.edu

T. Havryliuk, MD
Department of Emergency Medicine, University of Colorado
Denver, Denver, CO, USA
e-mail: tatiana.havryliuk@ucdenver.edu

© Springer Science+Business Media New York 2016
L. Ganti (ed.), *Atlas of Emergency Medicine Procedures*, DOI 10.1007/978-1-4939-2507-0_7

7.4   Procedure

1. Position patient in "sniffing" position.
2. Open the airway with chin-lift/head-tilt or jaw thrust maneuvers.
3. Place airway adjuncts to maintain airway patency. Use oral airway (Fig. 7.2) in unconscious patients. Use nasal airway (Fig. 7.3) in semiresponsive patients.
4. Attach oxygen tubing to high-flow oxygen (15 L/min).
5. Place appropriately sized mask on patient's face covering the nose and mouth.
   - For one-handed technique (Fig. 7.4), use nondominant hand to make a "C" with index finger and thumb on top of the mask and form an "E" with the rest of the fingers using them to pull up on the mandible (E–C technique). Use the dominant hand to provide bag ventilations.
   - For two-handed (Fig. 7.5), two-person technique (preferred), make two semicircles with index fingers and thumbs of both hands on top of the mask and use the rest of the fingers to pull up on the mandible.
6. Consider the Sellick maneuver (cricoid pressure) to compress the esophagus against the cervical vertebrae, preventing gastric insufflation.
7. Ventilate patient providing reduced tidal volume breaths (500 mL) at a rate of 10–12 breaths per minute.
8. Give each breath gently over 1–1.5 s to avoid high peak pressures, avoiding gastric insufflation.
9. Prepare for definitive airway as dictated by the clinical scenario.

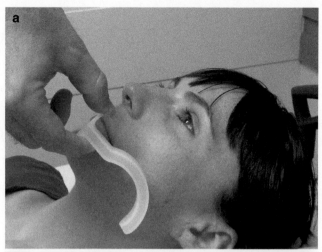

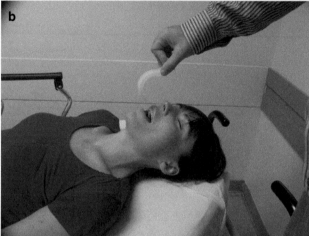

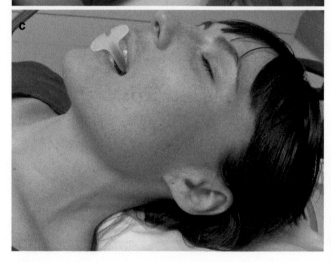

Fig. 7.2 (a–c) Oral airway insertion

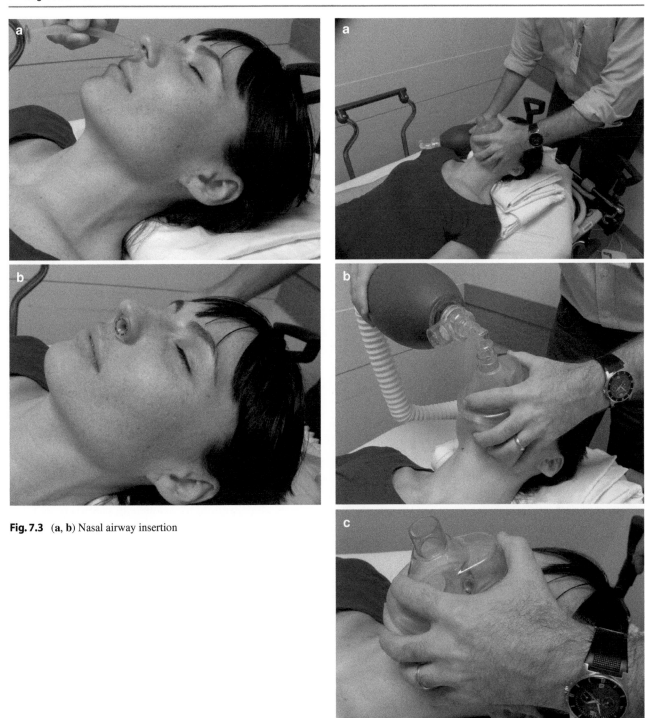

Fig. 7.3 (**a**, **b**) Nasal airway insertion

Fig. 7.4 (**a–c**) One-handed seal technique

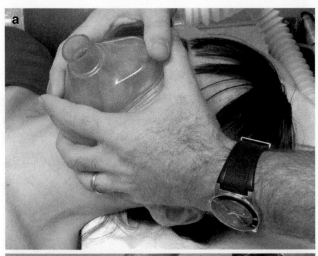

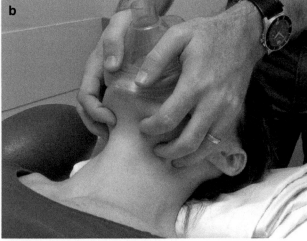

Fig. 7.5 Two-handed seal technique: (**a**) two semicircles, (**b**) alternative thumbs method

7.5   Complications

- Stomach inflation may lead to vomiting and aspiration.
- Increased positive thoracic pressure may cause decreased preload, worsening cardiac output, and/or hypotension.
- Hypoventilation (inadequate O_2 tidal volume, airway patency, or mask seal).

7.6   Pearls and Pitfalls

- Pearls
    - Use jaw thrust to open mouth for patients with possible cervical spine injury.
    - Use airway adjuncts whenever available, especially if prolonged BVM ventilation is anticipated.
    - Use lubricant jelly to insert nasal airway; do not insert in patients with severe facial trauma.
    - Mask should be placed on patient's face prior to attaching to bag.
    - Apply pressure to the bony part of the mandible only to avoid soft-tissue injury.
    - Provide just enough tidal volume to see a chest rise and deliver each breath gently over 1–1.5 s to prevent gastric insufflation.
    - Ensure good seal:
        - Select appropriate mask size.
        - Choose two-handed technique over one-handed, if possible.
        - Keep well-fitting dentures in place if present (and remove before intubation).
        - Lift the mandible toward the mask (as opposed to pushing the mask onto the face).
        - Rock the mask on face until no leak is present.
        - Apply K–Y jelly to beard to improve the seal.
- Pitfalls
    - Overcompression during the Sellick maneuver can compress the cricoid ring, preventing ventilation.
    - Cricoid pressure (Sellick maneuver) is not recommended during cardiac arrest resuscitation.
    - Difficult BVM ventilation: MOANS
        - *M*ask seal
        - *O*besity/obstruction
        - *A*ge
        - *N*o teeth
        - *S*tiff

Selected Reading

ECC Committee, Subcommittees and Task Forces of the American Heart Association. American heart association guidelines for cardiopulmonary resuscitation and emergency cardiovascular care. Circulation. 2010;122:S685–705.

Joffe AM, Hetzel S, Liew EC. A two-handed jaw-thrust technique is superior to the one-handed "EC-clamp" technique for mask ventilation in the apneic unconscious person. Anesthesiology. 2010;113:873–9.

Roberts JR, Hedges JR. Clinical procedures in emergency medicine. Philadelphia: Saunders Elsevier; 2010.

Walls RM, Murphy MF. Manual of emergency airway management. 3rd ed. Philadelphia: Lippincott Williams & Wilkins; 2008.

Awake Orotracheal Intubation

8

Benjamin M. Mahon, Justin Bennett, and Lars K. Beattie

8.1 Indications

- Urgent but not emergent endotracheal intubation is required in a patient who:
  - Is awake
  - Is currently protecting his airway
  - Is not a candidate for a supraglottic airway (LMA)
  - The patient
    - Is predicted to have a difficult airway
    - Has structural abnormalities of the airway
    - Will not tolerate a period of apnea
    - May lose his airway (anaphylaxis, angioedema, traumatic airway)
- Patients requiring urgent but not emergent intubation in whom paralytics are contraindicated (i.e., allergies, myasthenic crisis)

8.2 Contraindications

- Absolute
  - Surgical airway indicated
  - Emergent crash airway needed
  - Obtunded patient
  - Allergies to medications needed (lidocaine, glycopyrrolate)

B.M. Mahon, MD
Ponciana Medical Center,
Kissimmee, FL, USA
e-mail: drfaust2k9@aol.com

J. Bennett, MD
Department of Emergency Medicine, Wake Forest University
School of Medicine, Winston-Salem, NC, USA
e-mail: jubennet@wakehealth.edu

L.K. Beattie, MD, MS (✉)
Department of Emergency Medicine, University of Florida,
Gainesville, FL, USA
e-mail: lars.beattie@ufl.edu

- Relative
  - Inability to maintain airway or tolerate secretions

8.3 Materials and Medications

- Suctioning equipment
- Intravenous access equipment, cardiac monitor, pulse oximetry, blood pressure cuff
- 4 % lidocaine solution
- 2 % viscous lidocaine jelly
- Nebulizer
- Mucosal atomization device
- 4×4 gauze
- Tongue depressor
- Glycopyrrolate/atropine
- Sedation: ketamine, propofol, Versed, and/or fentanyl
- Intubation equipment
- Backup emergency airway adjuncts
- Bag valve mask
- Laryngoscope, fiber optics, oral airway, etc.

8.4 Procedure

1. Preparation
   (a) Establish IV access.
   (b) Place the patient on a cardiac monitor with continuous pulse oximetry.
   (c) Keep backup RSI emergency airway medication and equipment at the bedside.
2. Administer 0.2–0.4 mg of intravenous glycopyrrolate (or a small dose (0.5–1 mg) of atropine to decrease secretions) 15 min prior to procedure.
3. Nebulize 2 mL of 4 % lidocaine with oxygen at 5 l O2 per minute to anesthetize the pharynx (Fig. 8.1).

© Springer Science+Business Media New York 2016
L. Ganti (ed.), *Atlas of Emergency Medicine Procedures*, DOI 10.1007/978-1-4939-2507-0_8

4. Use Yankauer suction (with the patient's assistance) to dry out the mouth as much as possible. Dabbing the tongue with gauze can assist in this step.
5. Continue preoxygenation.
6. Immediately after the nebulized solution is applied, give the patient a "lidocaine lollipop" (Fig. 8.2).
   (a) A 2 ml dollop of 2 % viscous lidocaine is to be placed on the end of a tongue depressor and is given to the patient to place in his mouth (like a lollipop).
   (b) Have the patient copiously gargle, then swallow the viscous lidocaine.
7. Using a mucosal atomizer, spray 2 ml of 4 % lidocaine in the posterior oropharynx and as far down toward the glottis as possible (Figs. 8.3, 8.4, and 8.5).
8. Sedation
   (a) It is feasible to proceed with the awake intubation in an un-sedated, wide awake but cooperative patient.
   (b) Sedation can be initiated using institutional preferences, but some options include:

   (i) Midazolam 2 mg IV
   (ii) Ketamine 1 mg/kg IV
   (iii) Propofol 1 mg/kg IV
   (iv) Ketofol (ketamine and propofol both at concentrations of 10 mg/ml, 5 ml of each mixed in a 10 cc syringe) titrated at 1–3 ml aliquots
   (c) More atomized lidocaine can be provided prior to endotracheal tube (ETT) passage, but one must be aware of the upper lidocaine dose for your patient.
   (d) Adequate anesthesia is confirmed by the absence of a gag reflex upon direct palpation (Fig. 8.6).
9. Intubation, induction, and gentle direct laryngoscopy can be performed at this point to place the ETT (Fig. 8.7).
   (a) Induction (if no prior sedation) and paralytic agents should be available to immediately administer after ETT placement.
   (b) Thorough discussions on intubation techniques can be found in other chapters in the atlas.

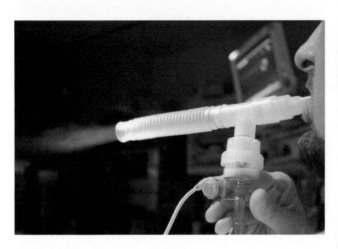

Fig. 8.1 Nebulization of 4 % lidocaine

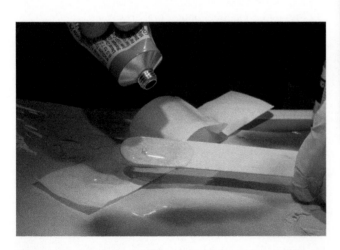

Fig. 8.2 Lidocaine lollipop

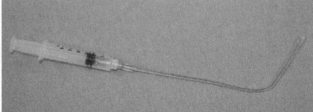

Fig. 8.3 Mucosal atomizer attached to syringe

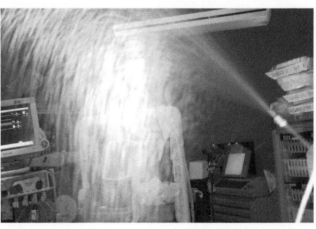

Fig. 8.4 Pushing syringe plunger atomizes lidocaine

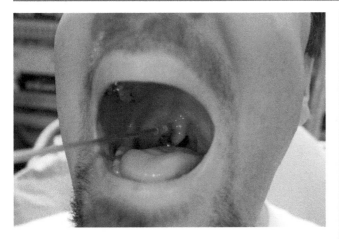

Fig. 8.5 Atomized lidocaine being administered to the posterior pharynx

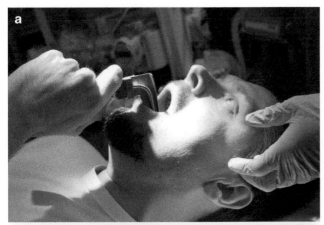

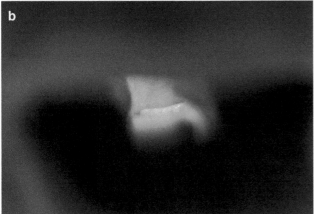

Fig. 8.6 (**a, b**) Adequately anesthetized awake patient with laryngoscopic view of epiglottis

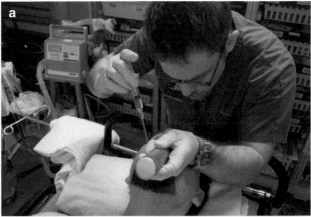

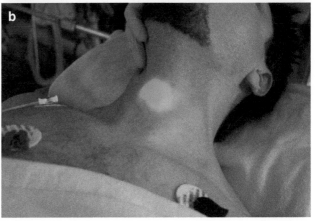

Fig. 8.7 (**a**) Final lidocaine atomization of deep structures and trachea, (**b**) intubation using a lighted stylet

8.5   Pearls and Pitfalls

- Pearls
  - Steps 3–7 should be done successively and as quickly as possible, to capitalize on the short half-life of lidocaine.
  - Simultaneous preoxygenation and anesthetization can be achieved by nebulizing the 4 % lidocaine through a face mask.
  - If the patient has been sedated, soft restraints may help prevent the patient from inadvertently grabbing the tube or your intubating equipment.
  - A nasotracheal intubation can be performed by simply anesthetizing the nares through which the ETT will be placed using lidocaine jelly and/or atomized lidocaine.
- Pitfalls
  - Failure to prepare all equipment beforehand may extend the procedure beyond the lidocaine half-life.

- The toxic dose of lidocaine is 300 mg or 3–5 mg/kg. The dosages listed are intended for a 70 kg patient and yields a total dose of 280 mg (4 mg/kg). This dose may need to be decreased in smaller individuals.

Selected Reading

Agro F, Hung OR, Cataldo R, Carassiti M, Gherardi S. Lightwand intubation using the Trachlight: a brief review of current knowledge. Can J Anaesth. 2001;48(6):592–9.

Rhee KY, Lee JR, Kim J, Park S, Kwon WK, Han S. A comparison of lighted stylet (Surch-Lite) and direct laryngoscopic intubation in patients with high Mallampati scores. Anesth Analg. 2009;108(4):1215–92.

Walls RM, Murphy MF. Manual of emergency airway management. 3rd ed. Philadelphia: Lippincott Williams and Wilkins, a Wolters Kluwer Business; 2008. Chap 11.

Rapid-Sequence Intubation

Ram A. Parekh

9

9.1 Indications

- Failure to oxygenate
- Failure to ventilate
- Unable to protect airway patency or reflexes
- Projected clinical course deterioration

9.2 Contraindications

- Absolute
  - Complete upper airway obstruction
  - Significant facial and airway trauma with loss of landmarks for orotracheal intubation
- Relative
  - Anticipated difficult intubation
    - Not an absolute contraindication.
    - Patient scenario requires a careful preintubation assessment and plan.
    - Consider an "awake" intubation.
    - Consider alternative airway adjuncts (e.g., extraglottic devices, video laryngoscopy, laryngeal mask airway [LMA]).

- Induction or paralytic agent-specific contraindications given clinical circumstances
  - Caution: induction agents that lower blood pressure in hypotensive patients
  - Caution: succinylcholine in potentially hyperkalemic patients
- Crash airway
  - Apneic, arrest, and periarrest situation

9.3 Materials and Medications

- Laryngoscope with appropriate blade (choice based on proceduralist's preference and patient anatomy) (Fig. 9.1)
- Intubating stylet
- Endotracheal tubes (ETTs)
- Syringe, 10 mL (to inflate ETT cuff)
- Surgilube
- Suction catheter
- Oral and nasal airways (Fig. 9.2)
- Ambu bag and mask attached to oxygen source
- Induction, pretreatment, and paralytic agents
- ETT confirmation device—EZ capnometry, quantitative end-tidal carbon dioxide concentration ($EtCO_2$) detection

R.A. Parekh, MD
Department of Emergency Medicine,
Icahn School of Medicine at Mount Sinai,
Elmhurst Hospital Center, Elmhurst, NY, USA
e-mail: ram.parekh@mssm.edu

© Springer Science+Business Media New York 2016
L. Ganti (ed.), *Atlas of Emergency Medicine Procedures*, DOI 10.1007/978-1-4939-2507-0_9

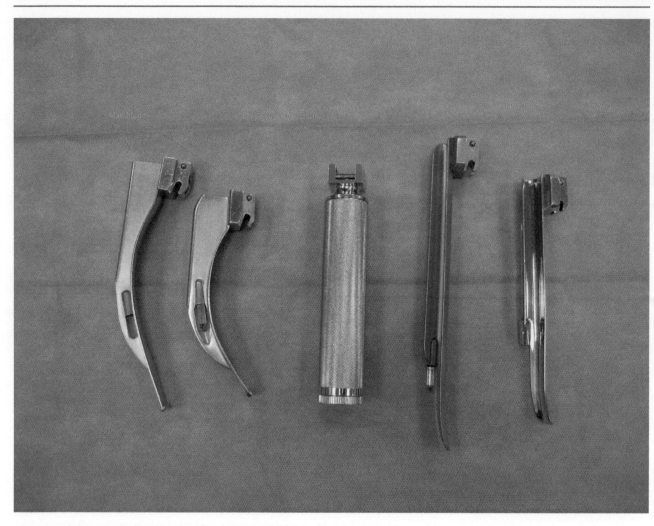

Fig. 9.1 Laryngoscope and blades

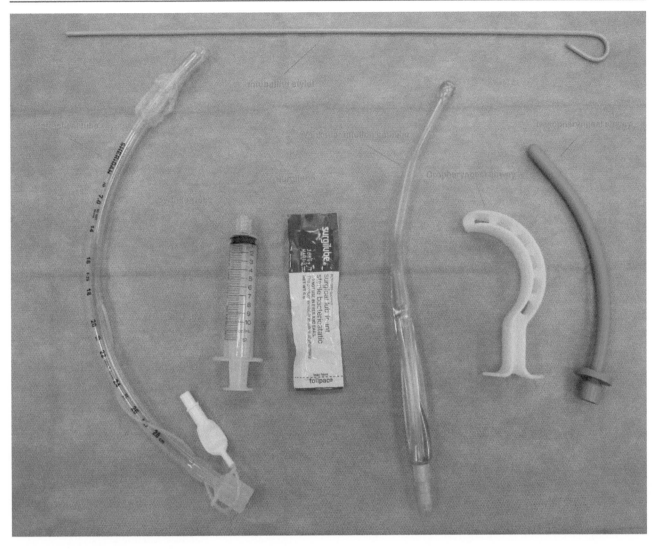

Fig. 9.2 Oral and nasal airways

9.4   Procedure

1. Preparation
   • Thoroughly assess patient for difficulty of intubation (Fig. 9.3).
   • Develop fallback plans for failed intubation attempt.
   • Establish at least one, but preferably two, secure intravenous (IV) lines.
   • Place on cardiac monitor with pulse oximetry, blood pressure monitoring, and continuous capnography.
   • Yankauer suction device attached to suction, suction on.
   • Pharmacological agents, drawn and labeled.
   • Laryngoscope and blades tested to ensure proper functioning of light source.
   • Desired ETT size, prepared for intubation:
     – Intubating stylet in position (tip at eye of ETT)
     – 10-mL syringe attached to ETT
     – ETT configured per proceduralist's preference (e.g., hockey stick, curved)
     – Cuff tested for air leak
2. Preoxygenation
   • Administer high-flow oxygen for 3–5 min (Fig. 9.4).
     – Nitrogen is exchanged for O_2 in the functional residual capacity of the lungs.
     – Establishes oxygen reservoir within lungs (primarily), blood, and body tissue.
     – Also known as nitrogen "washout."
   • This can be done using:
     – Non-rebreather masks—delivers 65–70 %
       • Difficult intubation not anticipated
     – Well-fitting bag-valve-masks (without positive-pressure ventilation)—delivers greater than 90 % oxygen (Fig. 9.5)
     – Noninvasive positive-pressure ventilation (NIPPV)—delivers 100 % oxygen
       • Consider NIPPV in high-risk patients with moderate to severe shunt physiology.

3. Pretreatment
   • Administer pharmacological agents to mitigate adverse physiological effects of intubation, induction, and paralysis, which may be undesirable in certain clinical circumstances (Table 9.1).
4. Induction and paralysis
   • Administer a rapidly acting induction agent to produce rapid loss of consciousness via IV push (Table 9.2).
   • Immediately follow induction agent with a neuromuscular-blocking agent via IV push (Table 9.3).
5. Positioning
   • If no cervical spine injury suspected, place the patient in the "sniff" position (Fig. 9.6):
     – Flex neck
     – Extend head
   • Ideally, the patient's pinna will be at the level of the sternum.
6. Direct laryngoscopy (see Chap. 10)
7. Proof of placement
   • Visualize ETT passing vocal cords
   • Confirm tube placement via $EtCO_2$:
     – Qualitative detection device—EZ Cap
     – Quantitative continuous $EtCO_2$ waveform on monitor (preferred) (Fig. 9.7)
   • Auscultation of breath sounds:
     – Lung fields bilaterally
     – Epigastric region (ensuring no breath sounds in the stomach)
8. Postintubation management
   • Secure ETT (Fig. 9.8)
   • Initiate mechanical ventilation.
   • Postintubation sedation and analgesia.
   • Postintubation chest x-ray.

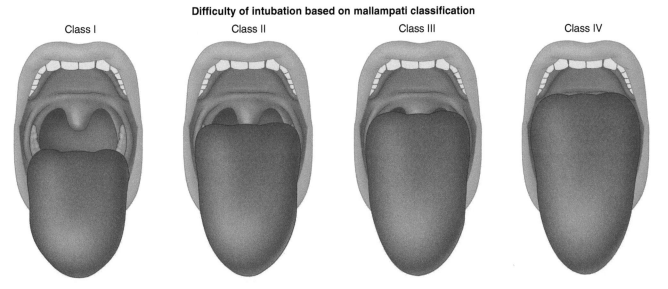

Fig. 9.3   Assess patient for difficulty of intubation

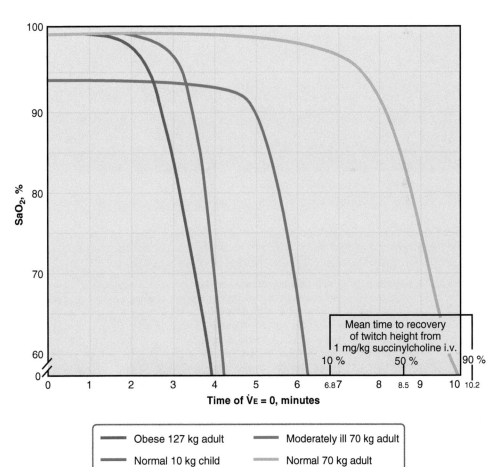

Fig. 9.4   *F*aO2 fractional concentration of alveolar oxygen, *Sa*O2 arterial oxygen saturation, *V*e expired volume per minute

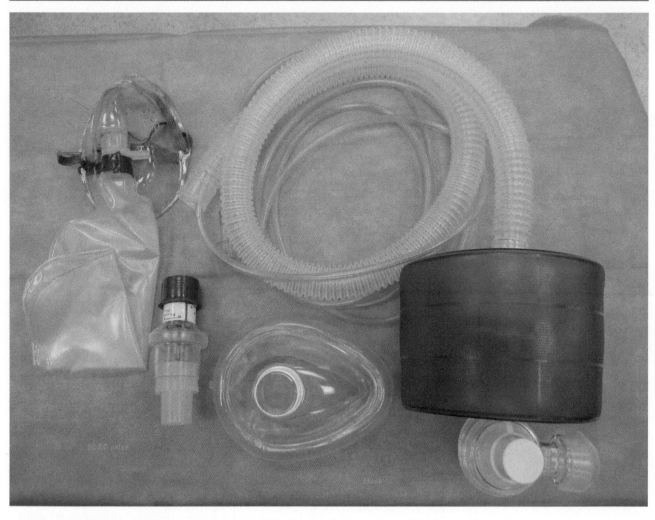

Fig. 9.5 Preoxygenation materials

Table 9.1 Pretreatment: pharmacological agents used to mitigate adverse physiological effects of intubation, induction, and paralysis

Agent	Dose (IV)	Indication
Lidocaine	1.5 mg/kg Rapid push	Use in tight brain to attenuate ICP increase from laryngoscopy/intubation; use in tight lungs to blunt bronchospastic response
Fentanyl	1–3 mcg/kg Slow push	Use in tight brain, tight heart, and tight vessels to blunt reflex sympathetic response to laryngoscopy

ICP intracranial pressure

Table 9.2 Induction: rapidly acting induction agents used to produce rapid loss of consciousness

Agent	Dose (IV) (mg/kg)	Onset (sec)	Duration (min)
Midazolam	0.2–0.3	60–90	15–30
Etomidate	0.3	15–45	3–12
Thiopental	3	<30	5–10
Ketamine	1.5–2.0	45–60	10–20
Propofol	1.5	15–45	5–10

Table 9.3 Paralysis: neuromuscular-blocking agents administered immediately after induction agent

Agent	Dose (IV)	Onset (sec)	Duration (min)
Succinylcholine	1.5 mg/kg	45	6–10
Rocuronium	1.0 mg/kg	60–75	40–60
Vecuronium	0.01 to prime, then 0.15 mg/kg	75–90	60–75

Fig. 9.6 Patient in the "sniff" position. *OA* oral axis, *LA* laryngeal axis, *PA* pharyngeal axis

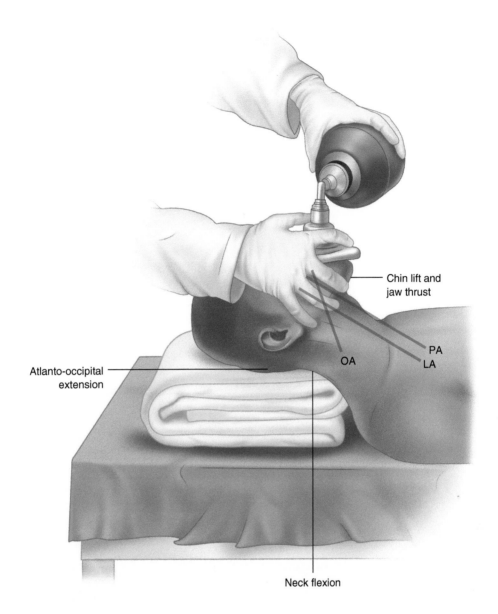

Chin lift and jaw thrust

PA
LA

OA

Atlanto-occipital extension

Neck flexion

Fig. 9.7 EtCO₂, end-tidal
carbon dioxide concentration:
a Qualitative detection
device—EZ Cap, *b*
quantitative continuous EtCO₂
waveform on monitor

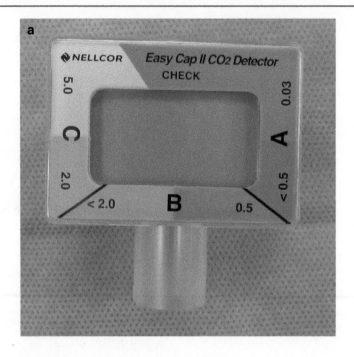

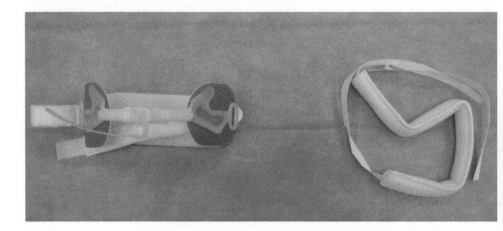

Fig. 9.8 Equipment used to
secure ETT

9.5   Complications

- Esophageal intubation
- Right mainstem intubation
- Pneumothorax from laryngeal trauma
- Aspiration
- Dental trauma
- Vocal cord injury
- Hypotension
  - Induction agent
  - Decreased venous return from positive pressure
  - Pneumothorax
- Hyperkalemia (succinylcholine used in mildly hyperkalemic patient)
- Iatrogenically obstructed airway
- Failure to intubate

9.6   Pearls and Pitfalls

- Utilization of oral and nasal airways will greatly increase the ease of preoxygenation and reoxygenation.
- Inadequate preoxygenation will cause premature desaturation, decreasing time for intubation.
- Suboptimal patient positioning can prevent vocal cord visualization during direct laryngoscopy.
- Consider alternative airway devices before intubation to have a plan in place if a difficult airway is encountered.

- Underdosing induction or paralytic agent will prevent adequate time to perform procedure or create patient discomfort.
- Inappropriately sized McIntosh laryngoscopic blades.
  - Too small—more difficulty in moving tongue and epiglottis out of way for vocal cord visualization
  - Too large—easier to overshoot and go past vocal cords into the esophagus
- Excessive cricoid pressure (Sellick maneuver) may lead to disrupted laryngoscopic view and difficulty passing the ETT.
  - Disrupted view: readjust larynx using dominant hand to allow cord visualization.
  - Difficulty passing ETT: ask for release of some cricoid pressure to allow for ETT passage.
- Inadequate postintubation sedation and analgesia, especially when long-acting paralytics are used.
- Acidic gastric contents can cause CO_2 qualitative capnometry to change to yellow, falsely indicating tracheal placement of the ETT.

Selected Reading

Walls R, Murphy M. Manual of emergency airway management. Philadelphia: Lippincott Williams & Wilkins; 2008.
Weingart SD. Preoxygenation, reoxygenation, and delayed sequence intubation. J Emerg Med. 2011;40:661–7.

Direct Laryngoscopy

Bharath Chakravarthy and Weston Seipp

10.1 Indications

- Orotracheal intubation
  - Maintenance of oxygenation/ventilation
  - Airway protection
- Visualization of laryngeal anatomy
- Foreign body retrieval

10.2 Contraindications

- Absolute
  - None
- Relative
  - Presumed difficult airway
    - Anatomical limitations
      - Small oral opening (less than three of the patient's fingers)
      - Small mandible (hyomental distance less than three fingers)
      - Hyoid-thyroid distance (less than two fingers)
    - Clinical limitations
      - Patient with unstable cervical spine
      - Patient with multiple facial or neck trauma
      - Patient with history of tracheal stenosis, irradiation, or history of tracheal mass or surgery

B. Chakravarthy, MD, MPH (✉)
Department of Emergency Medicine,
University of California Irvine,
Orange, CA, USA
e-mail: bchakrav@uci.edu

W. Seipp, MD
Department of Emergency Medicine,
University of California Irvine Medical Center,
Orange, CA, USA

© Springer Science+Business Media New York 2016
L. Ganti (ed.), *Atlas of Emergency Medicine Procedures*, DOI 10.1007/978-1-4939-2507-0_10

10.3   Materials and Medications (Fig. 10.1)

- Laryngoscope handle
- Laryngoscope blade with light
  - Macintosh blade ("Mac" or "curved blade")
  - Miller blade ("straight blade")
- Bag valve mask attached to 100 % O_2 source

- Endotracheal tube (ETT)
- 10-mL syringe
- Yankauer suction
- End-tidal CO_2 (EtCO_2) monitor (colorimetric or quantitative)
- McGill forceps (for foreign body retrieval)
- Postintubation chest radiograph

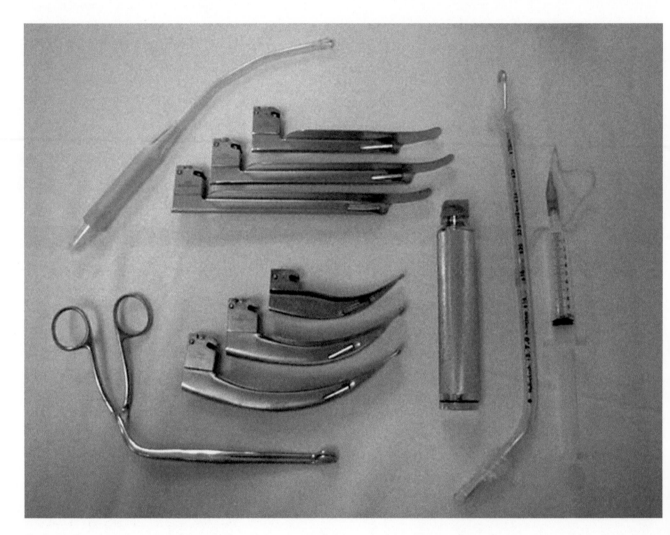

Fig. 10.1 Basic laryngoscopy supplies. *Clockwise from top left*: Yankauer suction, Miller Blades, endotracheal tube, 10-mL syringe, laryngoscope handle, Macintosh blades, and McGill forceps

10.4 Procedure

1. Check the laryngoscope handle and blades to ensure that the light is functioning.
2. Choose the appropriate blade based on patient size.
    (a) The Macintosh or Miller 3 size is appropriate for the majority of adults, and a 4 can be used for a larger body habitus.
    (b) The Macintosh blade is generally preferred in adults owing to increased space for ETT passage [1].
    (c) The Miller blade may be preferable in cases in which the patient has limited mouth opening (owing to its smaller vertical height), or in which the airway is particularly floppy (such as in infants and children) [1].
3. Position the patient (Fig. 10.2).
    (a) Raise the bed so that the patient's oral opening is at the level of the xiphoid process of the laryngoscopist.
    (b) The optimal laryngeal view is obtained in the neck flexion/head extension or "sniffing" position. To achieve this, place towels under the patient's occiput to raise it approximately 6–9 cm [2].
    (c) If patient is in cervical spine precautions, then an assistant must hold the cervical spine in midline immobilization throughout the laryngoscopy; elevation of the occiput is therefore contraindicated.
4. Provide 100 % O_2 via face mask to preoxygenate the patient before laryngoscopy.
5. After ensuring adequate anesthesia and neuromuscular blockade (if performing laryngoscopy for intubation), perform the scissor technique to open the patient's mouth and to lift the tongue base from the glottic opening.
6. Macintosh blade insertion (Fig. 10.3).
    (a) Insert the laryngoscope into the patient's mouth, starting from the right side, and slowly advance into the oropharynx, using the blade's vertical flange to "sweep" the tongue to the left and away from the glottic opening.
    (b) Advance the blade along the tongue toward the tongue base, until the epiglottis and posterior arytenoids are viewed.
    (c) In order to expose the cords, insert the Macintosh blade into the vallecula, which is the potential space anterior to the epiglottis and posterior to the tongue base. This will act as a fulcrum and raise the epiglottis, exposing the vocal cords.
    (d) To further expose the cords and/or expose the vallecula, exert force outward at a 45° angle to the patient. Do not "rock" the laryngoscope because this may cause injury to the teeth.
7. Miller blade insertion (Fig. 10.4).
    (a) Insert the blade into the right side of the mouth and slowly advance along tongue toward the tongue base. The Miller blade does not have a flange for isolating the tongue, and thus the Macintosh may be preferable in patients with large tongues.
    (b) Advance the blade along the right side of the tongue until the epiglottis and posterior arytenoids are visible.
    (c) In contrast to the Macintosh blade, the Miller blade is used to directly isolate the epiglottis and expose the vocal cords. Using the tip of the Miller, move the epiglottis anteriorly to expose the vocal cords.
    (d) As with the Macintosh, exert force outward at a 45° angle to the patient to increase the view of vocal cords. Do not "rock" the laryngoscope because this may cause injury to the teeth.
8. Assessing the glottic view (Fig. 10.5).
    (a) With the epiglottis either directly or indirectly lifted from the glottic opening, assess the Cormack-Lehane laryngeal view grade.
        (i) Grade I—view of entire laryngeal opening, including cords
        (ii) Grade II—view of posterior laryngeal cartilages
        (iii) Grade III—visualization of epiglottis only
        (iv) Grade IV—no structures visualized
    (b) A lower grade (higher quality, better) view is predictive of intubation success [3].
    (c) In the event of a higher grade view, the operator may request airway adjuncts, such as a bougie.
9. Improving the glottic view [4].
    (a) With the laryngoscope in the desired position, it is possible to improve the glottic view by exerting backward pressure on the thyroid cartilage either with the operator's right hand (bimanual laryngoscopy) or with an assistant applying BURP (backward-upward-rightward pressure) (Fig. 10.5a).
    (b) Backward pressure increases the vertical distance between the epiglottis and the posterior cartilages, thereby increasing the likelihood of vocal cord visualization.
10. Passing the ETT (Fig. 10.6).
    (a) With the optimal view of the cords obtained, pass the ETT from the right corner of the mouth through the vocal cords, to a depth of 21 cm at the incisors in females and 23 cm in males.
    (b) Inflate the ETT cuff with approximately 5 cc of air until the pilot balloon is firm to touch.
11. After completing intubation or after completion of laryngoscopy, slowly remove the blade from the mouth, taking care to avoid dental or lip trauma.
12. Attach the capnography device to the ETT tube to ensure $EtCO_2$ return.
    (a) Colorimetric devices will turn from purple to yellow in the presence of $EtCO_2$.
    (b) Quantitative devices will return a CO_2 waveform.
13. Attach the ETT to ventilator or bag-valve-mask connected to an oxygen source.

14. Auscultate breath sounds in both lung fields and ensure absence of breath sounds over the epigastrium (which could signify esophageal intubation).

15. Obtain a postintubation chest x-ray to ensure no right mainstem intubation or pneumothorax.

Fig. 10.2 Visualization axis and sniffing position: (**a**) The patient's occiput is not elevated and the neck is not in flexion, thereby creating a steep visual axis, (**b**) the occiput is correctly elevated 6–9 cm, placing the patient in sniffing position and allowing the visual axis to align with the airway axis

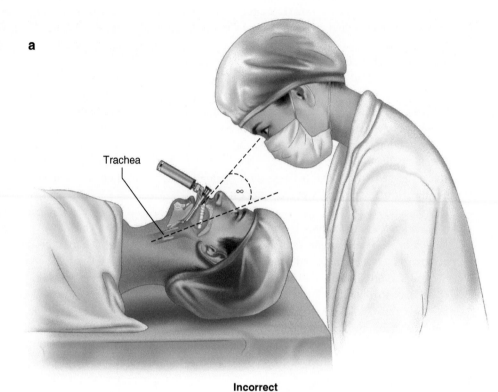

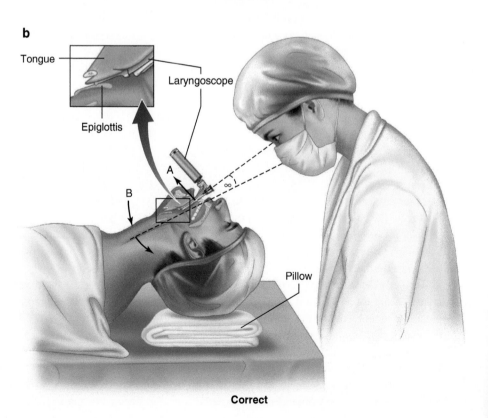

Fig. 10.3 Macintosh blade insertion. The blade is inserted into the vallecula, which raises the epiglottis and exposes the glottic opening

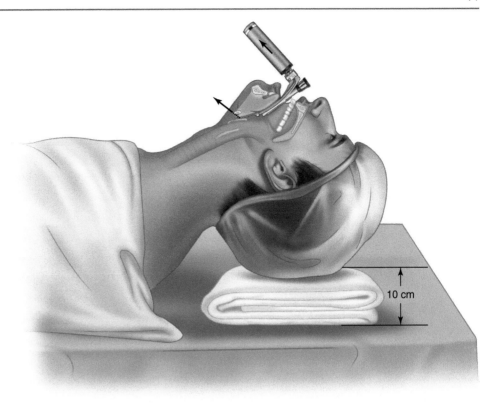

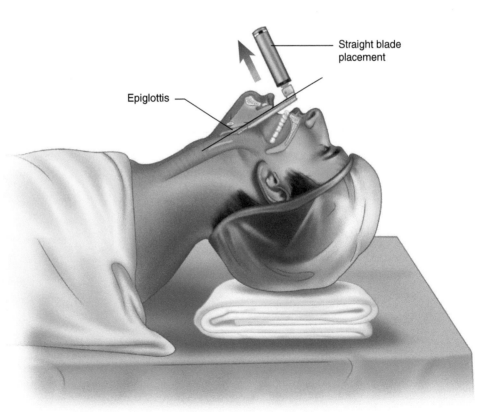

Fig. 10.4 Miller blade insertion. The blade is used to elevate the epiglottis directly, exposing the glottic opening

Fig. 10.5 (**a**) Bimanual laryngoscopy. The force on the neck is opposite the direction of lift by the laryngoscope, (**b**) laryngoscopy view, (**c**) Cormack and Lehane

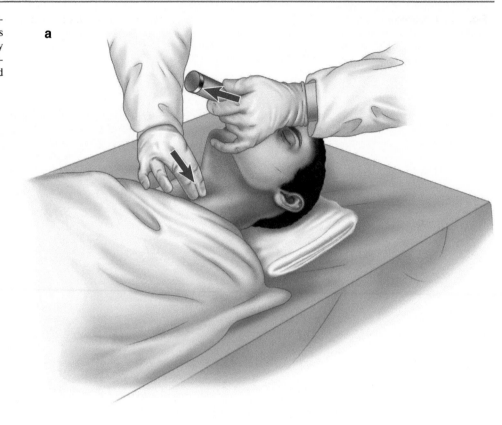

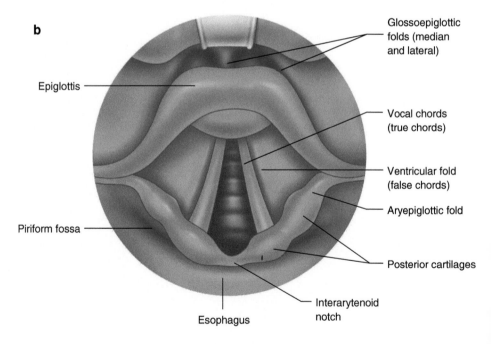

Fig. 10.5 (continued)   **Laryngoscopy view: cormack and lehane**

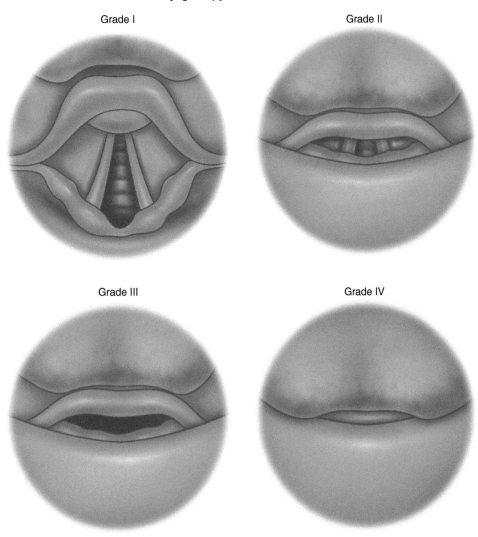

Grade I   Grade II

Grade III   Grade IV

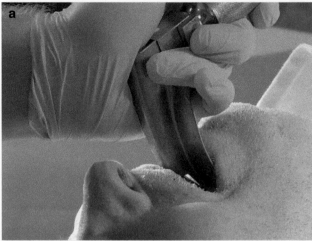

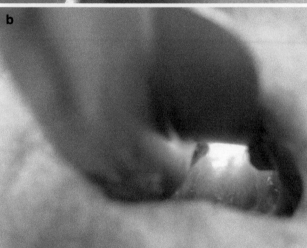

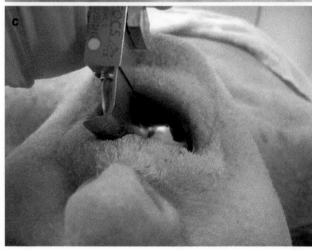

Fig. 10.6 (**a**) Insert the laryngoscope into the mouth, (**b**) sweep the tongue to the left, (**c**) advance the laryngoscope until the epiglottis is visible, and insert the blade into vallecula to expose the cords. When using the Miller blade, insert the blade until the epiglottis is seen. Slide the blade under the epiglottis and lift to expose the cords

10.5   Complications [3, 5]

- Common (1–4 %)
    - Esophageal intubation—*can be fatal if unrecognized*
    - Mainstem bronchus intubation
    - Tachycardia
    - Aspiration
    - Hypotension
- Uncommon (<1 %)
    - Dental/oral trauma
    - Oropharyngeal edema or bleeding
    - Laryngospasm
    - Dysrhythmia
    - Pneumothorax
    - Cardiac arrest

10.6   Pearls and Pitfalls

- Pearls
    - Positioning is of key importance—all patients with a stable cervical spine should be placed in the "sniffing" position to maximize view.
    - Consider the "ramping" position in obese patients with stable cervical spines—elevation of the head and shoulders allows redundant tissue to fall and gives an improved glottic view.
    - Always have suction readily available to remove blood, vomitus, or edema.
    - If structures are not readily visible, withdraw the blade gradually because it is common to insert the blade too deep.
- Pitfalls
    - "Rocking" the laryngoscope instead of lifting outward
    - Failure to recognize esophageal intubation
    - Failure to evaluate postintubation chest x-ray

References

1. Hagberg CA. Benumof's airway management. Maryland Heights, MO: Mosby; 2007. p. 363–5.
2. Park SH, Park HP, Jeon YT, Hwang JW, Kim JH, Bahk JH. A comparison of direct laryngoscopic views depending on pillow height. J Anesth. 2010;24:526–30.
3. Martin LD, Mhyre JM, Shanks AM, Tremper KK, Kheterpal S. 3,423 emergency tracheal intubations at a university hospital: airway outcomes and complications. Anesthesiology. 2011;114:42–8.
4. Levitan RM, Kinkle WC, Levin WJ, Everett WW. Laryngeal view during laryngoscopy: a randomized trial comparing cricoid pressure, backward-upward-rightward pressure, and bimanual laryngoscopy. Ann Emerg Med. 2006;47:548–55.
5. Walls RM, Brown CA 3rd, Bair AE, Pallin DJ, NEAR II Investigators. Emergency airway management: a multi-center report of 8937 emergency department intubations. J Emerg Med. 2011;41: 347–54.

Laryngeal Mask Airway

11

Sohan Parekh

11.1 Indications

- Rescue device in a failed intubation
- Initial device in a predictably difficult airway
- Temporizing airway prior to definitive endotracheal intubation or surgical airway

11.2 Contraindications

- Absolute
  - Inadequate mouth opening
- Relative
  - Neck trauma/injury/radiation
  - High risk of aspiration

S. Parekh, MD
Department of Emergency Medicine,
University of Texas at Austin Dell Medical School,
Austin, TX, USA

Department of Emergency Medicine,
University Medical Center Brackenridge,
Austin, TX, USA
e-mail: sohan.parekh@gmail.com

© Springer Science+Business Media New York 2016
L. Ganti (ed.), *Atlas of Emergency Medicine Procedures*, DOI 10.1007/978-1-4939-2507-0_11

11.3   Types (Fig. 11.1)

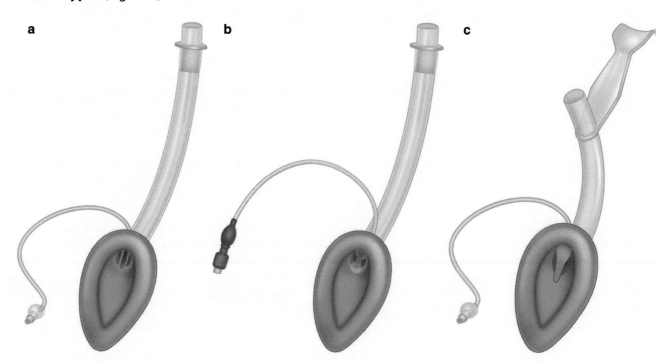

Fig. 11.1 Types of laryngeal mask airway: (**a**) LMA Unique, (**b**) LMA Classic Excel, (**c**) LMA Fastrach

11.4   Materials and Medications

- Appropriately sized laryngeal mask airway (LMA; LMA Unique/LMA Classic Excel/LMA Fastrach) and corresponding syringe (Table 11.1)
- Surgilube
- Bag valve mask
- Continuous end-tidal CO_2 (EtCO$_2$) or colorimetric EtCO$_2$ detector
- 8-mm or smaller endotracheal tube (ETT) (for Fastrach intubating LMA only)

Table 11.1 Laryngeal mask airway sizing

Size	Patient weight (kg)	Maximum cuff inflation volume (mL)	LMA product availability
1	<5	4	Unique
1½	5–10	7	Unique
2	10–20	10	Unique
2½	20–30	14	Unique
3	30–50	20	Unique, Classic Excel, Fastrach
4	50–70	30	Unique, Classic Excel, Fastrach
5	70–100	40	Unique, Classic Excel, Fastrach
6	>100	50	Unique

LMA laryngeal mask airway

11.5   Procedure

11.5.1 LMA Unique or Classic Excel

1. If using a reusable LMA Classic Excel, ensure that it is sterile and inspect it for any damage or wear.
2. Tightly deflate the cuff using a syringe such that it forms a spoon shape (Fig. 11.2).
3. Lubricate the posterior surface of the LMA with sterile lubricating jelly.
4. Stand behind the patient at the head of the bed as in direct laryngoscopy.
5. Place the patient's head in the sniffing position and ensure proper induction and paralysis.
6. Hold the LMA with the index finger of the dominant hand positioned at the juncture of the tube and cuff (Fig. 11.3).
7. Widely open the mouth with the nondominant hand and insert the LMA with the flattened tip flush with the palate.
   - Ensure that the tip of the device does not fold over during insertion.
8. Using the index finger, push the LMA along the curvature of the hard and soft palate (Fig. 11.4).
9. Continue to insert the LMA into the hypopharynx until resistance is felt. (At this point the tip of the LMA is in the esophagus.)
10. Stabilize the tube with the nondominant hand and remove index finger of the dominant hand from the LMA.
11. Inflate the cuff of the LMA to at least half of the maximum value using a syringe.
    - The LMA might move slightly outward during cuff inflation as the LMA positions itself in the hypopharynx.
12. Confirm placement and adequate gas exchange with continuous EtCO$_2$ capnography or colorimetry.

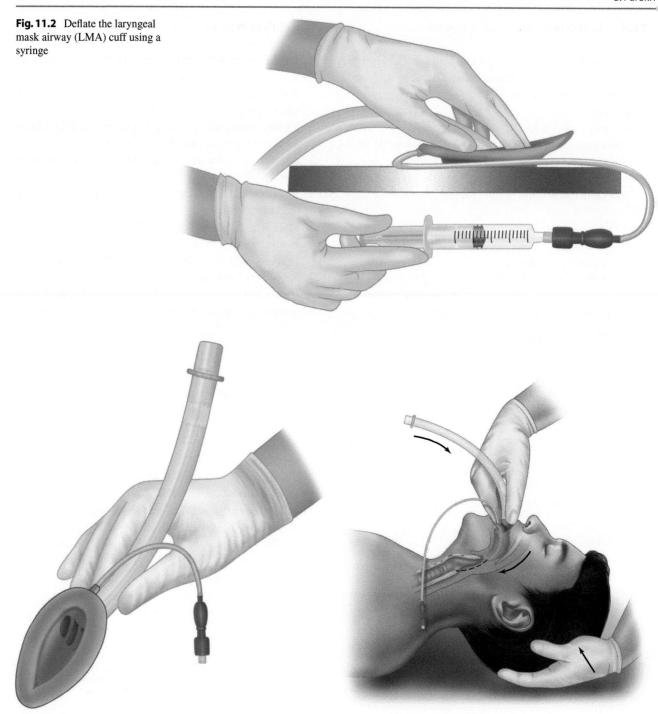

Fig. 11.2 Deflate the laryngeal mask airway (LMA) cuff using a syringe

Fig. 11.3 Hold the LMA with the index finger positioned at the juncture of the tube and the cuff

Fig. 11.4 Use the index finger to guide the LMA along the hard and soft palate

11.5.2 LMA Fastrach

1. If using a reusable LMA Fastrach, ensure that it is sterile and inspect it for any damage or wear.
2. Tightly deflate the cuff using a syringe such that it forms a spoon shape.
3. Lubricate the posterior surface of the LMA with sterile lubricating jelly.
4. The LMA Fastrach may be inserted from any position with respect to the patient's head.
5. Position the patient's head in the neutral position. Do not extend the head.
6. Widely open the mouth with the nondominant hand.
7. Holding the handle of the LMA Fastrach, insert the device into the mouth, placing the deflated cuff flush with the superior palate.
   - Distribute the lubricant over the superior palate using a side-to-side motion to allow for easier insertion.
   - Ensure that the tip of the device does not fold over during insertion.
8. Using the handle, gently advance the LMA Fastrach directly into the oropharynx until the curved portion of tube comes into the contact with the patient's chin (Fig. 11.5).
9. At this point use the handle to rotationally advance the device further into the oropharynx following the natural curvature of the palate and posterior pharynx (Fig. 11.6).
   - Do not initiate any rotation until the tube is in contact with the patient's chin.
10. Once resistance is felt, inflate the cuff of the device to at least half of the maximum value using a syringe.
    - Note that the tube is directed slightly caudally when properly inserted.
    - Confirm placement and adequate gas exchange with $EtCO_2$ capnography or colorimetry.

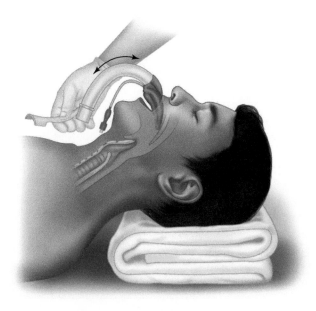

Fig. 11.5 Using the handle, insert the LMA Fastrach such that the posterior surface is in contact with the superior palate

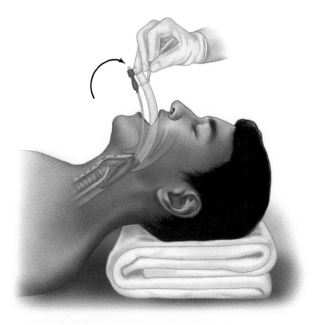

Fig. 11.6 Once the tube is in contact with the chin, use the handle to rotationally advance the device further into the oropharynx

11.5.3 Endotracheal Intubation through the LMA Fastrach

1. Ensure that the ETT will pass freely in the LMA.
2. Lubricate the cuff of the ETT.
3. Firmly hold the handle of the LMA Fastrach with the nondominant hand and insert the ETT to a depth of 15 cm (Fig. 11.7), which places the ETT tip at the point of emergency from LMA Fastrach.
   - Ensure that the tube does not pass beyond 15 cm at this point.

4. Using the handle of the LMA Fastrach, draw the device outward in order to displace the larynx slightly to accommodate insertion of the ETT (Fig. 11.8).
   - Use a lifting rather than a levering motion.
5. Carefully advance the ETT slightly further. If no resistance is felt, continue with insertion of the ETT (Fig. 11.9).
6. Confirm placement and adequate gas exchange with $EtCO_2$ capnography or colorimetry.
7. Once successful confirmation of intubation is established, deflate the cuff pressure on the LMA Fastrach.

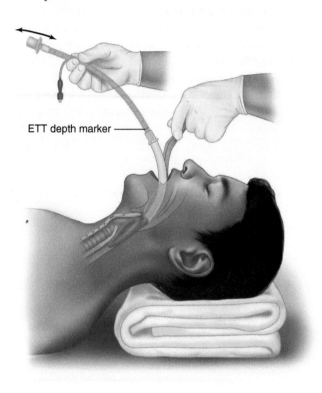

ETT depth marker

Fig. 11.7 While holding the handle of the LMA, insert the endotracheal tube (*ETT*) to the 15-cm mark

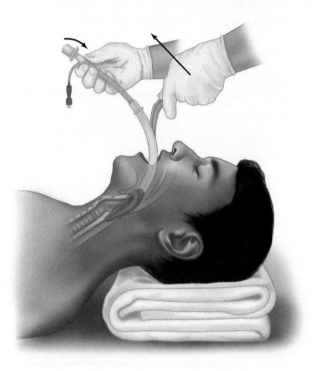

Fig. 11.8 Lift the handle outward to open the glottis for the ETT

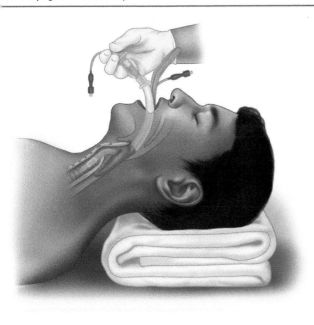

Fig. 11.9 If no resistance is felt during further insertion of the ETT, the ETT may be fully advanced

11.5.4 Removing the LMA Fastrach after Successful Intubation

1. The LMA Fastrach need not be removed immediately, but if this is desired, first adequately oxygenate the patient and then disconnect the patient from the circuit.
2. Remove the airway connector from the proximal end of the ETT.
3. Ensure that the cuff of the LMA Fastrach is entirely deflated.
4. Stabilize the ETT with the nondominant hand, and using the dominant hand, gently ease the LMA Fastrach out by rotating the handle caudally (Fig. 11.10).
5. Once the tube of the LMA Fastrach reaches the proximal end of the ETT, use the stabilizer rod to maintain the position of the ETT while continuing to remove the LMA Fastrach using the handle (Fig. 11.11).
6. After the cuff of the LMA Fastrach has been fully removed from the oral cavity, release the stabilizer rod and ensure stability of the ETT by grasping it distally at the mouth with the nondominant hand (Fig. 11.12).
7. Continue to ease the LMA Fastrach out from around the ETT, ensuring that the pilot balloon and inflation line of the ETT cuff pass through the device (Fig. 11.13).
   • Take care not to rupture the pilot balloon or tear the inflation line of the ETT.
8. Replace the airway connector on the proximal end of the ETT and reconnect the patient to the circuit.

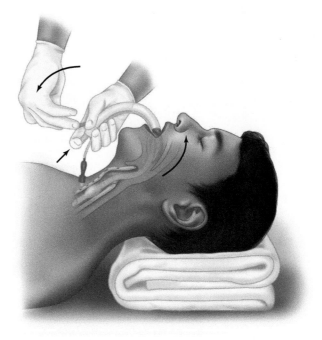

Fig. 11.10 Rotate the handle caudally to gently ease the LMA Fastrach out of the pharynx

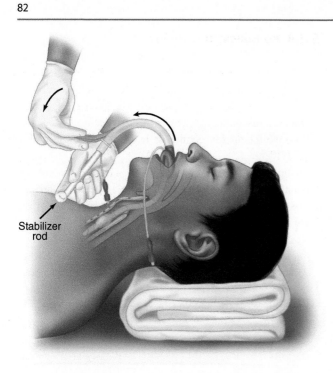

Stabilizer
rod

Fig. 11.11 Use the stabilizer rod to allow for further removal of the
LMA Fastrach

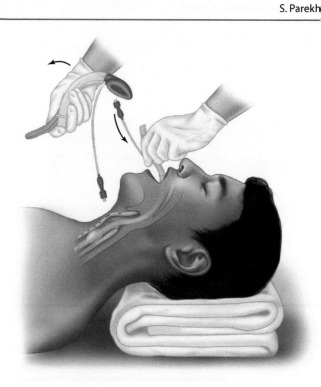

Fig. 11.13 Carefully pass the pilot balloon and inflation line of the
ETT cuff through the tube of LMA Fastrach as it is removed

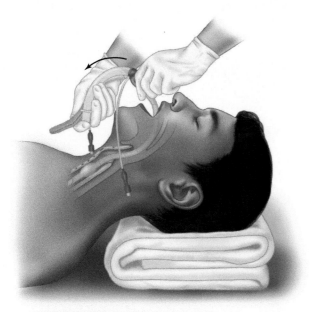

Fig. 11.12 Once the cuff of the LMA Fastrach is out of the mouth,
grasp the ETT distally and remove the LMA entirely

11.6   Complications

- Aspiration with resulting pneumonitis
- Ineffective seal resulting in insufficient ventilation
- Coughing, bucking, or breath holding
  - Ensure that the patient is adequately sedated.

11.7   Pearls and Pitfalls

- Cricoid pressure can push the tip of the LMA out of the esophagus and prevent optimal placement.

Selected Reading

Barata I. The laryngeal mask airway: prehospital and emergency department use. Emerg Med Clin North Am. 2008;24:1069–83.

LMA classic LMA flexible LMA classic single use LMA flexible single use instruction manual. Victoria: The Laryngeal Mask Company Limited; 2010.

LMA fastrach LMA fastrach single use instruction manual. Victoria: The Laryngeal Mask Company Limited; 2010.

Pollack CV. The laryngeal mask airway: a comprehensive review for the emergency physician. J Emerg Med. 2001;20:53–66.

Walls RW, Murphy MF, editors. Manual of emergency airway management. 3rd ed. Philadelphia: Lippincott Williams & Wilkins; 2008.

Combitube

12

Clint Masterson

12.1 Indications

- Need for ventilation and oxygenation in an unconscious, unresponsive, or paralyzed patient
- Rescue airway needed after failed intubation

12.2 Contraindications

- Absolute
  - Awake, responsive patient
  - Intact gag reflex
  - Known esophageal disease
  - Ingestion of caustic substances
  - Child (no Combitubes are made for children)
- Relative
  - D50 or naloxone about to be given
  - Facial trauma

12.3 Materials

- Combitube sized based upon height (Fig. 12.1)
  - >5 ft—size 41 French (cuff inflation 15 and 100 mL)
  - >4 ft to <5.5 ft—size 37 French (cuff inflation 12 and 85 mL)

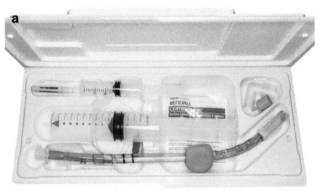

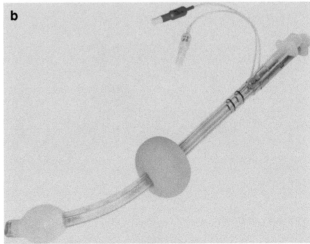

Fig. 12.1 (**a, b**) Combitube equipment

C. Masterson, MD
Department of Emergency Medicine,
Mayo Clinic Health System in Fairmont,
Fairmont, MN, USA
e-mail: clint@clintm.us

© Springer Science+Business Media New York 2016
L. Ganti (ed.), *Atlas of Emergency Medicine Procedures*, DOI 10.1007/978-1-4939-2507-0_12

12.4   Procedure

1. Test both balloons and cuffs for leaks as one would an endotracheal tube (ETT).
2. Open up the airway.
   (a) Use a laryngoscope to move the tongue and open the oropharynx.
      OR
   (b) Use the left hand to elevate the chin, elevating the tongue and pharyngeal tissue.
3. Insert Combitube blindly into the oropharynx until the teeth lie between the two black bands on the proximal Combitube (Fig. 12.2).
4. Inflate the proximal blue cuff until air pressure is produced or the manufacturer-recommended pressure is reached.
   (a) 85 mL for 37 French Combitube
   (b) 100 mL for 41 French Combitube
5. Identify placement and attach to oxygen.
   (a) Ventilate through tube #1 (blue).
   (b) Auscultate the stomach and lungs.
      (i) If breath sounds are heard, the Combitube is in its more common esophageal location.
      (ii) Attach tube #1 to bag valve mask and O_2.

   (c) ONLY IF gurgling is present over the stomach when tube #1 is ventilated:
      (i) Ventilate through tube #2.
      (ii) If breath sounds are heard, the Combitube is in the less common tracheal location.
      (iii) Attach tube #2 to bag valve mask and O_2.
6. If no breath sounds are heard in either location:
   (a) Consider obstruction—Combitube may be obstructing the glottis or collapsing the trachea owing to deep proximal cuff inflation.
      (i) Deflate the cuffs.
      (ii) Withdraw 3 cm.
      (iii) Reinflate and start from step 4.
   (b) Consider equipment failure.
      (i) Check that balloons are maintaining pressure and intact.
   (c) Consider reinsertion.
7. Confirm placement with capnogram and pulse oximetry.
8. Secure the Combitube in position (Fig. 12.3).

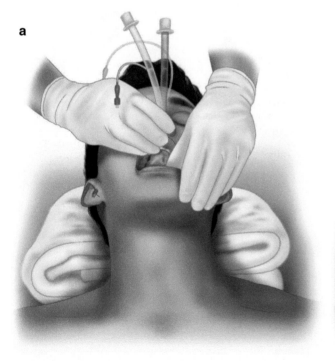
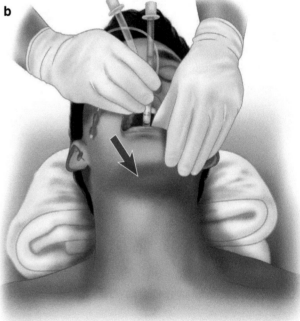

Fig. 12.2 (**a**) Insertion of Combitube. (**b**) Teeth should lie between the two black bands on the proximal Combitube

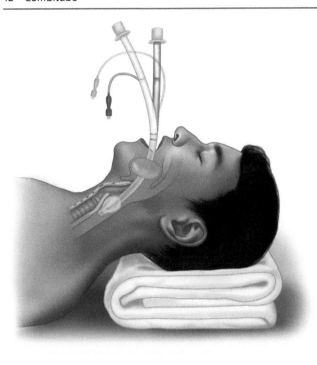

Fig. 12.3 Secure the Combitube in position

12.5 Pearls and Pitfalls

- Pearls
  - In an esophageal intubation situation, a suction tube may be threaded down using tube #2 to decompress the stomach.
  - The Combitube comes with an L-shaped piece that may also be attached to the end of tube #2 to deflect gastric contents away from practitioners.
- Pitfalls
  - After Combitube placement, a definitive airway should be placed when possible.
    - Gastric contents may aspirate despite placement of the Combitube.
    - Combitube should be considered a bridging airway device.
  - Combitubes are associated with a more pronounced hemodynamic stress response than ETTs or laryngeal mask airways (LMAs).
  - Balloon overinflation can lead to esophageal rupture (albeit rare).
  - Combitubes are associated with an increased incidence of sore throat, dysphagia, and upper airway hematomas than ETTs and LMAs.
  - Piriform sinus perforation.

Selected Reading

Agro F, Frass M, Beunmof JL, Krafft P. Current status of the Combitube: a review of the literature. J Clin Anesth. 2002;14:307–14.

Laurin E, Bair A. Devices for difficult airway management in adults. www.uptodate.com. Accessed 14 Mar 2014.

Liem EB. Combitube insertion. University of Florida Department of Anesthesiology, Center for Simulation, Advanced Learning and Technology, Virtual Anesthesia Machine Web site; 2006. http://vam.anest.ufl.edu/airwaydevice/combitube/index.html. Accessed 14 Mar 2014.

Walls R, Murphy M. Manual of emergency airway management. Philadelphia: Lippincott Williams & Wilkins; 2008.

Assessment of the Difficult Airway

13

Melinda W. Fernandez and Lars K. Beattie

13.1 Indications

- Should be performed on all patients that require airway management, conditions permitting
- Respiratory distress
- Airway protection

13.2 Materials and Medications

- None required

13.3 Procedure

1. Anticipating a difficult airway in emergency department patients is the first step to avoiding an unexpected surgical airway.
2. Two mnemonics can be applied quickly and easily to aid in an airway assessment: MOANS and LEMON.

13.3.1 Predicting Bag-Valve-Mask Difficulty

1. Use the mnemonic *MOANS* to assess for possible bag-valve-mask (BVM) difficulty.

   M—mask seal. Will you be able to get a good seal on the face? Predictors of difficulty include facial hair such as a beard, elderly, or emaciated owing to loss of muscle tone in the face.

O—obesity. Body mass index (BMI) >30.

A—age (>55 years). Loss of facial muscle tone can make bagging difficult.

N—no teeth. Although being edentulous makes for an easier intubation, it makes bagging more difficult.

S—stiff lungs. Acute or chronic lung disease can make a person difficult to bag. In the setting of Trauma, pulmonary contusion(s) and/or other direct lung injuries may increase BVM difficulty.

13.3.2 Predicting Difficult Laryngoscopy

1. Attempts should be made, if at all possible, to assess for a potentially difficult airway. This does not mean you cannot perform direct laryngoscopy if you are anticipating a difficult airway. It does, however, force you to consider all options and to have a solid backup plan in place with backup equipment readily available in the room.
2. Use the mnemonic *LEMON* to predict difficult direct laryngoscopy.

   L—look. A quick look at the patient will tell you a lot. Are there facial injuries; facial anomalies; obesity; short, thick neck; and small mouth or mandible?

   E—evaluate. Use the 3-3-2 rule to quickly assess for the strongest predictors of difficult laryngoscopy.
   - *3:* Open the patient's mouth and three vertically aligned fingers should fit between the incisors.
   - *3:* Three finger widths should fit along the length of the mandible from the mentum to the hyoid bone. Shorter or longer distances may make for a difficult intubation.
   - *2:* Thyromental distance should ideally be two fingers. Measure this from the hyoid to the thyroid.

M.W. Fernandez, MD
Department of Emergency Medicine, University of Florida Health, Gainesville, FL, USA
e-mail: mindyfernandez@ufl.edu

L.K. Beattie, MD, MS (✉)
Department of Emergency Medicine, University of Florida, Gainesville, FL, USA
e-mail: lars.beattie@ufl.edu

© Springer Science+Business Media New York 2016
L. Ganti (ed.), *Atlas of Emergency Medicine Procedures*, DOI 10.1007/978-1-4939-2507-0_13

M—Mallampati classification (Fig. 13.1). If patient's condition and situation allow, have the patient open the mouth wide, stick out the tongue, and say "Ahh." Evaluate for visible structures.

- *Class I:* Tonsillar pillars and the entire uvula are visible.
- *Class II:* More than the base of the uvula is visible but no pillars are visible.
- *Class III:* Only the base of the uvula is visible.
- *Class IV:* No uvula or soft palate is visible. Only the hard palate is visible.
- These classifications correlate with the Cormack-Lehane grading system for laryngoscopic views. A Mallampati class I will correlate with a grade 1 view about 99 % of the time, whereas a Mallampati IV will be a grade 3 or 4 view all of the time and a rescue plan with backup equipment immediately available should always be in place [1, 2].

O—obstruction. Observe for anything that can get in the way (e.g., the tongue, dentures, blood, vomit, foreign body, edema, redundant tissue).

N—neck mobility. If patient's condition and situation allow, have the patient flex and extend the neck to evaluate mobility. Many patients in the emergency department have limited neck mobility. Examples include the trauma patient who arrives in cervical collar immobilization or a patient with degenerative or rheumatoid arthritis.

3. The *"6-D"* method is another assessment tool that can be used to predict difficult laryngoscopy and intubation. This method can be remembered by the fact that the word "difficult" begins with the letter "D":

Disproportion
- Increased tongue size in relation to pharyngeal size
- Airway swelling or trauma

Distortion
- Neck mass, hematoma, abscess, previous surgical airway, arthritic neck changes

Decreased thyromental distance
- Anterior larynx and decreased mandibular space.
- Look for a receding chin or greater than three fingerbreadths from the mentum to the hyoid bone.

Decreased inter-incisor gap
- Reduced mouth opening.
- Look for less than two to three fingerbreadths placed vertically in the patient's open mouth.

Decreased range of motion in any joints of the airway
- Limited head extension
- Previous neck radiation and/or surgery
- Neck contractures

Dental overbite
- Oversized, angled teeth disrupt the alignment of airway axes.
- Can decrease the interincisor gap.

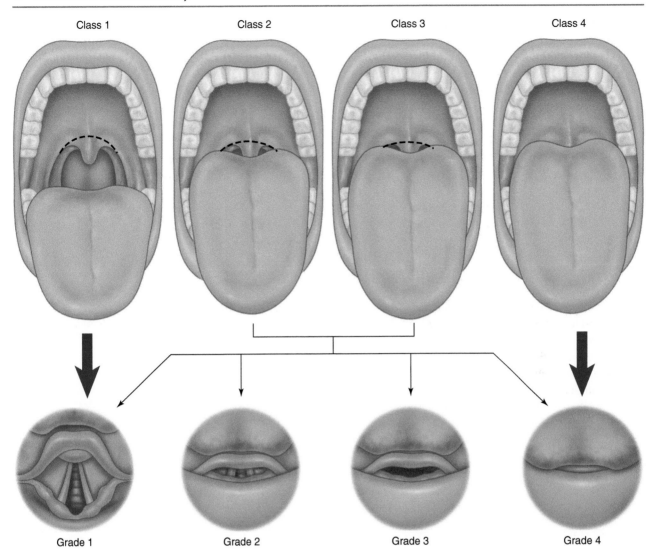

Fig. 13.1 Mallampati classification

13.3.3 Optimizing Laryngoscopy in the Obese Patient

- It is essential that emergency medicine physicians are able to successfully intubate the obese patient.
- Proper assessment and positioning will increase the success rate:
  - The goal is to ensure alignment of the oropharyngeal-pharyngeal-laryngeal (OA-PA-LA) airways by placing the patient in the head-elevated laryngoscopy position (Fig. 13.2a).
  - Align the external auditory meatus with the sternal notch along a horizontal line by positioning the patient on a "ramp."
  - The ramp can be created by stacking blankets/towels under the lower back ramping up to the neck and head (Fig. 13.2b).
- While the patient is in position on the ramp, the support is adjusted to minimize head flexion and allow for positioning in the sniffing position.
  - Because of the increased height, a step stool may be required to adequately visualize the airway from the head of the bed.

13.4 Pearls and Pitfalls

- Owing to time-sensitive patient care situations, emergency physicians are often not able to perform a thorough airway evaluation on every patient.
- With every airway that you manage and before pushing any drugs, always ask yourself:
  - Will I be able to ventilate this patient?
  - Will I be able to intubate this patient?
  - What is my difficult airway plan if I encounter trouble?
  - Will I be able to perform a surgical airway, if necessary?
- Be sure you have a solid backup plan A, B, and C before pushing any drugs.

References

1. Lee A, Fan LT, Gin T, Karmakar MK, Ngan Kee WD. A systematic review (meta-analysis) of the accuracy of the Mallampati tests to predict the difficult airway. Anesth Analg. 2006;102:1867–78.
2. Boschert S. Think L-E-M-O-N when assessing a difficult airway. ACEP News. Nov 2007.

Selected Reading

Murphy M. Bringing the larynx into view: a piece of the puzzle. Ann Emerg Med. 2003;41:338–41.
Rick J. Recognition and management of the difficult airway with special emphasis on the intubating LMA-Fastrach/whistle technique: a brief review with case reports. BUMC. 2005;18:220–7.
Roberts J, Hedges J. Clinical procedures in emergency medicine. 5th ed. Philadelphia: WB Saunders; 2009. p. 60–2.
Wilson W. Difficult intubation. In: Atlee J, editor. Complications in anesthesia. Philadelphia: WB Saunders; 1999. p. 138–47.

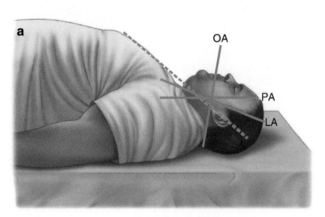

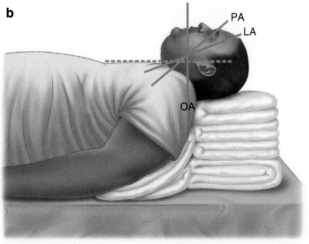

Fig. 13.2 (**a, b**) Ramping the obese patient will align the axes of the airway and allow easier direct laryngoscopy when viewed from the head of bed. (*LA* laryngeal airway, *OA* oropharyngeal airway, *PA* pharyngeal airway)

GlideScope

14

Sohan Parekh

14.1 Indications

- Initial device in a predictably difficult airway
- Rescue device in a failed intubation

14.2 Contraindications

- Absolute
  - Inadequate mouth opening
- Relative
  - Blood, vomit, or other secretions that can coat and obstruct the camera lens

14.3 Materials and Medications

- GlideScope video monitor with video cable (GlideScope Video Laryngoscope [GVL] system) (Fig. 14.1) or appropriate-size video baton (Cobalt System) (Fig. 14.2)
- Appropriate-size reusable video laryngoscope (GVL) or single-use laryngoscope blade (GVL Stat) (Table 14.1).
- Endotracheal tube (ETT)
- Malleable stylet or GlideRite rigid stylet
- 10 mL syringe
- End-tidal CO_2 (EtCO$_2$) capnography or colorimetry

S. Parekh, MD
Department of Emergency Medicine,
University of Texas at Austin Dell Medical School,
Austin, TX, USA

Department of Emergency Medicine,
University Medical Center Brackenridge,
Austin, TX, USA
e-mail: sohan.parekh@gmail.com

© Springer Science+Business Media New York 2016
L. Ganti (ed.), *Atlas of Emergency Medicine Procedures*, DOI 10.1007/978-1-4939-2507-0_14

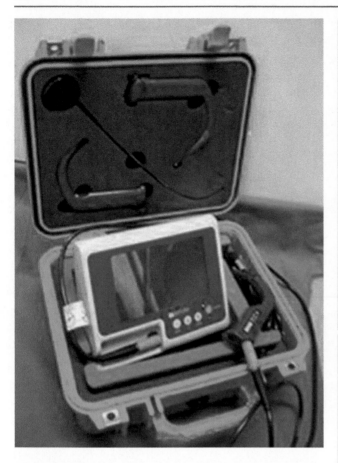

Fig. 14.1 GlideScope GVL system (With kind permission from Springer Science + Business Media: Noppens RR, Werner C, Piepho T. Indirekte Laryngoskopie. *Der Anaesthesist*. 2010;59(2):149–61)

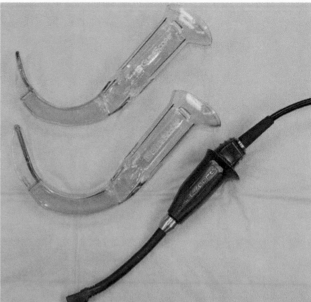

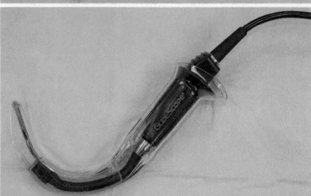

Fig. 14.2 GlideScope Cobalt system (With kind permission from Springer Science + Business Media: Jones PM, Turkstra TP, Armstrong KP, et al. Comparison of a single-use GlideScope® Cobalt videolaryngoscope with a conventional GlideScope® for orotracheal intubation. *Can J Anesthe/Journal canadien d'anesthésie*. 2010;57(1))

Table 14.1 GlideScope sizing

				Video Baton 1–2			Video Baton 3–4	
GVL 1	GVL 2	GVL 3	GVL 4	Stat 0	Stat 1	Stat 2	Stat 3	Stat 4
1.8–10 kg	10 kg—adult	40 kg—morbidly obese	40 kg—morbidly obese	<1.5 kg	1.5–3.6 kg	1.8–10 kg	10 kg—adult	40 kg—morbidly obese

14.4 Procedure

1. Insert the video cable (GVL system) or the video baton (Cobalt system) into the GlideScope video monitor (Fig. 14.3).
2. If using the GVL system, insert the distal end of the video cable into the port on the handle of the reusable video laryngoscope (GVL) (Fig. 14.4).
3. If using the Cobalt system, insert the video baton into the GVL Stat (Fig. 14.5).
   (a) Align the logo on the side of the video baton with the logo on the side of the single-use laryngoscope blade (GVL stat).

(b) The video baton should slide smoothly and click into the place.
4. Turn on the GlideScope at for at least 30–120 s before use to fully activate the antifog mechanism.
5. Insert a stylet into the ETT. If using a malleable stylet, shape the curvature of the distal end of the tube to conform to the 60° curvature of the laryngoscope blade.
6. Firmly hold the laryngoscope handle in the left hand and ensure that an image can be clearly seen on the video monitor.
7. After ensuring adequate sedation and paralysis, open the mouth wide and insert the laryngoscope blade in the midline underneath the tongue (Fig. 14.6).

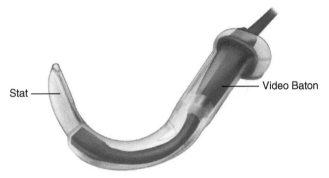

Fig. 14.5 Slide the video baton into the GVL Stat, Cobalt System

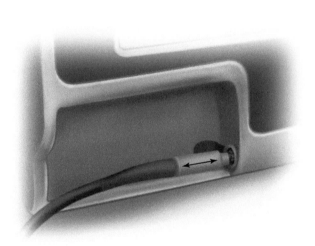

Fig. 14.3 Cable insertion into the video monitor

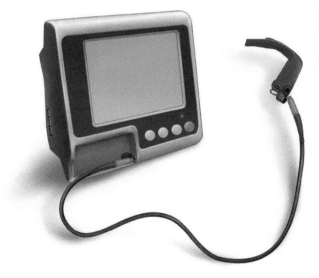

Fig. 14.4 Connect the distal end of the video cable the port on the handle of the GVL (GVL System)

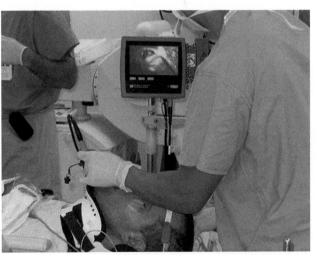

Fig. 14.6 Insert the laryngoscope blade in the midline beneath the tongue (with kind permission from Springer Science+Business Media: Osborn IP, Kleinberger AJ, Gurudutt VV. Chapter 8: Airway emergencies and the difficult airway. In: Levine AI, Govindaraj S, DeMaria S, editors. *Anesthesiology and otolaryngology*. 2013)

8. Looking at the video monitor, advance the laryngoscope blade further into the oropharynx in order to obtain a view of the epiglottis.
    (a) Do not look directly into the oropharynx.
    (b) Movements and adjustments should be guided by the image on the video monitor.
9. Place the laryngoscope blade in the vallecula (analogous to a Macintosh blade) and apply a gentle backward tilt to expose the glottis.
10. In the event that a satisfactory glottic view cannot be obtained, the laryngoscope blade may be advanced and used like a Miller blade to lift the epiglottis out of the way.
11. Directing attention back toward the patient, insert the ETT into the mouth adjacent to the laryngoscope blade.
12. Guide the ETT toward the tip of the laryngoscope such that the end of the ETT emerges on the video monitor.
13. Looking at the video monitor, advance the ETT toward the glottis, and maneuver the tip of the tube between the vocal cords by rotating and altering the angle of the ETT.
    (a) If the ETT tip is posterior to the arytenoids:
        (i) Pull the ETT superiorly, rotate it over the left arytenoid, and gently twist the tube over the epiglottic aperture.
        (ii) Apply external laryngeal manipulation.
        (iii) Withdraw the blade to reduce tilting of the laryngeal axis and lessen the angle of introduction.
    (b) If the ETT abuts the false vocal cords, turn the ETT in the clockwise direction while withdrawing the stylet (Fig. 14.7).
14. Using the thumb, partially withdraw the stylet a few centimeters from the ETT.
    (a) The distal end of the tube should be free of the stylet.
    (b) An assistant can perform this task to allow for greater control and stability of the ETT.
15. Insert the ETT to the desired depth.
16. Fully remove the stylet, inflate the cuff of the ETT using a syringe, and confirm placement with $EtCO_2$, capnography, or colorimetry.

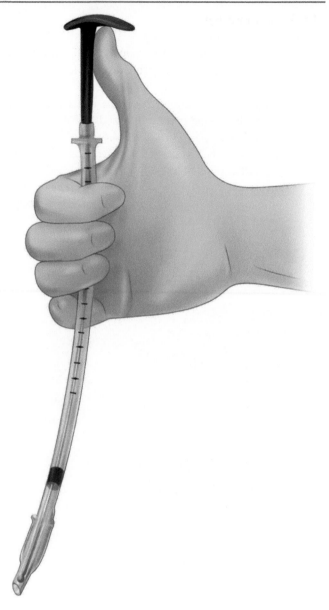

Fig. 14.7 Partially withdraw the stylet from the ETT to allow for passage through the vocal cords

14.5 Complications

- Dental injury
- Airway trauma

14.6 Pearls and Pitfalls

- Unlike conventional laryngoscopy, there is no need to displace the tongue.
- The greatest challenge when intubating with the GlideScope is maneuvering the ETT into the glottis aperture. Alternatives to the conventional technique are:
    - Make a 90° bend in the ETT just proximal to the cuff and insert it in the horizontal direction with the tip toward the right cheek. Once the tube is advanced past the flange of the laryngoscope, rotate it counterclockwise, at which point it should be pointed at the glottis. The tube can then be gently rotated into the glottis.
    - Consider inserting the laryngoscope slightly to the left of the midline upon initial insertion to allow greater space for advancement and maneuvering of the ETT.
- Do not overly lever the laryngoscope or use excessive lifting force after insertion into the vallecula. An adequate view of the glottis is generally easily obtained with minimal effort.
- Display settings can be adjusted using the menu button on the video monitor.

Selected Reading

Cho JE, Kil HK. A maneuver to facilitate endotracheal intubation using the GlideScope. Can J Anaesth. 2008;55:56–7.

GlideScope GVL and Cobalt user's manual & quick reference guide. Bothell: Verathon Inc; 2009–2011.

Kramer DC, Osborn IP. More maneuvers to facilitate tracheal intubation with the GlideScope. Can J Anaesth. 2006;53:737.

Lim HC. Utilization of a GlideScope videolaryngoscope for orotracheal intubations in different emergency airway management settings. Eur J Emerg Med. 2009;16:68–73.

Walls RW, Murphy MF, editors. Manual of emergency airway management. 3rd ed. Philadelphia: Lippincott Williams & Wilkins; 2008.

Endotracheal Tube Introducer (Bougie)

15

Joseph Rabinovich

15.1 Indications

- During orotracheal intubation, when only epiglottic visualization or partial glottic view is obtained during laryngoscopy.
- Particularly useful when neck mobility is limited, leading to inadequate visualization of the glottis (as in the case with cervical spine immobilization).
- When the glottic opening is narrowed either from pathological causes (burns, trauma, tumor, or other anatomical variation).
- When the direct view of the airway is very narrow, as with limited mouth opening or large tongue. In these scenarios, the endotracheal tube (ETT) can obstruct one's view of the cords during placement.

15.2 Contraindications

- When a failed airway occurs (three unsuccessful attempts at endotracheal intubation and inability to adequately oxygenate)

- When surgical airway is indicated (i.e., upper airway obstruction that prevents passage of the ETT via the orotracheal route)

15.3 Materials and Medications

- ETT introducer (bougie) (Fig. 15.1)
- Water-based lubricant
- Lubricated ETT 6 mm or larger *without* stylet (pediatric bougies are available that accommodate smaller ETTs)
- Standard orotracheal direct laryngoscopy (Miller or Macintosh blade) or video laryngoscopy setup
- Assistant

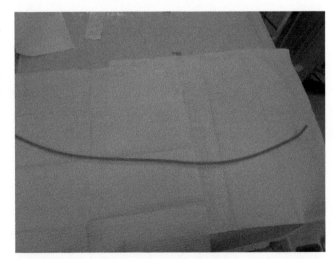

Fig. 15.1 Endotracheal tube introducer (bougie)

J. Rabinovich, MD
Department of Emergency Medicine,
Mount Sinai School of Medicine,
Elmhurst Hospital Center, Elmhurst, NY, USA
e-mail: joerab@gmail.com

© Springer Science+Business Media New York 2016
L. Ganti (ed.), *Atlas of Emergency Medicine Procedures*, DOI 10.1007/978-1-4939-2507-0_15

15.4   Procedure

1. The operator first optimizes airway visualization (Fig. 15.2). (Bougie use should not be a substitute for poor technique.)
2. Without losing sight of the airway, the operator asks the assistant to hand him or her the bougie with the coudé tip facing up.
3. The operator directs the bougie tip underneath the epiglottis (Fig. 15.3).
4. Confirmation of placement can be done visually or by tactile sensation:
   (a) A ratchet-like sensation may be felt as the bougie tip is advanced into the airway and slides over the tracheal rings.
   (b) As the bougie is further advanced, the operator may feel the bougie rotate as it enters the bronchus and/or will get a "hold up," the most reliable sign that the bougie is in the trachea [1]. (The "hold-up" sign occurs when the Bougie encounters a terminal bronchus [typically at around 35 cm] and stops advancing.) [2]

5. Once placement is confirmed, the bougie needs to be partially withdrawn to about 25 cm at the lip line.
   (a) Some brands will have a thick black indicator line.
   (b) A sufficient amount of the bougie needs to extend out beyond the proximal end of the ETT.
6. While the operator holds the bougie in place, the assistant threads the ETT over the bougie (Fig. 15.4).
7. The operator now grasps the ETT in her or his right hand and advances it over the bougie.
8. Simultaneously, the assistant holds and stabilizes the proximal end of the bougie.
9. The ETT should be advanced to approximately 23 cm in males and 21 cm in females. The assistant removes the bougie as the operator holds the ETT in place (Fig. 15.5).
10. As the operator holds the ETT firmly in position, the assistant inflates the ETT balloon and withdraws the bougie.
11. Confirmation of proper ETT placement is achieved through traditional means (end-tidal CO_2 detection, auscultation of breath sounds).

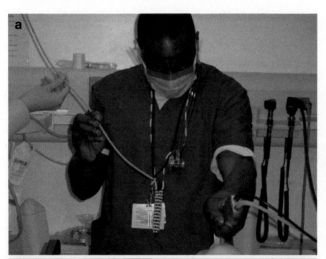

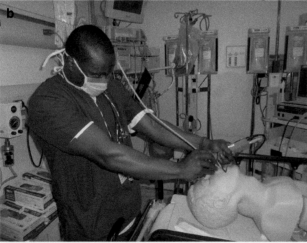

Fig. 15.2 (**a**) Assistant hands operator bougie with coudé tip directed upward, while operator maintains his focus on the target. (**b**) Bougie being placed, parallel with line of sight, underneath epiglottis

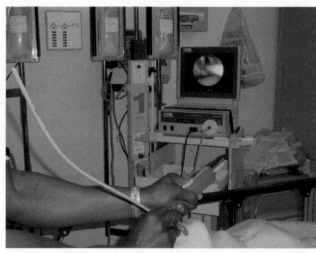

Fig. 15.3 Bougie can be placed into the glottis using direct laryngoscopy or video assistance

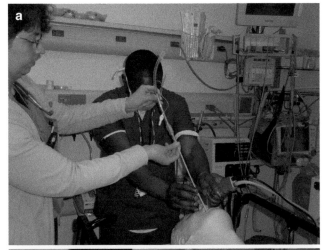

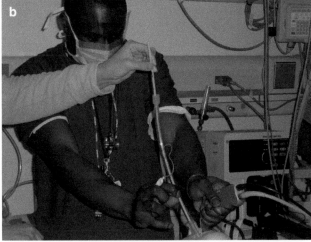

Fig. 15.4 (a) Assistant places ETT over bougie and operator withdraws bougie until it protrudes out the top of the ETT, (b) while assistant stabilizes the protruding portion of the bougie, the operator railroads the ETT into the airway. The operator continues to support the soft tissues with the laryngoscope blade to facilitate placement

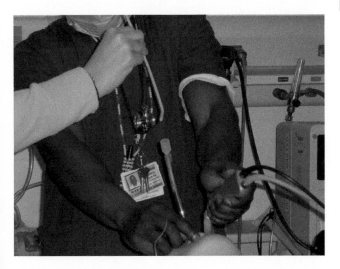

Fig. 15.5 The assistant removes the bougie while the operator stabilizes the endotracheal tube

15.5 Complications

- Trauma to the esophagus, larynx, trachea, or bronchus, including perforation [3, 4].
- In general, complications are rare.

15.6 Pearls and Pitfalls

- The line of sight should be as parallel as possible to the axis of the bougie as it is being passed, allowing better eye-hand coordination. This augments more accurate placement of the bougie tip.
- Maintain the view of the airway as the assistant hands the operator the bougie.
- Keep the laryngoscope in place to support the soft tissues, as the endotracheal tube is slid over the bougie, to facilitate placement.
- If resistance is met during passage, withdraw the ETT slightly (~2 cm) and rotate the ETT counterclockwise one-quarter turn (90°) and reattempt passage.
  - This changes the position of the leading edge of the ETT, which may catch on the posterior laryngeal inlet [2].
  - By rotating the ETT, the leading edge now is anterior facing and is less likely to catch on the arytenoid cartilage along with other laryngeal inlet structures.
- If encountering resistance to ETT placement, consider releasing cricoid pressure (if used).
- Measurement markings on the bougie are aligned with the coudé tip. If not sure of orientation and the loose site of the tip, use the markings to properly orient the tip.

References

1. Kidd JF, Dyson A, Latto IP. Successful difficult intubation. Use of the gum elastic bougie. Anaesthesia. 1988;43:437–8.
2. Murphy MF, Hung OR, Law JA. Tracheal intubation: tricks of the trade. Emerg Med Clin North Am. 2008;26:1001–14.
3. Kadry M, Popat M. Pharyngeal wall perforation – an unusual complication of blind intubation with a gum-elastic bougie. Anaesthesia. 1999;54:404–5.
4. Smith BL. Haemopneumothorax following bougie-assisted tracheal intubation. Anaesthesia. 1994;49:91.

Lighted Stylet Intubation

16

Benjamin M. Mahon and Lars K. Beattie

When lighted stylet intubation is done correctly, the procedure can be very safe, with very little difference in outcome from that of primary laryngoscopy. (*Note: several lighted stylet devices, such as the TrachlightTM and Light WandTM, are no longer being manufactured, but these devices are still in use.*)

16.1 Indications

- Difficult/impossible direct laryngoscopy [1, 2]
  - Congenital abnormalities of airway
  - High Mallampati grade [3]
  - Dental appliances
- Failed direct laryngoscopy

16.2 Contraindications

- Absolute
  - Morbid obesity
  - Airway foreign body
  - Expanding neck mass

- Relative
  - Abnormal airway anatomy
  - Airway lesions (e.g., abscess, mass, epiglottitis) that change oropharyngeal anatomy
  - Acute care where concomitant resuscitation requires a well-lit room
  - Lack of familiarity or experience with procedure
  - "Can't oxygenate, can't ventilate" situation

16.3 Materials and Medications

- Intravenous (IV) access, O_2, and monitor
- Ambu bag with supplemental oxygen
- Suction (Yankauer and tubing)
- Lighted stylet (LS)
- Endotracheal tube (ETT) 2.5-mm larger than LS with 10-cc syringe
- Surgilube
- Intubation medications (this procedure may be performed as an awake or a rapid-sequence intubation)

B.M. Mahon, MD
Ponciana Medical Center,
Kissimmee, FL, USA
e-mail: drfaust2k9@aol.com

L.K. Beattie, MD, MS (⊠)
Department of Emergency Medicine, University of Florida,
Gainesville, FL, USA
e-mail: lars.beattie@ufl.edu

© Springer Science+Business Media New York 2016
L. Ganti (ed.), *Atlas of Emergency Medicine Procedures*, DOI 10.1007/978-1-4939-2507-0_16

16.4 Procedure

1. Preoxygenate.
2. Positioning.
    (a) Sniffing position, pinna at the level of the sternal notch (Fig. 16.1).
    (b) Skip sniffing position if cervical spine injury is suspected.
3. LS-ETT unit preparation.
    (a) Insert the wire stylet into the device.
    (b) Check the LS light.
    (c) Lubricate the LS with K-Y Jelly.
    (d) Position the LS just distal to the Murphy eye.
    (e) Curve the LS to user preference at the line labeled "Bend Here."
4. Administer intubation medications.
5. Have an assistant to apply cricoid pressure.
6. Grasp and elevate the patient's jaw near the corner of the mouth with the operator's thumb, index, and middle fingers, elevating the tongue and epiglottis along with it.
7. Using the free hand, insert the LS-ETT unit into the oropharynx and advance (Fig. 16.2).
8. Use the midline glow in the neck to guide insertion of the LS-ETT (Fig. 16.3).
9. Bright light *below* the thyroid prominence indicates correct placement of the ETT tip.
10. Dim or blurred light or light at the thyroid prominence suggests incorrect positioning (Fig. 16.4).
11. If the transilluminated light is dim, off center, or not seen, esophageal positioning must be considered.
    (a) Withdraw the LS-ETT unit approximately 2–5 cm.
    (b) Reposition the patient's head and neck.
    (c) Reattempt according to steps 5–8.
12. Placement of the ETT (Fig. 16.5).
    (a) Hold the LS-ETT unit steady with one hand.
    (b) Check the depth of the ETT and adjust accordingly.
    (c) Release the LS latch that holds the ETT to the LS.
    (d) While holding the ETT in position, gently slide the LS out from the ETT.
    (e) Inflate the ETT balloon.
13. Confirm ETT placement (continuous end-tidal CO_2 [$EtCO_2$], colorimetric capnometry).
14. Secure the ETT.

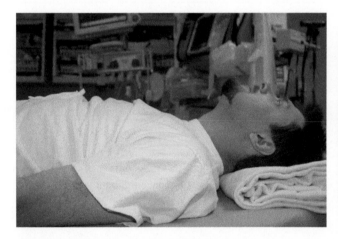

Fig. 16.1 Sniffing position, pinna at the level of the sternal notch

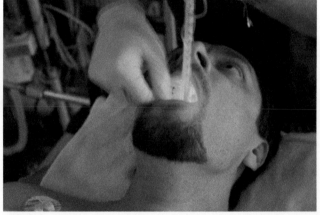

Fig. 16.2 Grasp and elevate the patient's jaw near the corner of the mouth with the operator's thumb, index, and middle fingers, elevating the tongue and epiglottis along with it. Using the free hand, insert the LS-ETT unit into the oropharynx and advance

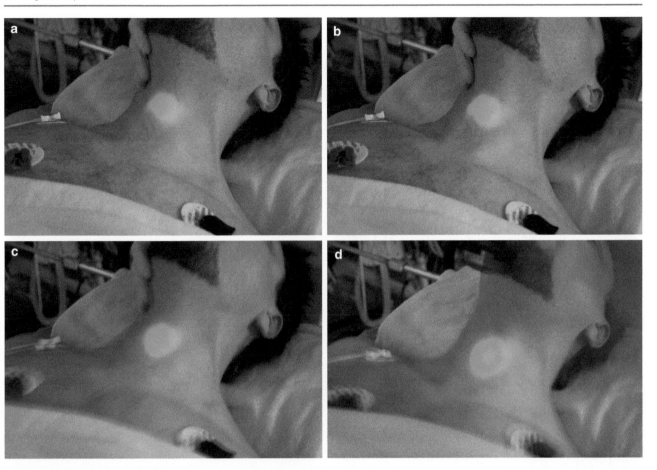

Fig. 16.3 (a–c) Use the midline glow in the neck to guide insertion of the LS-ETT. (d) Bright light *below* the thyroid prominence indicates correct placement of the ETT tip

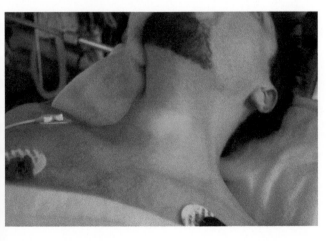

Fig. 16.4 Dim or blurred light or light at the thyroid prominence suggests incorrect positioning

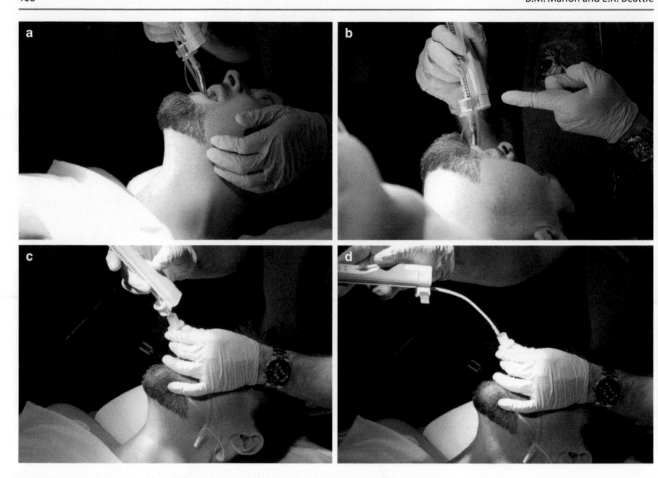

Fig. 16.5 (**a**) Hold the LS-ETT unit steady with one hand. (**b**) Check the depth of the ETT and adjust accordingly. (**c**) Release the LS latch that holds the ETT to the LS. (**d**) While holding the ETT in position, gently slide the LS out from the ETT

16.5 Pearls and Pitfalls

- Pearls
  - LS-ETT complex—Typically the classic "hockey-stick" shape with the 90° curve just proximal to the cuff is recommended [2].
  - Dimming the room lights will enhance transillumination.
  - Pulling the wire stylet out from the LS-ETT unit will make it more pliable and may facilitate its placement in the trachea and removal of the LS.
  - Some LS devices start to blink after 30 s to prevent bulb overheating.
  - The LS may be used with nasotracheal intubation, intubation through a laryngeal mask airway (LMA), or conventional laryngoscopy to enhance success.
- Pitfalls
  - LS intubation should not be used as an emergency airway alternative by a proceduralist unfamiliar with the technique:
    - It is technically complicated and more challenging than many other airway adjuncts in the standard difficult airway algorithm.
    - One study compared the use of four rescue airway devices in the difficult airway algorithm. A success rate of only 20 % was achieved with the Trachlight™ on the first attempt when in the hands of the novice physician when used as a rescue device in their difficult airway algorithm [4].

- In very thin patients, transillumination may be visualized quite well even when the LS-ETT unit is in the esophagus:
  - When the unit is in the esophagus, typically the light it will be more diffuse.
  - When the unit is in the trachea, the transilluminated area will be well circumscribed.
- In obese patients or patients with significant neck tissue, the transilluminated light from the LS-ETT unit may be dim despite correct positioning in the trachea.

References

1. Agro F, Hung OR, Cataldo R, Carassiti M, Gherardi S. Lightwand intubation using the Trachlight: a brief review of current knowledge. Can J Anaesth. 2001;48:592–9.
2. Davis L, Cook-Sather SD, Schreiner MS. Lighted stylet tracheal intubation: a review. Anesth Analg. 2000;90:745–56.
3. Rhee KY, Lee JR, Kim J, Park S, Kwon WK, Han S. A comparison of lighted stylet (Surch-Lite) and direct laryngoscopic intubation in patients with high Mallampati scores. Anesth Analg. 2009;108:1215–9.
4. Aikins NL, Ganesh R, Springmann KE, Lunn JJ, Solis-Keus J. Difficult airway management and the novice physician. J Emerg Trauma Shock. 2010;3:9–12.

Selected Reading

Langeron O, Birenbaum A, Amour J. Airway management in trauma. Minerva Anestesiol. 2009;75:307–11.
Walls RM, Murphy MF. Manual of emergency airway management. 3rd ed. Philadelphia: Lippincott Williams & Wilkins; 2008. Chap. 11.

Fiber-Optic Stylet Intubation (Rigid and Semirigid)

17

Joseph Rabinovich

17.1 Indications

- For use in routine and predicted difficult oral intubations.
- Similar to a flexible fiber-optic scope with the specific advantages of:
  - Less setup time
  - Less time to perform the procedure
  - Appropriate for routine intubations (and easier to accumulate experience)
  - Rigid enough to lift up the epiglottis
  - Easier to navigate through tissue
  - Less susceptible to being obscured by blood and secretions
  - More durable, more portable, easier to clean, and less expensive
- Particularly useful when neck mobility or mouth opening is restricted.
- Advantageous in awake intubations because it can minimize tissue contact, resulting in less stimulation to the patient's airway and better tolerance.
- Certain stylets can be used to intubate through supraglottic airways such as laryngeal mask airways (LMAs).

17.2 Contraindications

- Complete upper airway obstruction where surgical airway is indicated
- Oral pharyngeal swelling requiring a nasotracheal or surgical approach
- Failed airway and unable to adequately maintain oxygenation

17.3 Relative Contraindications

- Large amounts of blood and secretions may obscure visualization of the airway and cords.
- Very distorted airways. Compared with flexible endoscopy, this device is less maneuverable.

17.4 Materials and Medications

- Endotracheal tube (ETT) 5.5 mm or greater (Fig. 17.1) (Pediatric stylets are also available.)
- Water-soluble lubricant
- Defogging agent
- Optional: Swivel adaptor and meconium aspirator

J. Rabinovich, MD
Department of Emergency Medicine,
Mount Sinai School of Medicine, Elmhurst Hospital Center,
Elmhurst, NY, USA
e-mail: joerab@gmail.com

© Springer Science+Business Media New York 2016
L. Ganti (ed.), *Atlas of Emergency Medicine Procedures*, DOI 10.1007/978-1-4939-2507-0_17

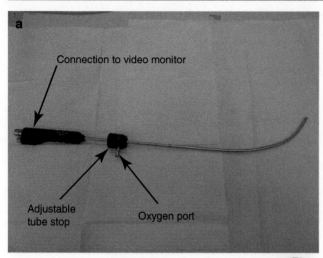

Connection to video monitor

Adjustable
tube stop

Oxygen port

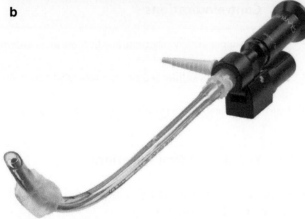

Fig. 17.1 (**a**) Bonfils rigid fiber-optic stylet, Karl Storz endoscopy, (**b**) Levitan FPS malleable fiber-optic stylet

17.5 Procedure

1. Use standard preparation for rapid sequence intubation (RSI) or for awake intubation.
2. Place the ETT over the stylet.
   (a) The ETT should extend slightly beyond the stylet tip.
   (b) If using the malleable stylet:
      (i) Without a laryngoscope: Bend tip to about 70° [1].
      (ii) With a laryngoscope: Bend tip to 35° [1].
   (c) Lubricate the tip of the ETT.
3. Depending on specific scope capability, connect oxygen tubing to the port on the scope.
   (a) This keeps secretions away from the tip while providing an oxygen source.
   (b) Keep flow less than 6 L/min [2].
4. Lens fogging prevention.
   (a) Warm the tip of the scope with the hand or immerse the tip in warm saline.
   (b) Apply the defogging agent.
   (c) Alternatively, chlorhexidine is an effective defogger.
5. Scope insertion.
   (a) Use the nondominant hand to pull the jaw forward while holding the tongue.
      (i) In an awake patient, have the patient protrude the tongue and the operator grasps it with 4×4 gauze. (Alternatively, a Macintosh laryngoscope blade can be used.)
      (ii) The goal is to move the base of the tongue off the posterior pharyngeal wall.
   (b) Initially position the scope horizontally and to the right of the patient's mouth.
   (c) Once the tip is in the oropharynx, reposition the scope vertically (Fig. 17.2a).
   (d) The scope tip should be in the midline or in the retromolar position (per scope design).
   (e) Position the scope and the tip of the ETT in front of the uvula.
   (f) Refer to the eyepiece or video screen to see if there is a clear image of the uvula (Fig. 17.2b).
   (g) Advance the scope very slowly to maintain a view of landmarks, avoiding tissue contact (Fig. 17.3).
6. Once the epiglottis is visualized:
   (a) Continue to advance slowly.
   (b) To get underneath the epiglottis, the tip of the scope may need to be moved posteriorly (by tilting the operator's hand slightly forward) (Fig. 17.4).

7. Once underneath the epiglottis, tilt the scope back, to advance into the more anterior directed airway.
   (a) Make sure the glottic opening is well centered on the screen to facilitate placement (Fig. 17.5).
   (b) If resistance is felt, operator may need to rotate the scope clockwise, or tip scope slightly forward, to prevent the ETT from abutting the anterior aspect of the trachea.
   (c) The ETT may need to be advanced off the rigid stylet to allow further advancement.

8. To remove scope:
   (a) Twist the proximal end of the ETT clockwise.
   (b) Stabilize the tube with the nondominant hand.
   (c) Use the dominant hand to pull the scope forward, following the curvature of the stylet (Fig. 17.6).
   (d) An assistant may be of use during this step.

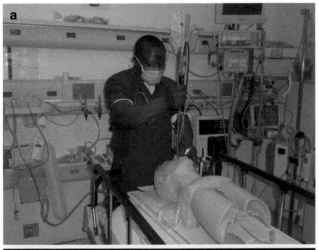

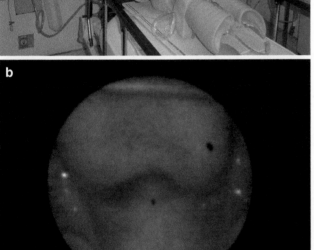

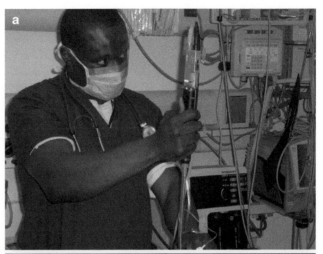

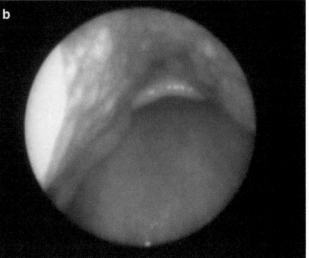

Fig. 17.2 (a) Initial placement of scope, under direct visualization; (b) tip is positioned in from the uvula

Fig. 17.3 (a) Using the video monitor, or through an eyepiece, the operator advances to the next landmark, (b) the epiglottis

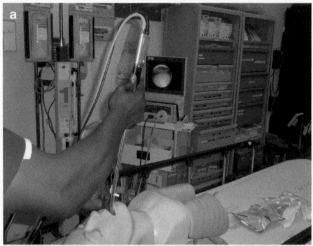

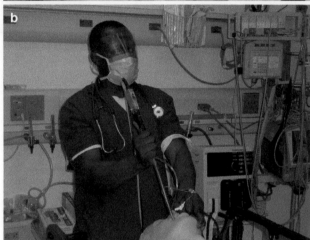

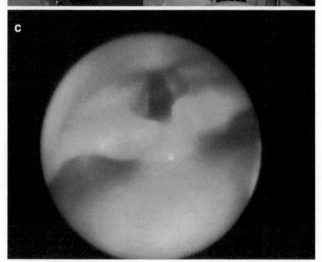

Fig. 17.4 (**a**) Operator tips scope forward to get underneath the epiglottis while advancing; (**b**) once under the epiglottis, the scope may need to be tipped back to advance to the glottic opening; (**c**) operator should try to keep the glottic opening in the center of the screen

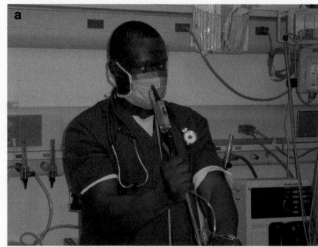

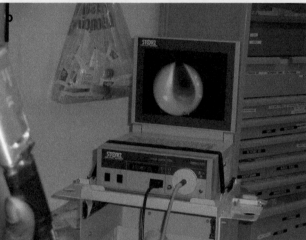

Fig. 17.5 (**a**) Operator is advancing the scope, (**b**) through the glottic opening keeping the image centered

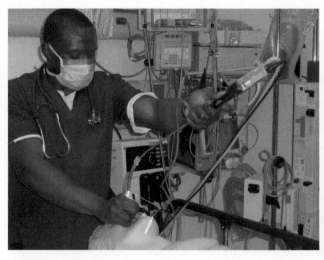

Fig. 17.6 To remove scope, operator must pull it forward while stabilizing the endotracheal tube

17.6 Pearls and Pitfalls

- Pearls
  - When the operator loses perspective or a clear view, withdraw the scope back to the point where identifiable structures are visualized and proceed.
  - The operator can suction through the scope by attaching a swivel adaptor and a meconium aspirator (Fig. 17.7) [3].
- Pitfalls
  - If the scope is advanced too quickly, orientation can be lost.
  - Structures that are too close to the scope will become blurred and unidentifiable.
  - If the scope tip abuts pharyngeal tissue, visualization can become blurred.
  - Flow greater than 6 L/min connected to the oxygen port may result in subcutaneous emphysema (single case report) [2].

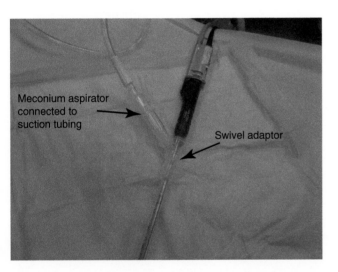

Fig. 17.7 By placing the stylet through the rubber valve of a swivel adaptor, which is then connected to suction via a neonatal meconium aspirator, the operator can now suction through the endotracheal tube

References

1. Levitan RM. Design rationale and intended use of a short optical stylet for routine fiberoptic augmentation of emergency laryngoscopy. Am J Emerg Med. 2006;24:490–5.
2. Hemmerling TM, Bracco D. Subcutaneous cervical and facial emphysema with the use of the Bonfils fiberscope and high-flow oxygen insufflation. Anesth Analg. 2008;106:260–2.
3. Weingart SD, Bhagwan SD. A novel set-up to allow suctioning during direct endotracheal and fiberscope intubation. J Clin Anesth. 2011;23:518–9.

Storz Video Laryngoscope

Joseph Rabinovich

18.1 Indications

- Orotracheal intubation for both routine and predicted difficult airways.
- Teaching traditional direct laryngoscopy to novice intubators.
- Ideal for unanticipated difficult airway with the option of intubating indirectly if an adequate direct view is unobtainable.
- An excellent tool when cervical spine precautions need to be taken: Because the video view of the airway is generated by a camera at the tip of laryngoscope blade, less manipulation is required for optimal glottic views.

18.2 Contraindications

- Absolute
  - When orotracheal intubation is contraindicated, e.g., for massive facial trauma, complete upper airway obstruction precluding orotracheal access to the airway
  - In a failed airway (three unsuccessful attempts with inability to maintain adequate oxygenation)
- Relative
  - Blood or copious secretions may prevent indirect viewing of the airway but does not always preclude the use of this device.

J. Rabinovich, MD
Department of Emergency Medicine,
Mount Sinai School of Medicine,
Elmhurst Hospital Center, Elmhurst, NY, USA
e-mail: joerab@gmail.com

© Springer Science+Business Media New York 2016
L. Ganti (ed.), *Atlas of Emergency Medicine Procedures*, DOI 10.1007/978-1-4939-2507-0_18

18.3   Materials and Medications (Fig. 18.1)

- Standard materials and medications for endotracheal intubation. Operator should have a backup laryngoscope in case of equipment failure.
- Endotracheal tube (ETT) with or without stylet.
- Water-based lubricant.
- Antifogging agent (not required for C-Mac).

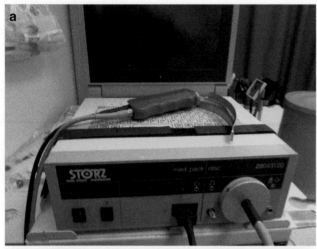

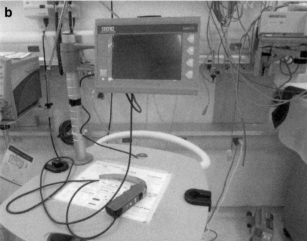

Fig. 18.1 (**a**) Storz video laryngoscope (older version), (**b**) Storz C-Mac (newer version)

18.4   Procedure

1. Standard preparation for orotracheal intubation. If there are no cervical spine precautions, then align the external auditory meatus with the sternal notch [1].
2. Apply antifogging drops to lens at tip of the blade, and/or hold the hand over the blade tip to warm it up to body temperature (older V-Mac model) (Fig. 18.2a).
3. Because blade geometry is the same as in standard laryngoscopes, the insertion technique is identical to that of standard laryngoscopy with a Macintosh blade (Fig. 18.2b).
4. Obtain the best direct view possible.
5. Consider the addition of the backward-upward-rightward pressure (BURP) maneuver [2].
6. Airway maneuvers may be performed by the operator or by the assistant using the video screen as a guide along with operator feedback (Fig. 18.3).
7. The operator has the option of intubating directly with adequate view or indirectly if visualization is improved.
8. Consider using an ETT introducer (bougie—see Chap. 15) if the view is inadequate.
9. Place the ETT, with or without a stylet, into the airway under direct or indirect visualization. If using a stylet, bend the distal end of the tube to approximately 35° as for a standard intubation (Fig. 18.4) [3].
10. Remove the stylet, inflate the cuff of the ETT using a syringe, and confirm placement with end-tidal CO_2, capnography, or colorimetry.

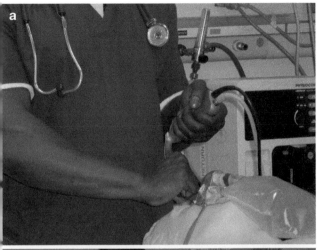

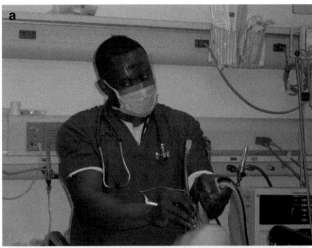

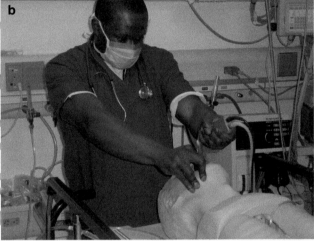

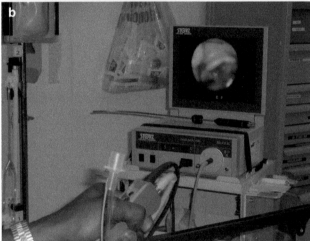

Fig. 18.2 (**a**) Operator warming the blade to prevent fogging, (**b**) laryngoscope blade insertion using the standard direct technique. Operator visually places the blade and optimizes the glottic view

Fig. 18.4 (**a**) Operator initially places the endotracheal tube (ETT) into the oropharynx using direct visualization to avoid injury; (**b**) the tip of the ETT passing through the cords can be confirmed by direct visualization or by watching the video image

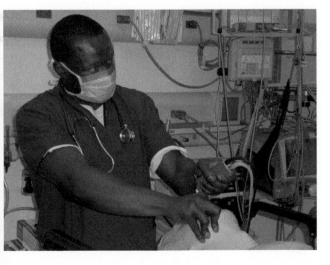

Fig. 18.3 Operator has the choice of using direct visualization (preferred when a novice intubator is learning laryngoscopy) or the indirect video view of the glottis

18.5   Complications (As with any Direct Laryngoscopy)

- Dental trauma
- Oropharyngeal trauma
- Vocal cord injury

18.6   Pearls and Pitfalls

- The initial placement of the laryngoscope blade and ETT should be done under direct visualization to avoid trauma to the oropharyngeal structures.
- As with direct laryngoscopy, the ETT should not be placed blindly, and the ETT must be seen to pass through the vocal cords to avoid placement in the esophagus.
- View can be obscured by secretions or fogging. If this occurs, the operator may need to remove the blade, wipe it down, and reinsert. The newer model, the C-Mac, is less likely to fog owing to design improvements.
- Observing the ETT pass through the vocal cords can sometimes be easier using the video image because the camera is angled to provide the most optimal view.
- Placement of the blade into the oropharynx can be awkward because the handle of laryngoscope is bulkier than a standard laryngoscope. Its handle is larger and has cables attached to its base. In patients with large anteroposterior diameter chests, the operator may need to rotate the laryngoscope handle toward the right corner of the mouth in order to introduce the blade into the oral cavity and then rotate it back to the proper position.
- These devices are ideal for teaching laryngoscopy. With same blade geometry, the technique is the same as with standard laryngoscopy. As the operator attempts intubation directly, the instructor can observe on the video screen and guide the student. The instructor will also be able to visually confirm that the ETT is entering the trachea.

References

1. Greenland KB, Edwards MJ, Hutton NJ, Challis VJ, Irwin MG, Sleigh JW. Changes in airway configuration with different head and neck positions using magnetic resonance imaging of normal airways: a new concept with possible clinical applications. Br J Anaesth. 2010;105:683–90.
2. Knill RL. Difficult laryngoscopy made easy with a "BURP.". Can J Anaesth. 1993;40:798–9.
3. Levitan RM, Heitz JW, Sweeney M, Cooper RM. The complexities of tracheal intubation with direct laryngoscopy and alternative intubation devices. Ann Emerg Med. 2011;57:240–7.

Selected Reading

Brown 3rd CA, Bair AE, Pallin DJ, et al. Improved glottic exposure with the video Macintosh laryngoscope in adult emergency department tracheal intubations. Ann Emerg Med. 2010;56:83–8.
Niforopoulou P, Pantazopoulos I, Demestiha T, Koudouna E, Xanthos T. Video-laryngoscopes in the adult airway management: a topical review of the literature. Acta Anaesthesiol Scand. 2010;54:1050–61.

Cricothyroidotomy

19

Henry Young II, Shannon Toohey, Bharath Chakravarthy, and Lars K. Beattie

Up to seven intubation attempts in 1000 end up in a "can't intubate/can't ventilate" situation in the emergency department. These are considered failed airways that may require a surgical airway to maintain ventilation and oxygenation.

19.1 Indications

- Endotracheal tube (ETT) placement attempts unsuccessful
- Failed bag valve mask, laryngeal mask airway, or Combitube ventilation
- Severe facial trauma affecting the upper airway
- Severe oropharyngeal hemorrhage or profound emesis
- Obstruction (foreign body, mass, mass effect)

19.2 Contraindications

- Airway protection achievable using a less invasive strategy

- Tracheal transaction
- Pediatric patients younger than 8 years

19.3 Techniques

- Scalpel-bougie – minimalist
- Scalpel-Trousseau – standard

19.3.1 Scalpel-Bougie

19.3.1.1 Materials and Medications (Fig. 19.1)

- Betadine or chlorhexidine
- Scalpel #11 blade
- ETT (≥ 6 cm)
- Bougie
- Surgilube
- Bag valve mask

H. Young II, MD
Department of Emergency Medicine, University of Florida Health, Gainesville, FL, USA
e-mail: hyoungii@ufl.edu

S. Toohey, MD
Department of Emergency Medicine, University of California Irvine Medical Center, Orange, CA, USA
e-mail: stoohey@uci.edu

B. Chakravarthy, MD, MPH
Department of Emergency Medicine,
University of California Irvine, Orange, CA, USA
e-mail: bchakrav@uci.edu

L.K. Beattie, MD, MS (✉)
Department of Emergency Medicine, University of Florida, Gainesville, FL, USA
e-mail: lars.beattie@ufl.edu

© Springer Science+Business Media New York 2016
L. Ganti (ed.), *Atlas of Emergency Medicine Procedures*, DOI 10.1007/978-1-4939-2507-0_19

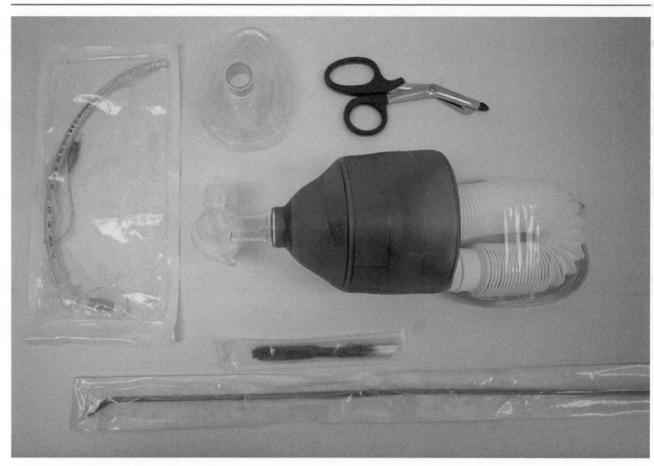

Fig. 19.1 *Right to left*, *top to bottom*: ETT (≥6 cm); bag valve mask; trauma shears; scalpel #11 blade; bougie

19.3.1.2 Procedure

1. Apply topical antiseptic.
2. Remove the 15-mm ETT ventilator connector from the ETT end.
3. Place copious Surgilube on the bougie and railroad over the end of the bougie.
4. Palpate the thyroid notch, cricothyroid membrane, and hyoid bone for orientation (Fig. 19.2a).
5. Stabilize the thyroid cartilage between the thumb and the middle finger of the nondominant hand.
6. Make a vertical skin incision (2–3 cm) over the cricothyroid membrane (Fig. 19.2b).
7. Use the index finger to palpate the cricothyroid membrane.
8. Turn the scalpel 90° and make a 1.5-cm horizontal incision through the lower half of the cricothyroid membrane (Fig. 19.3a).
9. With the scalpel still in the incision, turn it 90°, and insert the bougie into the incision, using the blade as a guide (Fig. 19.3b).
10. Advance the bougie caudally 5–6 cm. Stop if resistance is encountered.
11. Slide the ETT over the bougie into the incision (Fig. 19.4a).
12. Inflate the ETT cuff and ventilate the patient (Fig. 19.4b).
13. Verify the position of the ETT via auscultation, end-tidal CO_2 (EtCO$_2$), and chest radiograph.
14. Secure the ETT.

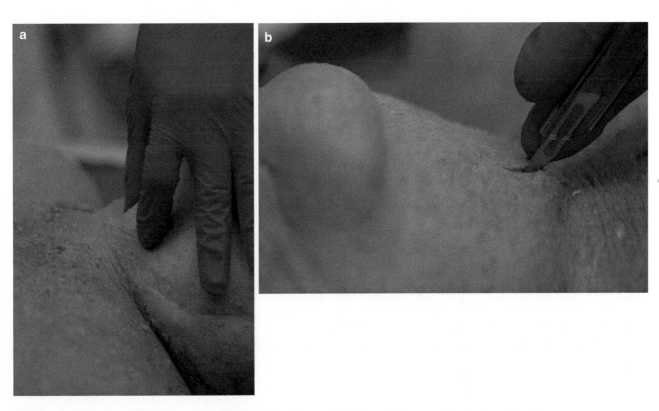

Fig. 19.2 (a) Palpate and stabilize the thyroid cartilage, (b) make a vertical 2–3 cm incision over the cricothyroid membrane

Fig. 19.3 (**a**) Make a horizontal incision into the cricothyroid membrane, (**b**) insert the bougie into the incision made in the cricothyroid membrane

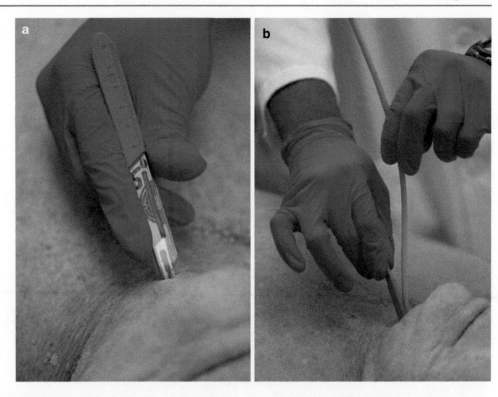

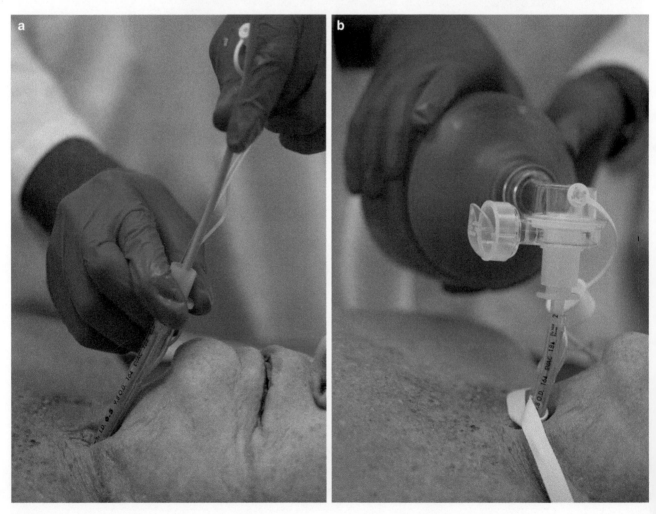

Fig. 19.4 (**a**) Slide the endotracheal tube (ETT) over the bougie into the trachea, (**b**) ventilate the patient

19.3.2 Scalpel-Trousseau

19.3.2.1   Materials and Medications (Fig. 19.5)
- Scalpel with #11 blade
- Tracheal hook
- Trousseau dilator
- Cuffed tracheostomy tube (TT) (6.5 or 7.0) or ETT (5.0, 5.5, or 6.0)
- Antiseptic preparation

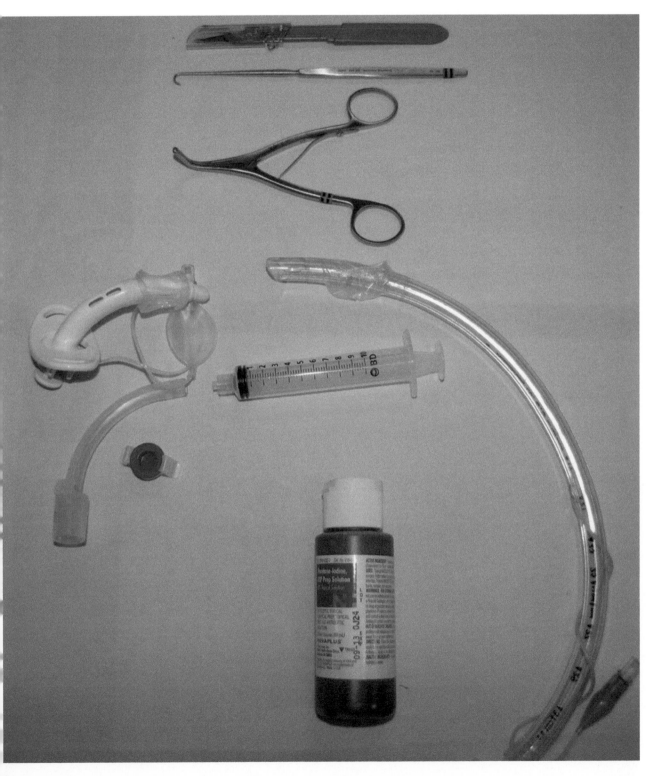

Fig. 19.5 *Top to bottom, right to left*: Scalpel with #11 blade; tracheal hook; Trousseau dilator; cuffed tracheostomy tube (TT) (6.5 or 7.0) or ETT (5.0, 5.5, or 6.0); antiseptic preparation

19.3.2.2 Procedure

1. Apply topical antiseptic.
2. Palpate the thyroid notch, cricothyroid membrane, and hyoid bone for orientation.
3. Stabilize the thyroid between the thumb and the middle finger of the nondominant hand (Fig. 19.6a).
4. Make a vertical skin incision (2–3 cm) over the cricothyroid membrane (Fig. 19.6b).
5. Palpate with the index finger to verify the cricothyroid membrane location.
6. Use stabilization of the thyroid and palpation to maintain orientation of the anatomy.
7. Make a 1.5-cm horizontal incision through the lower half of the membrane (Fig. 19.7a).
8. Insert a tracheal hook into the incision, then rotate such that hook faces superiorly (Fig. 19.7b).
9. Withdraw at a 45° angle in a cephalad direction, applying gentle traction to the thyroid cartilage.
10. Place the Trousseau dilator into the incision transversely and open the membrane incision vertically (Fig. 19.8a).
11. Insert a cuffed ETT (5.0–6.0) or TT (6.5–7.0) into the incision between the prongs of the dilator in the horizontal access (Fig. 19.8b).
12. Rotate both the dilator and the ETT toward the head of the patient and then direct the tube downward into the trachea while removing the dilator.
13. Inflate the ETT cuff and ventilate the patient.
14. Verify the position of the ETT via auscultation, $EtCO_2$, and chest x-ray.
15. Once placement of the tube has been verified, the tracheal hook can be removed.
16. Secure the ETT.

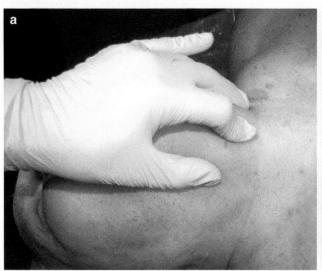
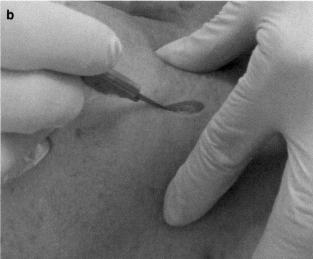

Fig. 19.6 (a) Stabilize the thyroid cartilage between the thumb and the middle finger of the nondominant hand; (b) make a vertical incision over the cricothyroid membrane

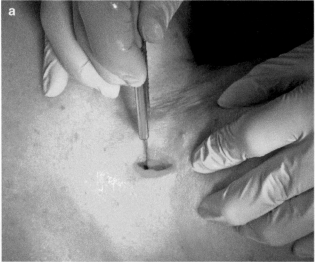
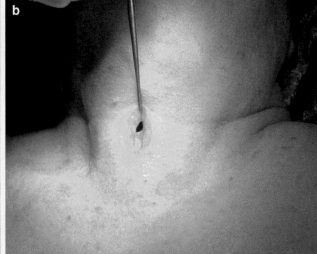

Fig. 19.7 (a) Make a horizontal incision in the lower half of the cricothyroid membrane. (b) Insert a tracheal hook and apply gentle traction superiorly at a 45° angle

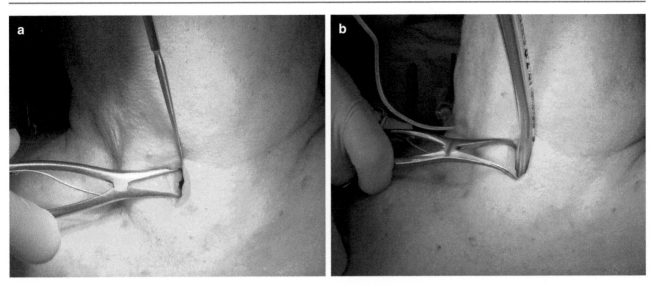

Fig. 19.8 (**a**) Insert the Trousseau dilator into the incision, and open the path for placement of the tracheostomy tube (TT) or the ETT. (**b**) Insert the TT or the ETT into the expanded incision between the Trousseau dilator prongs

19.4 Complications

- Bleeding
- ETT misplacement (false passage, through the thyrohyoid membrane, unintentional tracheostomy)
- Hoarseness, dysphonia, or vocal cord paralysis
- Subglottic or laryngeal stenosis
- Damage to thyroid cartilage, cricoid cartilage, or tracheal rings
- Perforated esophagus
- Infection
- Aspiration

19.5 Pearls

- Predictors of difficult cricothyrotomy: "SHORT" [1]
  - Prior *S*urgery or *S*car tissue
  - *H*ematoma
  - *O*bese
  - Prior *R*adiation
  - *T*umor/abscess
- The incision should cut through the skin and subcutaneous tissue down to the cricothyroid membrane and cartilages.
- Vertical incisions allow for extension in either direction if the cricothyroid membrane is above or below initial incision.
- Blood in the field may hinder visualization of the membrane, but the airway should be established before attempts to control any bleeding.
- Cricothyroid arteries are located cephalad to the cricothyroid membrane.

- Either a TT or an ETT can be used for the procedure.
  - ETTs are more ubiquitous.
  - TTs are easier to secure.
- If an ETT is used, a stylet can help direct placement.
- Cricothyroidotomy is preferred in the emergency setting over tracheostomy owing to the increased risks of bleeding, the mobility of the trachea, and the risk of lacerating the underlying thyroid gland [2].
- Ultrasound can be used to visualize landmarks in patients in whom landmarks are difficult to identify.

References

1. Walls RM, Murphy MF, editors. Manual of emergency airway management. 4th ed. Philadelphia: Wolters Kluwer; 2012.
2. Boon JM, Abrahams PH, Meiring JH, et al. Cricothyroidotomy: a clinical anatomy review. Clin Anat. 2004;17:478–86.

Selected Reading

DiGiacomo C, Neshat KK, Angus LD, et al. Emergency cricothyrotomy. Mil Med. 2003;168:541–4.
Hamilton PH, Kang JJ. Emergency airway management. Mt Sinai J Med. 1997;64:292–301.
Helm M, Gries A, Mutzbauer T. Surgical approach in difficult airway management. Best Pract Res Clin Anaesthesiol. 2005;19:623–40.
Sagarin MJ, Barton ED, Chng YM, Walls RM. Airway management by US and Canadian emergency medicine residents: a multicenter analysis of more than 6,000 endotracheal intubation attempts. Ann Emerg Med. 2005;46:328–36.
Walls RM. Cricothyroidotomy. Emerg Med Clin North Am. 1988;6: 725–36.

Tracheostomy Tube Malfunction

20

Deena Bengiamin and Bharath Chakravarthy

Tracheostomy tube (TT) malfunction is the source of airway compromise in patients requiring these airway devices. TT malfunction may create an airway emergency, and the timely replacement of TTs is a challenging procedure in the most experienced hands.

20.1 Indications

- Cuff rupture
  - Can lead to dislodgment
- Dislodgment
  - Most common emergency department TT complication
  - Can lead to air passage obstruction
- Obstruction
  - Caused by blood or thick, dry secretions (formed in the absence of nasopharyngeal air humidification).
  - Dried secretions or blood can act as a one-way valve, allowing air in but restricting outward flow.

20.2 Materials and Medications

- Airway suction catheter
- Oxygen humidifier
- Bougie/nasogastric (NG) tube (12 French)

D. Bengiamin, MD
Department of Emergency Medicine, University of San Francisco Fresno, Fresno, CA, USA
e-mail: dbengiamin@fresno.ucsf.edu

B. Chakravarthy, MD, MPH (✉)
Department of Emergency Medicine, University of California Irvine, Orange, CA, USA
e-mail: bchakrav@uci.edu

- Saline
- N-Acetyl-cysteine (NAC)
- Appropriately sized endotracheal tube (ETT) or TT

20.3 Procedure

1. Supply high-flow humidified oxygen through a bag valve mask (BVM), or a non-rebreather face mask.
2. Assess clinical indicators to determine TT problem.
   (a) Indicators of cuff rupture: Air leak with BVM and loose TT.
   (b) Indicators of dislodged TT (if TT is still in the stomal opening): Subcutaneous emphysema, crepitus, and diminished or absent breath sounds.
   (c) Indicators of an obstructed TT: ±stridor and diminished or absent breath sounds.
   (d) If time allows, chest radiograph, continuous capnography, and oxygen saturation can be helpful.
3. Obstruction
   (a) Remove the inner cannula and inspect for obstruction—clean if necessary.
   (b) If this fails, 5–10 mL of saline or NAC can be squirted directly down the TT to loosen secretions.
   (c) Suction thoroughly with a suction catheter (Fig. 20.1).
   (d) In refractory cases, the TT will need replacement.
4. Replacement
   (a) Ideally, the replacement tube should be of the same type and size as the original TT.
   (b) A smaller size TT or ETT can be helpful in settings of airway compromise.
   (c) A 6–7.5-cm ETT tube may be used if a TT is unavailable.
   (d) Remove the existing TT.
   (e) Hyperextend the patient's head and neck to maximize visualization of the stoma.

© Springer Science+Business Media New York 2016
L. Ganti (ed.), *Atlas of Emergency Medicine Procedures*, DOI 10.1007/978-1-4939-2507-0_20

(f) Note: Careful inspection of the area is paramount because the thyroid isthmus may obscure visualization of the tracheal stoma.

(g) Techniques

  (i) Direct insertion

   1. As soon as possible, insert the new TT or ETT into the stoma to prevent stomal narrowing (Fig. 20.2).
   2. Inflate the new TT/ETT cuff.

  (ii) Bougie or NG tube

   1. Lubricate the TT or ETT tube.
   2. Lubricate a bougie or 12-French NG tube.
   3. Insert the lubricated bougie or NG tube into the TT or ETT.
   4. Insert the bougie or NG tube into stoma and advance into the trachea (Fig. 20.3a).
   5. Direct the NG tube or bougie caudad toward the lower tracheobronchial tree.
   6. Do not advance more than 7 cm.

7. If resistance is noted:

   (a) Either the operator has reached a terminal bronchiole or is in a false passage.
   (b) Do not force bougie/NG tube farther at this point.
   (c) Use clinical judgment (bougie/ETT depth, palpation) to determine likely placement.

8. Advance TT or NG tube over bougie or NG tube is in trachea (Fig. 20.3b).

9. After the TT is in place, remove the bougie/NG tube.

  (iii) The fingertip technique

   1. Insert a gloved forefinger into tracheal stoma (Fig. 20.4a).
   2. Formulate a mental plan as to the direction and path of the stoma.
   3. Then place a TT or an ETT into the stoma as the finger is withdrawn (Fig. 20.4b).

5. If placement of a TT or ETT is not possible through the stoma, consider endotracheal intubation.

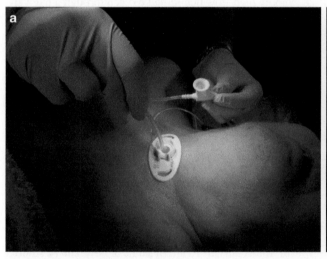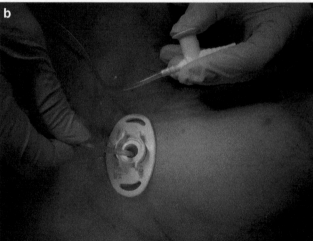

Fig. 20.1 (a) Insert the suction catheter to the appropriate depth, keeping the suction port open. (b) Slowly withdraw the catheter in a circular motion, keeping the suction port closed

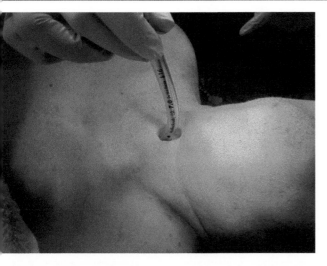

Fig. 20.2 Insertion of the endotracheal tube (ETT) directly into the stoma

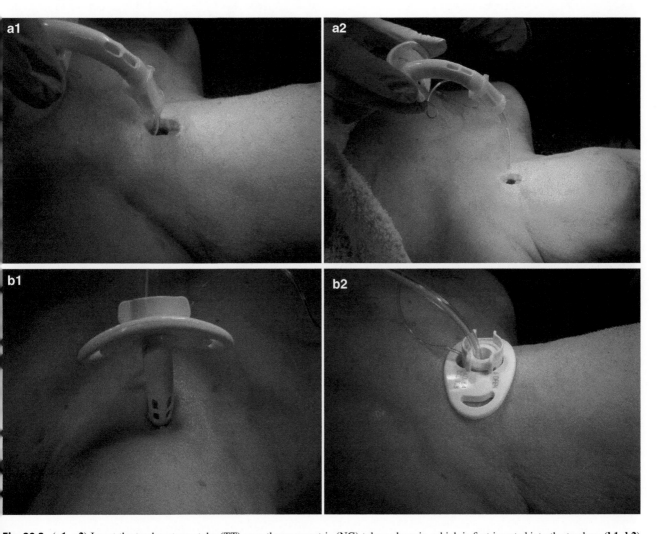

Fig. 20.3 (**a1, a2**) Insert the tracheostomy tube (TT) over the nasogastric (NG) tube or bougie, which is first inserted into the trachea. (**b1, b2**) Advance the TT over the NG tube or bougie, which serves as a guidewire

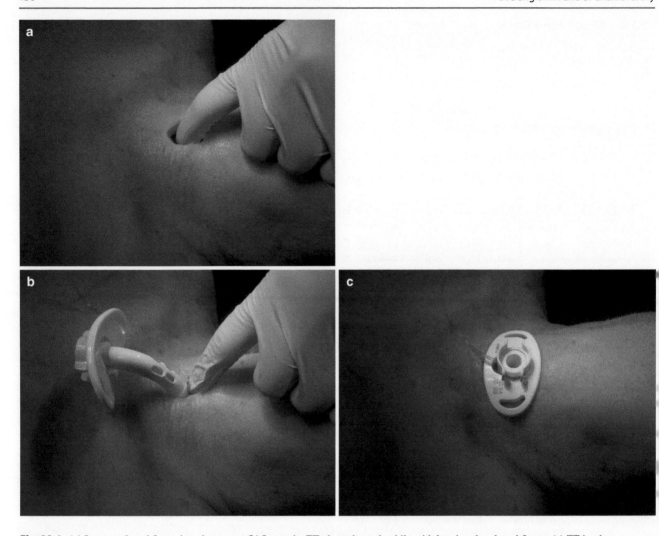

Fig. 20.4 (a) Insert a gloved finger into the stoma. (b) Insert the TT along the path while withdrawing the gloved finger. (c) TT in place

20.4 Pearls and Pitfalls

- Stomal closing
  - Stomal constriction begins as soon as the TT is removed or displaced.
  - Forceful attempts to replace a large TT may result in false passages and trauma.
- Tracheal stenosis
  - Constant TT cuff pressure may cause necrosis, ulceration, and granulation tissue formation, leading to tracheal narrowing.
  - Complicates TT replacement in the setting of dislodgment or obstruction.
  - Bougie use can be helpful to place a small(er) ETT until surgical dilation and/or resection can be achieved.
- Creation of a false lumen during recannulation
  - Subcutaneous emphysema will be an early indicator of this.
  - Early confirmation of correct placement of TT by confirming:
    - Continuous end-tidal CO_2 monitoring
    - Equal chest rise
    - Bilateral breath sounds

- Unrecognized trachea–innominate artery fistula (Fig. 20.5)
  - Usually occurs within 3–4 weeks of placement
  - Presentation: Bleeding around the tracheostomy tube (>10 mL) or massive hemoptysis
  - Requires
    - ETT cuff overinflation to compress the fistula.
    - Digital pressure on stoma may be helpful to tamponade the bleeding.
    - Place stomal ETT deep to bleeding fistula to protect airway.
    - Definitive surgical intervention in operating room.
  - Associated with high mortality
- Unrecognized tracheoesophageal fistula
  - Usually iatrogenic injury from TT placement or NG tube erosion
  - Presentation: Dyspnea, copious TT secretions, recurrent food aspiration, and gastric distention
  - Requires
    - Bronchoscopy or swallowing studies to confirm diagnosis
    - Surgical repair or stenting

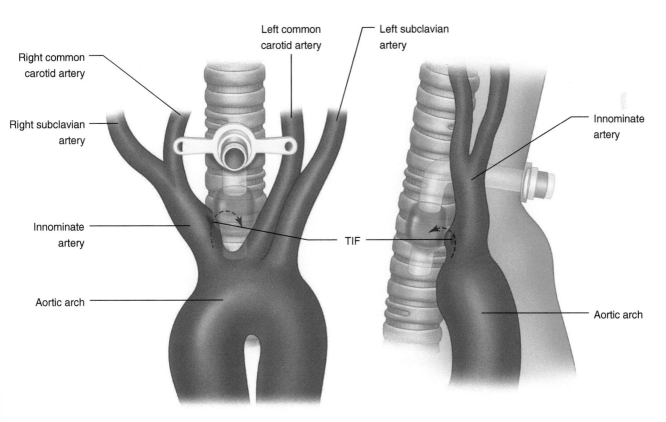

Fig. 20.5 Anatomical relationship between the trachea and the innominate artery. *TIF* trachea–innominate artery fistula

Selected Reading

De Leyn P, Bedert L, Delcroix M, et al. Tracheotomy: clinical review and guidelines. Eur J Cardiothorac Surg. 2007;32:412–21.

Dobiesx VA, Miller SA, Pitzele MJ. Complications of tracheostomies. In: Wolfson AB, Hendey GW, Ling LJ, Rosen CL, Scheider JJ, Sharieff GQ, editors. Harwood-Nuss' clinical practice of emergency medicine. 5th ed. Philadelphia: Lippincott Williams & Wilkins; 2009.

Epstein SK. Late complications of tracheostomy. Respir Care. 2005;40:542–9.

Friedman M, Ibrahim H. The dislodged tracheostomy tube: "fingertip" technique. Oper Technol Otolaryngol. 2002;13:217–8.

Young JS, Brady WJ, Kesser B, Mullins D. A novel method for replacement of the dislodged tracheostomy tube: the nasogastric tube "guidewire" technique. J Emerg Med. 1996;14:205–8.

Percutaneous Transtracheal Jet Ventilation

21

Clint Masterson

21.1 Indications

- Failure to control the airway by other means
- As a temporary measure while preparing for definitive airway control
- Securing the airway in crash airways in infants and small children

21.2 Contraindications

- Absolute
  - Transection of the trachea below the cricothyroid membrane
- Relative
  - Inability to identify the cricothyroid landmarks
  - Anatomical distortion to the cricothyroid membrane
  - Supraglottic obstruction (preventing gas exhalation)

21.3 Materials and Medications (Fig. 21.1)

- Betadine, chlorhexidine, or similar skin sterilization solution
- 12- to 16-gauge angiocatheter or transtracheal jet ventilation (TTJV) purpose-specific catheter
- 10-mL syringe filled with 4 mL of normal saline, 2 % lidocaine, or viscous lidocaine
- Hand-operated regulator valve
- Attach oxygen supply.
  - Connect kit tubing to wall oxygen OR.
  - Connect 7–0 endotracheal connector to bag valve mask (BVM) attached to oxygen.

C. Masterson, MD
Department of Emergency Medicine, Mayo Clinic Health System in Fairmont, Fairmont, MN, USA
e-mail: clint@clintm.us

© Springer Science+Business Media New York 2016
L. Ganti (ed.), *Atlas of Emergency Medicine Procedures*, DOI 10.1007/978-1-4939-2507-0_21

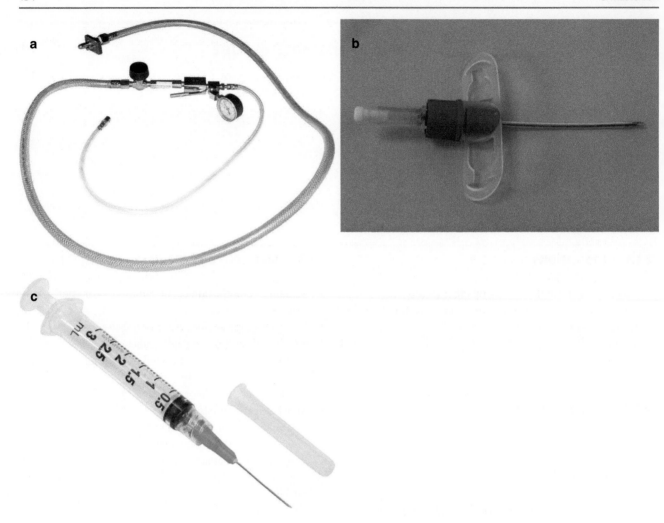

Fig. 21.1 (**a**) Tubing and regulator valve, (**b**) commercially available catheter, (**c**) 3-mL or 10-mL syringe

21.4   Procedure

1. Attach the tubing and the hand-operated regulator valve to wall oxygen (Fig. 21.2a), and place the distal end of the tubing near the patient in preparation for ventilation.
2. Adjust regulator to maximum pressure, 50 psi if possible (Fig. 21.2b).
3. Palpate the cricothyroid membrane just distal to the thyroid prominence (Fig. 21.3).
   (a) Sterilize the area with a suitable cleansing agent.
   (b) Use the thumb and index finger of the nondominant hand to stabilize the trachea for the procedure.
4. Attach the TTJV catheter (or angiocatheter) to the syringe (Fig. 21.4).
5. Advance the catheter through the cricothyroid membrane at a 30–45° caudal direction while aspirating with the syringe (Fig. 21.5).

6. Return of air confirms entry into the trachea.
7. If lidocaine is utilized, it can then be injected to prevent spasm during the procedure.
8. Fully advance the angiocatheter and secure it while the needle and syringe are withdrawn.
9. Remove the needle, secure it to the skin, and connect it to the regulator hose.
10. Secure the distal end of the oxygen tubing (distal to the hand-operated valve) to the catheter (Fig. 21.6).
11. If a BVM is used as the oxygen source:
    (a) Attach a 3-mL syringe to the angiocatheter.
    (b) Attach the BVM with the 7–0 endotracheal tube (ETT) connector to the end of the plungerless 3-mL syringe (Fig. 21.7).
12. Operate the valve 12–20 times a minute with long periods to allow gas exhalation and exchange (Fig. 21.8).
13. Preparations should be made for a definitive airway as soon as possible—preferably within 15 min.

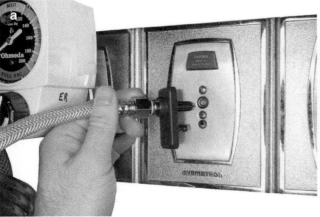
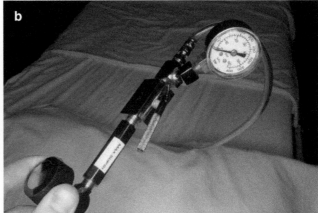

Fig. 21.2 (a) Attach tubing and the hand-operated regulator valve to wall oxygen, and (b) adjust regulator to maximum pressure (50 psi if possible)

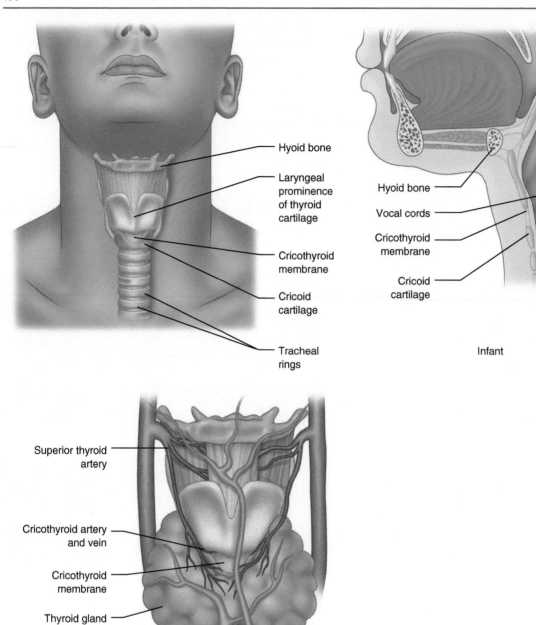

Fig. 21.3 Airway anatomy

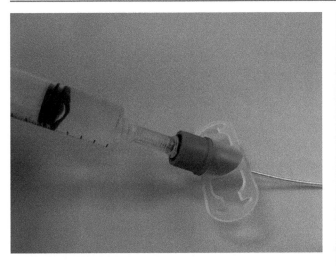

Fig. 21.4 Attach the TTJV catheter to the syringe

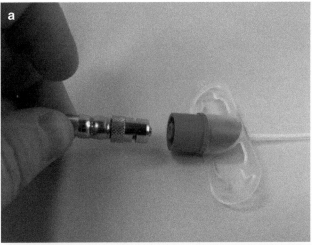

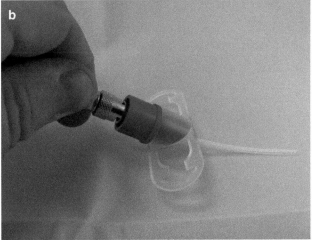

Fig. 21.6 Secure the distal end of the oxygen tubing to the catheter

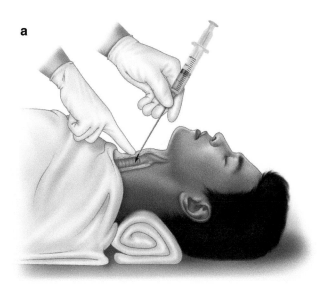

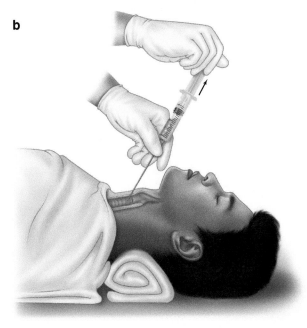

Fig. 21.5 (**a**) Advance the catheter through the cricothyroid membrane at a 30–45° caudal direction (**b**) while aspirating with the syringe

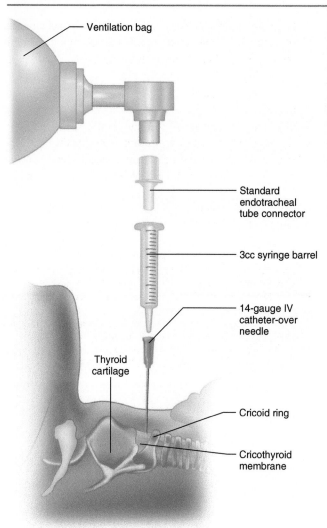

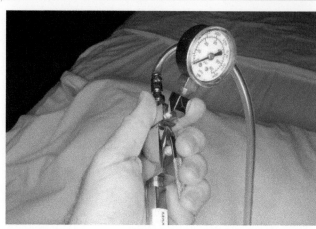

Fig. 21.8 Operate the valve 12–20 times a minute with long periods to allow gas exhalation and exchange

Fig. 21.7 Attach the BVM with the 7–0 endotracheal tube (ETT) connector to the end of the plungerless 3-mL syringe

21.5 Complications

- Pneumothorax
- Pneumomediastinum
- Subcutaneous emphysema
- Catheter kink or misplacement
- Hypercarbia and respiratory acidosis
    - Use of TTJV for prolonged periods of time without adequate ventilation will elevate CO_2.
- Barotrauma
- Coughing in conscious patients
- Aspiration
- Persistent stoma

21.6 Pearls and Pitfalls

- If the wall connector does not have a pressure regulator, it can still be used although the risk of barotrauma is greater. Use the endpoint of chest rise to determine the end of each ventilation burst in this case.

- Higher pressures and lack of supraglottic air exchange are risk factors for pneumothorax. If the supraglottic area is obstructed, a Y catheter can be attached to allow gas to escape before the next insufflation.
- TTJV may or may not allow sufficient gas exchange to prevent hypercarbia. Preparations should be made to obtain a definitive airway as soon as possible.
- Endotracheal intubation may be facilitated by the high pressures insufflated in the trachea, and a repeat attempt may be performed after the transtracheal ventilation is achieved.

Selected Reading

Patel R. Percutaneous transtracheal jet ventilation. A safe, quick and temporary way to provide oxygenation and ventilation when conventional methods are unsuccessful. Chest. 1999;116:1689–94.

Roberts JR, Hedges JR. Clinical procedures in emergency medicine. Philadelphia: Saunders Elsevier; 2010.

Tintinalli J. Tintinalli's emergency medicine: a comprehensive study guide. 7th ed. New York: McGraw Hill; 2010.

Walls R. Manual of emergency airway management. 3rd ed. Philadelphia: Lippincott Williams & Wilkins; 2008.

Part III

Thoracic Procedures

Needle Thoracostomy

22

Lucas McArthur and Christian Fromm

22.1 Indications

Needle decompression thoracostomy is a procedure used in the emergent treatment of a tension pneumothorax. Tension pneumothorax is a clinical diagnosis. Decompression treatment should not be delayed in order to obtain radiographic confirmation. The following scenarios illustrate some of the clinical signs that *may* be present in such patients:

- *Awake patient* with suspected or confirmed tension pneumothorax
  - Chest pain
  - Respiratory distress
  - Decreased breath sounds with hyperresonance and/or subcutaneous emphysema
  - Trachea deviated away from the side of the pneumothorax
  - Tachycardia
  - Falling pulse oximetry (SpO_2)
  - Shock
- *Ventilated patient* with suspected or confirmed pneumothorax (often insidious)
  - Increased resistance to ventilation
  - Hypotension
  - Elevated central venous pressure
  - Tachycardia

  - Decreased breath sounds with hyperresonance and/or subcutaneous emphysema
  - Trachea deviated away from the side of the pneumothorax
  - Falling SpO_2
  - Shock
- *Injured patient* (especially with penetrating chest trauma) with suspected or confirmed tension pneumothorax
  - In arrest
  - Unexplained hypotension
  - Apnea
  - Decreased breath sounds with hyperresonance and/or subcutaneous emphysema

22.1.1 Absolute Indications

- Patient in acute respiratory distress with rapid decompensation secondary to suspected or confirmed tension pneumothorax
- Injured patient in extremis with apnea, unexplained hypotension, or arrest

22.2 Contraindications

- No absolute contraindications.

22.3 Materials

- Large-bore needle/angiocatheter (minimum of 16 gauge)
- 10-mL syringe (optional)
- One-way valve (optional)
- Betadine (povidone-iodine) swab/chlorhexidine scrub
- Tape

L. McArthur, MD (✉)
Department of Emergency Medicine, Maimonides Medical Center, New York, NY, USA
e-mail: LMcarthur@jfkhealth.org

C. Fromm, MD
Department of Emergency Medicine, Maimonides Medical Center, SUNY Downstate College of Medicine, New York, NY, USA
e-mail: cfromm@maimonidesmed.org

© Springer Science+Business Media New York 2016
L. Ganti (ed.), *Atlas of Emergency Medicine Procedures*, DOI 10.1007/978-1-4939-2507-0_22

22.4 Procedure

1. Expose the anterior chest at the level of the second intercostal space on the affected side (Fig. 22.1). Alternatively, expose the chest wall at the level of the anterior axillary line in the fourth or fifth intercostal space on the affected side.
2. Cleanse the area with a Betadine swab or chlorhexidine scrub (Fig. 22.2).
3. Using a gloved hand, locate the second intercostal space at the midclavicular line.
   (a) The first rib is normally not felt.
   (b) The second rib is felt just below the clavicle.
   (c) The second intercostal space is the area between the second and the third ribs.
   Note: Alternatively, this procedure may also be performed on the midaxillary line in the fourth intercostal space of the affected side. The same general steps listed later are employed in this approach and care is taken to avoid the neurovascular bundles inferior to the fourth rib.
4. Insert the needle/angiocatheter perpendicular to the chest wall into the second intercostal space just above the superior edge of the third rib to avoid the intercostal neurovascular bundle (Fig. 22.3).
   (a) This step may be done with or without a syringe attached.
   (b) Local anesthesia is usually unnecessary but may be used if the patient is not in extremis.
5. Carefully walk the needle over the third rib and advance until the pleural space is entered.
   (a) Entry into the pleural space is accompanied by a "popping" sound or a sensation of "giving way."
6. If you are able to withdraw air with the syringe or hear a "hiss" of air escaping through the angiocatheter during expiration and inspiration, then placement is considered successful.
7. After removing the needle, secure the angiocatheter in place with tape (Fig. 22.4).
   Caution: Do not reinsert needle into the angiocatheter owing to the danger of sheering the angiocatheter.
8. Assess the patient and evaluate the effectiveness of the procedure.
   (a) The patient should exhibit immediate and obvious improvement in respiratory status including improved lung sounds and vital signs.
   (b) The procedure may be repeated if the patient is not improving.
   (c) Excess pleural air may be aspirated through the angiocatheter with a syringe.
9. Obtain a chest radiograph to confirm success.
   (a) Repeat in 6 h.
10. Because needle decompression is only a temporizing measure, tube thoracostomy (see Chap. 23) must be performed for definitive management of the pneumothorax.

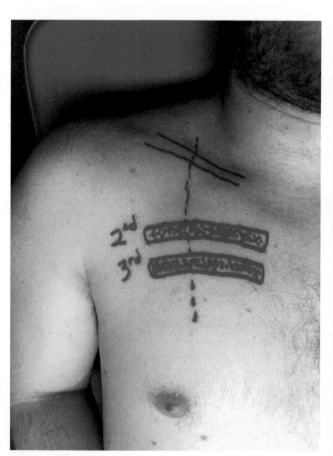

Fig. 22.1 The preferred site for needle thoracostomy is the second intercostal space in the midclavicular line

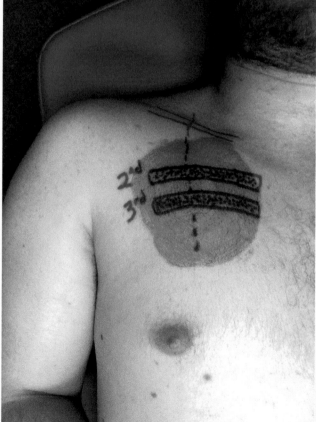

Fig. 22.2 Prepare the skin with povidone-iodine or chlorhexidine

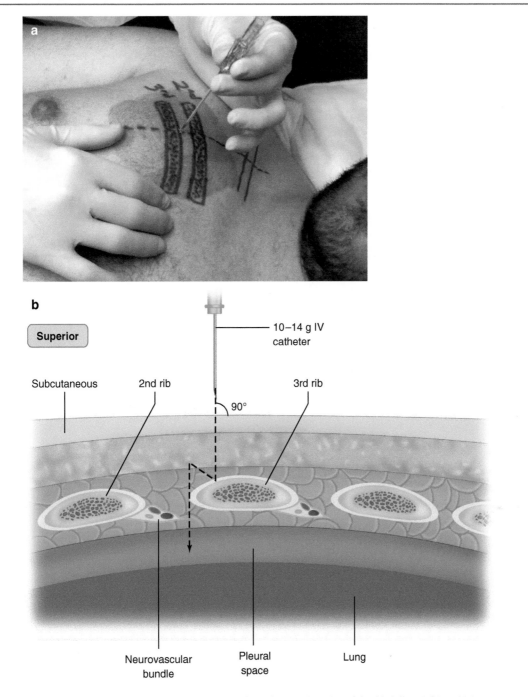

Fig. 22.3 (a) Insert the needle into the second intercostal space just above the superior edge of the third rib and (b) avoid the neurovascular bundle by approaching the skin with the needle perpendicular to the chest wall just above the superior edge of the third rib

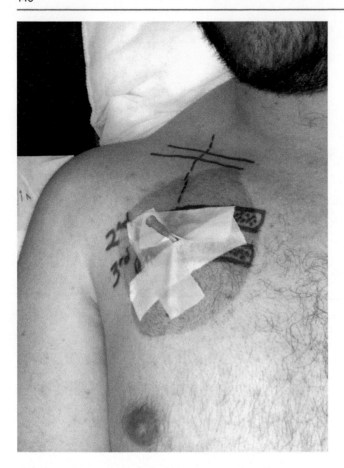

Fig. 22.4 After removing the needle, secure the angiocatheter in place with tape

22.5   Complications

- Failure to resolve the tension pneumothorax.
  - Obese or muscular patients may require a longer needle and catheter to reach the pleural space or, alternatively, may require proceeding immediately to tube thoracostomy.
- Iatrogenic pneumothorax.
- Laceration of intercostal artery or nerve.
- Rapid re-expansion may result in the development of pulmonary edema.
- Infection.

22.6   Pearls and Pitfalls

- Use the sternum as a landmark to more easily locate the second and third ribs.
- The same procedure may also be done on the midaxillary line in the fourth intercostal space, which is usually landmarked with the nipple.

- Primary pneumothorax is unusual in those older than 40 years. Consider the presence of underlying disease in this population.

Acknowledgments We would like to thank Antonios Likourezos, MA, MPH, and Abraham Lederman for assisting with the photographs.

Selected Reading

Britten S, Palmer SH. Chest wall thickness may limit adequate drainage of tension pneumothorax by needle thoracocentesis. Emerg Med J. 1996;13:426–7.

Custalow CB. Color atlas of emergency department procedures. Philadelphia: Saunders; 2005.

Leigh-Smith S, Harris T. Tension pneumothorax—time for a re-think? Emerg Med J. 2005;22:8–16.

Roberts JR, Hedges JR. Clinical procedures in emergency medicine. 3rd ed. Philadelphia: Saunders; 1998.

Chest Tube Thoracostomy

23

Brandon R. Allen and Latha Ganti

23.1 Indications

- Spontaneous pneumothorax (large and/or symptomatic)
- Tension pneumothorax (or suspected)
- Iatrogenic pneumothorax
- Penetrating chest injuries
- Hemopneumothorax in acute trauma
- Patient in extremis with evidence of thoracic trauma
- Complicated parapneumonic effusions (empyema)
- Chylothorax/hemothorax
- Post-thoracic surgery
- Bronchopleural fistula

23.2 Contraindications

- Absolute
  - Emergent thoracotomy
- Relative
  - Coagulopathy
  - Pulmonary bullae
  - Pulmonary, pleural, or thoracic adhesions
  - Loculated pleural effusion or empyema
  - Skin infection over the chest tube insertion site

23.3 Materials and Medications

- Tube thoracostomy tray
  - #10 scalpel; 18-, 22-, and 25-gauge needles; 10-mL syringes; forceps; clamps; scissors; drape; abdominal pads; 0 or 1–0 silk suture; needle driver; curved clamp (Fig. 23.1a)
- Betadine (povidone-iodine) or other skin antiseptic preparation solution
- Lidocaine (1 % or 2 % with epinephrine)
- Appropriate chest tube size (approximate)
  - Adult male: 28–36 French
  - Adult female: 28 French
  - Child: 12–24 French
  - Infant: 12–16 French
  - Neonate: 10–12 French

Vaseline gauze
Chest drainage system (Fig. 23.1b)

B.R. Allen, MD
Department of Emergency Medicine, University of Florida Health Shands Hospital, Gainesville, FL, USA
e-mail: brandonrallen@ufl.edu

L. Ganti, MD, MS, MBA (✉)
Professor of Emergency Medicine, University of Central Florida, Orlando, FL, USA

Director, SE Specialty Care Centers of Innovation, Orlando Veterans Affairs Medical Center, Orlando, FL, USA
e-mail: lathagantimd@gmail.com

© Springer Science+Business Media New York 2016
L. Ganti (ed.), *Atlas of Emergency Medicine Procedures*, DOI 10.1007/978-1-4939-2507-0_23

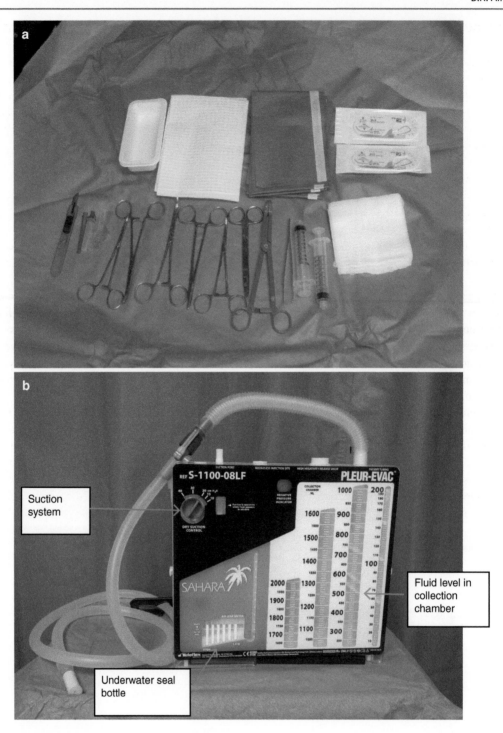

Fig. 23.1 (**a**) Tube thoracostomy tray, (**b**) chest drainage system

23.4 **Procedure** (Fig. 23.2)

1. Sterile skin preparation with sterile drape.
2. Anesthetize the appropriate area subcutaneously up to and including the rib periosteum with 5 mL of 1 % lidocaine with epinephrine (Fig. 23.2a).
3. Using a #10 or #11 blade, make an approximately 4-cm skin incision over the desired intercostal level of entry (most often the fourth or fifth intercostal space in the midaxillary line) (Fig. 23.2b, c).

   If the incision is placed *below* the fifth intercostal space, the risk of subdiaphragmatic placement into the abdominal space is increased.
4. Bluntly dissect with a hemostat or Kelly clamp through the subcutaneous tissue to the level of the intercostal muscles with intermittent opening of the dissection instrument during advancement (Fig. 23.2d, e).
5. Digitally palpate the selected intercostal space and the superior margin of the inferior rib (pay careful attention to avoid the neurovascular bundle lying inferiorly) (Fig. 23.2f).
   - If time permits, additional analgesia is recommended at this point of the procedure.
6. Guiding the closed Kelly clamp over the upper margin of the rib, enter the chest wall into the pleural cavity. (This will require some controlled force and a twisting motion.) Once the pleural space is entered, a rush of air or fluid should occur (Fig. 23.2g).

   Uncontrolled force and a lunging motion can result in penetration to the lung, heart, liver, or spleen.
7. Open the Kelly clamp while still inside the pleural space and then withdraw while the clamp is still open to enlarge the dissected tract of entry and allow easier passage of the thoracostomy tube (TT).
8. Explore the dissected tract with a sterile finger to appreciate lung tissue and possible adhesions.
9. To estimate the length the TT is to be inserted, measure the distance between the skin incision and the apex of the lung. If preferred, place a clamp over the tube at the estimated length (Fig. 23.2h).
10. Grasp the proximal end of the TT with the large Kelly clamp and pass the tube through the thoracic cavity along the previously dissected tract.
11. Release the Kelly clamp and continue to advance the tube posteriorly and superiorly.

    Make sure all of the fenestrated holes of the TT are within the thoracic cavity to prevent unnecessary manipulation and/or replacement of the TT.
12. Once the TT is in the desired position, connect the tube to the drainage device (Fig. 42.1b). Once connected, release the cross clamp on the distal end of the TT.
13. Secure the TT to the skin with 0 or 1–0 silk or nylon suture. A simple, interrupted suture above and below the TT with each stitch wrapped tightly around the TT is recommended.

    Incomplete security of the TT leads to dislodging of the tube with routine patient movements.
14. Apply petrolatum gauze over the skin closure surrounding the TT and then apply a support dressing with 4 × 4 gauze and adhesive tape (4 in.).
15. Obtain a chest radiograph to confirm placement of the TT.

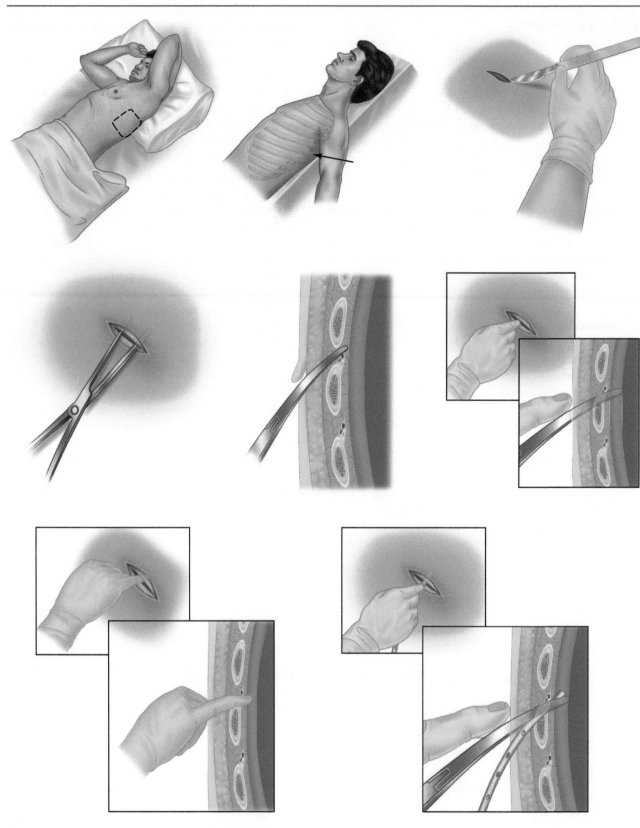

Fig. 23.2 Chest tube thoracostomy procedure

23.5 Complications

- Improper placement for pneumothorax
  - Reposition if:
    - Horizontal (over diaphragm)
    - Subcutaneous
    - Placed too far into the chest (against apical pleura)
  - Remove if:
    - Placed into the abdominal space
- Bleeding (local vs. hemothorax)
- Hemoperitoneum (liver or spleen injury)
- Tube dislodgment
- Empyema (TT introduces bacteria into the pleural space)
- Retained pneumothorax (may require second TT)
- Re-expansion pulmonary edema
- Subcutaneous emphysema

23.6 Pearls and Pitfalls

- Water seal acts as a one-way valve; if the system bubbles, there is an air leak.
- In the Pleur-evac® systems, there is an orange floater which, when static, means the desired suction pressure (usually 20 cmH$_2$O) has been reached.
- The negative pressure in the chest cavity equals the amount of water in water seal plus amount of suction.
- A chest tube can be removed when there is no air loss or blood for 24 h.
- When removing the tube, have the patient exhale and remove as quickly as possible.
- Leave petrolatum gauze in place for 48 h before changing it (allows wound to heal better).

Selected Reading

Ball CG, Lord J, Laupland KB, et al. Chest tube complications: how well are we training our residents? Can J Surg. 2007;50:450.

Collop NA, Kim S, Sahn SA. Analysis of tube thoracostomy performed by pulmonologists at a teaching hospital. Chest. 1997;112:709.

Dalbec DL, Krome RL. Thoracostomy. Emerg Med Clin North Am. 1986;4:441.

Miller KS, Sahn SA. Chest tubes. Indications, technique, management and complications. Chest. 1987;91:258–64.

Millikan JS, Moore EE, Steiner E, et al. Complications of tube thoracostomy for acute trauma. Am J Surg. 1980;140:738.

Thoracentesis

Lee Richard Donner and Michael Anana

24.1 Indications

- *Therapeutic thoracentesis* is performed to relieve dyspnea, hypoxia, or otherwise compromised respiratory function due to a large pleural effusion.
- *Diagnostic thoracentesis* is performed to aid in the diagnosis and workup of:
  - Pleural effusions of unknown cause
  - Unilateral pleural effusions
  - Pleural effusions originally determined to be due to heart failure but persisting after 3 days of diuresis

24.2 Contraindications

- Absolute
  - None
- Relative:
  - Coagulopathy, thrombocytopenia.
  - Small or loculated pleural effusion. These will increase the risk of missing the effusion and causing lung injury.
  - Positive-pressure ventilation.
  - Skin infection over the needle insertion site.

24.3 Materials and Medications

- Thoracentesis tray (commercially available kits generally include the items in the following list) (Fig. 24.1)
  - (1) Fenestrated drape
  - (1) 25-gauge × 1-in. needle
  - (1) 21-gauge × 1.5-in. needle
  - (1) 8-French catheter over 18-gauge needle
  - (1) Small plastic syringe, 5 mL
  - (1) Small plastic syringe, 10 mL
  - (1) Large plastic syringe, 50–60 mL
  - (1) Three-way stopcock
  - Specimen vials and caps
  - (1) Collection bag, 1500 mL, or vacuum container
  - (1) Tubing set
  - (1) Hemostat
  - Betadine (povidone-iodine) or other skin antiseptic preparing solution
  - 10-mL lidocaine 1 % without epinephrine

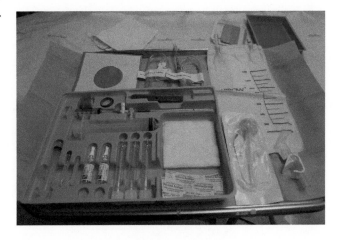

Fig. 24.1 Typical commercial thoracentesis tray

L.R. Donner, MD (✉)
Emergency Medicine Department, Lincoln Medical and Mental Health Center, New York, NY, USA
e-mail: LeeDonnerMD@gmail.com

M. Anana, MD
Emergency Department, University Hospital, Rutgers New Jersey Medical School, Newark, NJ, USA
e-mail: ananami@njms.rutgers.edu

© Springer Science+Business Media New York 2016
L. Ganti (ed.), *Atlas of Emergency Medicine Procedures*, DOI 10.1007/978-1-4939-2507-0_24

24.4 Procedure

1. Place patient in seated position with arms at rest on a bedside table (Fig. 24.2).
2. The location and height of the pleural effusion are confirmed by physical examination. Auscultation of decreased or absent breath sounds, dullness to percussion, and decreased tactile fremitus are physical findings to confirm the location and height of the effusion (Fig. 24.3).
3. Determine and mark the site of needle insertion. This will be at the midscapular line one or two intercostal spaces below the maximum height of the effusion as determined by a combination of imaging and physical examination (Fig. 24.4).
   - *Do not* attempt thoracentesis inferior to the eighth intercostal space because respiratory cycle and anatomical variation place the diaphragm and intraabdominal organs at risk.
4. Prepare the skin with the sterile skin preparation and sterile drape.
5. Anesthetize the appropriate area subcutaneously using a 25-gauge needle on a 10-mL syringe. Create a wheal in the skin and then infiltrate up to and including the periosteum of the rib inferior to the landmarked space with 5 mL of 1 % lidocaine.
   - Remember that the neurovascular bundle is found at the inferior border of each rib. Keep this in mind as you approach the rib and throughout the rest of the procedure to avoid injury to these structures (Fig. 24.5).
6. Using a 22-gauge needle, slowly walk the needle up and over the superior border of the rib. Continue to advance the needle along the superior border of the rib with the syringe withdrawn and infiltrating lidocaine intermittently along the way.
7. Pleural fluid will be aspirated once the pleural space is reached. Do not advance the needle further. Deposit 1–2 mL more lidocaine. A hemostat can be placed on the needle at the level of the skin to mark the depth of the pleural space and the needle can be removed.

8. Some commercial kits may come with an adjustable depth guard to be positioned at the determined depth. On an 18-gauge catheter-over-needle device, position the depth guard to the appropriate depth determined from the prior step. If a depth guard is not available, use the index finger and thumb on the catheter at the appropriate depth. With the 5-mL syringe attached, advance the device over the superior border of the rib while aspirating, expecting pleural fluid to return again at the determined depth (Fig. 24.6).
9. When the pleural space is reached, do not advance the needle further. Advance the catheter over the needle until the hub reaches the skin. Remove the needle during expiration and immediately cover the open hub with a gloved finger to prevent development of pneumothorax. Some kits provide catheters with one-way valves to prevent air entry.
10. Attach the 50–60-mL syringe to the catheter via the three-way stopcock. Pleural fluid can be drained and transferred to appropriate collection vials for diagnostic thoracentesis. A collection bag may be attached with tubing to the third port of a three-way stopcock for larger volume evacuation in the case of a therapeutic thoracentesis. Employ a syringe pump method to drain 50–60 mL of fluid at a time to the collection bag. Fill the syringe by withdrawing the plunger while the stopcock is closed to the bag. Then, close the stopcock to the patient and pump the contents of the syringe to the bag. Next, close the syringe closed to the bag, and repeat the cycle until the desired volume is drained. A vacuum container is an alternative that simply attaches via tubing to the stopcock (Fig. 24.7).
    - If using a three-way stopcock and a device that does not have a one-way valve on the catheter, be sure to always keep the stopcock closed to the patient unless withdrawing fluid in order to decrease the risk of pneumothorax.
11. When the desired amount of pleural fluid is obtained, remove the catheter during expiration and apply an occlusive dressing.

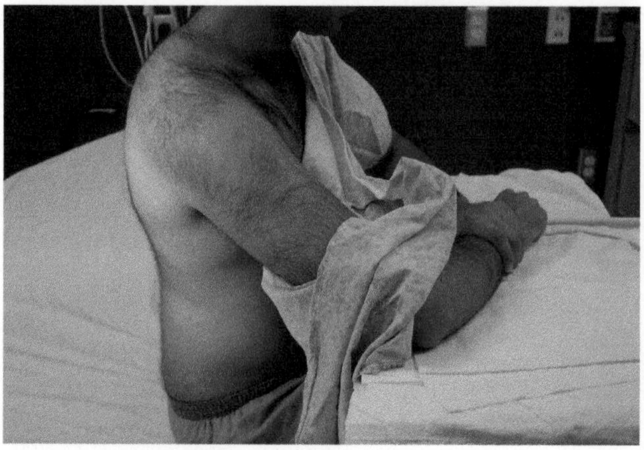

Fig. 24.2 Patient in upright, seated position

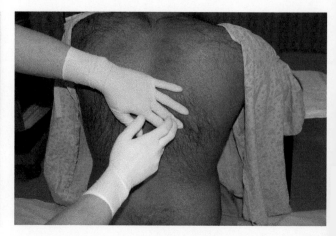

Fig. 24.3 Determining the location and height of the pleural effusion

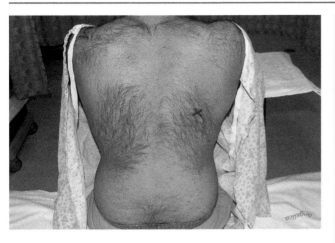

Fig. 24.4 Marked site for needle insertion

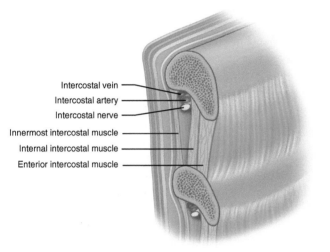

Fig. 24.5 The intercostal neurovascular bundle

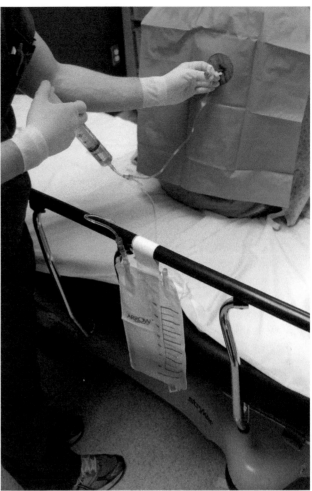

Fig. 24.7 Pleural fluid collection via syringe pump method

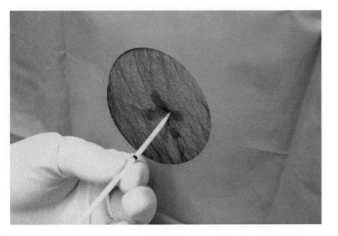

Fig. 24.6 Needle and catheter insertion, thumb and index finger at desired depth

24.5 Complications

- Pneumothorax
- Re-expansion pulmonary edema
- Hemothorax, hematoma
- Intra-abdominal organ injury
- Air embolism
- Empyema

24.6 Considerations

- If available, the use of bedside ultrasound is highly recommended because ultrasound guidance has been shown to substantially reduce the risk of pneumothorax. Before the procedure, the height, width, and depth of the effusion can be appreciated by scanning the chest and viewing the effusion through the intercostal spaces. The use of ultrasound aids in selecting the needle insertion site by:
  - Visualizing the distance the needle must pass to reach the parietal pleura
  - Confirming the thickness of the effusion in the site selected is at least a minimum of 1.5 cm
  - Providing the clinician with a view of the effusion and surrounding structures through the complete respiratory cycle

  With these items in mind, the needle insertion site can be selected with confidence and marked before beginning the procedure.
- In addition, the use of bedside ultrasound in real time will allow the clinician to visualize the needle as it passes toward and enters the pleural space. This use requires sterile probe covers.
- Re-expansion pulmonary edema is a rare but feared complication of thoracentesis. The cause is not fully understood. Historically it was thought that re-expansion pulmonary edema was caused by removing too large a volume of fluid from the pleural space (>1–1.5 L). Another theory is that re-expansion pulmonary edema is caused when great negative intrapleural pressures (<20 cmH$_2$O) are generated during the procedure. The low incidence of this complication has yielded inconclusive evidence.
  - In light of this, it is prudent to continue to limit the volume of pleural fluid removed to no more than 1–1.5 L. Pleural manometry is not widely available for use in the emergency department, but should also be

considered if available to maintain intrapleural pressures from reaching more negative values.

24.7 Pearls and Pitfalls

- Bedside ultrasound reduces the risk of complications.
- Never attempt thoracentesis below the eighth intercostal space.
- Thoracentesis should not be performed on pleural effusions demonstrated to be less than 1–1.5 cm thick by ultrasound or on a lateral decubitus film.
- Positive-pressure ventilation mandates extreme care while performing thoracentesis because the lungs can be punctured during inflation. In addition, ventilated patients will not be able to sit upright and will need to have the procedure performed in lateral decubitus position with the effusion side down and the posterior axillary line as the needle insertion site. Alternatively, the patient can be placed supine with the head of the bed elevated to 45° and the midaxillary line as the needle insertion site.
  - Routine post-procedure radiographs are not necessary to exclude pneumothorax. Indications for post-procedure imaging include onset of chest pain during the procedure, persisting cough or chest discomfort after the procedure, air aspiration along any step of the procedure, or positive-pressure ventilation.
  - Pneumothorax rates are higher for inexperienced providers. Although an effusion compromising respiratory function is considered a clear indication for therapeutic thoracentesis, the performance of nonurgent diagnostic thoracentesis might best be delayed for those more practiced in the procedure.

Selected Reading

Dewitz A, Jones R, Goldstein J. Additional ultrasound-guided procedures. In: Ma OJ, Mateer JR, Blavias M, editors. Emergency ultrasound. 2nd ed. New York: McGraw-Hill; 2008. p. 546–50.

Feller-Kopman D, Berkowitz D, Boiselle P, Ernst A. Large-volume thoracentesis and the risk of reexpansion pulmonary edema. Ann Thorac Surg. 2007;84:1656–61.

Gordon CE, Feller-Kopman D, Balk EM, Smetana GW. Pneumothorax following thoracentesis: a systematic review and meta-analysis. Arch Intern Med. 2010;170:332–9.

Light RW. Pleural effusion. N Engl J Med. 2002;346:1971–7.

Thomsen TW, DeLaPena J, Setnik G. Videos in clinical medicine. Thoracentesis. N Engl J Med. 2006;355, e16.

Open Chest Wounds and Flail Chest

25

Jacob J. Glaser and Carlos J. Rodriguez

25.1 Background

Thoracic injuries are commonly associated with penetrating and blunt abdominal trauma and are implicated in 50–70 % of trauma deaths [1]. Cardiac tamponade, tension pneumothorax, massive hemothorax, airway obstruction, flail chest, and open pneumothorax represent the six immediately life-threatening injuries attributed to chest trauma [2]. Accordingly, they must be accurately identified and dealt with urgently.

Open pneumothorax ("sucking" chest wound) is seen in penetrating chest injuries. If the associated chest wound is greater than 2/3 the diameter of the trachea (generally anything greater than 1.5–2 cm), air can preferentially enter the intrapleural space, via the trachea, with each inspiration [3]

(Fig. 25.1). This allows equilibration of pressure between the pleural space and the atmosphere, causing the lung to collapse and leading to profound hypoventilation and hypoxia.

Flail chest results from high-energy blunt, crushing chest trauma causing two or more fractures in two or more contiguous ribs. Classically, the fractures are lateral or sternal. Posterior rib fractures rarely cause flail physiology (Fig. 25.2). Flail chest has been reported to have mortality as high as 16 % [4]. This injury pattern is associated with a high incidence of underlying pneumothorax, hemothorax, pulmonary contusion, and chest wall instability. Mortality from flail chest is thought to be correlated with the degree of underlying pulmonary contusion and attendant hypoxia [2].

Both open pneumothorax and flail chest are immediately life threatening and require early appropriate management.

J.J. Glaser, MD (✉)
Combat Casualty Care Directorate, Naval Medical Research Unit,
San Antonio, TX, USA
e-mail: Jacob.glaser1@gmail.com

C.J. Rodriguez, DO
Division of Trauma Surgery, Surgical Critical Care, Walter Reed
National Military Medical Center, Bethesda, MD, USA
e-mail: Carlos.J.Rodriguez.mil@health.mil

© Springer Science+Business Media New York 2016
L. Ganti (ed.), *Atlas of Emergency Medicine Procedures*, DOI 10.1007/978-1-4939-2507-0_25

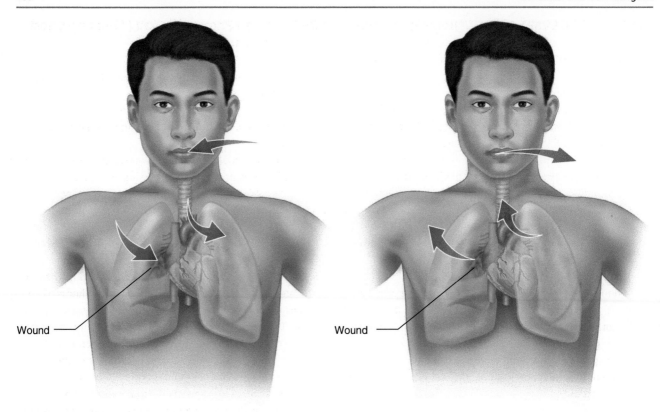

Fig. 25.1 Air preferentially will enter the chest via the wound, collapsing the lung on the affected side

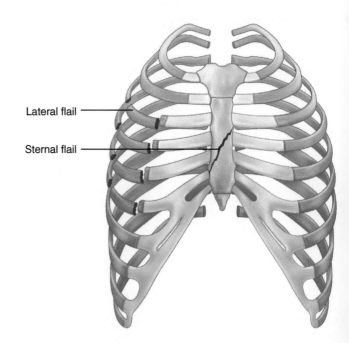

Fig. 25.2 Flail chest: two or more rib fractures in two or more segments. Lateral flail (most common) and sternal flail segments represented below

25.2 Initial Evaluation of Thoracic Trauma

- To the best extent possible, obtain good patient handover from the prehospital caregivers.
- Initial physical evaluation.
  - Appropriate attention should be given to the ABCs (airway, breathing, circulation) of ATLS (Advanced Trauma Life Support) management.
  - Evaluation and resuscitation are to be *concurrent* with diagnostic procedures and immediate interventions.
  - Maintain a high degree of suspicion for open chest wound in impalement injury and destructive penetrating trauma (blast injury or shotgun).
  - Maintain a high degree of suspicion for flail chest in high-energy direct impact trauma (motor vehicle crash, fall, crush injury).
- Administer high-flow O_2 with a non-rebreather mask.
  - If patient is in respiratory distress, is unstable, or has an obvious chest wall defect, consider early intubation to secure the airway.
  - Inspect the chest wall for occlusive dressings.
- Decompress the chest if tension physiology is present or suspected.
  - Immediate decompression of a suspected tension pneumothorax can be readily accomplished by removing any existing occlusive dressings *or*
  - Place a large-bore cannula over the rib, second intercostal space, or midclavicular line.
- Specific immediate management appropriate to open chest wound and flail chest (see later).
- Monitor continuous pulse oximetry and electrocardiogram.
- Initiate crystalloid resuscitation via large-bore intravenous (IV) access.
  - Early mobilization of blood products if ongoing hemorrhage or expectation of excessive blood loss.
  - Placement of resuscitative lines concurrent with management of respiratory parameters.
- Early surgical consultation for management of intrathoracic injuries and management of chest wall defect.

25.3 Open Pneumothorax ("Sucking Chest Wound")

- Immediate management requires attention to airway and respirations.
  - If in respiratory distress, *intubate*.
- Close the chest wall defect with an occlusive three-sided dressing.
  - This includes a valve mechanism that allows trapped air to escape, preventing tension (Fig. 25.3).
  - An IV bag cut to fit the wound and then taped on three sides can be useful in an emergent situation.
  - Commercial products are available and appropriate for smaller wounds, including the Asherman Chest Seal and HyFin Vent.
- A completely occlusive dressing may quickly convert an open chest wound into a tension pneumothorax [2, 3, 5] and therefore should *never* be done.
  - The patient and dressing must be serially checked to ensure that trapped air is allowed to escape.
  - If there is any doubt, immediately remove the dressing and replace it with an appropriate dressing.
- These maneuvers are a bridge to definitive care.
- When the timing is appropriate (i.e., time and resources are available), perform a formal tube thoracostomy and convert to a completely occlusive dressing over the wound.
  - Avoid placing the tube through the open wound.
- Once tube thoracostomy, placement of occlusive dressing, and the airway are secured, the pathophysiology of the open pneumothorax becomes inconsequential.
- Immediate consultation with surgery for definitive care of associated intrathoracic injuries is required.
  - The patient may need urgent thoracotomy to treat associated injuries.
  - Irrigation and debridement should take place in the operating room.
  - Depending on injury severity, the patient may need chest wall reconstruction.

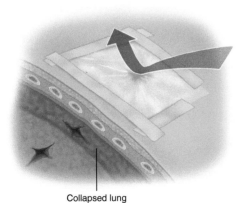
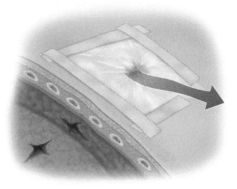

Collapsed lung

Fig. 25.3 Three-sided dressing, allowing a valve to decompress tension in the chest

25.4 Flail Chest

- Diagnosis is made from mechanism and examination, not radiographically.
  - With inspiration, the affected chest will move inward with negative pressure.
  - With expiration, the affected chest will move outward.
  - Patients who are intubated on positive pressure (and not spontaneously breathing) will often not show this paradoxical chest movement.
- Attention *must* be paid to presumed underlying blunt lung injury and contusion.
  - The degree of underlying contusion (not the flail segment itself) is directly related to the degree of hypoxia and associated morbidity and mortality [2, 3].
  - There should be a low threshold for intubation to manage respiratory distress, hypoxemia, or hemodynamic instability.
  - The patient is at high risk for hemothorax and pneumothorax requiring tube thoracostomy.
- Abdominal injuries may be present in up to 15 % of patients [2].
- After initial stabilization, treatment is supportive.
  - Intensive care unit admission for management of underlying pulmonary contusion.
  - Pain control in the form of epidural or regional block for excellent pain control.
  - Close attention to pulmonary toilet and lung re-expansion.
  - Patients require observation and treatment in a monitored setting until ensured that respiratory parameters and oxygenation are improving.
- Surgical stabilization of the chest wall is rarely performed.
  - Early surgical consultation for chest wall fixation in questionable cases is warranted.

References

1. LoCicero J, Mattox KL. Epidemiology of chest trauma. Surg Clin North Am. 1989;69:15–9.
2. Pietzman AB, Schwab CW, Yealy DM, editors. The trauma manual. 2nd ed. Philadelphia: Wolters Kluwer Health; 2000.
3. Weinberg JA, Croce MA. Chapter 33: Chest wall injury. In: Flint L, Meredith JW, Schwab CW, editors. Trauma: contemporary principles and therapy. 1st ed. Philadelphia: Lippincott Williams & Williams; 2007.
4. Clark GC, Schecter WP, Trunkey DD. Variables affecting outcome in blunt chest trauma: flail chest vs. pulmonary contusion. J Trauma. 1988;28:298–304.
5. Borden Institute Walter Reed Army Medical Center. Emergency war surgery. 3rd ed. Washington: Office of the Surgeon General U.S. Army, Borden Institute; 2004.

Emergent Resuscitative Thoracotomy, Open Cardiac Massage, and Aortic Occlusion

Kevin M. Jones and Jay Menaker

26.1 Indications

- Penetrating chest trauma with recent or immanent loss of vital signs
- Consider in blunt trauma with pericardial tamponade or exsanguination where aortic occlusion may provide proximal control

26.2 Contraindications

Absolute
- Prolonged cessation of vital signs
- Injury profile obviously incompatible with life
- Absence of surgical services to whom care can be transferred

Relative
- None

26.3 Materials and Medications (Fig. 26.1)

- Betadine (povidone-iodine) for rapid skin preparation
- #10 Scalpel
- Mayo or long Metzenbaum scissors
- Finochietto retractor (rib spreader)
- Long DeBakey or other tissue forceps (2)
- Satinsky vascular clamp and/or straight vascular clamp
- Long needle holders (2)
- Lebsche knife or sternal osteotome with hammer
- Lap sponges or gauze pads

K.M. Jones, MD (✉)
Trauma and Surgical Critical Care, R Adams Cowley Shock
Trauma Center, University of Maryland Medical Center,
Baltimore, MD, USA
e-mail: KJones12@umm.edu

J. Menaker, MD
Departments of Surgery and Emergency Medicine, R Adams
Cowley Shock Trauma Center, University of Maryland Medical
Center, Baltimore, MD, USA
e-mail: jmenaker@umm.edu

© Springer Science+Business Media New York 2016
L. Ganti (ed.), *Atlas of Emergency Medicine Procedures*, DOI 10.1007/978-1-4939-2507-0_26

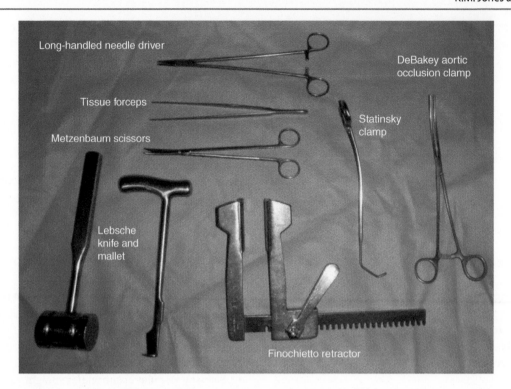

Fig. 26.1 Basic components of an emergency thoracotomy tray: Lebsche knife and mallet for crossing sternum (bone-cutting forceps or sternal osteotome would also suffice), Finochietto retractor, atraumatic vascular clamps (a Satinsky clamp and a DeBakey aortic occlusion clamp), long-handled needle driver, tissue forceps, and Metzenbaum scissors. *Not illustrated* Scalpel with #10 or #20 blade, Mayo scissors

26.4 Procedure

26.4.1 Resuscitative Thoracotomy and Open Cardiac Massage

1. Rapidly prepare the entire anterior and bilateral chest with Betadine.
2. Using a scalpel, incise the skin and subcutaneous tissue from just right of the sternum to the anterior margin of the left latissimus dorsi, following the curvature of the inframammary crease or the fourth or fifth intercostal space (Fig. 26.2).
   - This incision is often made too low on the patient's chest. It should extend across the sternum, not at the level of the xiphoid. Upward retraction of the breast may help provide access to the fourth or fifth intercostal space, where the incision should be located.
3. Bluntly enter the right pleural space through the fourth or fifth intercostal space.
4. Using scissors, cut the intercostal muscles, dividing between the fourth and the fifth ribs from the sternum to the posterior axillary line.
5. If better exposure to the heart is desired, some practitioners advocate extending the incision across the sternum using a Lebsche knife, sternal osteotome, or bone-cutting forceps at this time (Fig. 26.3).
   - If the thoracotomy incision extends to or through the sternum, tie off the internal mammary arteries before closing the chest should the patient be successfully resuscitated, because these will have been divided with the incision.
6. Insert a Finochietto retractor and retract the ribs in order to gain access to the left chest and expose the pericardium (Figs. 26.4 and 26.5).
   - Insert a Finochietto retractor with the rack and pinion bar down and lateral, as in Fig. 26.4, so as not to interfere with extension of the thoracotomy across the sternum into a clamshell maneuver if needed.

7. If massive left pleural hemorrhage is encountered, investigate and control the source at this time.
8. Using tissue forceps, raise a portion of the pericardium anterior to the phrenic nerve, and enter the pericardium using scissors (Fig. 26.6).
9. Widely open the pericardium with scissors, cutting in a cranial-caudal direction anterior to the phrenic nerve and deliver the heart (Fig. 26.7).
10. If hemopericardium is encountered, investigate for and initiate appropriate repair of identified cardiac injuries.
11. Initiate open cardiac massage by cupping the heart between the flattened palmar aspect of the fingers of both hands and rhythmically compressing the heart from apex to base, relaxing completely between compressions to allow filling (Fig. 26.8).

26.4.2 Aortic Occlusion

1. Expose the posterior aspect of the left mediastinum by having an assistant retract the left lung superomedially, dividing the inferior pulmonary ligament if necessary (Fig. 26.9).
2. Bluntly dissect the pleura separating the pleural and mediastinal space just anterior to the vertebral bodies, exposing the aorta (Fig. 26.9).
3. Completely encircle the aorta with the finger of the nondominant hand (Fig. 26.10).
   - Differentiating the aorta from the esophagus when the patient is in a state of profound shock is very difficult. Having an assistant pass an orogastric tube may help distinguish the two. The aorta should be the most posterior structure, lying immediately on the anterior aspect of the vertebral bodies.
4. With the aorta completely encircled, place a vascular clamp across the aorta and verify by sight and feel that the complete vessel is occluded within the clamp (Fig. 26.11).

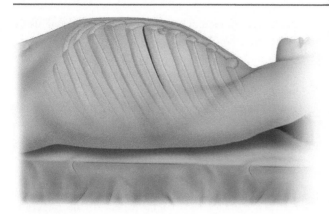

Fig. 26.2 Raise the left arm above the head. Make an incision along the left fourth intercostal space, just below the nipple in a male or at the inframamillary crease in a female

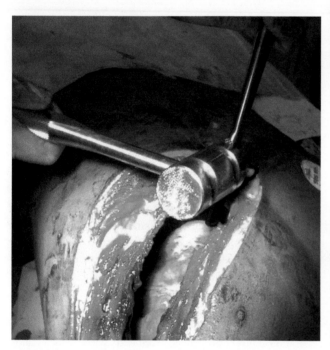

Fig. 26.3 Use a Lebsche knife to extend the incision across the sternum to improve exposure to the heart

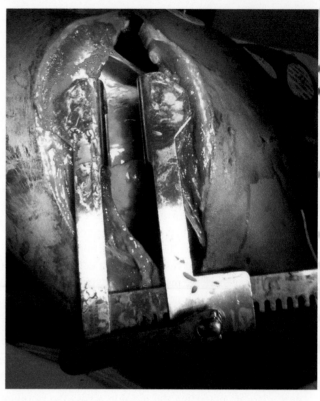

Fig. 26.4 Finochietto retractor placed through the fourth intercostal anterolateral incision. Note the rack and pinion bar placed posterolaterally, where it will not impede access to the midline

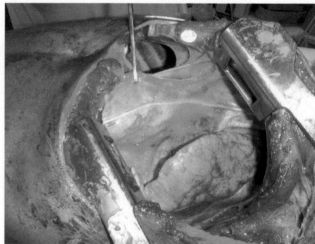

Fig. 26.5 Finochietto retractor extended, exposing the left pleural space and the pericardium. In this case the sternum has been divided as above, and the resultant window into the right pleural space is seen anterior to the pericardium. The lung is deflated in this postmortem picture but would be far more an obstacle in the actively ventilated patient. The clamp seen in the upper portion of the picture is reapproximating the pericardium, which has previously been divided, for the sake of illustration

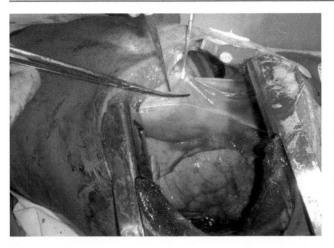

Fig. 26.6 The pericardium is lifted with tissue forceps and opened with a nick using scissors. The phrenic nerve is easily visualized running cranial-caudal just below the scissors in this picture

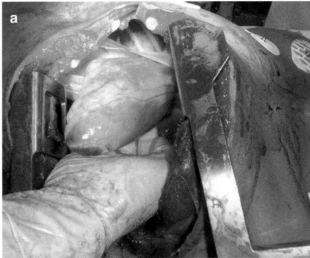

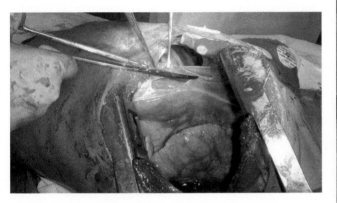

Fig. 26.7 Open the pericardium widely in the cephalad-caudad plane anterior to the phrenic nerve, taking care not to damage the phrenic nerve

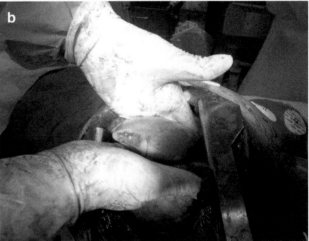

Fig. 26.8 (**a**) Deliver the heart from the pericardium, rapidly assess for cardiac injury requiring damage-control repair; (**b**) initiate open cardiac massage

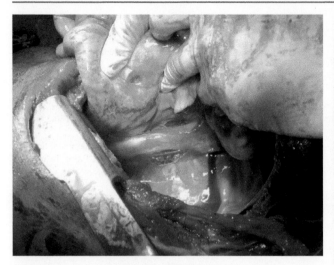

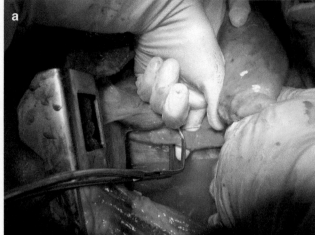

Fig. 26.9 The heart and lung are retracted superomedially, allowing visualization of the left posterior mediastinal pleura; the aorta lies just anterior to the vertebral bodies and has been previously isolated through the pleural interruptions seen here. The heart and lung are assertively retracted here for the benefit of illustration of the posterior mediastinum. Such retraction would completely occlude venous return

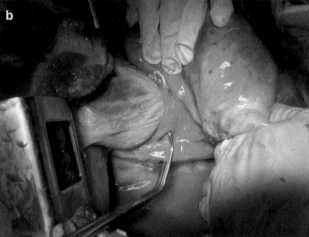

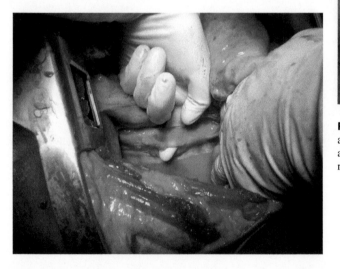

Fig. 26.11 (**a**) A vascular clamp (a Satinsky clamp is used here, although any large atraumatic vascular clamp can be used) is applied across the descending aorta, (**b**) followed by visual and tactile confirmation that the aorta is completely occluded

Fig. 26.10 After bluntly dissecting the mediastinal pleura, the aorta is looped using a finger of the nondominant hand

26.5 Complications

- Injury to care providers, by means of scalpel, needlestick, or sharp foreign body, is the principal concern.
- Post-emergency department thoracotomy infections are rare, even given the less than optimal sterile conditions.
- Damage to lung parenchyma during the initial incision is common and often leads to air leak in survivors.
- Neglect of the mammary arteries, often divided during emergent thoracotomy and not briskly bleeding in the shock state, will result in intrathoracic hemorrhage if not tied off.

Selected Reading

Bartlett RL. Resuscitative thoracotomy. In: Roberts JR, Hedges JR, editors. Clinical procedures in emergency medicine. 3rd ed. Philadelphia: WB Saunders; 1998.

Feliciano DV, Mattox KL. Indications, technique, and pitfalls of emergency center thoracotomy. Surg Rounds. 1981;4:32.

Siemans R, Polk Jr MC. Indications for thoracotomy following penetrating thoracic injury. J Trauma. 1977;17:493.

Wall Jr MJ, Huh J, Mattox KL. Indications and techniques of thoracotomy. In: Feliciano DV, Mattox KL, Moore EE, editors. Trauma. 6th ed. New York: McGraw Hill; 2008.

Lung Ultrasonography

27

Ali H. Dabaja, L. Connor Nickels, and Rohit Pravin Patel

27.1 Indications

Evaluation of respiratory failure and insufficiency due to pneumothorax, pleural effusion, pulmonary edema, acute respiratory distress syndrome (ARDS), and alveolar consolidation (atelectasis, pneumonia, aspiration)
- Monitoring progress of diseases such as pulmonary edema and pneumothorax
- Procedural guidance during pleural fluid removal or pneumothorax treatment
- Procedural guidance for chest tube placement for complex pleural effusions, hemothorax, pneumothorax, and other pleural diseases

27.2 Contraindications

- None

27.3 Materials

- Ultrasound equipment/machine, ultrasonography gel
- Microconvex or phased-array cardiac probe for sufficient evaluation of lung artifact (use abdominal preset). Linear-array probes, or vascular probes, can be used for more detailed evaluation of the pleura, although this is insufficient for penetration to deeper structures.
- Sterile materials and equipment where appropriate

27.4 Preparations

- Clean ultrasound equipment and use sterile operating procedures and ultrasound conductive gel whenever adequate.
- Ultrasound positioning. Place ultrasound device where it is easily accessible and in adequate view.
- Proper environment. Minimize light interference. Close shades and lights where appropriate.
- Position the patient. This helps optimize and expedite the examination. Supine position should be adequate for critically ill patients. Upright positioning is best for all others, with arms abducted above the head or spaced away from the chest to allow space for the probe. Patients should be moved to the edge of the bed. Uncover appropriate areas, including anterior and lateral chest walls.
- Equipment use. Turn on equipment, enter patient data, and select proper probe (cardiac probe or abdominal probe with abdomen presets). Depth and gain should be adjusted accordingly, where depths in the range of 4–10 cm give proper evaluation of more superficial and deeper structures, respectively.

A.H. Dabaja, DO
Division of Critical Care, Department of Anesthesia, University of Florida Health, Gainesville, FL, USA
e-mail: ali.dabaja@gmail.com

L.C. Nickels, MD, RDMS (⊠) • R.P. Patel, MD
Department of Emergency Medicine, University of Florida Health Shands Hospital, Gainesville, FL, USA
e-mail: cnickels@ufl.edu; rohitpatel@ufl.edu

© Springer Science+Business Media New York 2016
L. Ganti (ed.), *Atlas of Emergency Medicine Procedures*, DOI 10.1007/978-1-4939-2507-0_27

27.5 Procedure

1. Probe position (Fig. 27.1). Start examination at the mid-clavicular level at the space between the second and the third ribs. Probe positioning should be perpendicular to the ribs (longitudinal positioning) with the ultrasound marker pointed cephalad. This should place the most superficial structures at the top, with deeper structures at the bottom of the monitor. Upon completion, probe positioning can be mapped to evaluate three or four additional areas, typically between the anterior and the posterior axillary lines. Lateral views with the probe should be most posterior, typically along the posterior axillary line, tracking caudad toward the diaphragm. PLAPS (posterolateral alveolar and/or pleural syndrome) pointed posteriorly should also be evaluated, specifically in supine patients. PLAPS is lateral to the scapula and typically requires that the patient be lifted off the bed from one side.

2. Identify the "bat sign" (Fig. 27.2). The initial view observed should be a window of lung flanked by two rib shadows. This view, termed the "bat sign," should now allow evaluation of the parietal and visceral pleura, seen most superficial as echogenic line (approximately 0.5 cm below start of rib shadows), subsequent lung sliding, and other findings such as "A" and "B" lines, as well as abnormal lung tissue.

3. Identify "A lines" (Fig. 27.3). A lines indicate air. These are multiple echogenic lines appearing horizontally in sequence deep to the pleural line. This artifact represents reverberations of the pleura and can be found in aerated lungs, which can be normal or abnormal (e.g., pulmonary embolism, chronic obstructive pulmonary disease [COPD]). The first true A line, denoted "A1," is found equidistant from the chest wall to the pleural line. Many other A lines might be seen and are denoted "A'" lines. Subsequent equidistant A lines are "A2," "A3," and so on.

4. Identify "B lines" (Fig. 27.4). These artifacts appear in well-aerated lung and are vertical echogenic lines (ray, flashlight, lung rockets) transmitted from the pleura to the deeper parts of the lung on the ultrasound monitor field. They are due to thickened interlobular septa and represent alveolar fluid surrounded by air. True B lines arise from the pleural line and shoot all the way down to the far lung fields, whereas "comet tails" are seen only close to the pleural and are sometimes referred to as "shimmering" or "glimmering" during movement of the pleural line. When multiple B lines are seen in a patient, it is sometimes referred to as "lung rockets" or "flashlights" because many rays are shooting from the pleura.

Even though most of the time B lines represent pulmonary edema, they can be seen in other conditions such as aspiration, pulmonary fibrosis, acute respiratory distress syndrome (ARDS), and pneumonia.

5. Identify lung sliding (Fig. 27.5). Lung sliding identifies movement of a normal parietal-visceral interface. Patient breathing causes a rhythmic movement of parietal against the visceral pleura appearing as movement of the hyperechoic line. M-mode can be used to show a timed clip of this through a still image and should only be used as a method of reporting or saving for documentation purposes. A "lung point" is an area adjacent to lung sliding (parietal pleura) that is devoid of movement. This is highly specific for pneumothorax. If one suspects a pneumothorax, quantification of the size can be made by evaluation at the anterior lung points and movement toward the lateral wall of the chest. The more rib spaces found to have absent lung sliding, the larger the pneumothorax. Lung sliding (Fig. 27.5) can be evaluated with M-mode which can help identify a normal parietal-visceral interface at that level. Obtain an adequate two-dimensional view ("bat sign") and press the "M-mode" option on the equipment. A normal interface appears as multiple hyperechoic lines, the pleura (termed "seashore"; Fig. 27.5a), followed by a sandlike pattern, the lung tissue. This pattern together is termed a "seashore sign." Air that disrupts the parietal-visceral interface, as found within a pneumothorax, is identified as horizontal repeating echogenic lines, similar to a barcode (Fig. 27.5b), and is termed "stratosphere sign." M-mode can be discontinued.

   - Lung sliding can be absent in conditions other than pneumothorax: apnea, right or left bronchial intubation, lung collapse (blebs), pneumonia, and pulmonary fibrosis.

6. Identify lung pulse. This appears as a shimmering of the pleural line due to cardiac activity. This is most apparent on the left side of the chest, closest to the heart. This helps to exclude pneumothorax as well.

7. Move posteriorly. Move the ultrasound probe laterally and posteriorly to the PLAPS point. The transducer can be directed toward the center of the patient's body in supine patients. Pleural effusions and consolidations are found in the dependent areas of the lung.

8. Move caudally. With the marker still pointing cephalad, move along the posterior axillary line in two or three additional rib spaces. Identification of pleural disease and other pathology requires multiple views and will aid in evaluating the extent of the disease. This will also allow for identification of boundaries of the lung, such as the diaphragm. Identification of the diaphragm is most critical to determine location of fluid.

9. Identify the diaphragm and liver and/or spleen (Fig. 27.6). Along the posterior axillary line, or the posterior chest wall, move the probe caudad to identify the diaphragm. This appears as an echogenic curvilinear structure, with the liver or spleen being subdiaphragmatic and typically of different echogenicity than the lung. Many times the diaphragm is very high in the supine critically ill patient. Massive edema and obesity may also degrade image quality in this location.

   - Always identify the diaphragm. Hypoechoic fluid surrounding the liver or spleen can appear as a pleural effusion and must not be mistaken as such. In addition, lung tissue may mimic hepatic tissue in certain diseases such as dense consolidations termed "hepatization" of the lung. Proper probe positioning, clear identification of the diaphragm, subdiaphragmatic structures, and lung are crucial. This is a common error in novice operators owing to the confusion of the hepatorenal or splenorenal recess for the diaphragm.
   - Identifying the diaphragm can be technically difficult depending on patient position, size, and clinical condition. It maybe useful to start below the diaphragm, first identifying the hepatorenal recess (liver and kidney view interface) and then moving cephalad until the lung and diaphragm are visualized. In addition as ribs change their orientation anatomically, the probe may need to be adjusted while still in the longitudinal axis. Moving the probe clockwise and counterclockwise may be of benefit to bring into view the lung, the diaphragm, and the subdiaphragmatic structures.

10. Identify pleural effusions (Figg. 27.6). Confirming the presence of pleural effusions requires identifying anechoic material between the pleura and the lung. This can be seen as lung movement in an undulating pattern, which typically is facilitated by cardiac activity and respirations. This is termed "jellyfish sign," where the lung flaps as it freely floats in the effusion. Floating debris can also confirm effusion, termed "plankton sign." It is also important to identify the depth of the chest wall to the pleural fluid in order to determine the best location/depth of needle insertion when attempting thoracentesis or chest tube insertion. The challenge is to find a safe path for needle insertion. The key when using ultrasound as guidance is that the angle of the needle/syringe assembly must duplicate the angle of the probe. The time between scan and needle insertion must also be minimized. Real-time guidance is not required. In patients who are obese or edematous, skin indentation during probe placement can result in underestimation of depth of needle insertion required and must be taken into account. Safety margin of thoracentesis is thought to be 10 mm of visceral-parietal distance. Dry taps may be due to loculations the blocking needle, needle plugs, patient movement from scan to tap, and poor angle selection.

   - Exudates, empyemas, and hemothoraces may appear more echogenic, unlike, for example, a transudative effusion that could be anechoic. Complex effusions can also appear as heterogeneous and echogenic. The consistency of the effusion can make identification technically difficult because this can limit lung motion. Sometimes the operator may think there is no effusion when there is an echo-dense effusion.

11. Identify consolidations (Fig. 27.7). Compressed lung appears with alveolar consolidation pattern (tissue-like sign). Alveolar consolidations are devoid typically of air and appear as tissue density; these can be atelectasis, pneumonia, aspiration, or other diseased lung. "Hepatization" of the lung is typical, where the images mimic liver tissue. Images may also have hyperechoic foci representing air bronchograms, which would indicate pneumonia. Probe location should be correlated with an anatomical lobular or segmental area.

   - Lung may slide into the effusion during the respiratory cycle and can be problematic during needle insertion, causing pneumothorax or abnormal wire placement during the performance of pigtail chest tube catheters. This is called a "curtain sign."

12. Sinusoid sign (Fig. 27.8). M-mode is placed in the center of the visible lung when a large amount of pleural fluid is seen. A sinusoid sign strengthens the operator's determination that pleural fluid is present and that the pleural fluid is not necessarily compromising lung dynamics. If the sinusoid sign is absent, it may indicate a "trapped" lung dynamic.

13. Assessment and clinical decision making. Upon completion of ultrasonography of bilateral lung fields, clinical decision-making tools may be of benefit, especially in undifferentiated respiratory failure. A protocol has been developed to organize the exam of a respiratory failure patient (on noninvasive or invasive ventilation only). The BLUE protocol assesses patients based on findings (e.g., A lines, B lines, lung sliding) of both lungs and incorporates them into an algorithm. With acceptable sensitivities and specificities, practitioners can diagnose pulmonary edema, pneumonia, pneumothorax, and COPD/asthma with the BLUE protocol.

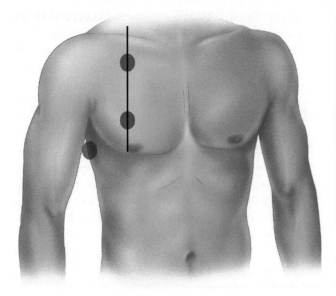

Fig. 27.1 *Black circles* indicate possible ultrasound view points. These are just guides, and one may view a few interspaces left/right and cephalad/caudad from each point to obtain better views

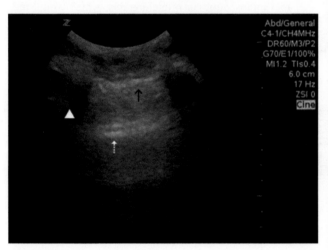

Fig. 27.2 Typical bat sign with rib shadows (*arrowhead*) that surround the pleura (*black arrow*) and lung tissue. Incidentally, A lines (*white arrow*) are seen

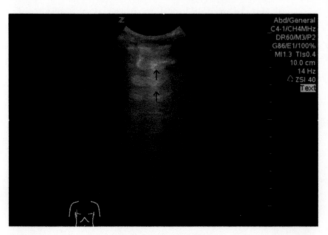

Fig. 27.3 Rib shadows can be seen, with multiple A lines (*arrows*)

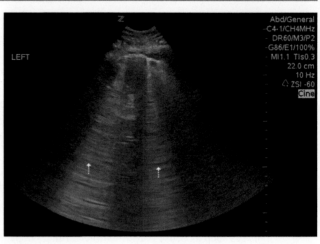

Fig. 27.4 Two B lines can be appreciated (*arrows*)

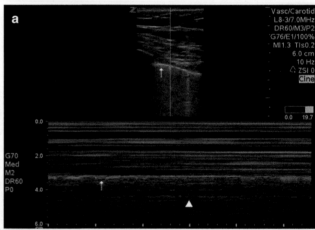

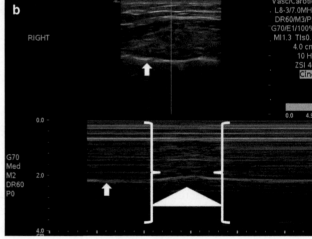

Fig. 27.5 (**a**) M-mode identifies the seashore sign, with the pleura (*arrows*) and the lung parenchyma (*arrowhead*) together producing an image similar to a seashore. (**b**) M-mode shows the stratosphere or barcode sign. *White arrows* indicate the pleura, and the *large triangle* shows an area of artifact from movement. Artifact from movement can be distinguished by a similar pattern change above and below the pleural line. On either side of the bracket is a continued horizontal line pattern typical of absent lung sliding

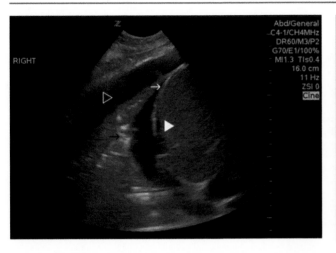

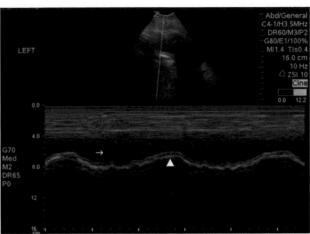

Fig. 27.6 Diaphragm (*white arrow*), liver (*white arrowhead*), lung (*black arrow*), and anechoic fluid, likely an effusion (*open arrowhead*). Incidentally, hyperechoic foci in the lung tissue, likely representing air bronchograms, can be seen

Fig. 27.8 In M-mode, identification of pleural effusion becomes evident with the sinusoidal sign (*arrowhead*) and identification of pleural fluid (*arrow*)

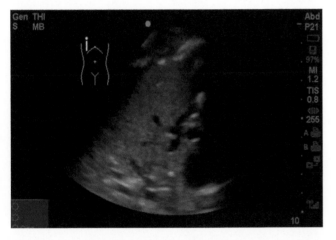

Fig. 27.7 Lung here appears as tissue density, likely representing the alveolar consolidation pattern seen in pneumonia, and is termed "hepatization" and "tissue-like sign"

Selected Reading

Levitov A, Mayo PH, Slonim AD. Ultrasound evaluation of the lung. In: Critical care ultrasonography. New York: McGraw-Hill; 2009.

Lichtenstein DA, Menu Y. A bedside ultrasound sign ruling out pneumothorax in the critically ill. Lung sliding. Chest. 1995;108: 1345–8.

Lichtenstein DA, Meziere GA. A lung ultrasound sign allowing bedside distinction between pulmonary edema and COPD: the comet-tail artifact. Intensive Care Med. 1998;24:1331–4.

Lichtenstein DA, Meziere GA. Relevance of the lung ultrasound in the diagnosis of acute respiratory failure: the BLUE protocol. Chest. 2008;134:117–25.

Mayo PH, Doelken P. Pleural ultrasonography. Clin Chest Med. 2006;27:215–27.

Mayo PH, Goltz HR, Tafreshi M, Doelken P. Safety of ultrasound-guided thoracentesis in patients receiving mechanical ventilation. Chest. 2004;125:1059–62.

Part IV

Cardiac Procedures

Repair of Cardiac Injuries

Ronald Tesoriero

Whether performed by an emergency physician or a surgeon, the majority of cardiac repairs performed at emergency department thoracotomy will be temporary in nature and require further revision in the operating room. This chapter's main focus is the temporary control of cardiac injuries.

28.1 Indications

- Wounds to the heart in patients presenting with pulseless electrical activity (PEA) or asystole with evidence of cardiac tamponade
  - Penetrating wounds: <15 min of prehospital cardiopulmonary resuscitation (CPR)
  - Blunt wounds: <10 min of prehospital cardiopulmonary resuscitation (CPR)

28.2 Contraindications

- Absolute
  - Presenting rhythm of asystole and no evidence of pericardial tamponade on Focused Assessment with Sonography for Trauma (FAST)
- Relative
  - None

28.3 Materials and Medications

- Diagnostic ultrasound
- Emergency department thoracotomy tray (Fig. 28.1)
  - Sterile drapes, #10 scalpel, curved Mayo scissors, Finochietto retractor, Lebsche sternal knife and mallet, forceps, curved Metzenbaum scissors, surgical skin stapler, Foley catheter, clamps, needle driver, 2–0 and 3–0 polypropylene suture on MH or SH (noncutting) needle, Satinsky vascular clamps
- Betadine (povidone-iodine) or other skin antiseptic preparing solution
- Defibrillator and internal cardiac panels
- Epinephrine

R. Tesoriero, MD
Department of Surgical Critical Care,
University of Maryland School of Medicine,
R Adams Cowley Shock Trauma Center,
Baltimore, MD, USA
e-mail: rtesoriero@umm.edu

© Springer Science+Business Media New York 2016   179
L. Ganti (ed.), *Atlas of Emergency Medicine Procedures*, DOI 10.1007/978-1-4939-2507-0_28

Fig. 28.1 Emergency
department thoracotomy tray.
Left to right: Scalpel, curved
Mayo scissors, Finochietto rib
spreader, DeBakey forceps,
Metzenbaum scissors, needle
driver, Lebsche knife and mallet,
Satinsky vascular clamp, aortic
clamp, bone cutter

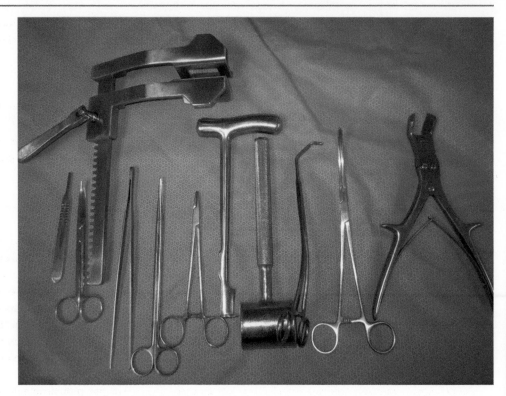

28.4   Procedure

1. Identify the pericardium anterior to the phrenic nerve, pinch it between the fingers, and enter it by making a nick with the Metzenbaum scissors. Then open the pericardium longitudinally anterior to the phrenic nerve.
2. If the heart is not contracting effectively (PEA, asystole, fibrillation), immediately begin internal cardiac massage.
   - Unless the injury is so large that it cannot be controlled, taking time out at this point to repair the injury may lead to significant acidosis and inability to reestablish a perfusing rhythm.
3. While continuing internal cardiac massage, identify the area of injury and attempt to control it with manual pressure; if a larger wound, use a Foley catheter to prevent continued bleeding.
4. If necessary owing to the location of injury, extend the incision to a bilateral anterolateral thoracotomy and transect the sternum with a Lebsche knife and mallet or heavy shears.
5. If, after several minutes of internal massage and appropriate red blood cell and plasma transfusion, the patient remains in PEA or asystole, irrigate the heart with warmed saline and administer intravenous (IV) or intracardiac epinephrine.
6. If the heart enters ventricular fibrillation or ventricular tachycardia, cardiovert with internal paddles applied directly to the heart with an energy between 10 and 30 J.
7. Once a perfusing rhythm is reestablished, or if on initial evaluation the wound is so large that it cannot be controlled and will require immediate repair before internal massage can be effective, proceed to cardiac repair.

8. Choose the simplest method that will allow control of the injury until definitive repair can be performed in the operating room.
   (a) Injuries to the atrium: The pliable nature of the atria will often allow placement of a Satinsky clamp for control followed by repair with a running 3–0 polypropylene suture (Fig. 28.2).
   (b) Small injuries to the ventricles: Control the injury with direct manual pressure and close with either interrupted 3–0 polypropylene suture or a surgical skin stapler (Figs. 28.3 and 28.4).
   (c) Medium to large injuries to the ventricle: Attempt to control the wound by placing a Foley catheter through it, then blow up the balloon and apply gentle traction. Either staple or suture the wound closed before deflating the balloon and removing the catheter (Fig. 28.5).
      - Place an occluding clamp on the open end of the catheter or blood loss will continue through the catheter
      - Avoid excessive traction on the Foley because it will pull through the ventricle and make the hole larger
   (d) Extensive or inaccessible injury: Perform temporary inflow occlusion to the heart by manually compressing the right atrium against the heart so that it cannot fill. The heart will likely immediately enter PEA, fibrillation, or asystole giving the physician a couple of minutes to gain control of the injury before the patient becomes unrecoverable.
   (e) Injuries in proximity to coronary vessels: To avoid compression of the vessel, perform a horizontal mattress suture that passes beneath the artery. Teflon pledgets may assist in the repair (Fig. 28.6).

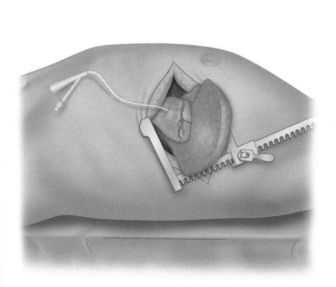

Fig. 28.2 Position the Finochietto retractor with the closed end toward the axilla. A Foley catheter may be used for initial control of large cardiac lacerations

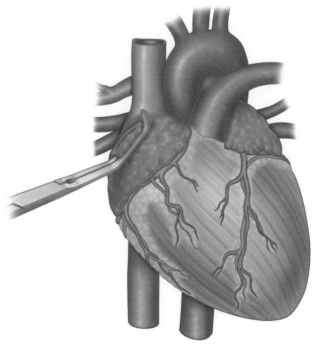

Fig. 28.3 Atrial injuries may be quickly controlled with a Satinsky clamp followed by repair with a 3–0 polypropylene suture

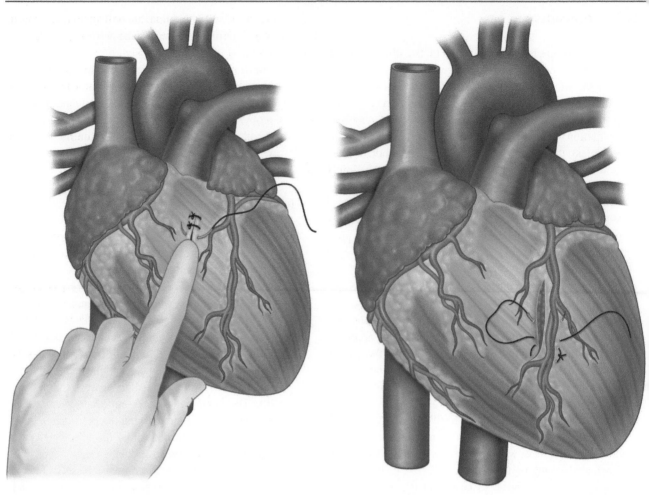

Fig. 28.4 Injuries may be controlled with direct manual pressure and closed with interrupted 3–0 polypropylene suture

Fig. 28.6 Lacerations in close proximity to coronary vessels can be controlled with horizontal mattress sutures passed beneath the artery to avoid coronary arterial compression

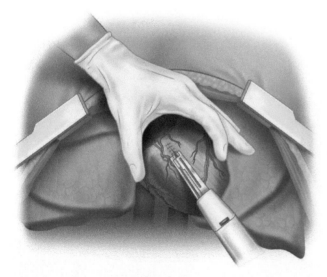

Fig. 28.5 A surgical skin stapler is a quick way to gain initial control of simple cardiac lacerations with minimal risk to the provider

28.5   Complications

Cardiac and/or pulmonary laceration during entry into the chest

Bleeding

Delayed hemorrhage (failure to control internal mammary artery, disruption of sutures or staples)

Infections: empyema and sternal infection

Missed intracardiac valvular or septal injury (echocardiography should be performed after repair is complete)

Air embolus

28.6   Pearls and Pitfalls

Pearls

– There may be more than one wound to the heart (especially with gunshot wounds). Look for them. However, if the wound is posterior and not bleeding with the heart in its natural position, it will be more prudent to leave the injury alone until the patient can be transported to the operating room. Elevating the heart can cause both inflow and outflow obstruction, leading to dysrhythmia that may be difficult to recover from.

– To avoid sutures pulling through in patients with thin, edematous, or friable myocardium, consider horizontal mattress rather than simple sutures. These may be buttressed with Teflon pledgets for added security.

- Pitfalls
  – The myocardium tears easily. When tying sutures, take care to not tighten them too forcefully.

Selected Reading

Asensio JA, Trunkey DD. Current therapy of trauma and surgical critical care. Philadelphia: Mosby/Elsevier; 2008.

Feliciano DV, Mattox KL, Moore EE. Trauma. 6th ed. New York: McGraw-Hill Medical; 2008.

Hirshberg A, Mattox KL. Top knife: the art & craft of trauma surgery. Castle Hill Barns: TFM; 2005.

Moore EE, Knudson MM, Clay CB, et al. Defining limits of resuscitative emergency department thoracotomy: a contemporary Western Trauma Association perspective. J Trauma. 2011;70:334–9.

Wall MJ, Mattox KL, Chen CD, et al. Acute management of complex cardiac injuries. J Trauma. 1997;42:905–12.

Synchronized Electrical Cardioversion

29

Jason Jones, Ann Tsung, and Marie-Carmelle Elie

Tachycardia is defined as >100 beats per minute

29.1 Indications

- Non-sinus-rhythm tachycardias with a pulse including:
  - Atrial fibrillation
  - Atrial flutter
  - Monomorphic ventricular tachycardia (VT)
  - Refractory or unstable supraventricular tachycardia (SVT)
- Unstable signs and symptoms including acute coronary syndrome, decreased level of consciousness, chest pain, dyspnea, pulmonary edema, and hypotension

29.2 Contraindications

- Absolute
  - Ventricular fibrillation and pulseless or polymorphic (irregular) VT require unsynchronized electrical cardioversion (defibrillation), not synchronized cardioversion.
  - Known atrial thrombus.
  - Sinus tachycardia.
- Relative
  - Digitalis toxicity-related tachycardia
  - Atrial fibrillation of greater than 48 h duration without anticoagulation

- Multifocal atrial tachycardia
- Electrolyte abnormalities
- Left atrial diameter greater than 4.5 cm
- Patients with low probability of maintaining sinus rhythm and readily return to atrial fibrillation
- Patients with sick sinus syndrome or sinoatrial blockage who will require a pacemaker for maintenance of stable rhythm

29.3 Materials and Medications

- Airway management equipment (laryngoscopes, endotracheal tubes)
- Cardiac monitoring, pulse oximetry, end-tidal CO_2 monitoring
- Cardioverter/defibrillator
- Sedation and analgesic medications

29.4 Procedure

1. Obtain a 12-lead electrocardiogram (ECG) and intravenous (IV) access.
2. If possible, correct underlying electrolyte abnormalities that may cause or contribute to the patient's arrhythmia.
3. Discuss risks, benefits, and alternatives (including pharmacological cardioversion) with the patient and obtain consent.
4. Prepare airway equipment and Advanced Cardiac Life Support (ACLS) code drugs.
5. Consider IV sedation (e.g., propofol, midazolam).
6. Provide IV analgesia (e.g., fentanyl, morphine).
7. Place defibrillator adhesive pads (8- to 12-cm diameter in adults) or paddles on the patient. Pediatric-sized pads/paddles should be used if the patient is less than 10 kg.

J. Jones, MD • M.-C. Elie, MD, RDMS (✉)
Department of Emergency Medicine, University of Florida Health Shands Hospital, Gainesville, FL, USA
e-mail: jasonjones@ufl.edu; elie@ufl.edu

A. Tsung, MD
Department of Emergency Medicine, University of Florida Health, Gainesville, FL, USA
e-mail: TSUNGANN@UFL.EDU

© Springer Science+Business Media New York 2016
L. Ganti (ed.), *Atlas of Emergency Medicine Procedures*, DOI 10.1007/978-1-4939-2507-0_29

8. The first paddle/pad is placed to the right of the sternum at the second/third intercostal space. The second paddle/pad can be placed in one of two equally efficacious positions:
   (a) Anterolateral position—left fourth/fifth intercostal space in the midaxillary line (Fig. 29.1)
   (b) Anteroposterior position—between the spine and the edge of the left scapula (Fig. 29.2)
9. Turn the defibrillator/cardioverter into synchronized mode—marker above R-waves will be present (Fig. 29.3).
10. Select the energy level to be delivered based on the underlying rhythm
    (a) Regular VT (with pulses)—Adults: 100 J (monophasic or biphasic), 200 J for subsequent shocks

(b) Atrial fibrillation—120–200 J (biphasic), 200 J (monophasic), 360 J for subsequent shocks
(c) Atrial flutter and paroxysmal SVT—50–100 J (biphasic), 100 J for subsequent shocks
(d) Pediatric dosage (regular and pulsed VT or SVT)—0.5–1 J/kg, up to 2 J/kg for subsequent shocks (Fig. 29.4)
11. Announce that you are going to deliver the shock on the count of three, and ensure that everyone is clear of the patient.
12. Deliver the shock by pressing button marked "SHOCK."
    • If using paddles, apply firm pressure and keep paddles in place until shock is delivered.
13. Reassess the patient's pulse and cardiac rhythm.
14. Repeat with escalating energy in a stepwise fashion if cardioversion is unsuccessful.

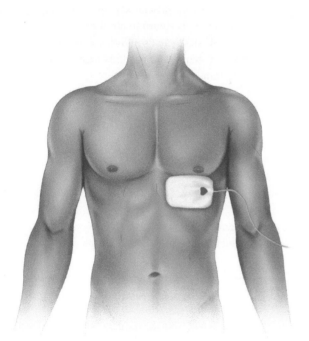

Fig. 29.1 Anterolateral pad placement

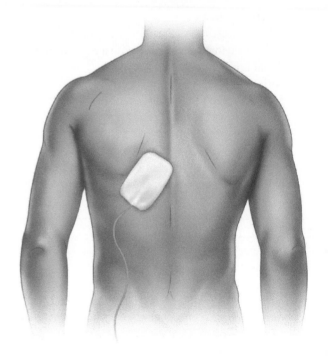

Fig. 29.2 Anteroposterior pad placement

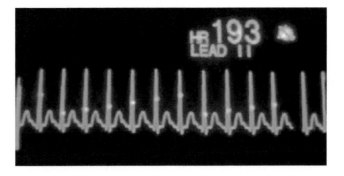

Fig. 29.3 Synchronized cardioversion—mark on R wave

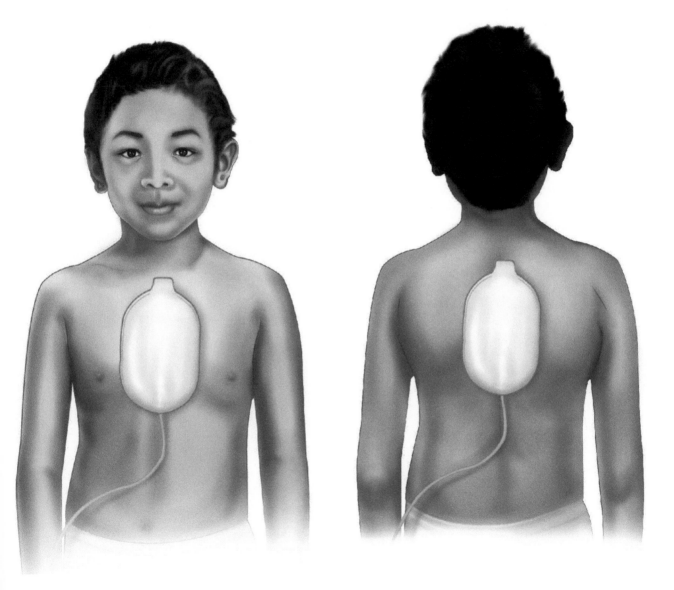

Fig. 29.4 Pediatric pad placement

29.5 Complications

- Superficial burns if there is inadequate gel.
- Induced arrhythmias (bradycardia in patients with previous inferior myocardial infarction, atrioventricular block, VT, ventricular fibrillation, asystole).
- Improperly synched cardioversion may rarely induce ventricular fibrillation.
  - Ectopy of the atria or ventricle in first 30 min after cardioversion
  - Atrial clot embolization in patients without adequate anticoagulation
- Apnea, hypoxia, hypercarbia, or hypotension may occur from sedation/analgesia.
- Medical professionals who incidentally touch the patient during shock delivery may be shocked or burned.
- Rarely, fire has occurred as a consequence of poor pad placement and a hyperoxygenated environment.

29.6 Pearls and Pitfalls

- Hirsute males should be shaved at the pad/paddle placement sites.
- Placing the cardioverter in "synchronized" mode avoids delivering a shock during the relative refractory segment, which could induce ventricular fibrillation.

- Cardioversion of pregnant patients is performed as in the general adult population.
- Keep pacemakers and implantable cardioverter-defibrillators at least 10 cm away from contact with paddles.
- If patient has implanted pacemaker, position pads so that they are not directly over the device.

Selected Reading

Gowda SA, Shah A, Steinberg JS. Cardioversion of atrial fibrillation. Progr Cardiovasc Dis. 2005;48:88–107.

Kleinman ME, Chameides L, Schexnayder SM, et al. Part 14: pediatric advanced life support. 2010 American Heart Association Guidelines for Cardiopulmonary Resuscitation and Emergency Cardiovascular Care. Circulation. 2010;122 Suppl 3:S876–908.

Link MS, Atkins DL, Passman RS, et al. Part 6: electrical therapies: automated external defibrillators, defibrillation, cardioversion, and pacing. 2010 American Heart Association Guidelines for Cardiopulmonary Resuscitation and Emergency Cardiovascular Care. Circulation. 2010;122 Suppl 3:S706–19.

Mayeaux EJ. The essentials guide to primary care procedures. Philadelphia: Lippincott Williams & Wilkins; 2012. p. 88–92.

Sirna SJ, Ferguson DW, Charbonnier F, et al. Factors affecting transthoracic impedance during electrical cardioversion. Am J Cardiol. 1988;62:1048–52.

Trohman RG, Parrillo JE. Direct current cardioversion: indications, techniques, and recent advances. Crit Care Med. 2000;28: 170–3.

Unsynchronized Cardioversion (Defibrillation)

30

Matthew R. Tice, Zachary B. Kramer,
and Marie-Carmelle Elie

Unsynchronized cardioversion or defibrillation is the delivery of a *high-energy* shock as soon as the button is pushed on defibrillator. This means it can be delivered anywhere in the cardiac cycle. By contrast, synchronized cardioversion (see Chap. 29) delivers a low-energy shock at the peak of the R wave in the cardiac (QRS) cycle.

30.1 Indications

Ventricular fibrillation (VF)
Pulseless ventricular tachycardia (VT)
Cardiac arrest due to or resulting from VF

30.2 Contraindications

Absolute
- Conscious patient
- Presence of a pulse
- Pulseless electrical activity (PEA)
- Asystole
- Multifocal atrial tachycardia
- Defibrillation without knowing the rhythm
- A second defibrillation before 2 min (or five cycles) of CPR
- Advanced Directive, Physician Order for Life-Sustaining Treatment (POLST) indicating no cardiopulmonary resuscitation (CPR) or do not resuscitate (DNR)

- Relative
  - Potential electrical catastrophe (explosive environment [i.e., operating rooms])
  - Dysrhythmias due to enhanced automaticity such as in digitalis toxicity and catecholamine-induced arrhythmia (because mechanism of tachycardia remains after the shock)
- Factors that are not contraindications
  - Pregnancy.
  - Chest trauma.
  - Automatic implantable cardiac defibrillators (AICDs).
  - The patient is on a wet or moist surface.
  - Piercings on the chest.

30.3 Materials and Medications

- Electrocardiogram (ECG) monitor/defibrillator.
- Self-adhesive defibrillation pads or defibrillation paddles (paddles may be more successful than self-adhesive pads, but they have more complications and pose more danger to operators).
- Conductive gel for defibrillation paddles (not ultra sound gel).
- ECG electrodes.
- Supplemental oxygen.
- Intubation equipment as needed.

M.R. Tice, MD • Z.B. Kramer, MD • M.-C. Elie, MD, RDMS (✉)
Department of Emergency Medicine,
University of Florida, Gainesville, FL, USA
e-mail: mtice@ufl.edu; kramer@ufl.edu; elie@ufl.edu

© Springer Science+Business Media New York 2016
.. Ganti (ed.), *Atlas of Emergency Medicine Procedures*, DOI 10.1007/978-1-4939-2507-0_30

30.4 Procedure

Defibrillation is an emergent maneuver and, when necessary, should be promptly performed in conjunction with or before administration of induction or sedative agents to facilitate intubation.

1. Assess the ABCs (airway, breathing, circulation).
   - Open the airway with a head tilt/chin lift (or jaw thrust in a suspected traumatic patient). If the patient is apneic, provide breaths with a bag-valve-mask (BVM) and observe chest rise.
   - Check for pulses. If absent, start CPR.
   - CPR should be initiated before any shock while getting all equipment ready for at least 2 min to provide adequate circulation to the brain and heart.
2. Wipe off the patient's chest if moist or wet.
3. Remove transdermal patches, jewelry, and piercings if possible.
4. Attach ECG electrodes to the patient.
   - The self-adhesive defibrillation pads or defibrillation paddles can be used as ECG electrodes to access the rhythm.
5. Paddles: With conductive gel applied to the metal surface, place one paddle on the patient's right chest, just below the clavicle, near the sternal border. The other should be on the left chest, midaxillary line above the fifth or sixth intercostal space (Fig. 30.1).
   - The long axis of the paddles should be perpendicular to the ribs to allow for better transduction of current through the chest.
   - Pads: Same placement as paddles except that pads can be placed in any orientation as long as they are in full contact with the chest.

- If a lot of breast tissue is present, push the tissue to one side or lift it away and place the paddles or pads underneath.
- An error in pad or paddle placement can distort the rhythm into looking like a rhythm that does not require defibrillation.

6. Place the ECG monitor/defibrillator into a mode to acquire a rhythm from the pads or paddles.
   - Steps 1–3 can be done simultaneously.
7. Stop CPR and assess the rhythm and pulse for no longer than 10 s.
8. If VF or pulseless VT is observed, then switch the defibrillator to charge mode.
9. Charge to 200 J.
   - Continue CPR while the defibrillator is being charged.
10. When the defibrillator indicates that it is charged, clearly order that everyone stop touching the patient and observe that there is no physical contact before defibrillating the patient.
    - If using the paddles, apply extra force to the chest through the paddles to deflate the lungs to allow for better defibrillation.
    - The operator should observe a muscle twitch during defibrillation.
11. Restart CPR for 2 min or five cycles.
    - Another operator may charge (but not fire) the defibrillator while CPR is being performed to expedite the time between pulse/rhythm check and the initiation of a shock.
12. After 2 min or five cycles of CPR, assess the rhythm and pulse and repeat steps 6–8 and give appropriate Advanced Cardiac Life Support (ACLS) medications.
13. If successful return of spontaneous circulation (ROSC) occurs, initiate the hypothermia protocol per hospital guidelines.

Fig. 30.1 Proper placement
of defibrillation paddles

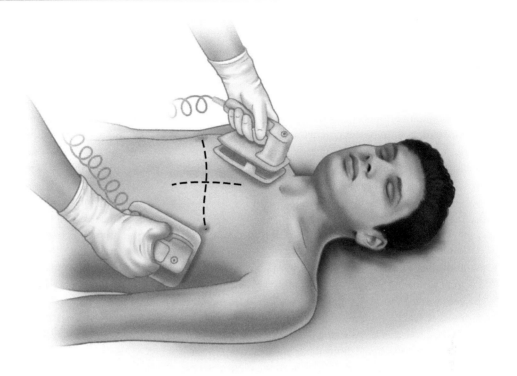

30.5   Complications

- Skin burns (most common and likely due to improper technique).
- Injury to cardiac tissue (myocardial necrosis secondary to burn).
  - ST segment elevation that lasts longer than 2 min usually indicates myocardial injury unrelated to the shock.
- Abnormal heart rhythms (usually benign like atrial, ventricular, and junctional premature beats).

30.6   Pearls and Pitfalls

- Pearls
  - Post-defibrillation cardiac dysrhythmias are more common following prolonged VF and higher-energy-level countershocks. Early defibrillation at the recommended energy levels minimizes this complication. Follow ACLS protocols to manage the resulting dysrhythmias.
  - The presence of liquid (body fluids, medications, or intravenous fluids) may cause electrical arcing thermal burns to the skin and soft tissue and produce ineffective defibrillation by allowing the current to pass across the trunk rather than transthoracically. To minimize this potential complication, ensure that any body fluids or liquids are wiped away from the skin before defibrillation attempts.
- Pitfalls
  - Myocardial and epicardial injury (not direct thermal injury) may result from the electrical current applied in defibrillation. Use the minimal recommended energy levels to minimize injury.
  - Electrical injuries to health-care providers can result if participants remain in contact with the patient during delivery of a countershock because they can serve as a ground for the current discharged.
    - This can be minimized by wearing gloves and using biphasic machines and electrode pads.
  - Fires that can result from sparks in the presence of nitroglycerin patches or ointment, flammable gases, or an oxygen-rich environment can also be a source of injury to the patient or health-care providers. Ensure "all clear" from the patient before delivery of shock to avoid these complications.

Selected Reading

Advance cardiovascular life support: provider manual. Dallas: American Heart Association; 2011.

Deakin CD, Sado DM, Petley GW, Clewlow F. Is the orientation of the apical defibrillation paddle of importance during manual external defibrillation? Resuscitation. 2003;56:15–8.

Pagan-Carlo LA, Spencer KT, Robertson CE, Dengler A, Birkitt C, Kerber RE. Transthoracic defibrillation: importance of avoiding electrode placement directly on the female breast. J Am Coll Cardiol. 1996;27:449–52.

Walker C, Callies F, Langenfeld H. Adverse effects of direct current cardioversion on cardiac pacemakers and electrodes: is external cardioversion contraindicated in patients with permanent pacing systems? Eur Soc Cardiol. 2004;6:165–8.

Transcutaneous Pacing

31

Nour Rifai and Christian Coletti

31.1 Indications

- Hemodynamically unstable (i.e., hypotension, pulmonary edema, chest pain, shortness of breath, or evidence of decreased cerebral perfusion) bradyarrhythmias refractory to medical therapies
- As a bridge to a transvenous or permanent pacemaker
- As an overdrive pacer in tachyarrhythmias
- Controversially, within the first 10 min of a witnessed asystolic cardiac arrest
- In children only with bradycardia associated with a known congenital cardiac defect or after cardiac surgery

31.2 Contraindications

- Absolute
  - None
- Relative
  - Bradyarrhythmia associated with hypothermia (ventricles are more prone to defibrillation-resistant fibrillation)
  - Prolonged cardiac arrest (>20 min)
  - Bradyarrhythmia in children (usually secondary to hypoxia or a respiratory issue)
  - Patient is unable to tolerate the procedure despite sedation and analgesia

31.3 Materials and Medications

- Pacemaker device (modern units offer combined pacer and defibrillator functions) (Fig. 31.1)
- One set of standard electrocardiogram (ECG) electrodes
- One set of pacer pads
- Code cart and airway equipment (prophylactically)
- Sedation and analgesia (typically a short-acting benzodiazepine and an opioid)
  - Midazolam: 0.2–0.10 mg/kg intravenous (IV) push and may repeat with 25 % of initial dose after 3–5 min. Do not exceed 2.5 mg/dose or a cumulative dose of 5 mg.
  - Fentanyl: 1–2 mcg/kg IV slow push over 1–2 min, may repeat dose in 30 min. (Fentanyl is the opioid of choice because it is less likely to exacerbate any hypotension.)

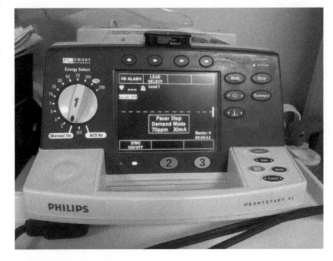

Fig. 31.1 Pacemaker device

N. Rifai, MBCHB • C. Coletti, MD (✉)
Department of Emergency Medicine,
Christiana Care Health System,
Newark, DE, USA
e-mail: nourifai@gmail.com; chris.coletti@gmail.com

© Springer Science+Business Media New York 2016
L. Ganti (ed.), *Atlas of Emergency Medicine Procedures*, DOI 10.1007/978-1-4939-2507-0_31

31.4   Procedure

1. Time permitting, clean and dry the skin, and shave any excess hair off the chest.
2. Administer any appropriate sedation and analgesia.
3. Attach the ECG electrodes to both the input port of the pacemaker unit and the patient. On the patient, the white lead is placed just above the right clavicle, the black lead is just above the left clavicle, and the red lead is around the left midaxillary line.
4. Attach the pacer pads either in the anteroposterior or anterolateral positions as pictured (avoid placement over an implanted pacemaker or defibrillator; Fig. 31.2).
5. Turn the machine on and switch it to synchronous (or on-demand) mode.
   - Asynchronous (or fixed) mode fires impulses with no regard to the intrinsic cardiac cycle, increasing the likelihood of an R on T phenomenon, which could result in ventricular tachycardia or fibrillation.
   - Synchronous (or on-demand) mode will not fire an electrical impulse when a QRS complex is sensed; this is the preferred mode for transcutaneous pacing.
6. Set the desired heart rate: typically 60–80 beats/min to achieve adequate perfusion.
7. Select a lead on the pacemaker unit and then press Start.
8. Slowly increase the output current until electrical capture is denoted by a visible pacemaker spike, which will precede every QRS complex on the ECG monitor (Fig. 31.3).
   - Electrical capture is usually achieved between 50 and 100 mA.
   - If a patient is unconscious or truly deteriorating quickly or in cardiac arrest, it may be prudent to set the initial currents at maximum to ensure rapid capture and then decrease the current to just above that at which electrical capture was achieved.
9. After electrical capture is appreciated on the monitor, assess for mechanical capture by palpation of a pulse at a rate that corresponds to that which the machine is set at. An improved blood pressure or resolution of chest pain, shortness of breath, or altered mental status also suggests that the heart rate has improved and perfusion has been restored.
10. When pacing in overdrive for tachyarrhythmias, the pacer rate is set 20–60 beats/min faster than the detected tachycardic rate.
    - Bear in mind that rhythm acceleration or the induction of ventricular fibrillation is a possibility with pacing, hence the recommendation of having a code cart and airway equipment in the room at all times.

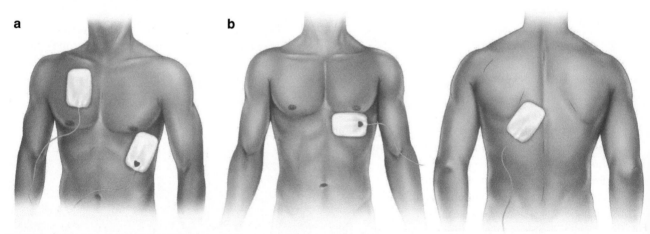

Fig. 31.2 Pacer pads attached in the anterolateral (**a**) or anteroposterior positions (**b**)

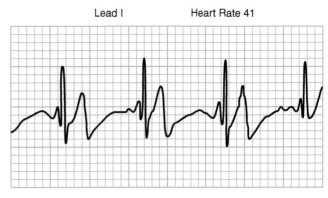

Lead I   Heart Rate 41

Bradycardia prepacing attempt

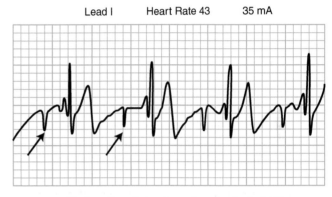

Lead I   Heart Rate 43   35 mA

Pacing attempted, note pacing stimulus indicator
(arrow) which is below threshold, no capture

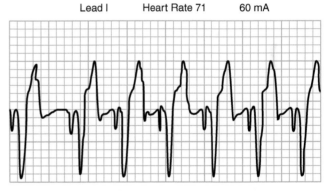

Lead I   Heart Rate 71   60 mA

Pacing above threshold (60mA), with capture (QRS
complex broad and ventricular, T wave opposite QRS)

Fig. 31.3 A visible pacemaker spike will precede every QRS
complex on the ECG monitor

31.5   Pearls and Pitfalls

- Pearls
  - Pacer pads can be prophylactically placed on brady-cardic but stable patients in preparation for potential decompensation.
  - It may be prudent to discuss with a stable but brady-cardic patient the option of trying the pacemaker not only to ensure that the machine and pads are working but also to gauge an idea of the output current that will be needed to electrically capture for quicker, more efficient, and potentially lifesaving pacing that may prove necessary.
  - When palpating for mechanical capture, the femoral pulse may be easier because carotid palpation may prove difficult with muscular contractions induced by the pacer impulses.
  - If impulses are not capturing, try slightly readjusting the pacer pads, making sure the leads are still on, the settings were not changed, the machine's battery did not die, or that the machine is plugged in.
  - If electrical capture is achieved but mechanical is not, increase the rate until adequate pulses are palpated.
  - Be careful to not miss an underlying ventricular fibrillation if the monitor is not blanked or dampened by an ECG screen.
  - Cardiopulmonary resuscitation (CPR) can be continued even while transcutaneous pacing is taking place because the pacer pads are insulated and the power delivered in each impulse is minimal, making the risk of injury to health-care workers very low.
- Pitfalls
  - Certain factors including a large body habitus, the presence of large pericardial effusions, scarring secondary to intrathoracic surgeries, or large amounts of intrathoracic air associated with obstructive pulmonary diseases may not only increase the threshold for capture but also may even cause a failure to capture, in which case transvenous pacing should immediately be considered.
  - Be aware that long-term pacing and pacing in children increases the likelihood for cutaneous and soft tissue damage.

Selected Reading

Bonow JS, Mann DL, Zipes DF, editors. Braunwald's heart disease: a textbook of cardiovascular medicine. 9th ed. Philadelphia: Saunders Elsevier; 2008.

Pfenninger JL, Fowler GC, editors. Pfenninger and Fowler's procedures for primary care. Philadelphia: Saunders Elsevier; 2010.

Roberts JR, Hedges JR, editors. Clinical procedures in emergency medicine. 5th ed. Philadelphia: Saunders Elsevier; 2010.

Tintinalli JE, Stapczynski JS, Cline DM, Ma OJ, Cydulka RK, Meckler GD, editors. Tintinalli's emergency medicine: a comprehensive study guide. 7th ed. New York: McGraw-Hill Medical; 2011.

Transvenous Cardiac Pacing

Katrina John, Jeffrey Kile, and Amish Aghera

32.1 Indications

Hemodynamic compromise in the presence of:

- Sinus node dysfunction
- Second- and third-degree heart block
- Atrial fibrillation with slow ventricular response
- New left bundle branch block (LBBB)
- Right bundle branch block (RBBB)
- Bifascicular block
- Alternating bundle branch block (BBB)
- Implanted pacemaker malfunction

32.2 Contraindications

- Absolute
  - Prosthetic tricuspid valve
- Relative
  - Bradycardia in the presence of severe hypothermia

K. John, MBBS • J. Kile, MBBS, PhD, MPH (✉)
Department of Emergency Medicine, Eisenhower Medical Center,
Rancho Mirage, CA, USA
e-mail: trenjohn@me.com; jeffrey.kile@gmail.com

A. Aghera, MD
Department of Emergency Medicine, Maimonides Medical Center,
New York, NY, USA
e-mail: aaghera@maimonidesmed.org

© Springer Science+Business Media New York 2016
L. Ganti (ed.), *Atlas of Emergency Medicine Procedures*, DOI 10.1007/978-1-4939-2507-0_32

32.3   **Materials and Medications** (Fig. 32.1)

- Sterile gloves
- Sterile gown and drapes
- Face mask and surgical cap
- Two 10-mL syringes
- One 3-mL syringe
- Local anesthetic (1 or 2 % lidocaine without epinephrine)
- 22-gauge needle
- Povidone-iodine or chlorhexidine/isopropyl alcohol
- Several 4×4-in. gauze sponges
- Sterile dressing pack
- 4-0 nylon or silk sutures

- Scalpel (#11 blade)
- Needle holder
- Scissors
- Introducer needle
- Guidewire
- Dilator
- Introducer sheath
- Collapsed sterile extension sheath
- Balloon-tipped pacing catheter
- Pacing generator with working battery
- Insulated cable with alligator clamps or other suitable connectors
- Electrocardiogram (ECG)/cardiac monitor

Fig. 32.1 Materials and medications

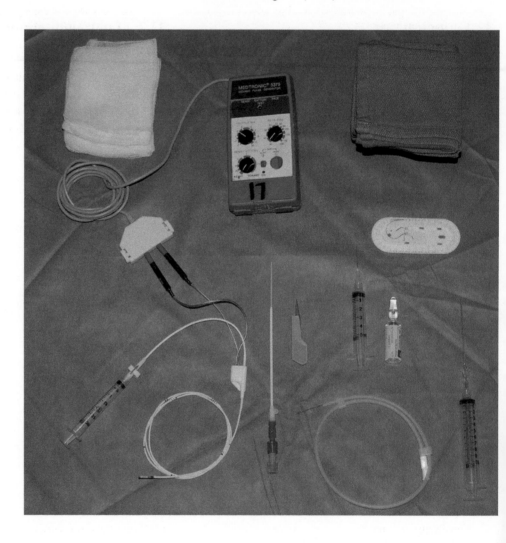

32.4   Procedure

1. Select appropriate catheterization site.
   - Four sites provide superior access to right atrium: brachial, femoral, internal jugular, and subclavian veins. The right internal jugular and left subclavian veins, respectively, are the most direct routes and, thus, the most commonly used in the emergency department setting.
2. If clinical situation permits, explain the procedure fully to the patient and obtain consent.
3. Sterilize the skin and apply sterile drapes.
4. Anesthetize the intended insertion site with lidocaine.
5. Prepare the pacing wire by inflating and deflating the balloon with 1–1.5 mL of air using a 3-mL syringe, and confirm that locking lever functions correctly to maintain balloon inflation (Fig. 32.2).
6. Using ultrasound guidance by means of a probe covered in a sterile sheath, insert the introducer needle into the vein while applying negative pressure to the attached 10-mL syringe (as with standard central line placement) (Fig. 32.3).
7. When flashback of blood is visualized in the syringe, remove the syringe, stabilizing the introducer needle firmly in place.
8. Pass the guidewire through the needle to a depth of 10–15 cm.
9. Holding the guidewire securely in place, remove the introducing needle.
10. Using a scalpel, make a small incision (approximately the width of the catheter to be used) through the dermis at the insertion site of the guidewire.
    - Avoid severing the guidewire by facing the sharp edge of the scalpel *away* from the guidewire.
11. Pass a dilator over the guidewire to make a tract in the skin and then remove the dilator.
12. Pass the introducer catheter over the guidewire until the hub is in contact with the skin and then remove the guidewire (Fig. 32.4).
13. Attach the collapsible sterile sheath to the hub of the introducer catheter.
14. Attach the positive and negative connectors of the pacing wire to their respective terminals on the cable(s) connected to the generator.
15. Set generator rate at 80 beats/min, output to 5 mA, and sensitivity to 3 mV.
16. Insert the free end of the pacing wire into introducer catheter with the balloon deflated and slowly advance the wire.
17. When the tip of the wire is within the superior vena cava, inflate the balloon, lock the valve to ensure that the balloon remains inflated, and continue to advance the pacing wire.
18. Closely watch the cardiac monitor for signs of capture (i.e., a wide QRS preceded by a pacing spike).
    - Markings on the pacing wire indicate its depth of insertion. At 20 cm, the wire should be in the right ventricle. If there is no capture observed by 25 cm, then the wire should be slowly withdrawn and advanced again.
19. Once capture is achieved, deflate the balloon.
20. Advance the wire a further 1–2 cm.
21. Coil the wire that remains outside the extended sterile sheath and suture it loosely but securely to the skin.
22. Suture the introducer hub to the skin.
23. Reduce generator output to zero and then increase it slowly to determine the minimum pacing threshold (i.e., the minimum voltage at which capture is achieved) and then set the output to twice this value.
24. Set the generator rate.
25. Stabilize the generator near the catheterization site.
    - For example, the generator can be attached to an intravenous (IV) fluid stand to the right of the patient's head if the pacing wire has been placed via the patient's right internal jugular vein.
26. Obtain a chest x-ray to confirm pacing wire position and absence of potential complications (e.g., pneumothorax) (Fig. 32.5).
27. Obtain a 12-lead ECG (Fig. 32.6).

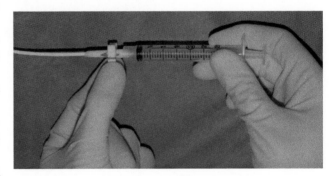

Fig. 32.2 Pacing wire balloon locking lever

Fig. 32.3 Insertion of introducer needle into internal jugular
vein with ultrasound guidance

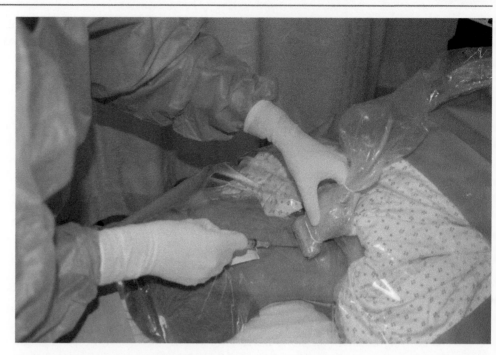

Fig. 32.4 Placement of
introducer catheter over
guidewire

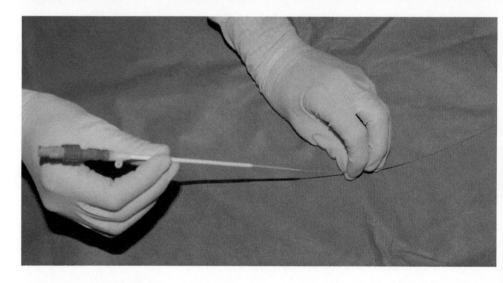

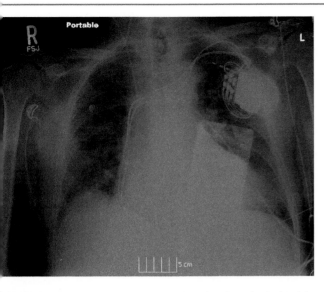

Fig. 32.5 X-ray displaying correct position of pacing wire in the right ventricle

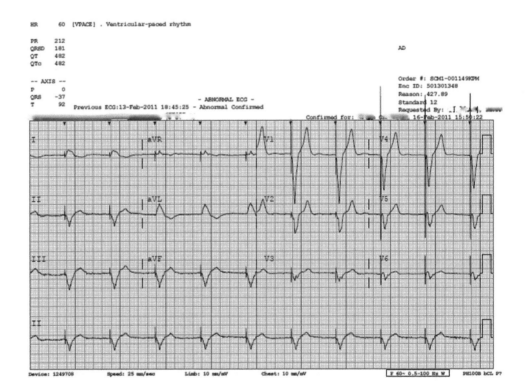

Fig. 32.6 Cardiac monitor displaying wide-complex QRS and pacing spike

32.5 Complications

- Arterial puncture
- Venous thrombosis
- Thrombophlebitis
- Pulmonary embolus
- Pneumothorax
- Fracture of guidewire with embolization
- Hemothorax
- Thoracic duct laceration
- Indwelling line infection (local or systemic)
- Dysrhythmias/premature ventricular contractions (PVCs)
- Insertion of pacing wire into coronary sinus/pulmonary artery
- Left (rather than right) ventricular pacing through atrial septal defect/ventricular septal defect (ASD/VSD)
- Septal perforation
- Ventricular perforation
- Entrapment/twisting of preexisting permanent pacing wires by the temporary pacing wire
- Balloon rupture
- Chordae tendineae rupture
- Pacing wire fractures
- Loss of capture owing to wire displacement or fracture
- Generator failure

32.6 Pearls and Pitfalls

- Confirm all necessary equipment is present and functional before beginning the procedure. If a dedicated transvenous pacing set is unavailable, individual components required (e.g., pacing catheter, connector cables, introducer catheter, guidewire) may need to be "cannibalized" from several different procedure kits in an emergency department.
- Become familiar with the locking valve for the pacing wire balloon before beginning the procedure. This small

part is essential for inflating and deflating the balloon but is frequently difficult to adjust owing to stiffness (and all the more so if covered in blood).
- The ideal position for the pacing wire tip is against the diaphragmatic aspect of the right ventricle between its midpoint and its apex. This position is confirmed by development of an LBBB pattern with left axis deviation on the cardiac monitor. If difficulty is encountered achieving this position, the tip of the pacing wire can be moved to the right ventricular outflow tract, where the wire is less stable, but adequate pacing can still be achieved. In this latter position, the threshold will need to be kept relatively high and the monitor should display an LBBB pattern with an inferior axis.
- The use of balloon-tipped catheters enables the catheter tip to be directed with blood flow and its position (and successful capture) to be confirmed with a cardiac monitor. Nonballoon-tipped catheters, however, have typically required insertion with guidance of either constant ECG monitoring or fluoroscopy.

Selected Reading

Aguilera PA, Durham BA, Riley DA. Emergency transvenous cardiac pacing placement using ultrasound guidance. Ann Emerg Med. 2000;36(3):224–7.

Birkhahn RH, Gaeta TJ, Tloczkowski J, Mundy T, Sharma M, Bove J, Briggs WM. Emergency medicine-trained physicians are proficient in the insertion of transvenous pacemakers. Ann Emerg Med. 2004;43(4):469–74.

Dalsey WC, Syverud SA, Hedges JR. Emergency department use of transcutaneous pacing for cardiac arrests. Crit Care Med. 1985;13(5):399–401.

Harrigan RA, Chan TC, Moonblatt S, Vilke GM, Ufberg JW. Temporary transvenous pacemaker placement in the Emergency Department. J Emerg Med. 2007;32(1):105–11.

Silver MD, Goldschlager N. Temporary transvenous cardiac pacing in the critical care setting. Chest. 1988;93(3):607–13.

Pericardiocentesis (Optional: Ultrasound Guidance)

33

Katrina Skoog Nguyen, L. Connor Nickels, and Rohit Pravin Patel

33.1 Indications

- Treatment of hemodynamic compromise from cardiac tamponade
- To diagnose the cause or presence of a pericardial effusion

33.2 Contraindications

- Absolute
  - Aortic dissection
  - Need for immediate surgery for trauma patients
- Relative
  - Coagulopathy
  - Anticoagulant therapy
  - Thrombocytopenia

33.3 Materials and Medications

- Antiseptic (e.g., Chloraprep)
- 1 % lidocaine
- 25-gauge needle, 5/8-in. long
- 18-gauge catheter-type needle, 1½-nch long
- Syringes (10, 20, and 60 mL)
- Ultrasound (US) machine and cardiac/phased array probe
- Sterile US probe cover
- Cardiac monitor

33.4 Procedure

1. Identify the point of maximal effusion with US. Evaluate for hypoechoic or anechoic (dark) effusion around the heart, between the pericardial sac and the myocardium. A patient with hemodynamic compromise from a pericardial effusion or tamponade will have right ventricular collapse, septal bulging, and dilation of the inferior vena cava. Diastolic collapse of the right ventricular free wall can be absent in elevated right ventricular pressure and right ventricular hypertrophy or in right ventricular infarction.
2. Measure the distance from the skin surface to the effusion border to assess the expected needle depth.
3. Choose the needle trajectory based on the point of maximal effusion in the path with the fewest intervening structures. The most commonly used approaches are left parasternal, apical, and subxiphoid. For complex loculated posterior pericardial effusions, optional techniques such as transatrial and transbronchial may be performed by specialists. These types of loculated effusions can occur in autoimmune diseases, infective pericarditis, after cardiac surgery, and after radiotherapy.
4. Sterile preparation: prepare the skin of the entire lower xiphoid and epigastric area with antiseptic. Prepare the US transducer with a sterile sleeve.
5. Local anesthetic: if the patient is awake, anesthetize the skin and planned route of the needle.
6. Pericardial needle insertion: depends on approach used.

K.S. Nguyen, DO
Northwest Community Hospital, Arlington Heights, IL, USA
e-mail: katrinaskoog@hotmail.com;

L.C. Nickels, MD, RDMS (✉) • R.P. Patel, MD
Department of Emergency Medicine, University of Florida
Health Shands Hospital, Gainesville, FL, USA
e-mail: cnickels@ufl.edu; rohitpatel@ufl.edu

© Springer Science+Business Media New York 2016
L. Ganti (ed.), *Atlas of Emergency Medicine Procedures*, DOI 10.1007/978-1-4939-2507-0_33

33.4.1 Subxiphoid Approach (Fig. 33.1)

- The US transducer is placed just inferior to the xiphoid process and left costal margin.
- Insert the needle between the xiphoid process and the left costal margin at a 30–45° angle to the skin.
- Aim for the left shoulder.

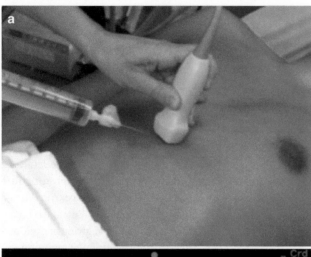

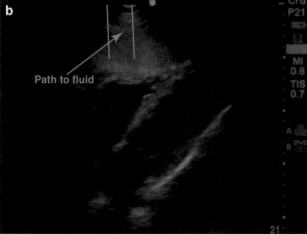

Fig. 33.1 Subcostal approach (**a**) and corresponding ultrasound image (**b**). *Red line* through liver to obtain fluid (no fluid present on ultrasound image)

33.4.2 Apical Approach (Fig. 33.2)

- The US transducer is placed at the patient's point of maximal impulse and aimed at the patient's right shoulder for a four-chamber view of the heart.
- Insert the needle in the fifth intercostal space 1 cm lateral to and below the apical beat, within the area of cardiac dullness.
- Aim for the right shoulder.
- A Mayo Clinic review showed, in 80 % of total effusions, that the distance to the effusion was least and the size was maximal in the apical approach [1].

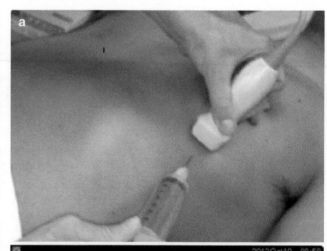

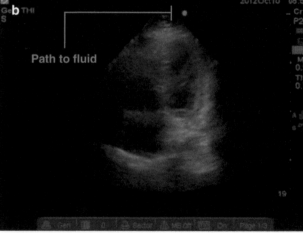

Fig. 33.2 Apical approach (**a**) and corresponding ultrasound image (**b**). *Red line* with minimal distance to fluid if present (no fluid present on ultrasound image)

33.4.3 Parasternal Long-Axis Approach

- The US transducer is placed obliquely on the left sternal border between the fourth and fifth ribs with the transducer indicator aimed at the right shoulder.
- Insert the needle perpendicular to the skin in the fifth intercostal space medial to the border of cardiac dullness.
  - Visualize and feel a giving way as the needle penetrates the pericardium. Removal of fluid confirms successful entry. Remove fluid with the goal of restoring hemodynamic stability. Aspiration of fluid should result in improvement in blood pressure and cardiac output.
  - Remove the catheter and apply a dressing. Optional: Place a pigtail catheter using the Seldinger technique for continued drainage.

33.5 Complications

- Blind techniques are associated with 20 % morbidity and 6 % mortality. The complication rate with US-guided approaches is less than 5 % [2].
- Any vital structure within reach of the pericardial needle has the potential for injury: pneumothorax; hemothorax; coronary vessel laceration; hemopericardium; heart chamber lacerations; intercostal vessel injury; dysrhythmias; ventricular tachycardia; puncture of the liver, diaphragm, or gastrointestinal tract; bacteremia; purulent pericarditis; air embolisms; and pleuropericardial fistulas.

33.6 Pearls and Pitfalls

- Pearls
  - A scoring index is available that can be obtained at initial presentation in patients without hemodynamic compromise that identifies those who require pericardial effusion drainage later in the course of treatment.

The scoring index uses echocardiographic findings, etiological information, and the size of the effusion at end-diastole [3].
  - Take care to avoid the left internal mammary artery, which travels in a cephalad-to-caudad direction 3–5 cm lateral to the left sternal border [4].
- Pitfalls
  - Tamponade should always be considered in the differential diagnosis of shock or cardiac arrest owing to pulseless electrical activity (PEA). Complications of acute coronary syndrome, aortic dissection, and decompensations in chronic advanced constriction may also need treatment [5].
  - When cardiac compensation mechanisms are exhausted, small increases in pericardial volume can lead to an increase in ventricular diastolic pressure, systemic and pulmonary congestion, and decrease preload and cardiac output.
  - Use US-guidance rather than a blind or an electrocardiogram (ECG)-alone-guided approach for pericardiocentesis to significantly decrease the risk of injury to vital structures [4].
  - Do not delay patient transport to the operating room to perform pericardiocentesis on a traumatically induced effusion unless the patient is hemodynamically unstable and on the verge of cardiac arrest.

References

1. Tsang TS, Enriquez-Serano M, Freeman WK, Barnes ME, Sinak LJ, Gersh BJ, et al. Consecutive 1127 therapeutic echocardiography guided pericardiocentesis: clinical profile, practice patterns, and outcomes spanning 21 years. Mayo Clin Proc. 2002;77:429–36.
2. Guo K, Ding ZP, Tan J. Trans-pleural pericardiocentesis: revisiting an old technique. Catheter Cardiovasc Interv. 2011;78:815–8.
3. Halpern DG, Argulian E, Briasoulis A, Chaudhry F, Aziz EF, Herzog E. A novel pericardial effusion scoring index to guide decision for drainage. Crit Pathw Cardiol. 2012;11:85–9.
4. Seferović PM, Ristić AD, Imazio M, et al. Management strategies in pericardial emergencies. Herz. 2006;31:891–901.
5. Sagristà-Sauleda J, Mercé AS, Soler-Soler J. Diagnosis and management of pericardial effusion. World J Cardiol. 2011;3:135–43.

Ultrasound Evaluation of Pulmonary Embolism and Heart Strain

34

Giuliano De Portu, L. Connor Nickels, and Marie-Carmelle Elie

34.1 Indications

- Undifferentiated respiratory distress
- Unexplained hypotension
- Evaluation for cardiac tamponade, pericardial effusion

34.2 Contraindications

- Relative
  - Morbidly obese patients
  - Patients with chest wall deformities
  - Patient with subcutaneous emphysema, pneumopericardium
  - Combative or altered patients

34.3 Materials and Medications

- Portable ultrasound machine with appropriate probes (phased array)
- Ultrasonic gel for the probe
- Drapes for the patient (if the condition allows)

34.4 Procedure

1. Begin with the parasternal long-axis view. If possible have the patient turn to the left decubitus side (that helps "move" the heart closer the chest wall).

2. Find the phased array probe, select the "cardiac examination" on the machine, and make sure the orientation marker is pointed toward the right shoulder of the patient.
3. Place the probe along the left side of the sternum over the fourth to sixth intercostal space. This should produce the image shown in Fig. 34.1.
4. Measure the diameter of the ventricle during the end of diastole (normal values, 21 mm ± 1 mm; any measurement >25–30 mm is abnormal).
5. Using the aorta as a landmark, evaluate the structures starting with the pericardium (bright white line around the heart), making sure there is no fluid around it. (Fluid above the aorta indicates a pericardial effusion. Fluid below the aorta indicates a pleural effusion.) If a hypoechoic or anechoic stripe appears in the anterior side of the heart, it is most likely a fat pad. Fluid seen "all around" categorizes it as an effusion.
6. While keeping the probe in the same place, rotate the probe marker 90° clockwise toward the left shoulder to obtain the parasternal short-axis view (Fig. 34.2).

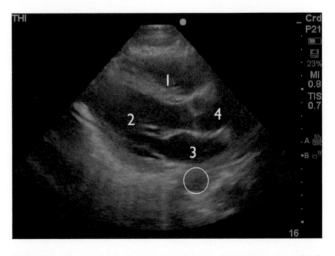

Fig. 34.1 Parasternal long-axis view (PSLA). *1* right ventricle, *2* left ventricle, *3* left atrium, *4* aortic outflow track; *circle* descending aorta (right atrium is not visualized in the PSLA)

G. De Portu, MD • L.C. Nickels, MD, RDMS
M.-C. Elie, MD, RDMS (✉)
Department of Emergency Medicine, University of Florida Health Shands Hospital, Gainesville, FL, USA
e-mail: gdeportu@ufl.edu; cnickels@ufl.edu; elie@ufl.edu

© Springer Science+Business Media New York 2016
L. Ganti (ed.), *Atlas of Emergency Medicine Procedures*, DOI 10.1007/978-1-4939-2507-0_34

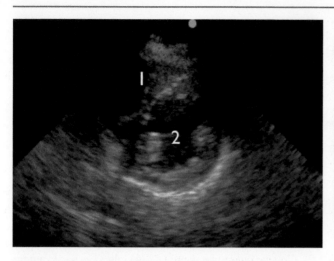

Fig. 34.2 Parasternal short-axis view (PSSA). *1* right ventricle, *2* left ventricle

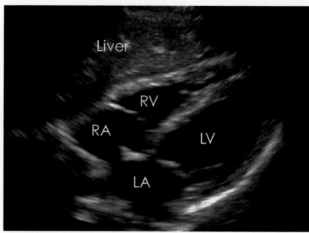

Fig. 34.4 Subcostal/subxiphoid view. *RV* right ventricle, *RA* right atrium, *LV* left ventricle, *LA* left atrium

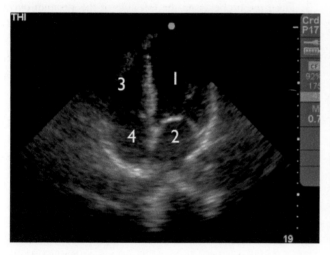

Fig. 34.3 Four-chamber view (4C). *1* left ventricle, *2* left atrium, *3* right ventricle, *4* right atrium

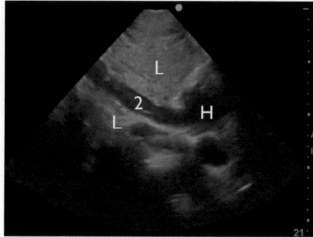

Fig. 34.5 Inferior vena cava. *L* liver, *2* inferior vena cava, *H* heart

7. The parasternal short-axis view will give information on the contractility of the heart. The right ventricle should be anterior and to the left and the left ventricle to the right. The normal position of the septum bows slightly toward the right ventricle.

8. Obtain a four-chamber view. Place the orientation marker to the patient's left.

9. Palpate for the point of maximum impulse (PMI) and place the transducer. All four chambers should appear in one view (Fig. 34.3).

10. Compare the sizes of the ventricles and note any difference. Notice also the interventricular septum. The normal right-to-left ventricular ratio is less than 0.5. (In an unstable patient, this is probably the most useful because both ventricles can be quickly visualized and the ratio compared.)

11. A subxiphoid approach is also possible. Make sure the orientation marker is toward the right side of the patient (Fig. 34.4).

12. Use the liver for orientation. The right side of the heart will be nearest to the liver (think that the liver is on the right of the body); again note for any differences in the size ratio.

13. Next take a look at the inferior vena cava (IVC) by placing the curved array transducer just inferior to the xiphoid in a longitudinal fashion. (Switch from the subxiphoid view to the IVC by rotating the probe counterclockwise until the IVC is seen.) Evaluate the IVC. During normal physiological inspiration, the drop in intrathoracic pressure "pulls" blood into the heart, thus decreasing the relative IVC size. If something is preventing venous return, such as a massive PE, collapse will not be as evident and the suspicion for PE increases (fluid overload and increased central venous pressure [CVP] will also account for this finding). Normal IVC diameter is 1.2–2.3 cm, and total collapse and greater than 50 % collapse are normally visualized. An increase in IVC size and less than 50 % or no change has been correlated with increased right atrial pressures (11 to >20 cm Hg) (Fig. 34.5).

34.5 Findings

A right heart that is "strained" or pumping against a higher resistance owing to a PE will show some or all of these changes:

1. Right ventricular dilation (Fig. 34.6).
2. Right ventricular hypokinesis (especially of the middle segment), McConnell's sign but normal motion of the apex.
3. Tricuspid regurgitation.
4. Abnormal septal motion: deviated toward the left ventricle (normally it relaxes during diastole toward the right ventricle); as pressure increases, the right ventricle will not empty properly and septal flattening can be seen.
5. Dilated IVC with little or complete loss of changes in diameter with respiration (variability); the IVC collapses less than 50 % during inspiration.

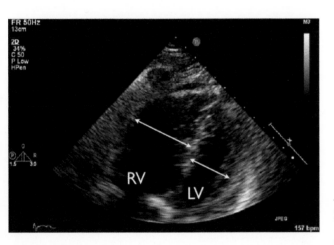

Fig. 34.6 Four-chamber view that shows right ventricular dilatation due to pulmonary embolism. Normally, the LV is greater than the RV during diastole, but in the case of increased pressure, the RV will be enlarged. *RV* right ventricle, *LV* left ventricle

34.6 Complications

- Ultrasound per se has been shown to cause no direct complications with proper use unless it is interfering with advanced airway or life-saving procedures.

34.7 Pearls and Pitfalls

- Pearls
  - Proper interpretation of the images is necessary because some normal anatomy could be confused with a positive finding. Make sure to properly identify the structures because a common mistake is to identify the aorta thinking it is the IVC.
  - Depth: increase to be sure to visualize all structures.
- Pitfalls
  - Ultrasound is user dependent, and the acquisition of images will vary with each user, creating the possibility of false-negatives if images not properly acquired.
  - Reversal of the orientation owing to transducer misplacement could "reverse" the anatomy and allow mistakenly identification of structures.
  - An enlarged right ventricular wall (>5 mm) is considered hypertrophied and would indicate a more chronic etiology of a right ventricular dilation.
  - Gain problems: adjust so the heart chambers are anechoic and the walls are echogenic.

Selected Reading

Kline JA. Thromboembolism In: Tintinalli J, Stapczynski J, Ma OJ, Cline D, Cydulka R, Meckler G, editors. Tintinalli's emergency medicine. 7th ed. New York: McGraw Hill; 2012.

McConnell MV, Solomon SD, Rayan ME, Come PC, Goldhaber SZ, Lee RT. Regional right ventricular dysfunction detected by echocardiography in acute pulmonary embolism. Am J Cardiol. 1996;78:469–73.

Reardon RF, Joing SA. Cardiac. In: Ma OJ, Mateer J, Blaivas M, editors. Emergency ultrasound. 2nd ed. New York: McGraw Hill Professional; 2007. p. 109–44.

Vanden Hoek TL, Morrison LJ, Shuster M, et al. Part 12: cardiac arrest in special situations: 2010 American Heart Association Guidelines for Cardiopulmonary Resuscitation and Emergency Cardiovascular Care. Circulation. 2010;122(18 Suppl 3):S829–61.

Pacemaker Evaluation in the Emergency Department

35

Joseph D. Romano and Christian Coletti

35.1 Pacemaker Function

There are approximately 500,000 implanted cardiac pacemakers in the USA and another 100,000 are implanted each year [1]. In the emergency department, a physician may be faced with a pacemaker that is not functioning appropriately. To understand the ways in which a pacemaker can malfunction or lead to medical complications, first it is important to understand how pacemakers work when they do so appropriately.

A common pacemaker system is composed of a pulse generator and insulated wire leads that originate in the pulse generator and end within the myocardium. The pulse generator is implanted in the pectoral region. It contains circuitry and the battery and creates the electrical impulses that depolarize the myocardium. The leads leave the pulse generator and are directed to the heart by following the venous system. Leads may terminate in the right atrium, the interventricular septum of the right ventricle, or biventricular pacing; a third lead navigates the coronary sinus to the left ventricular wall (Figs. 35.1 and 35.2).

Early pacemakers produced impulses only at a set rate. Today, however, virtually all pacemakers have sensing leads that detect intrinsic activity and react with electrical impulses when the intrinsic intervals fall outside of a set time threshold. Some pacemakers are programmed to allow for rate changes based on physical activity. To simplify the classification of different pacemaker types, the North American Society of Pacing and Electrophysiology and British Pacing and Electrophysiology Group (NASPE/BPEG) developed a five-letter code to describe each pacemaker (Table 35.1) [2].

J.D. Romano, MD (✉) • C. Coletti, MD
Departments of Emergency Medicine and Internal Medicine,
Christiana Care Health System,
Newark, DE, USA
e-mail: jromano@christianacare.org; chris.coletti@gmail.com

© Springer Science+Business Media New York 2016
L. Ganti (ed.), *Atlas of Emergency Medicine Procedures*, DOI 10.1007/978-1-4939-2507-0_35

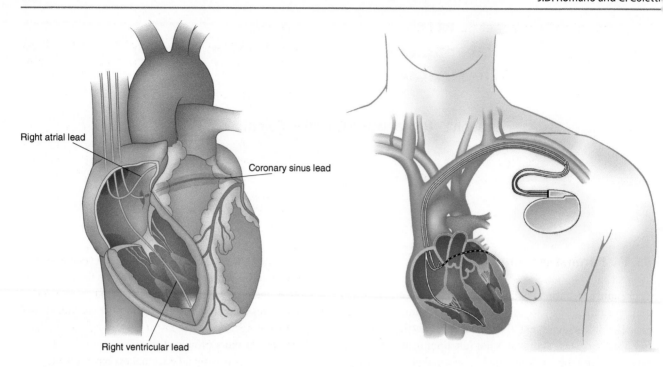

Fig. 35.1 Common pacemaker lead insertion sites

Fig. 35.2 Common generator location and path of pacemaker leads

Table 35.1 NASPE/BPEG five-letter pacemaker code

Paced chamber	Sensed chamber	Response to sensing	Rate modulation	Multisite pacing
A=atrium	A=atrium	T=triggered	R=rate modulation	A=atrium
V=ventricle	V=ventricle	I=inhibited	O=none	V=ventricle
D=dual	D=dual	D=dual		D=dual
O=none	O=none	O=none		O=none

Reproduced with permission from Bernstein et al. [2]

35.2 Common Pacemaker Codes [3]

- VVI: ventricular paced and sensed, inhibited by normal intrinsic pacing; used for patients with a need for pacing if bradycardia occurs
- VVIR: ventricular paced and sensed, inhibited by normal intrinsic pacing; adaptive to changes in intrinsic rate for physically active patients
- DDD: dual-chamber paced and sensed, inhibited by normal intrinsic atrial and ventricular electrical activity; used in third-degree atrioventricular (AV) block to allow for more physiological conduction
- DDDR: dual-chamber paced and sensed, inhibited by normal intrinsic atrial and ventricular electrical activity; adaptive to changes in intrinsic rate; used primarily in sinoatrial (SA) node dysfunction to closely mimic normal, adaptable heart conduction

35.3 Pacemaker Malfunction

Malfunctioning pacemakers can have complicated programming that is best altered after thorough "interrogation" by a trained electrophysiologist. This type of evaluation is beyond the scope of this chapter and, in many clinical settings, subspecialty support is not readily available. In the emergency department, it is vital to stabilize the patient and identify common pacemaker system issues. Pacemaker system malfunctions can be identified as a failure to sense, failure to pace, failure to capture, or pacing at an inappropriate rate [4]. Another common abnormality associated with pacing is the "pacemaker syndrome" [3].

- Failure to sense:
  - Oversensing: The sensor interprets external stimuli as a normal ventricular rate leading to inappropriate inhibition. This may be due to lead fracture, fibrosis of the lead tip, or lead dislodgment. Cross talk is present when the atrial stimulus is sensed on the ventricular lead causing inappropriate inhibition. Oversensing is rarely due to failure of the generator.
  - Undersensing: Present when there is constant pacing despite cardiac activity that has not exceeded threshold. This can be due to low-amplitude intrinsic cardiac activity, lead dislodgment, battery depletion, or metabolic abnormalities.

- Failure to pace:
  - Lack of pacing despite appropriate sensing of the intrinsic electrical activity or activity below the threshold rate.
  - Typically caused by lead fracture, battery depletion, or fibrosis of the lead tip.
  - It is rare for any specific part of the device to fail, but suspicion should be high if the patient had recent radiation therapy, electrocautery, defibrillation, electroshock therapy, magnetic resonance imaging (MRI), lithotripsy, or transcutaneous electrical nerve stimulation (TENS) treatments.
  - Rarely due to battery depletion.
- Failure to capture:
  - A lack of cardiac response despite appropriate sensing and subsequent pacer stimuli.
  - Commonly due to lead dislodgement, but can be due to myocardial perforation, lead fracture, fibrosis of the lead tip, poor lead placement, battery depletion, and antiarrhythmic medications.
  - Functional failure to capture occurs when pacer stimuli fall within the refractory period of previous depolarization.
- Pacing at an inappropriate rate:
  - Likely due to an endless-loop reentry tachycardia known as pacemaker-mediated tachycardia.
    - More common in DDD pacemakers.
    - Initiated by a premature ventricular stimulus, which is carried retrograde through the intrinsic conduction system to the atrioventricular node (AVN) and then the atria. This conduction is sensed by the atrial lead and causes triggering of pacing back in the ventricle. The ventricular depolarization is then sensed again in the atria, forming a loop. The intrinsic conduction system acts as a retrograde limb and the pacer circuit acts as the anterograde limb of a reentry tachycardia.
- The "pacemaker syndrome":
  - Constellation of symptoms found in 20 % of patients with pacemakers.
  - Symptoms include syncope, near-syncope, dizziness, fatigue, weakness, pain, shortness of breath, and cough.
  - Ventricular rates are poorly timed with atrial activity such that atrial contraction occurs against closed mitral and tricuspid valves.
  - Ventricles lose the benefit of the atrial kick, the atria enlarge, and signs and symptoms similar to congestive heart failure ensue.

35.4   Initial Evaluation of the Patient with a Pacemaker [4]

- History:
    - Symptoms of syncope, near-syncope, chest pain, palpitations, and irritation at the generator pocket
    - Brand and NASPE/BPEG code
    - Date of implantation
    - Location of generator pocket and any previous locations
    - Most recent electrophysiological interrogation
    - Medications that interfere with function, such as flecainide or lidocaine
    - Recent procedures, such as MRI, lithotripsy, or defibrillation
- Physical examination:
    - Check vital signs, listen for heart sounds (paradoxically split S2 is normal).
    - Inspect generator pocket; turning of the leads is associated with Twiddler's syndrome, in which a patient compulsively touches the skin around the device.
    - Look for jugular venous distension.
- Laboratory studies and electrocardiogram (ECG):
    - Obtain a chest x-ray to determine effusions, infiltrates, generator placement, and lead placement or fracture.
    - Electrolyte imbalances must be detected and corrected.
    - ECG: The following are examples of appropriate ECG patterns in patients based on type of pacing [3]:
        - VOO (asynchronous pacing): Regular pacer spikes lead to immediate QRS waveforms. Left bundle branch block (LBBB) is a normal finding in a right ventricular lead location.
        - VVI: Pacer spikes and an LBBB waveform should be seen if the intrinsic rate is below the threshold rate.
        - DDD: Various patterns are possible. If the intrinsic rhythm and intervals are normal, then no pacer spikes will be seen. If the atrial rate is slow and AV delay is normal, then an atrial spike will cause a P wave and a normal QRS. If AV delay is prolonged, then two spikes may be observed: a P wave and a QRS with an LBBB waveform.
- If malfunction is suspected:
    - Obtain intravenous (IV) access, place the patient on a heart monitor, and, if possible, consult cardiology for interrogation and reprogramming.
    - Obtain a ring magnet:
        - Positioning over the generator causes the pacing stimuli to revert to an asynchronous ventricular pacing mode at a set rate [5].

35.5   Interpreting the Type of Malfunction Based on ECG

The first step in evaluating the ECG of a malfunctioning pacemaker is to determine the presence of pacing spikes [6]:

- If pacing spikes are noted on the ECG, determine whether capture is present by ensuring that an appropriate waveform follows each pacer spike and that there is an associated pulse.
    - If capture is present, check the rate:
        - If the rate is appropriate, the pacer is functioning normally.
            - If the rate is slow, suspect oversensing.
            - If the rate is rapid, suspect undersensing or pacemaker-mediated tachycardia.
    - If capture is not present, consider metabolic effects or component failure.
- If pacing spikes are not noted on the ECG, determine whether the patient is in an intrinsic rhythm:
    - If the patient is in an intrinsic rhythm and the rate is appropriate, application of a ring magnet will cause pacer spikes to show up at a set rate. This is normal functioning.
        - If application of the magnet does not cause pacing, suspect mechanical failure.
    - If the patient is not in an intrinsic rhythm, place a magnet over the generator.
        - If magnet application causes pacing, consider oversensing.
        - If it does not, consider mechanical failure.
- If a patient is hemodynamically unstable and application of a magnet leads to stability, keep the magnet in place until the patient is able to have the pacemaker interrogated.

35.6   Management of Pacemaker-Mediated Tachycardia

- After ensuring adequate IV access, placing a heart monitor, and interpreting a baseline ECG, put a ring magnet over the generator [5].
    - If a normal rhythm results, keep the magnet on the chest.
    - If it does not change the rate, attempt isometric pectoral exercises by having the patient press the left hand against the right shoulder.
        - This is an attempt to overstimulate the pacemaker sensor and precipitate inhibition of pacer output.
        - If this is unsuccessful, consider transcutaneous pacing.
        - If transcutaneous pacing is unsuccessful, then the leads may require surgical adjustment or removal.

References

1. Ford-Martin PA, Spiwak AJ. Pacemakers. In: Gale encyclopedia of surgery: a guide for patients and caregivers. 2004. Encyclopedia. com: http://www.encyclopedia.com/doc/1G2-3406200337.html. Accessed 01 Apr 2011.

2. Bernstein A, Daubert J, Fletcher R, et al. The revised NASPE/BPEG generic code for antibradycardia, adaptive-rate, and multisite pacing. North American Society of Pacing and Electrophysiology/ British Pacing and Electrophysiology Group. Pacing Clin Electrophysiol. 2002;25:260–4.

3. Marx JA, Hockberger RS, Walls RM, Adams J, editors. Rosen's emergency medicine. 7th ed. Philadelphia: Mosby; 2009.

4. Bonow RO, Mann DL, Zipes DP, Libby P, editors. Braunwald's heart disease: a textbook of cardiovascular medicine. 9th ed. Philadelphia: Saunders; 2011.

5. Roberts JR, Hedges JR, editors. Clinical procedures in emergency medicine. 4th ed. Philadelphia: Saunders; 2004.

6. Kaszala K, Huizer JF, Ellenbogen KA. Contemporary pacemakers: what the primary care physician needs to know [review]. Mayo Clin Proc. 2008;83:1170–86.

Part V

Spine Evaluation

Cervical Collar Placement

Justin Bennett and Lars K. Beattie

The cervical spine (C-spine) accounts for the majority of all spinal injuries. In the US prehospital setting, patients are often transported using cervical collars (C-collars) and rigid backboards in trauma and when spinal cord injuries are suspected. After airway, breathing, and circulation, every effort must be made to secure the C-spine.

There are two main subcategories of C-collars: the one-piece and the two-piece. One-piece C-collars include the Stifneck and the Ambu Perfit. Two-piece C-collars have posterior and anterior pieces, with the anterior piece usually the larger of the two. Examples of two-piece collars include the Aspen collar, the Philadelphia collar, and the Miami J collar. The basic features of a C-collar include:

- Adjustable circumference with fasteners (usually Velcro straps)
- Adjustable height with a locking device of different sizes
- Hooks for a nasal cannula
- Exposure of the anterior neck for pulse checks and advanced airway procedures
- Posterior access for cervical palpation
- Padding to protect the soft tissues of the neck

36.1 Indications

- Prehospital suspicion for spine trauma:
  - Emergency department patients or trauma patients who fail clinical rule-out criteria such as NEXUS (National Emergency X-Radiography Utilization Study) and Canadian C-spine rules (see Chap. 37)

36.2 Contraindications

- Absolute:
  - Cervical dislocation with fixed angulation
  - Impaled foreign object in the neck
  - Massive soft tissue swelling in the neck
- Relative:
  - Unsecured airway
  - Surgical airway
  - Vomiting
  - Mandible or soft tissue injuries with potential for airway compromise
  - Preexisting anatomical abnormalities

36.3 Materials and Medications

- Properly fitting C-collar
- Consider:
  - Head blocks, if needed for lateral stabilization
  - Towels or backboard pads for custom support
    - Under shoulders – pediatric patients
    - Under occiput – adults with poor C-spine mobility

J. Bennett, MD
Department of Emergency Medicine, Wake Forest University School of Medicine, Winston-Salem, NC, USA
e-mail: jubennet@wakehealth.edu

L.K. Beattie, MD, MS (✉)
Department of Emergency Medicine, University of Florida, Gainesville, FL, USA
e-mail: lars.beattie@ufl.edu

36.4   Procedure (Aspen Collar)

1. Address airway, breathing, and circulation while maintaining in-line immobilization, before placing a C-collar.
2. Gather personnel:
    (a) One person is needed to apply the collar to an awake patient.
    (b) Two or more people may be required when a patient has an altered level of consciousness:
        (i) One to maintain in-line immobilization in the neutral position
        (ii) One to place the C-collar
3. While the C-spine is being held in neutral position, assess the airway before placing the C-collar:
    (a) Anticipate and prepare for airway compromise early to avoid a crash intubation.
    (b) Place airway if necessary.
4. Palpate and inspect the C-spine, head, and shoulders for evidence of trauma *before* placing the C-collar.
5. While maintaining the neutral position of the C-spine, place the C-collar:
    (a) Remove loose clothing, jewelry, and earrings that may cause soft tissue pressure wounds.
    (b) Begin with the piece of C-collar that fits under the occiput (Fig. 36.1).
    (c) Fold the Velcro straps behind the C-collar.
    (d) Gently hold back the hair (Fig. 36.2).
    (e) Slide the occipital section or piece of the C-collar behind the occiput (Fig. 36.3). (Use in-line C-spine stabilization in patients with an altered level of consciousness.)
    (f) Wrap (one-piece) or place (two-piece) the anterior section of the C-collar around the circumference of the patient's neck and snugly under the chin (Fig. 36.4).

(g) Once the Velcro fasteners are in place, ensure that the height is properly adjusted on the C-collar to minimize C-spine mobility.
    (i) Most C-collars have height adjustments that utilize a locking device that requires releasing a locking mechanism by pulling out.

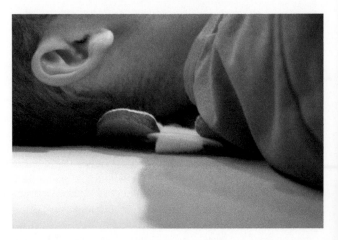

Fig. 36.2 Slide occipital section of collar behind occiput flat against stretcher

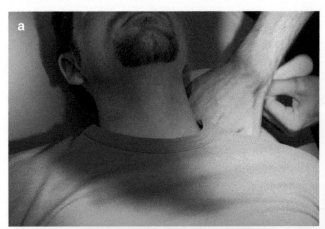

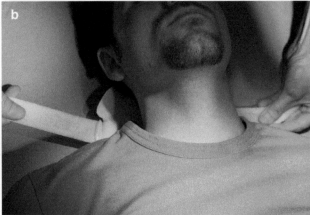

Fig. 36.3 (**a**) Use of hand to guide C-collar behind occiput; (**b**) unfold Velcro strap and position collar behind cervical spine

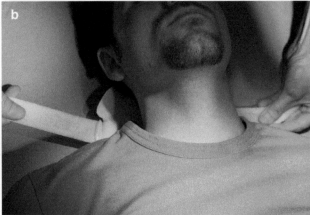

Fig. 36.1 Fold Velcro strap of C-collar posteriorly

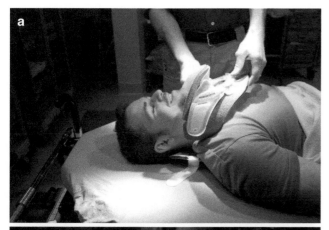

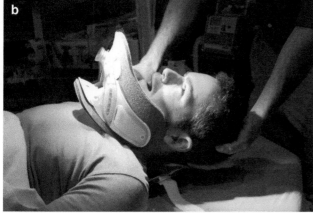

Fig. 36.4 (**a**) Correct orientation of anterior portion of C-collar; (**b**) incorrect orientation of anterior portion of C-collar may cause injury

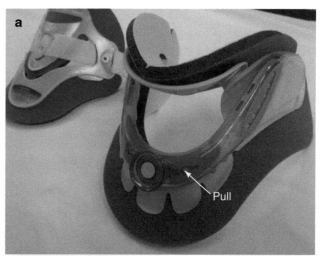

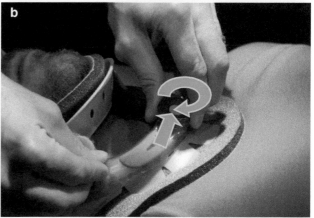

Fig. 36.5 Aspen collar is adjusted with a combination of (**a**) pulling out while (**b**) twisting a round knob at the sternal notch

   (ii) The Aspen collar is adjusted with a combination of pulling out while twisting a round knob at the sternal notch (Fig. 36.5).

   (iii) Pull out (away from patient) and twist for height adjustment of the Aspen two-piece collar.

   (iv) Adjust the height of the Ambu Perfit one-piece collar by simultaneously pulling (away from the patient) the two locking pins out and adjusting the height of the collar before pushing the pins back in (toward the patient) to lock the collar at the desired height (Fig. 36.6).

6. Special cases:

  (a) Depending on the age of the patient, it may be necessary to place towels under the shoulder blades to keep the neck in a neutral position.

  (b) Children:

   (i) Head-to-body ratios are relatively larger than that of adults.

  (ii) Placement on a backboard may cause significant neck flexion because the occiput rests on a flat board.

  (iii) Towels can be placed under a child's shoulders to minimize flexion.

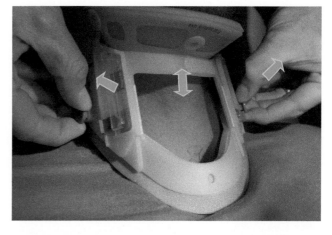

Fig. 36.6 Adjustment the height of the Ambu Perfit one-piece collar by simultaneously pulling (away from the patient) the two locking pins out and adjusting the height of the collar before pushing the pins back in (toward the patient) to lock the collar at the desired height

(c) Adults with excess soft tissue or degenerative changes that prevent C-spine straightening:
  (i) A towel or pad is placed behind the occiput to prevent hyperextension.

36.5 Pearls and Pitfalls

- Pearls
  - Airway, breathing, and circulation should be assessed before placement of the C-collar.
  - A high index of suspicion of C-spine injury is needed in intoxicated or comatose patients and the elderly.
  - Always remember to adjust the height and circumference of a C-collar for a snug fit.
- Pitfalls
  - Spinal immobilization increases the risk of aspiration in vomiting patients.
  - Failure to palpate and inspect the C-spine, head, and shoulders before C-collar placement may delay recognition of an impending airway emergency and conceal signs of critical injury needing rapid assessment and care.

- Lateral C-spine motion is unsecured unless tape, rubber blocks, or towels are used for support.
- Overlooking C-spine stabilization during C-collar placement leaves the C-spine at risk of further injury in patients with an altered level of consciousness.
- C-collars that are too tight may decrease venous return from the head and may increase intracranial pressure.

Selected Reading

American College of Surgeons Committee on Trauma. Advanced trauma life support for doctors. 8th ed. Chicago: American College of Surgeons; 2004.

Hankins DG, Boggust A. Prehospital equipment and adjuncts. In: Tintinalli JE, Stapczynski JS, Cline DM, Ma OJ, Cydulka RK, Meckler GD, editors. Tintinalli's emergency medicine: a comprehensive study guide. 7th ed. New York: McGraw Hill; 2012.

Hoffman JR, Wolfson AB, Todd K, Mower WR. Selective cervical spine radiography in blunt trauma: methodology of the National Emergency X-Radiography Utilization Study (NEXUS). Ann Emerg Med. 1998;32:461–9.

Roberts JR, Hedges JR. Clinical procedures in emergency medicine. 5th ed. Philadelphia: Saunders Elsevier; 2009.

Stiell IG, Clement CM, McKnight RD, et al. The Canadian C-spine rule versus the NEXUS low-risk criteria in patients with trauma. N Engl J Med. 2003;349:2510–8.

Cervical Spine Clearance

Braden Hexom and Tatiana Havryliuk

37.1 Indications

- Assessment of the need for radiological imaging in trauma

37.2 Contraindications

- Known unstable cervical spine (C-spine) fracture
- Known unstable ligamentous injury
- Intoxication/altered mental status
- Presence of distracting injury

37.3 National Emergency X-Radiography Utilization Study (NEXUS) and Canadian C-Spine Rules (CCR) to Assess the Need for Imaging

- *The NEXUS clinical criteria*
  1. Tenderness at the posterior midline of the C-spine
  2. Focal neurological deficit
  3. Decreased level of alertness
  4. Evidence of intoxication
  5. Clinically apparent pain that might distract the patient from the pain of a C-spine injury

- The presence of any one of the above findings is considered to be clinical evidence that a patient is at increased risk for C-spine injury and requires radiographic evaluation.
- *CCR*
  For alert (Glasgow Coma Scale [GCS] 15) and stable trauma patients
  1. Any high-risk factor that mandates radiography? *YES → Radiography*
     - Age older than 65 years
     - Dangerous mechanism (Table 37.1)
     - Paresthesias in extremities
     ↓ *NO*
  2. Any low-risk factor that allows safe assessment of range of motion? *NO → Radiography*
     - Simple rear-end motor vehicle crash (MVC)
     - Sitting position in emergency department
     - Ambulatory at any time
     - Delayed onset of neck pain
     - Absence of midline C-spine tenderness
     ↓ *YES*
  3. Able to actively rotate neck? *NO → Radiography*
     - 45° left and right
     ↓ *ABLE*
     No radiography
- CCR found to have higher sensitivity (99.4 % vs. 90.7 %) and specificity (45.1 % vs. 36.8 %) and a lower rate of imaging (55.9 % vs. 66.6 %) than NEXUS criteria for C-spine clearance of low-risk alert trauma patients.

B. Hexom, MD (✉)
Department of Emergency Medicine, Mount Sinai Hospital, New York, NY, USA
e-mail: braden.hexom@mssm.edu

T. Havryliuk, MD
Department of Emergency Medicine, University of Colorado Denver, Denver, CO, USA
e-mail: tatiana.havryliuk@ucdenver.edu

Table 37.1 Dangerous Mechanism

Fall from elevation ≥3 ft/5 stairs
Axial load to head (e.g., diving)
Motor vehicle crash at high speed (>100 km/h), rollover, ejection
Motorized recreational vehicles
Bicycle crash

© Springer Science+Business Media New York 2016
L. Ganti (ed.), *Atlas of Emergency Medicine Procedures*, DOI 10.1007/978-1-4939-2507-0_37

37.4 Type of Imaging

- Bones
  - C-spine computed tomography (CT)—the new gold standard.
  - Plain X-rays—less sensitive than CT; in one study X-rays missed 45 % of injuries that were picked up by CT [1].
- Ligaments
  - C-spine magnetic resonance imaging (MRI)—consider for possible ligamentous injuries and for further evaluation of obtunded patients.
  - Flexion-extension X-rays—less sensitive than MRI for detection of ligamentous injuries in the acute phase. Delayed flexion-extension films are more sensitive for ligamentous injury than those done the day of injury, but less sensitive than MRI.

37.5 Materials

- Cervical collar (C-collar) (Fig. 37.1)

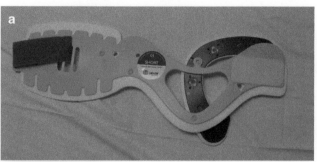
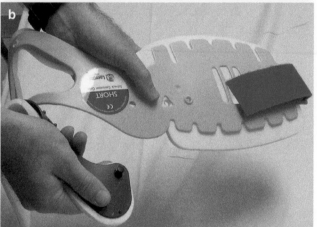
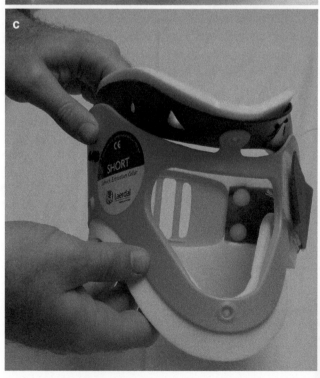

Fig. 37.1 Assembly of C-collar: Select appropriate size (**a**). Invert chinstrap and snap into place (**b**). Assembled C-collar (**c**)

37.6 Procedure (Fig. 37.2)

1. Apply C-collar to stabilize spine. Select appropriate size.
2. Perform a brief neurological examination and assess the patient's mental status; proceed only if both are normal.
3. Loosen the collar to palpate the midline while the patient holds his or her head still. If spinal tenderness exists replace the C-collar and proceed to imaging (Fig. 37.3).
4. Instruct the patient to rotate the neck 45° to each side and flex the neck. If the patient is pain free and with no neurological comprise, the C-collar may be removed and no imaging of the C-spine is required (Fig. 37.4).

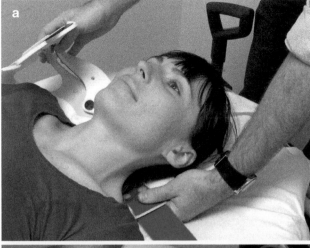

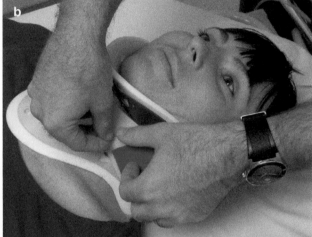

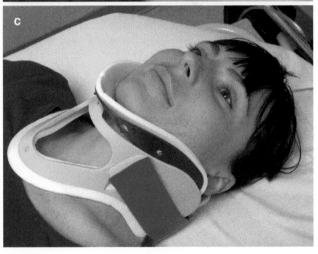

Fig. 37.2 Proper placement of C-collar: Slide C-collar under the neck while keeping neck immobilized (**a**). Secure the collar (**b**). Correct C-collar placement (**c**)

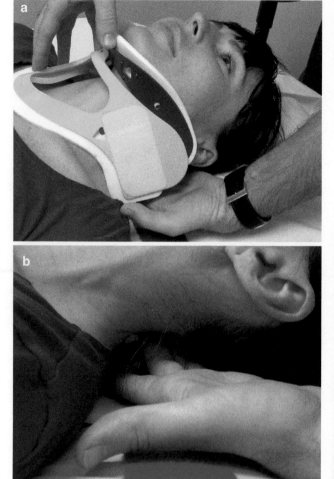

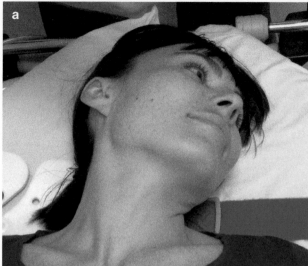

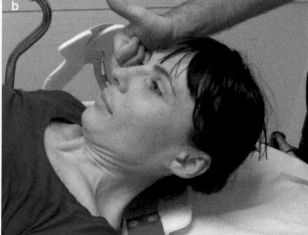

Fig. 37.3 Assessment of C spine tenderness: Loosen C-collar while keeping neck immobilized (**a**). Palpate midline of C spine (**b**)

Fig. 37.4 C-spine clearance: Instruct patient to rotate neck 45° each way (**a**). Instruct patient to flex neck (**b**)

37.7 Complications

- Missing clinically important C-spine injury
- Pressure ulcer from prolonged use of C-collar

37.8 Pearls and Pitfalls

- *Pearls*
  - Select appropriate size of C-collar.
  - Ensure adequate mental status because further imaging might be required in obtunded/intoxicated patients.
- *Pitfalls*
  - Avoid prolonged use of C-collar because this can lead to a pressure ulcer.

Reference

1. Schenarts PJ, Diaz J, Kaiser C, Carrillo Y, Eddy V, Morris Jr JA. Prospective comparison of admission computed tomographic scan and plain films of the upper cervical spine in trauma patients with altered mental status. J Trauma. 2001;51:663–8; discussion 668–9.

Selected Reading

Hoffman JR, Schriger DL, Mower W, Luo JS, Zucker M. Low-risk criteria for cervical-spine radiography in blunt trauma: a prospective study. Ann Emerg Med. 1992;21:1454–60.

Platzer P, Jaindl M, Thalhammer G, et al. Clearing the cervical spine in critically injured patients: a comprehensive C-spine protocol to avoid unnecessary delays in diagnosis. Eur Spine J. 2006;15:1801–10.

Stiell IG, Clement CM, McKnight RG, et al. The Canadian C-spine rule versus the NEXUS low-risk criteria in patients with trauma. N Engl J Med. 2003;349:2510–8.

Stiell IG, Wells GA, Vandemheen K, et al. The Canadian C-spine rule for radiography in alert and stable trauma patients. JAMA. 2001;286:1841–8.

Log Roll

38

Justin Bennett and Lars K. Beattie

38.1 Indications

- Any patient arriving on a rigid backboard in the emergency department
- Assessment of posterior traumatic injuries
- Performed as early as possible after arrival to prevent skin breakdown from pressure ulcers

38.2 Contraindications

- Improperly fitted cervical collar (C-collar) or unsecured cervical spine (C-spine) before log roll
- Unsecured endotracheal tube before log-rolling intubated patients

38.3 Materials and Medications

- Personnel: three or four people
  - One to stabilize the C-spine
  - One or two to roll the patient
  - One to palpate the length of the spine
- Properly fitting hard C-collar
- Trauma shears for removing transport straps

38.4 Procedure

1. Ensure that the airway, breathing, and circulation (ABCs) are established before attempting to remove the patient from the backboard.
2. Gather personnel, at least three, but preferably four people. Larger patients will often require additional assistance.
3. For intubated patients an additional person will be needed to secure the endotracheal tube during the log roll.
4. Ensure the height is properly adjusted on the C-collar to minimize C-spine mobility (Fig. 38.1).
5. Position the stretcher at an ergonomic lifting position for the person responsible for stabilizing the C-spine.
6. Clothing and transport straps should be removed before the log roll to improve visualization of injuries.
7. The patient is asked to cross his or her hands over the chest.
8. C-spine stabilization (at head of bed)
   - Grasp the patient's trapezoids at the midclavicular line.
   - Secure the sides of the patient's head between the operator's forearms.
   - Stabilize the patient's head in neutral anatomical position relative to the body using the operator's forearms (Fig. 38.2).

J. Bennett, MD
Department of Emergency Medicine, Wake Forest University
School of Medicine, Winston-Salem, NC, USA
e-mail: jubennet@wakehealth.edu

L.K. Beattie, MD, MS (✉)
Department of Emergency Medicine, University of Florida,
Gainesville, FL, USA
e-mail: lars.beattie@ufl.edu

© Springer Science+Business Media New York 2016
L. Ganti (ed.), *Atlas of Emergency Medicine Procedures*, DOI 10.1007/978-1-4939-2507-0_38

9. Thoracic and lumbar spine stabilization
   - One or two (preferably two) people should stand next to the patient on the side to which the patient will be rolled.
     - One person: Place hands over the patient's shoulder and hip.
     - Two people
       - First person places hands on the patient's shoulder and hip.
       - Second person places hands on the patient's hip and knees.
   - The decision to roll to the left or right side is determined by injury sites, to minimize injury exacerbation and pain, and to minimize risk of endotracheal tube dislodgment.

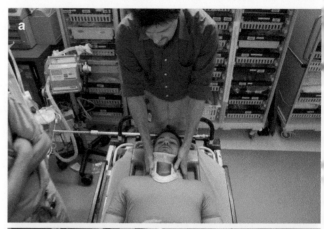

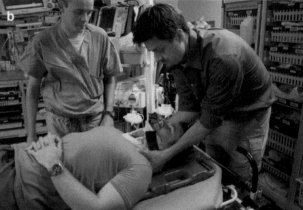

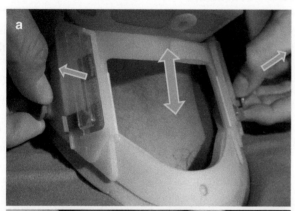

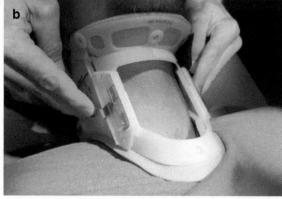

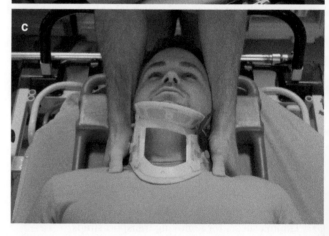

Fig. 38.1 (**a**) The height of the Ambu Perfit one-piece collar is adjusted by simultaneously pulling the two locking pins out (away from the patient) and adjusting the height of the collar, (**b**) then pushing the pins back in (toward the patient) to lock the collar at the desired height

Fig. 38.2 (**a**) Incorrect: Single-point stabilization does not keep head and C-spine in line with torso (**b**, **c**). Correct: The two-point stabilization technique keeps the head and C-spine in line with the torso during the log roll

10. The person at the head of the bed signals the initiation of a synchronized log roll when everyone is in position.

11. Attention should be directed at maintaining a neutral axis along the anatomical line of symmetry during the roll (Fig. 38.3).

12. While the patient is on her or his side, the rigid backboard should be removed and secured to prevent injury of caretakers.

13. The patient's entire posterior should be exposed and examined, taking care to note lacerations and obvious deformities.

14. The entire length of the spine is examined by inspection and then by palpation to assessed for tenderness, step-offs, and deformities (Fig. 38.4).

15. Before returning the patient back onto the stretcher, ensure that any debris, glass, lumps of clothing, or blankets are removed.

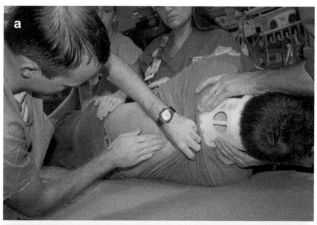

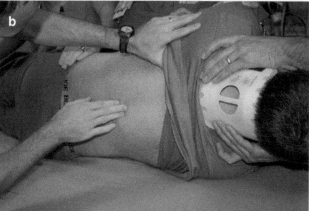

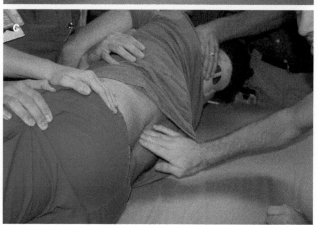

Fig. 38.4 (**a–c**) After backboard has been removed, the entire length of the of the spine can be appropriately palpated and assessed for injury to the thoracic and lumbar spine

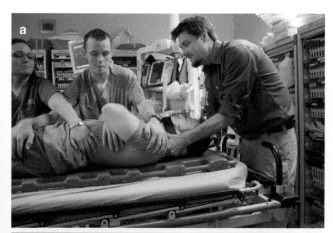

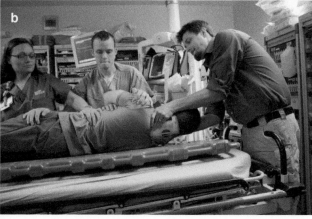

Fig. 38.3 (**a**) The interlocking hands of operators performing lateral log roll help maintain spine immobilization and minimize twisting. (**b**) Two-point cervical spine stabilization is maintained in neutral axis relative to the anatomical line of symmetry during the roll. Appropriate bed height adjustment will increase the ease of the procedure

38.5 Pearls and Pitfalls

- Pearls
  - The log roll should be performed in unison to avoid segmental rotation.
  - The ABCs should be established before initiating the log roll, which is part of the secondary survey in the trauma evaluation.
  - A proper log roll begins with stabilization of the C-spine because it is the most freely mobile part of the spine and, therefore, most frequently injured.
  - Take the patient off the backboard as soon as possible to prevent formation of pressure sores.
- Pitfalls
  - Failure to establish a two-point stabilization between the patient's body and the head leaves the C-spine at risk of further injury during the log roll.
  - Patients should not be left on the backboard for spinal precautions.
  - Failure to ensure that the ABCs are established before attempting a log roll.

Selected Reading

American College of Surgeons Committee on Trauma. Advanced trauma life support for doctors. 8th ed. Chicago: American College of Surgeons; 2008. ISBN 1880696312.

Roberts JR, Hedges JR. Clinical procedures in emergency medicine. 5th ed. Philadelphia: Saunders Elsevier; 2009.

Part VI

Neurologic and Neurosurgical Procedures

Burr Hole Craniotomy

Latha Ganti

39.1 Indications

- Extradural hematoma (EDH) or subdural hematoma (SDH) with Glasgow Coma Scale (GCS) <8 and unavailability of timely neurosurgical intervention in the face of increased intracranial pressure
- Signs of increased intracranial pressure [1]
  - Deteriorating level of consciousness
  - Slowing of the pulse
  - Dilating pupils
  - Focal seizures
  - Hemiparesis
  - Extensor posturing of the limbs

39.2 Contraindications

- Absolute
  - GCS >8
  - Immediate availability of neurosurgeon
- Relative
  - Lack of imaging (in this case, decision is guided by neurologic findings and signs of increased intracranial pressure or impending herniation)

39.3 Materials and Medications

- Razor to shave area
- 2 % lidocaine with epinephrine to numb scalp
- 10 % povidone-iodine or chlorhexidine prep
- Light, suction, cautery, dressing tray
- Gelfoam
- Penrose drain
- 3-0 silk
- #10 scalpel blade and #3 handle
- Small self-retractors or rakes
- Drill and drill bits: can be manual (Fig. 39.1) or automatic stopping variety (Fig. 39.2)
- Bone wax or electric cautery apparatus
- Suction apparatus
- Saline irrigation (IV tubing connected to a saline bag with clamp set so flow is low, or a saline syringe flush)

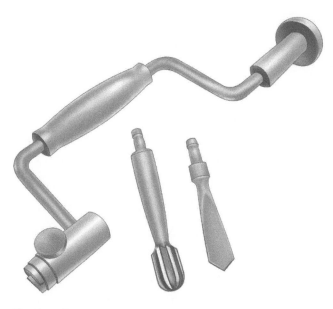

Fig. 39.1 Hudson brace, burr, and perforator

L. Ganti, MD, MS, MBA
Professor of Emergency Medicine, University of Central Florida, Orlando, FL, USA

Director, SE Specialty Care Centers of Innovation, Orlando Veterans Affairs Medical Center, Orlando, FL, USA
e-mail: lathagantimd@gmail.com

© Springer Science+Business Media New York 2016
L. Ganti (ed.), *Atlas of Emergency Medicine Procedures*, DOI 10.1007/978-1-4939-2507-0_39

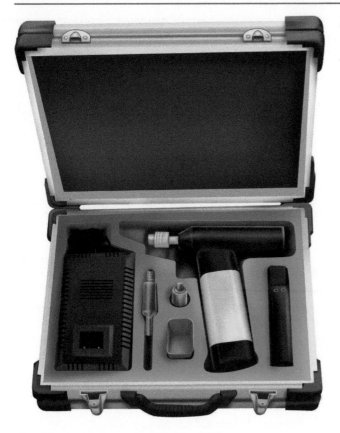

Fig. 39.2 Automatic stopping craniotomy drill set

39.4 Procedure

Preparation

1. Patient should be supine, intubated, with appropriate C-spine precautions
   - Hypertonic saline and/or mannitol can be considered for medical management of increased ICP if/as directed by neurosurgery
2. Determine location and depth for burr hole placement (Figs. 39.3 and 39.4):
   - Have CT images immediately available for viewing
   - Most common location for EDH or SDH is temporal
     - Temporal burr hole placement: 2 fingerbreadths above the ear, 2 fingerbreadths forward (Fig. 39.5)
     - Parietal burr hole placement: 2 fingerbreadths above the ear, 3 fingerbreadths backward (behind the ear)
     - Frontal burr hole placement: 3 fingerbreadths from midline, 3 fingerbreadths above hairline
   - Estimate depth of hematoma by counting the number of slices the hematoma is as seen on CT scan and multiplying by the slice thickness [2]
3. Shave hair around area of hematoma.
4. Prep skin with betadine and chlorhexidine.
5. Anesthetize scalp skin with lidocaine and epinephrine.
   Accessing hematoma
6. Make a vertical incision approximately 4 cm long down to bone.s
7. Use periosteal elevator or end of scalpel blade to scrape muscle and periosteum away from bone.
8. Place self-retaining retractors (or rakes) to keep field open (Fig. 39.6).
9. Using a drill with a clutch mechanism [2], drill through outer table (resistance), diploic space (no resistance), then inner table.
   - Burr hole needs to be placed over the *center* of the hematoma (Fig. 39.7).
10. Control bone bleeding with bone wax; control bleeding from veins and/or muscle with gelfoam sponge or cautery (diathermy).
    - Wound edges may also be cauterized or tamponaded with manual pressure +/− epinephrine gauze.
11. Once in the inner table, separate dura from bone
12. Enlarge opening by switching to a conical or cylindrical burr or use a rongeur
    Evacuating hematoma
13. EDH blood will be visible at this point and should be gently suctioned out.
14. SDH blood will be seen as a tenting of the dura and may be clotted: lift the dura with a hook or make an incision with a fresh scalpel through it to expose the clot and drain.

15. Irrigate with saline (this can be via a hand syringe or via IV tubing connected to a saline bag at low sped flow).
16. Repeat gentle suction.
    Closure
17. For temporal burr holes, ligate middle meningeal artery (if visible) or cauterize.
18. Place Penrose drain (Fig. 39.8) and close the dura first with a 3-0 absorbable suture, ensuring there is no dural leak (will lead to infection if present).
    • A watertight seal of the duraplasty is essential to minimize cerebrospinal fluid leakage.
19. Loosely suture scalp using 3-0 silk.

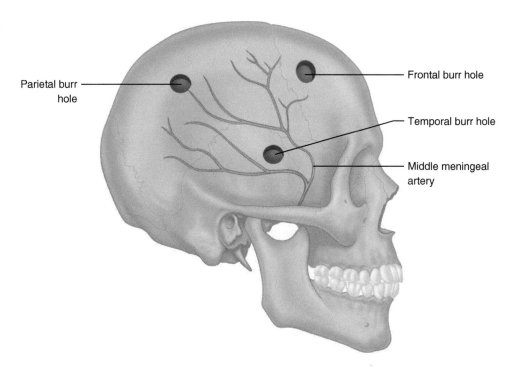

Fig. 39.3 Positions of burr hole placement

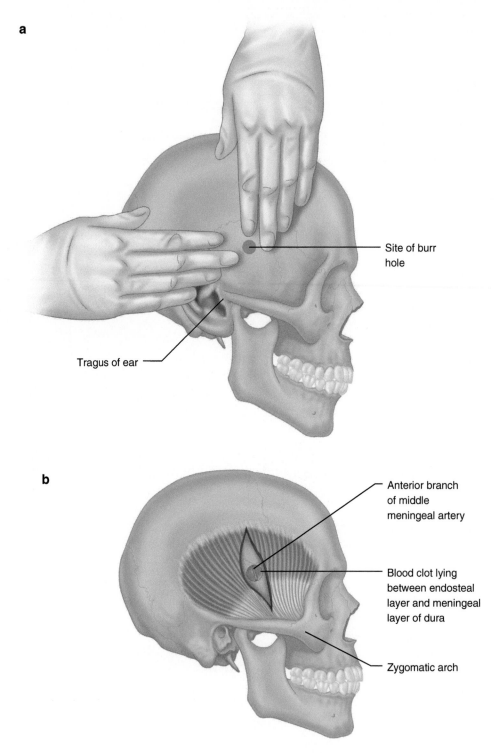

a

Site of burr hole

Tragus of ear

b

Anterior branch of middle meningeal artery

Blood clot lying between endosteal layer and meningeal layer of dura

Zygomatic arch

Fig. 39.4 (**a**, **b**) Anatomy for temporal burr hole placement (most common location)

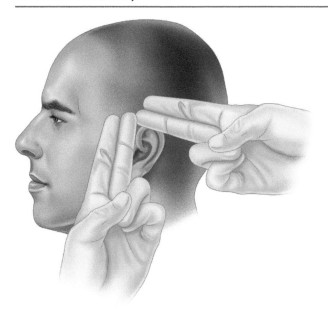

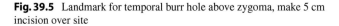

Fig. 39.7 Use penetrator drill to get through outer table. Follow up with a burr to get through the rest of the layers. Can also use an automatic stop craniotomy drill

Fig. 39.5 Landmark for temporal burr hole above zygoma, make 5 cm incision over site

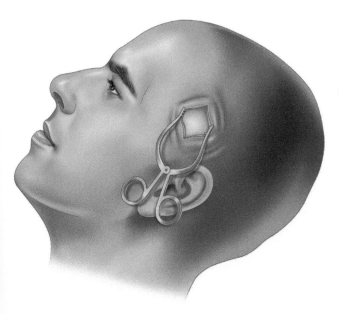

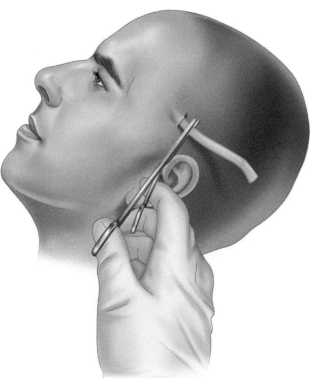

Fig. 39.6 After incision is made, use retractors (preferably self-retaining) to visualize field

Fig. 39.8 Suture in Penrose drain and close the wound

39.5   Complications

- Brain laceration/perforation
- Temporal artery laceration
- Wrong location (minimized when viewing images during procedure)
- Facial artery laceration
- Meningitis
- Brain abscess

39.6   Pearls and Pitfalls

- Pearls
    - If brain herniates through the burr hole, there is likely a hematoma at another location.
    - Remember this is only a lifesaving procedure that is to be done when timely neurosurgical intervention is not possible. *Do not delay transfer* of the patient

- Pitfalls
    - Bone in temporal area is quite thin; if not using an automatic stop drill, be very careful not to go too far and perforate the brain.

References

1. Wilkinson DA, Skinner MF. The primary trauma care manual for trauma management in district and remote locations. World Health Organization (WHO). http://www.steinergraphics.com/surgical/006_17.6.html. Accessed 22 May 2014.
2. Wilson MH, Wise D, Davies G, Lockey D. Emergency burr holes: "how to do it.". Scand J Trauma Resusc Emerg Med. 2012;20:24. doi:10.1186/1757-7241-20-24.

Selected Reading

http://www.viewmedica.com/vm/pages/library/L_df8516c9#vm_A_ac54d3a1. Accessed 29 June 2014.

External Ventricular Drain Placement

Latha Ganti

An external ventricular drain (EVD; also known as a ventriculostomy tube) is placed via a burr hole in one of the ventricles of the brain (Fig. 40.1) to drain excess cerebrospinal fluid (CSF) that causes elevated intracranial pressure.

40.1 Indications

- Emergent need for intracranial pressure (ICP) monitoring and or management
- Enlarged ventricles on neuroimaging with Glasgow coma scale <12
- Subarachnoid hemorrhage with Hunt-Hess grade ≥3 (Table 40.1)
- Coma
- Obstructive hydrocephalus
- Intraventricular hemorrhage
- Signs of increased intracranial pressure

40.2 Contraindications

- Absolute
  - Immediate availability of a neurosurgeon who can do the procedure
- Relative
  - Coagulopathy
  - Scalp infection

L. Ganti, MD, MS, MBA
Professor of Emergency Medicine, University of Central Florida, Orlando, FL, USA

Director, SE Specialty Care Centers of Innovation, Orlando Veterans Affairs Medical Center, Orlando, FL, USA
e-mail: lathagantimd@gmail.com

40.3 Materials and Medications

- Intubation equipment and medications for sedation as needed
- Sterile gloves, gown, mask
- Ruler
- Surgical marking pen
- 1–2 % lidocaine with epinephrine to numb scalp
- 5 cc syringe and needles to give anesthetic
- 10 % povidone-iodine solution and swabs
- Razor to shave area
- Fenestrated clear drape
- Scalpel #11 blade (for scalp) and #15 blade (for periosteum) with #3 handle (Fig. 40.2a)
- 4×4 sterile gauze
- Adson forceps
- Mosquito forceps
- Self-retaining eyebrow retractor (Fig. 40.2b)
- 3-0 nylon suture and needle holder and/or skin stapler
- Scissors
- A hand drill with variable chuck
- One or more drill bits with depth guards in 5/32″ (3.97 mm), 13/64″ (5.31 mm), and 1/4″ (6.35 mm) sizes
- A hex wrench for depth guard adjustment
- Ventricular catheter
- Primed ventricular drainage collection system

40.4 Procedure

Patient preparation

1. Patient is intubated and placed supine in neutral position with head of the bed elevated 30–45°.
2. Administer one dose of intravenous antibiotics that covers skin flora.
3. Make precise measurement of where the hole and incision will be made. Most commonly, EVDs are placed in

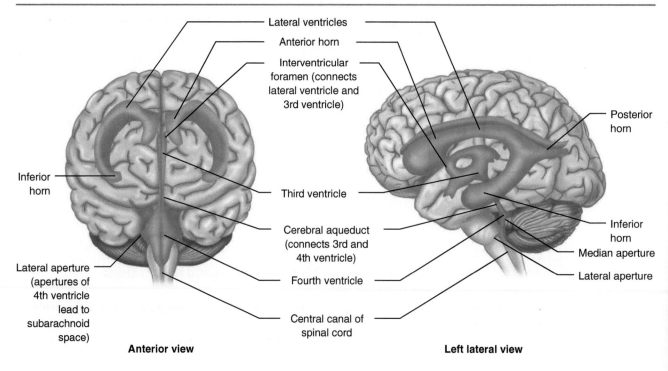

Fig. 40.1 Ventricles of the brain that contain CSF

Table 40.1 Hunt and Hess scale for subarachnoid hemorrhage [1]

Grade	Signs and symptoms
1	Alert and oriented, mild headache, slight or no nuchal rigidity
2	Alert and oriented, moderate to severe headache, nuchal rigidity, no neurologic deficit
3	Drowsiness, confusion, mild focal neurologic deficit
4	Stupor, moderate-severe hemiparesis
5	Coma, decerebrate posturing

the right frontal scalp, as this is the nondominant hemisphere in >95 % of the population.

4. Using a sterile skin/surgical marker, draw a line 11 cm back from nasion and then a point 3 cm to the right of that, which corresponds to the mid-pupillary line. This is called Kocher's point (Fig. 40.3).

5. Once Kocher's point is marked, shave skin and remove loose hairs so field is wide enough for subcutaneous catheter placement and tunneling.

6. Prep area with povidone-iodine.

7. Place sterile clear drape over field.

8. Prep area of incision once more.

9. Infiltrate scalp with 1–2 % lidocaine with epinephrine (the epinephrine acts as a hemostatic agent, keeping surgical field clean) (Fig. 40.4).

10. Make a 2 cm linear stab incision and extend incision to skull (Fig. 40.5).

11. Use eyebrow self-retaining retractors to hold skin edges back.

12. Drill burr hole with hand drill (Fig. 40.6).

13. Irrigate burr hole with sterile saline.

14. Put on a new pair of sterile gloves (prior to handling ventriculostomy catheter).

15. Remove ventricular tubing from sterile package. It has markings on it that are 1 cm apart.

16. Insert ventriculostomy catheter perpendicular to the skull at the point of insertion. Catheter is aimed at the ipsilateral medial canthus of the eye (anteroposterior plane) and tragus of ear (lateral plane).

17. Advance ventriculostomy tube 5–6 cm with stylet from outer skull table so it sits in the anterior horn of the lateral ventricle (Fig. 40.7).

18. Ensure ventriculostomy catheter is draining CSF.

19. Attach metal trocar to tip of ventriculostomy catheter and tunnel the trocar and catheter under the galea approximately 3–5 cm to the right of the original incision. Bring trocar out through separate stab incision in scalp.

20. Remove trocar, make sure ventriculostomy catheter is still draining CSF.

21. Place temporary cap on ventriculostomy catheter to prevent overdrainage of CSF.

22. Close the original incision with either sutures or staples.
23. Secure catheter to the scalp using staples.

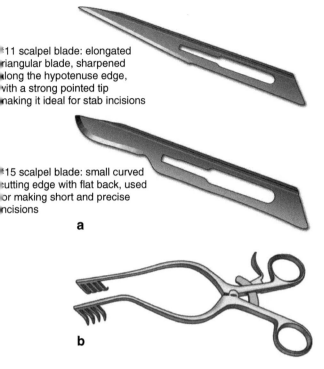

#11 scalpel blade: elongated triangular blade, sharpened along the hypotenuse edge, with a strong pointed tip making it ideal for stab incisions

#15 scalpel blade: small curved cutting edge with flat back, used for making short and precise incisions

a

b

Fig. 40.2 (**a**) Surgical scalpel blades. (**b**) Self-retaining eyebrow retractors

24. Cover incision with sterile transparent dressing.
25. Suture stopcock to ventricular catheter to ensure it does not come off (take care not to make suture too tight or it will occlude ventriculostomy catheter).
26. Remove blind end of stopcock, attach ventricular catheter to ventricular drain system once it is primed.

Priming, setup, and maintenance of ventricular drainage system

27. Prepare drainage system by priming system with sterile, preservative-free saline.
28. Place zero point of drainage system at midbrain (level of patient's ear tragus) or above midbrain at 15–20 cm of H_2O (target ICP set by neurointensivist and will change depending on patient's situation) (Fig. 40.8).
29. Attach drainage tubing.
30. Patients who require an EVD should be closely monitored by nurses trained and competent in assessment and management of the drain and in recognizing signs of increased ICP in the patient.
31. Assessment of the drainage system should be done a minimum of every 4 h, which includes inspecting the EVD from the insertion site along the entire drainage system, checking for cracks in the system or fluid leaking from the insertion site [2].

Post-procedure

32. Obtain CT scan of brain to verify placement (Fig. 40.9).

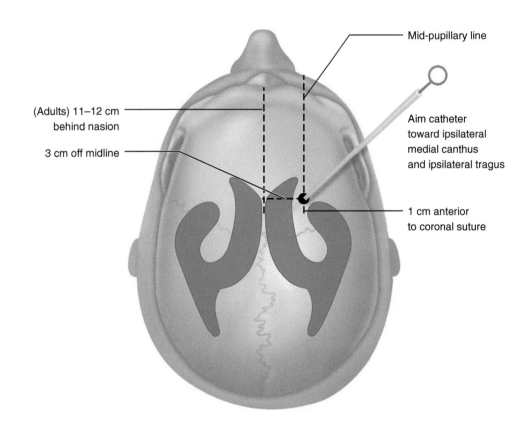

Mid-pupillary line

(Adults) 11–12 cm behind nasion

3 cm off midline

Aim catheter toward ipsilateral medial canthus and ipsilateral tragus

1 cm anterior to coronal suture

Fig. 40.3 Kocher's point for frontal EVD placement

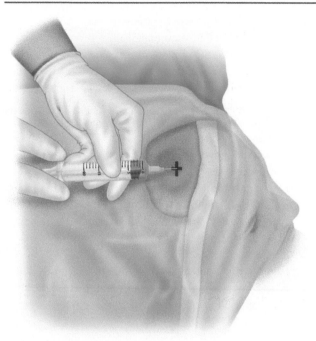

Fig. 40.4 Anesthetize skin

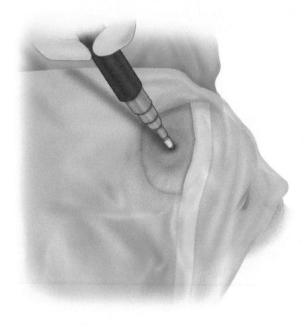

Fig. 40.6 Make burr hole

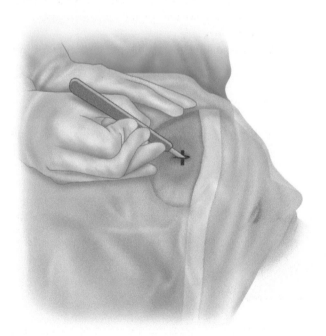

Fig. 40.5 Make stab incision

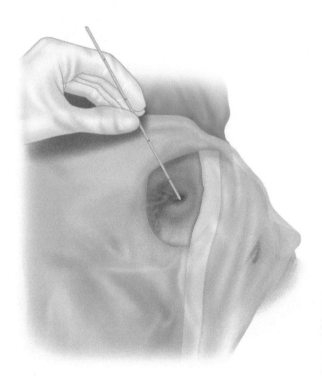

Fig. 40.7 Advance ventriculostomy catheter with stylet

40.5 Complications

- Hemorrhage
- Infection: meningitis, ventriculitis
- Tract hematoma
- Migration/dislodgement

40.6 Pearls and Pitfalls

- Pearls
  - EVD needs to be re-leveled every time the patient moves. Family and all visitors must be informed that any patient movement or change in elevation of head

Fig. 40.8 Zero point of drainage system placed at midbrain (level of patient's ear tragus)

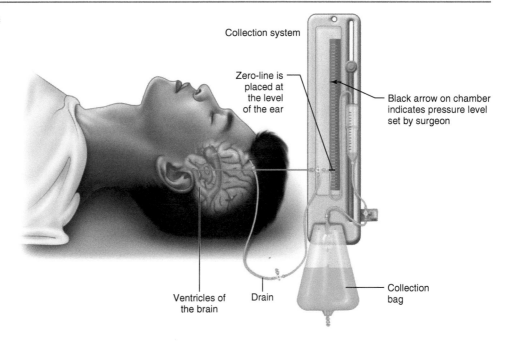

Collection system

Zero-line is placed at the level of the ear

Black arrow on chamber indicates pressure level set by surgeon

Ventricles of the brain

Drain

Collection bag

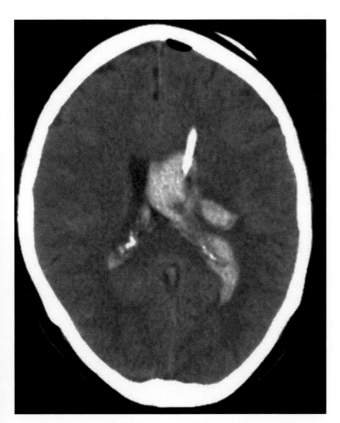

Fig. 40.9 CT scan demonstrating typical placement of ventriculostomy catheter in ipsilateral anterior horn of lateral ventricle [3] (Reproduced with permission from National Institutes of Health: Jaffe et al. [3])

of bed will require re-leveling of EVD in order to ensure it is a the appropriate level for CSF drainage.

– CSF collection chamber should remain upright to prevent reflux/leakage.

– EVD placement in the parieto-occipital scalp or frontotemporal or trans-sylvian locations is generally not done at the bedside due to higher rate of complications. This is performed in the operating room.

• Pitfalls

– If the drain is leveled too low: CSF will drain too easily, which can lead to re-rupture of an unrepaired ruptured cerebral aneurysm or cause a subdural hematoma due to shearing of bridging veins.

– If the drain is leveled too high, CSF will not drain or will not drain at desired rate, leading to hydrocephalus. The ICP will need to be higher in order for the CSF to drain.

References

1. Hunt WE, Hess RM. Surgical risk as related to time of intervention in the repair of intracranial aneurysms. J Neurosurg. 1968; 28(1):14–20.
2. Care of the patient undergoing intracranial pressure monitoring/external ventricular drainage or lumbar drainage. AANN clinical practice guideline series. 2011. http://www.aann.org/uploads/AANN11_ICPEVDnew.pdf. Accessed 27 Sept 2014.
3. Jaffe J, Melnychuk E, Muschelli J, et al. Ventricular catheter location and the clearance of intraventricular hemorrhage. Neurosurgery. 2012;70(5):1258–64.

Lumbar Puncture in Adults

41

Kevin Tench, L. Connor Nickels, and Rohit Pravin Patel

41.1 Indications

- Diagnostic
  - Evaluation for the possibility of a central nervous system (CNS) infection: viral, bacterial, and fungal meningitis and encephalitis
  - Evaluation for inflammatory processes: multiple sclerosis, Guillain-Barré syndrome
  - Evaluation for spontaneous subarachnoid hemorrhage (SAH)
  - Suspicion of CNS diseases: oncological and metabolic processes
- Therapeutic
  - Therapeutic reduction of cerebrospinal fluid (CSF) pressure
  - Procedures requiring lower body analgesia or anesthesia
  - Intrathecal antibiotic administration for some types of meningitis
  - Chemotherapy and methotrexate for some forms of leukemia and lymphomas

41.2 Contraindications

- Presence of infection in tissues at or around puncture site.
- Increased intracranial pressure (ICP) from a space-occupying lesion; patients with signs of cerebral herniation or with potential of increased ICP and focal neurological signs.
- Bleeding diathesis (thrombocytopenia, anticoagulant therapy, hemophilia); may increase risk of spinal hematoma, but level of coagulopathy that increases risk is unclear.
- Patients with cardiorespiratory compromise may worsen owing to position.

Patients with prior history of lumbar surgery, osteoarthritis, ankylosing spondylitis, kyphoscoliosis, or degenerative disk disease might have more success if lumbar puncture is performed by an interventional radiologist using imaging techniques and should be considered.

41.3 Materials and Medications
(See Fig. 123.1)

- Spinal needle(s) with stylet
  - Adults: 3.5-in. 20-gauge needle; obese may require 5.0-in. 22- to 24-gauge needle
  - Children: 2.5-in. 22-gauge needle
  - Infants: 1.5-in. 22-gauge needle
- Three-way stopcock (optional: drainage catheter)
- Manometer (optional: extension tube for higher opening pressures)
- Specimen tubes (# may vary, but in general labeled 1–4, important to obtain from 1, 2, 3, 4 owing to cell count obtained from tubes 1 and 3)
- Local anesthetic (lidocaine 1 or 2 %), 5- to 10-mL syringe and needle (25-gauge) for local anesthesia
- Sterile drapes and gauze
- Mask, sterile gown, sterile gloves
- Antiseptic solution for skin preparation (Chloroprep or iodine)

K. Tench, MD
Department of Emergency Medicine, Banner Boswell Medical Center, Sun City, AZ, USA

L.C. Nickels, MD, RDMS (✉) • R.P. Patel, MD
Department of Emergency Medicine, University of Florida Health Shands Hospital, Gainesville, FL, USA
e-mail: cnickels@ufl.edu; rohitpatel@ufl.edu

© Springer Science+Business Media New York 2016
L. Ganti (ed.), *Atlas of Emergency Medicine Procedures*, DOI 10.1007/978-1-4939-2507-0_41

41.4   Procedure

1. Positioning
   - Determined by practitioner preference or patient capability.
   - Options: lateral recumbent position, upright sitting position (Fig. 41.1).
   - Lateral recumbent position is preferred to obtain accurate opening pressure and to reduce the risk of postpuncture headache.
   - Both positions require the patient to arch the lower back toward the practitioner in order to open up the intervertebral spaces (obtain the "fetal position" or arch "like a cat").
   - Shoulders and hips should remain aligned during process.

2. Landmarks
   - Determined by palpation.
   - Draw a visual line between the superior aspects of the iliac crests that intersects the midline at the L4 interspace. The L3–4 and L4–5 spaces are preferred because these points are below the termination of the spinal cord.
   - Palpate the posterosuperior iliac crests with the midpoint of a visual line that connects the two crests representing the L4 spinous process.
   - Palpate the space between the L3–4 or the L4–5 spinous processes and mark where the needle will be placed.

3. Ultrasound guidance (optional)
   - Helpful in obese patients, patients with previous surgical scarring, or anyone in whom palpation of the spinous processes is not easily done.
   - Sonographic measurement of the dura mater strongly correlates with needle depth needed to obtain CSF.
   - Identify the spinal process in the short and long axis to determine the midline and the interspinous space.
   - Identify the interspinous ligament for estimation of the depth of needle insertion.

     Commonly only the spinous processes are well visualized, and the interspinous ligament, ligamentum flavum, and subarachnoid space are less clearly seen.
   - High-frequency (5–10 MHz) linear probe to best evaluate anatomy.
   - A marking pen can be used to create a cross-hair-type figure (Fig. 41.1).
   - After placing the patient as described, locate the midline at the lumbar spine in transverse and longitudinal orientations.
   - Bright echogenic structures with shadowing posteriorly identify the spinous processes.
   - Transverse probe positioning to identify midline (Fig. 41.2), and then longitudinal probe positioning to identify interspinous space (Fig. 41.3).

4. Sterile preparation
   - After positioning and palpating the appropriate landmarks, the practitioner should then dress in the appropriate protective gear: mask, gown, and sterile gloves.
   - After dressing, the practitioner can then sterilely prepare the patient.
   - Make sure the patient's back is completely exposed.
   - Clean the patient's back with an antiseptic solution (Chloroprep should be scrubbed in an up/down and side/side fashion; iodine in a circular motion starting from the center of the anticipated insertion point).
   - Apply sterile drapes with the puncture site exposed.

     This is an optimal time to make sure all equipment in a standard lumbar puncture tray connects properly and that the stopcock for opening pressure measurement is assembled. Make sure the stopcock is closed away from the patient so that CSF can flow from the patient to the manometer. If the assembly is done, it will decrease the amount of CSF lost after the puncture.
   - Local anesthesia
     - 1 % Lidocaine or anesthetic cream topically before preparing skin
     - For injection, form a skin wheal over the insertion site.
     - Inject into the deep tissues below the wheal in all directions while only breaking the skin once.
     - Systemic sedatives and analgesics may also be used.

5. Needle insertion
   - Needle should be inserted in the midline between the L3–4 or the L4–5 spinous process, and the stylet should be firmly in place.
   - Initially parallel to the bed, but once into the subcutaneous tissue, the needle should be angled toward the umbilicus (slightly cephalad, 15°) with the bevel facing upward (Fig. 41.4). This sagittal plane orientation spreads rather than cuts the fibers of the dural sac, which run parallel to the spinal axis.
   - If properly positioned, the needle passes through the skin; subcutaneous tissue; supraspinous ligament; interspinous ligament between the spinous processes; ligamentum flavum; epidural space including the internal vertebral venous plexus, dura, and arachnoid; into the subarachnoid space and between the nerve roots of the cauda equina.
   - In most cases, a "pop" will be felt when the needle penetrates the ligamentum flavum, entering into the subarachnoid space; then intermittent withdrawal should be done in 2-mm intervals to assess for CSF flow.
   - If bone is encountered during insertion, the needle should be withdrawn partially without exiting the skin and readjusted to a different angle more cephalad.

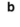
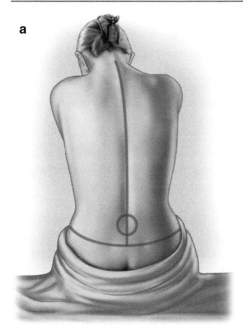
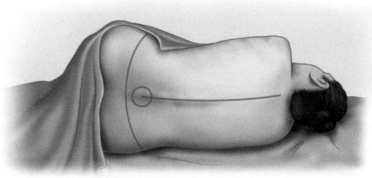

Fig. 41.1 Sitting position (**a**) left lateral decubitus position, (**b**) with general areas of insertion of needle

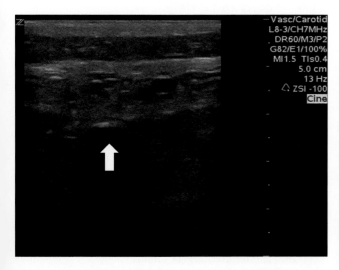

Fig. 41.2 Transverse view, *white arrow* indicates spinous process. Place in middle of ultrasound view to locate appropriate midline access point

- If the tap is traumatic, CSF may be blood tinged but should clear as more is collected. If it does not clear, it may indicate intracranial hemorrhage or subarachnoid blood. Also in traumatic patients, clotting will be seen in the tubes; clotting does not occur in SAH owing to defibrinated blood being present in the CSF. Blood-tinged CSF can also be seen in herpes simplex virus (HSV) encephalitis.
- A dry tap is usually due to incorrect positioning and misdirection of needle, often due to a superior direction of the needle with obstruction by the lamina or

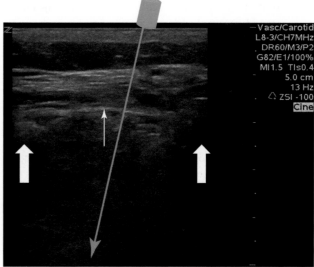

Fig. 41.3 Longitudinal view of lumbar spine. *Thick white arrows* indicate vertebral shadows; *thin white arrow* indicates supraspinous ligament. *Red arrow* indicates trajectory of needle

spinous process of the superior or inferior vertebra. If the needle is too lateral, an inferior or superior articular process may be hit.

  If flow slows down, rotate the needle 90° because a nerve root may be obstructing the opening.

6. Opening pressure measurement
- Must be performed in the lateral recumbent position. Although there are some conversion formulas from the sitting position, these are not standard of care.

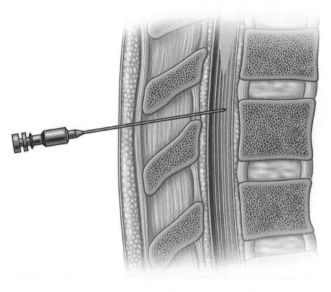

Fig. 41.4 Angle of insertion of needle, cephalad with bevel up

- Once the needle is in the subarachnoid space and CSF is flowing from the needle, the three-way stopcock should be attached to the needle and the manometer should be attached to the stopcock to take a measurement. Use the flexible tube to connect the manometer to the hub of the needle.
- Note the height of fluid in the manometer after it stops rising (normal opening pressure, <20 cm Hg); it may be possible to see pulsations from cardiac or respiratory motion.
  - Elevated CSF pressure is seen with meningeal inflammation, hydrocephalus, pseudotumor cerebri, SAH, and CHF.
  - Decreased CSF pressure is seen in leakage of CSF and severe dehydration.
7. Collecting CSF fluid
  - Collect at least 1–2 mL of CSF fluid in each tube, going from 1 to 4 and never aspirate because this can cause hemorrhage.
  - After collecting the fluid, replace the stylet and remove the needle, clean the skin, and place a bandage over the puncture site.
  - General recommendations
    - Tube 1: glucose, protein, protein electrophoresis
    - Tube 2: Gram stain, bacterial and viral cultures
    - Tube 3: cell count and differential
  - When ruling out SAH, cell count should be performed in tubes 1 and 3 or 1 and 4 to differentiate between SAH and traumatic tap.
    - Tube 4: Any special tests: myelin basic proteins, lactate, pyruvate, and smear on cell concentrates all depend on suspicion.

41.5   Complications

- Implantation of epidermoid tumors: from introducing skin plug into the subarachnoid space and can be avoided by using stylet when advancing.
- Postlumbar puncture headache: most common, occurring in 36.5 % of patients within 48 h
- CSF leak: causes headache when CSF leak through puncture site exceeds rate of production
- Bleeding: most common in patients with bleeding diathesis; may result in spinal cord compression
- Epidural hematoma
- Infection: local cellulitis, abscess (local or epidural), or meningitis
- Herniation syndromes: high risk can be identified by computed tomography but may not completely identify all patients with increased ICP
- Backache: local or referred pain
- Cardiorespiratory compromise

41.6   Pearls and Pitfalls

- Pearls
  - Positioning the patient is key to a successful procedure.
  - In adults the spinal cord may terminate higher than previously thought and it may be okay to go one interspace higher than recommended; but in infants owing to the differential in longitudinal growth of the spinal canal and cord, the spinal cord usually ends in L3. So in children the tap must go L4–5 or L5–S1.
  - Always keep the stylet in place until after the skin barrier is penetrated because this will avoid introduction of epidermoid tissue.
- Pitfalls
  - Postspinal headaches can be avoided with smaller needles and intravenous (IV) fluids.
    - Having the patient lie on the back for 1 h after the procedure has no change in incidence of headache.
    - Treatment consists of IV fluids initially, then caffeine, and, ultimately, if the headache persists, a blood patch.

Selected Reading

Boon JM, Abrahams PH, Meiring JH, Welch T. Lumbar puncture: anatomical review of a clinical skill. Clin Anat. 2004;17:544–53.

Ellenby MS, Tegtmeyer K, Lai S, Braner DA. Videos in clinical medicine. Lumbar puncture. N Engl J Med. 2006;355:e12.

Ferre RM, Sweeney TW, Strout TD. Ultrasound identification of landmarks preceding lumbar puncture: a pilot study. Emerg Med J. 2009;26:276–7.

Peterson MA, Abele J. Bedside ultrasound for difficult lumbar puncture. J Emerg Med. 2005;28:197–200.

Reflex Eye Movements (Doll's Eyes and Caloric Testing)

42

Thomas T. Nguyen, Tina Dulani, and Saadia Akhtar

42.1 Doll's Eyes (Oculocephalic Reflex Testing)

42.1.1 Indications: Doll's Eyes

- To assess brain stem function of a comatose patient
- To assess cerebral function in a comatose patient if brainstem function is intact

42.1.2 Contraindications: Doll's Eyes

- Absolute
  - Occult cervical spine injury; rule out radiographically and clinically
  - Basilar skull fracture
- Relative
  - Rheumatoid arthritis; increased risk of atlantoaxial subluxation resulting in spinal cord compression
  - Osteoporosis; increased risk of cervical spine injury
  - Cervical spine ankylosis; increased risk of cervical spine injury

42.1.3 Procedure: Doll's Eyes (Fig. 42.1)

1. Stand at the head of bed and grasp the patient's head with both hands.

T.T. Nguyen, MD (✉) • S. Akhtar, MD
Department of Emergency Medicine, Mount Sinai Beth Israel, New York, NY, USA
e-mail: tnguyen@chpnet.org

T. Dulani, MD
Department of Emergency Medicine, New York Methodist Hospital, Brooklyn, NY, USA
e-mail: tdulani@gmail.com

2. Use the thumbs of both of hands to open the patient's eyelids.
3. Rapidly move the patient's head to one side and hold.
4. Simultaneously observe for the presence or absence of horizontal movements.
   (a) Head movement to one side should result in conjugate eye movement to the opposite side and then in spontaneous return of the eyes to the midline (normal test).
   (b) Normal oculocephalic reflex is the observation of conjugate eye movements to the opposite side of head turning. This indicates a functionally intact brainstem in a comatose patient.
   (c) Abnormal oculocephalic reflex: incomplete or absent horizontal eye movements. The eyes remain in the midline. This indicates impairment of the brainstem; caloric testing should be done if not contraindicated.
   (d) A partially abnormal oculocephalic reflex: conjugate eye movement opposite to head turning but does not return to the midline means the brainstem is intact but cerebrum function is not.
5. Repeat by rotating the head to the opposite side.
6. Vertical oculocephalic response can be tested by moving the patient's head up and down. A compensatory vertical eye movement should be observed.
   (a) This test is useful only if the horizontal oculocephalic reflex is negative. An intact vertical oculocephalic reflex with a negative horizontal oculocephalic reflex suggests a pontine lesion.
7. Document the observations.

42.1.4 Pearls and Pitfalls: Doll's Eyes

- Oculocephalic reflex may not be present in the first 10 days of life and is unreliable until 2 years of age.
- Do not attempt the doll's eye maneuver in patients with cervical spinal injuries.

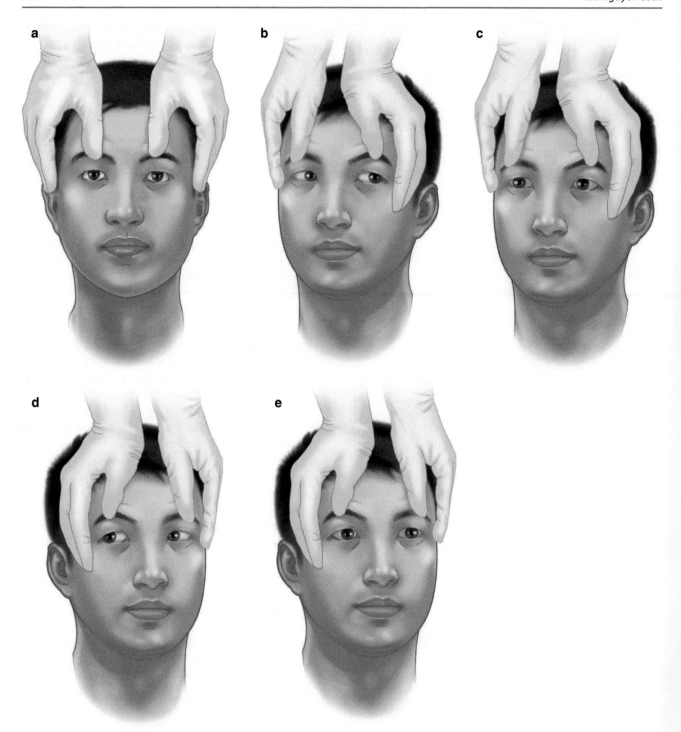

Fig. 42.1 The oculocephalic (doll's eyes) reflex in a patient with an intact brainstem. (**a**) Start with the head facing upright and grasp as depicted using both thumbs to keep the eyes open. (**b**) Rotate the head 90° to the right and the eyes deviate to the left (opposite side). (**c**) The eyes will spontaneously return to the midline. (**d**) Then rotate the head 180° to the left and the eyes should deviate to the right (opposite side). (**e**) The eyes will spontaneously return to the midline

- The doll's eye reflex can be absent or partial in patients with ocular muscle nerve palsy (e.g., cranial nerve [CN] 6).
- Make sure the patient does not have a neuromuscular blockade agent or other toxins present.
- A conscious person can suppress the doll's eye or oculocephalic reflex.

42.2 Caloric Reflex Testing (Vestibuloocular Reflex)

42.2.1 Indications: Caloric Reflex Testing

- In any comatose patient with abnormal doll's eye or if it cannot be performed
- To assess brainstem function of a comatose patient
- To assess asymmetrical function in the peripheral vestibular system

42.2.2 Contraindications: Caloric Reflex Testing

- Absolute
  - Perforated tympanic membrane
  - Presence of tympanostomy tubes
  - Basilar skull fracture, petrous bone fracture
  - Suspicion of cerebrospinal fluid (CSF) otorrhea

42.2.3 Materials and Medications: Caloric Reflex Testing

- Otoscope
- 60-mL syringe
- 16- to 18-gauge angiocatheter
- Thermometer
- Ice-cold water (30–33 °C)
- Warm water (44 °C)
- Emesis basin (to collect water)
- Towels or Chux

42.2.4 Procedure: Caloric Reflex Testing (Fig. 42.2)

1. Place the patient supine and elevate the head to 30° to bring the lateral semicircular canal into the upright position.
   (a) Careful otoscopic examination should be done before caloric testing to make sure there are no contraindications.

(b) Remove any cerumen from the external auditory canal (EAC); the irrigation fluid should be able to reach the tympanic membrane.

2. Get a 60-mL syringe with an 18-gauge angiocatheter. Remove the plastic angiocatheter from the needle and discard the needle.
3. Place the angiocatheter on the 60-mL syringe and fill it with ice water (30 °C).
4. Place the angiocatheter in the EAC and squirt the water in over a period of 30–40 s. The water should freely enter and exit the auditory canal.
   (a) The stimulus depends upon the temperature of the water and not on water pressure.
   (b) Reflex horizontal movements may be delayed for up to 1 min after irrigation of the EAC.
5. Observe: Have an assistant hold the eyelids open with the head still and facing forward.
   (a) Normal test: Cold water induces slight deviation of the eyes to the side being irrigated followed by a latent period of approximately 20 s and then nystagmus to the opposite side (direction of the fast phase).
   (b) Abnormal test: Eyes do not deviate; this implies brainstem problems.
   (c) The quick phase may return in patients in a persistent vegetative state. Search for the slow, full eye deviation in response to caloric stimulation and not nystagmus when assessing a comatose patient.
6. Pause at least 5 min so the auditory canal can warm up.
   (a) The same EAC can be irrigated with warm water if the contralateral side cannot be tested for any reason.
7. Repeat steps 3–5 in the opposite ear.
   (a) Warm water testing can be used if there is no response to cold water testing. Use warm water (44 °C) and repeat testing, starting with one ear and then, after 5 min, with the other ear.
   (b) Warm water induces nystagmus to the same side (direction of the fast phase).
   (c) COWS: Cold opposite, warm same (referring to the compensatory fast phase of eye movement, the nystagmus).
8. Dry the patient off and reexamine the tympanic membranes to assess for testing-related injury.

42.2.5 Complications: Caloric Reflex Testing

- If contraindications are excluded, no significant complications are expected.
- Tympanic membrane injury or EAC injury can occur from the angiocatheter, forceful irrigation, or injury during cerumen removal.
- Potential complications from caloric testing include meningitis, otitis media, and vomiting.

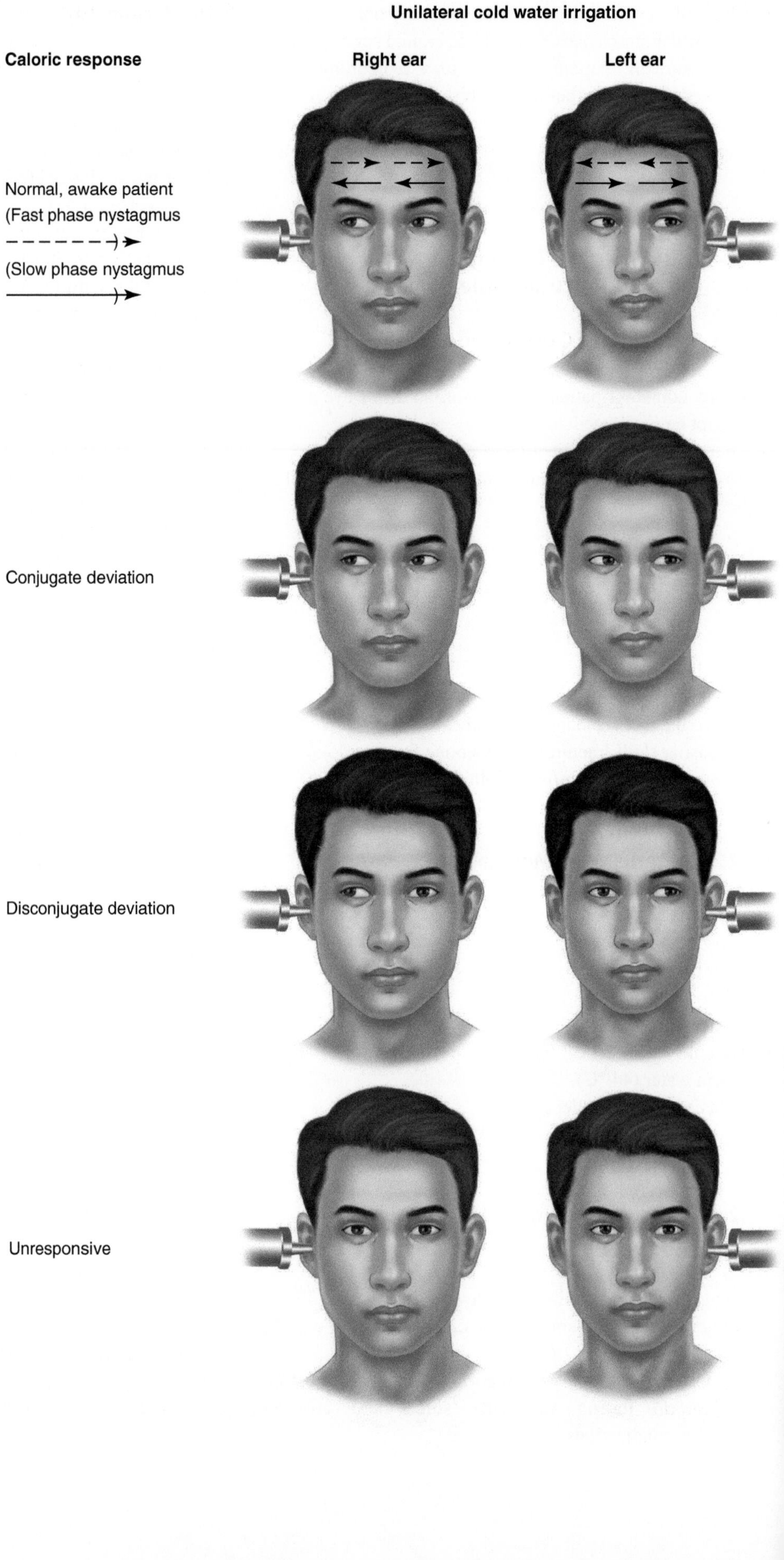

Fig. 42.2 Depiction of the vestibuloocular reflexes with unilateral cold-water irrigation

Unilateral cold water irrigation

Caloric response

Right ear   **Left ear**

Normal, awake patient
(Fast phase nystagmus
– – – – – –⟶➤
(Slow phase nystagmus
——————⟶➤

Conjugate deviation

Disconjugate deviation

Unresponsive

42.2.6 Pearls and Pitfalls: Caloric Reflex Testing

- A positive response to caloric testing indicates intact brainstem function.
- In an awake patient, excessive reflex vagal activity may occur (i.e., nausea, vomiting, dizziness).
- Absence of horizontal eye movement means comatose brainstem injury.
- Disconjugate or impaired reflex horizontal eye movements indicate impaired brainstem function at or below the level of the oculomotor nucleus.
- A comatose patient with intact full-reflex horizontal eye movements indicates that the lesion causing coma is in the cerebral hemisphere.

Selected Reading

Gomella LG. Central nervous system. In: Clinician's pocket reference. 11th ed. New York: McGraw-Hill; 2007.

McCann J, et al. Rapid assessment: a flowchart guide to signs and symptoms. Philadelphia: Lippincott William & Wilkins; 2004.

Reeve A, Swensen R. Auditory and vestibular function. In: Disorders of the nervous system: a primer. Hanover, NH: Dartmouth Medical School; On Line; 2009.

Reichman EF, Simon RR. Chapter 103. Reflex eye movements (caloric testing and doll's eyes). In: Emergency medicine procedures. New York: McGraw Hill Education; 2004.

Ropper AH, Samuels MA. Chapter 15. Deafness, dizziness, and disorders of equilibrium. Chapter 17. Coma and related disorders of consciousness. In: Adams and Victor's principles of neurology. 9th ed. New York: McGraw Hill; 2009.

Simon RP, Greenberg DA, Aminoff MJ. Chapter 3. Disorders of equilibrium. In: Clinical neurology. 7th ed. New York: McGraw Hill; 2009. http://www.accessmedicine.com.elibrary.einstein.yu.edu/content.aspx?aID=5146162.

Dix-Hallpike Maneuver

43

Rui Domingues and Muhammad Waseem

The Dix-Hallpike maneuver, also termed the "head-hanging positioning maneuver," is helpful in confirming the clinical suspicion of benign paroxysmal positional vertigo (BPPV). This maneuver provokes abnormal nystagmus, which is a characteristic feature of BPPV.

43.1 Indications

- BPPV is one of the most common types of vertigo.
  - The pathophysiology of BPPV, in brief, is believed to be due to free-moving densities (canaliths/otoliths) in the posterior semicircular canal; with head movement, the particles would alter the flow of the endolymph and cause the stimulation of the ampulla. The particles in the canal cause slow or even reversal of the movement of the cupula and create signals that do not correlate with the actual head movements, therefore causing the sensation of nystagmus.
  - This maneuver locates the cause of vertigo as either the inner ear or the brain; if the problem is in the ear, this maneuver helps localize which ear is affected.
- This maneuver is indicated for patients presenting with vertigo, which is evoked by a change in position and has no symptoms at rest.
- This maneuver is inexpensive, easily done, and part of the physical examination when a patient presents with the complaint of dizziness or vertigo.

R. Domingues, MD • M. Waseem, MD (✉)
Department of Emergency Medicine, Lincoln Medical and Mental Health Center, New York, NY, USA
e-mail: rbdomingues@hotmail.com; waseemm2001@hotmail.com

43.2 Contraindications

- Severe cervical spine disease.
- Unstable spinal injury.
- High-grade carotid stenosis.
- Unstable heart disease.
- Elderly patients may not tolerate this maneuver.
- There is no need to perform this test in the presence of nystagmus at rest.

43.3 Materials

- Examination table
- Flat cushion
- Frenzel goggles: These high-powered (+20 diopters) magnifying glasses can be placed on a patient during the performance of the maneuver and have shown to increase the sensitivity of the Dix-Hallpike maneuver by preventing the patient from visually fixating on an object, thereby preventing suppression of nystagmus. They are not required to perform the maneuver; they usually are used by specialists.

43.4 Procedure (Fig. 43.1)

1. Have the patient sit at the edge of a bed. The patient is instructed to maintain eye contact with the physician throughout the maneuver.
2. With the patient seated, the examiner will extend the neck, approximately 20°, and turn the head to one side, approximately 30–45°.
3. The examiner then assists the patient by lowering the patient quickly into a supine position, so that the head hangs over the edge of the bed or table, with the neck in a hyperextended position. A flat cushion can be placed

© Springer Science+Business Media New York 2016
L. Ganti (ed.), *Atlas of Emergency Medicine Procedures*, DOI 10.1007/978-1-4939-2507-0_43

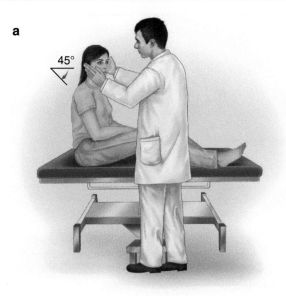

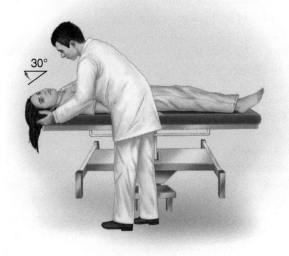

Fig. 43.1 (a) With the patient seated, the doctor will extend the neck, approximately 20°, and turn the head to one side, approximately 30–45°. (b) The physician then assists the patient by lowering the patient quickly into a supine position, so that the head hangs over the edge of the bed or table, with the neck in a hyperextended position

beneath the person's back in the shoulder blade area to assist with obtaining head extension.

4. This position is held, and the examiner observes for nystagmus for up to 60 s.
   (a) Nystagmus is a rapid, rhythmic movement of the eyes and usually appears after a brief period and lasts less than 30 s.
   (b) The direction of the nystagmus is usually up and twisted; therefore, the eyes will beat toward the ground.

(c) If the patient becomes dizzy or the doctor sees nystagmus, the test is positive for the ear that is pointed to the floor.
5. The patient is then returned to the upright position and is again observed for nystagmus for 30 s.
6. If nystagmus is not provoked, the maneuver is repeated with the head turned to the opposite direction.
7. If nystagmus is provoked, the patient should have the maneuver repeated to the same side.
   (a) With each repetition, the intensity and duration of nystagmus should decrease.

43.5 Complications

- Vertigo
- Nausea

43.6 Pearls and Pitfalls

- The maneuver can be uncomfortable to the patient because it can cause vertigo and nausea.

Selected Reading

Brandt T, Steddin S, Daroff RB. Therapy for benign paroxysmal positioning vertigo, revisited. Neurology. 1994;44:796–800.

Buckingham RA. Anatomical and theoretical observations on otolith repositioning for benign paroxysmal positional vertigo. Laryngoscope. 1999;109:717–22.

Fife TD, Iverson DJ, Lempert T, et al. Practice parameter: therapies for benign paroxysmal positional vertigo (evidence-based review): report of the Quality Standards Subcommittee of the American Academy of Neurology. Neurology. 2008;70:69–74.

Halker RB, Barrs DM, Wellik KE, Wingerchuck DM, Demaerschalk BM. Establishing a diagnosis of benign paroxysmal positional vertigo through the Dix-Hallpike and side-lying maneuvers: a critically appraised topic. Neurologist. 2008;14:201–4.

Herdman SJ. Treatment of benign paroxysmal vertigo. Phys Ther. 1990;70:381–8.

Lanska DJ, Remler B. Benign paroxysmal positioning vertigo: classic descriptions, origins of the provocative positioning technique and conceptual developments. Neurology. 1997;48:1167–77.

Li JC, Meyers AD. Benign paroxysmal positional vertigo. http://emedicine.medscape.com/article/884261-overview. Accessed December 20, 2015.

Von Brevern M, Radtke A, Lezius F, et al. Epidemiology of benign paroxysmal positional vertigo: a population based study. J Neurol Neurosurg Psychiatry. 2007;78:710–5.

Epley Maneuver for Vertigo (Particle Repositioning or Canalith Repositioning Procedure)

44

Rui Domingues and Muhammad Waseem

During the Dix-Hallpike test (see Chap. 43), the particles move in the canal and trigger a burst of upbeat-torsional nystagmus. The Epley maneuver causes resolution of positional nystagmus. This maneuver is effective in about 80 % of patients with benign paroxysmal positional vertigo (BPPV).

44.1 Indications

- Performed to alleviate the symptoms of posterior canal BPPV

44.2 Contraindications

- Back or spine injuries or other problems
- Presence of detached retina

44.3 Materials

- Pillow or pad
- Padded table or bed

44.4 Procedure (Fig. 44.1)

1. The patient is positioned on the bed with the head slightly extended and turned 45° to the affected side; hold this position for 60 s.

- The patient may hold the physician's arm for support.
2. The patient is then assisted by the physician to a supine position, with the head in extension, with a pillow or pad placed at the shoulder level allowing for extension; this position is held for a 60 s. This position will likely provoke transient dizziness and vertigo.
3. The head is then turned 90° to the opposite side; this position is held for 60 s. This position will likely provoke transient dizziness and vertigo.
4. The head is then turned through a further 90° while the patient rolls onto the unaffected side; this position is held for 60 s.
5. The patient then sits up slowly, by rolling up from lying on the unaffected side; this position is held for 60 s.
6. The patient should wait for 10–15 min before discharge.
7. Discharge instructions are then provided. Home instructions:
   - Instruct the patient to sleep in a semi-recumbent position for the next two nights; the patient should sleep at a 45° angle, which is most easily done by sleeping in a recliner or with several pillows arranged on a couch.
   - Sleep on the nonaffected side.
   - During the day, try to keep the head in a vertical position; no sudden head movements to the right, left, up, or down.
   - When men shave under their chins, they should bend their bodies forward in order to keep their heads vertical.
   - Do not go to the hairdresser or dentist because these require head movements.
   - Care should be taken when putting in eye drops because it requires head extension.
   - No vacuuming or mopping the floor.
   - Try not to wear clothing that needs to be pulled over the head. Try to avoid bending down to tie shoes.

R. Domingues, MD • M. Waseem, MD (✉)
Department of Emergency Medicine, Lincoln Medical and Mental
Health Center, New York, NY, USA
e-mail: rbdomingues@hotmail.com; waseemm2001@hotmail.com

© Springer Science+Business Media New York 2016
L. Ganti (ed.), *Atlas of Emergency Medicine Procedures*, DOI 10.1007/978-1-4939-2507-0_44

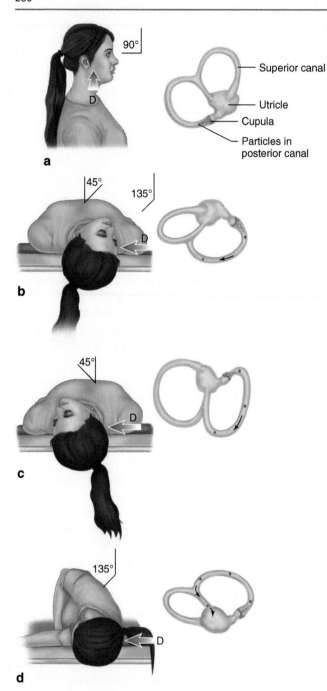

Fig. 44.1 (**a**) Patient seated on the table. (**b**) Patient in supine position, with the head turned 45° to the affected side. (**c**) Head then turned to the unaffected side (45°). (**d**) Head turned additional 90° on the unaffected side. *D* direction of view of labyrinth

44.5   Complications

When performing the previous maneuver, caution is advised should neurological symptoms occur. Occasionally such symptoms are caused by compression of the vertebral arteries; if it persists for a long period of time, a stroke can occur.

44.6   Pearls and Pitfalls

- Pearls
    - This maneuver should initially be performed by a trained therapist or medical physician.
    - It is best to perform the Epley maneuver before going to bed at night.
- Pitfalls
    - The patient should not drive herself or himself home after the procedure.
    - Avoid rapid changes in head position that might provoke BPPV.

Selected Reading

Harvey SA, Hain TC, Adamiec LC. Modified liberator maneuver: effective treatment for benign paroxysmal positional vertigo. Laryngoscope. 1994;104:1206–12.

Herdman SJ. Treatment of benign paroxysmal vertigo. Phys Ther. 1990;70:381–8.

Massoud EA, Ireland DJ. Post-treatment instructions in the nonsurgical management of benign paroxysmal positional vertigo. J Otolaryngol. 1996;25:121–5.

Parnes LS, Price-Jones RG. Particle repositioning maneuver for benign paroxysmal positional vertigo. Ann Otol Rhinol Laryngol. 1993;102:325–31.

Radtke A, Neuhausen H, von Brevern M, Lempert T. A modified Epley's procedure for self-treatment of benign paroxysmal positional vertigo. Neurology. 1999;53:1358–60.

Smouha EE. Time course of recovery after Epley maneuvers for benign paroxysmal positional vertigo. Laryngoscope. 1997;107:187–91.

Welling DB, Barnes DE. Particle repositioning maneuver for benign paroxysmal positional vertigo. Laryngoscope. 1994;104:946–9.

Clinical Brain Death Examination in Adults

45

Eric S. Papierniak, Hassan M. Alnuaimat, Tracy Timmons, and Deborah M. Stein

45.1 Indications

- Deep coma without any identifiable reversible causes
- Suspected brain death in a mechanically ventilated patient

45.2 Contraindications

- Metabolic derangements
- Acid-base disorders
- Electrolyte abnormalities sufficient to cause the coma
- Profound hypotension
- Hypothermia (core body temperature <36°C)
- Drug overdose or toxic exposure
- Locked-in syndrome

E.S. Papierniak (✉)
Division of Pulmonary, Critical Care, and Sleep Medicine,
Department of Medicine, University of Florida Health,
Gainesville, FL, USA

Malcom Randall VA Medical Center, Gainesville, FL, USA
e-mail: eric.papierniak@medicine.ufl.edu

H.M. Alnuaimat, MD
Department of Medicine, University of Florida, University of
Florida Health Shands Hospital, Gainesville, FL, USA
e-mail: Hassan.Alnuaimat@medicine.ufl.edu

T. Timmons, MD
Department of Trauma/Surgical Critical Care, R Adams Cowley
Shock Trauma Center, University of Maryland Medical Center,
Baltimore, MD, USA
e-mail: ttimmons1@umm.edu

D.M. Stein, MD, MPH
Department of Surgery, University of Maryland School of
Medicine, R Adams Cowley Shock Trauma Center, University of
Maryland Medical Center, Baltimore, MD, USA
e-mail: dstein@umm.edu

45.3 Materials and Medications

- A bright light
- Intravenous (IV) catheter
- 30-mL syringe
- 50-mL of ice water
- Endotracheal suction catheter
- Long swab or tongue depressor
- Gauze 4×4 or saline eye drops

45.4 Procedure

1. Evaluate the motor response to pain.
   - Apply pressure to the supraorbital nerve and nail beds. No motor response is consistent with brain death (Figs. 45.1 and 45.2).
2. Test for the absence of brainstem function.
   - Check pupillary response to bright light.
   - Check the oculocephalic reflex. With the eyelids held open, quickly turn the head to the side. The normal response is for the eyes to move in the opposite direction, maintaining the focus forward. Failure of the eyes to deviate during head rotation is consistent with brain death (Fig. 45.3).
   - Check the oculovestibular reflex with cold caloric testing. Elevate the head of the bed to 30°. Attach an IV catheter to the tip of a 30-mL syringe. Inject 50 mL of cold water into the external ear canal. Observe the pupils for 1 min for deviation toward the ear with the cold stimulus. Wait 5 min before testing the other side. No deviation of the pupils is consistent with brain death (Figs. 45.4 and 45.5).
   - Check for bulbar paralysis.
     - Check for a cough response to bronchial suctioning.

© Springer Science+Business Media New York 2016
.. Ganti (ed.), *Atlas of Emergency Medicine Procedures*, DOI 10.1007/978-1-4939-2507-0_45

- Stimulate the posterior pharynx with a long swab or tongue depressor and observe for a gag.
- Check the corneal reflex by lightly touching the cornea with a cotton swab, corner of gauze, or drops of sterile saline and observe for blinking of the eyelids (Fig. 45.6).

3. Check for respiratory effort by performing an apnea test. Before starting the apnea test, the following conditions must be met:

(a) The patient must not be hypothermic. The core temperature must be greater than 36°C.

(b) The patient must be hemodynamically stable with a systolic blood pressure greater than 90 mmHg.

(c) The arterial blood gas (ABG) must demonstrate a normal arterial partial pressure of carbon dioxide ($PaCO_2$). The arterial partial pressure of oxygen (PaO_2) may be elevated with preoxygenation to minimize the risk of hypoxemia prematurely ending the examination.

- Monitor the patient with a pulse oximeter.
- Disconnect the ventilator and deliver oxygen at 6 L/min by cannula into the endotracheal tube.
- Alternately the patient can remain connected to the ventilator with no applied support, which allows for an in-line negative pressure monitor to be attached to the circuit. Note: Most ventilators are too sensitive to be used as the sole method of sensing respiratory effort as they can produce false-negative results.
- Watch the chest and abdomen for respiratory motion, or monitor for negative inspiratory force on the pressure gauge. Check an ABG every 10 min and when the test ends.
- If the $PaCO_2$ increases by 20 mmHg or the $PaCO_2$ is greater than 60 mmHg and there was no respiratory effort, the test is consistent with brain death.

- The test must be aborted and the patient reconnected to mechanical ventilation if the patient becomes hypotensive, desaturates, or develops cardiac arrhythmias.
- If there is respiratory effort, the patient must be reconnected to mechanical ventilation (Figs. 45.7 and 45.8).

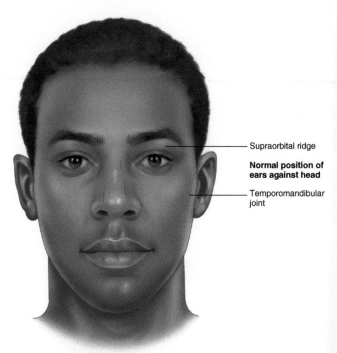

Supraorbital ridge

Normal position of ears against head

Temporomandibular joint

Fig. 45.1 Motor response to pain 1. Temporomandibular joint and supraorbital ridge test supraorbital nerve function

Fig. 45.2 Motor response to pain 2: Firm pressure can be applied to the nail beds with a penlight or similar instrument

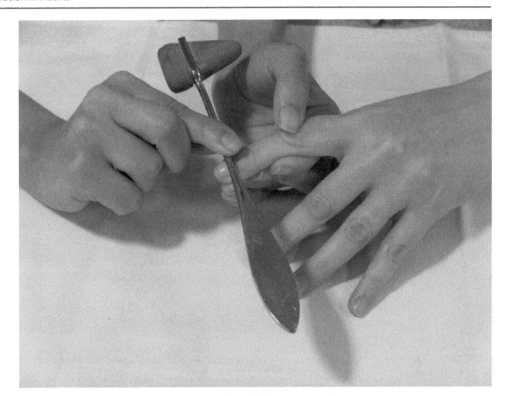

a Normal reaction: Eyes move side to side when head is turned

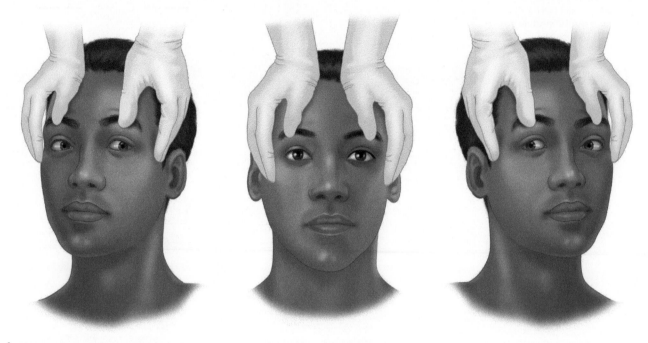

b Abnormal reaction: Eyes remain in fixed position in skull when head is turned

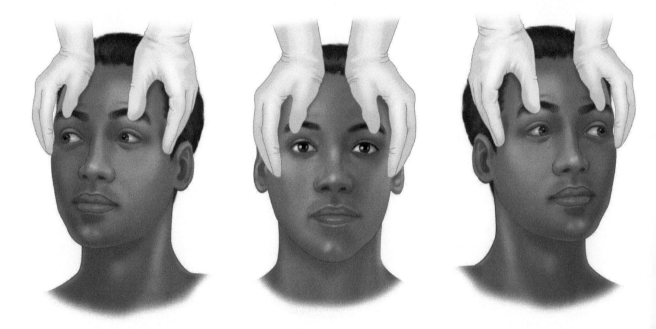

Fig. 45.3 (**a, b**) Oculocephalic reflex or "Doll's eyes." Movement of the eyes away from the direction of head turning (i.e., to keep the gaze forward) indicates intact functioning

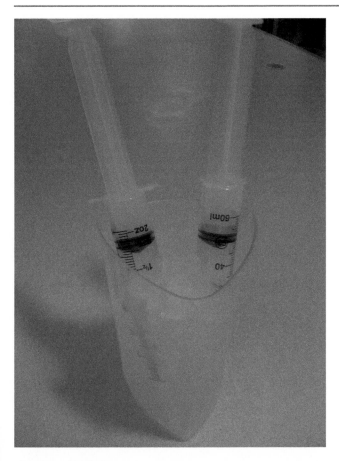

Fig. 45.4 Preparation of cold saline for testing of the oculovestibular reflex or "cold calorics"

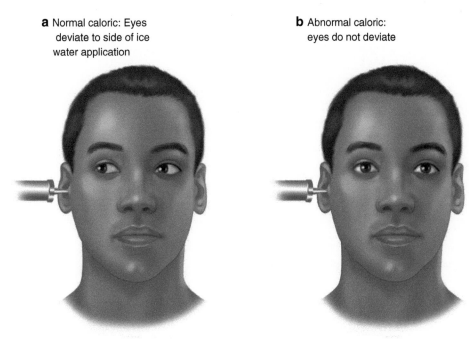

a Normal caloric: Eyes deviate to side of ice water application

b Abnormal caloric: eyes do not deviate

Fig. 45.5 (**a**, **b**) Oculovestibular reflex. Intact functioning is demonstrated by deviation of the gaze toward the side being tested

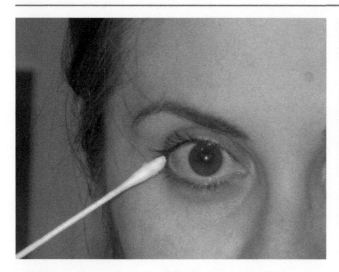

Fig. 45.6 Use of a cotton ball or unwound tip of a cotton swab for testing of the corneal reflex. A piece of sterile gauze ("4×4") is also commonly used

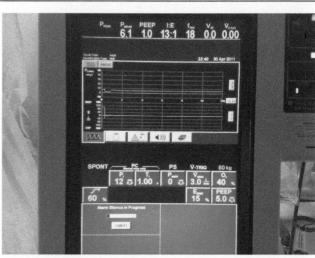

Fig. 45.8 Ventilator waveform in a patient without spontaneous respirations during the apnea test

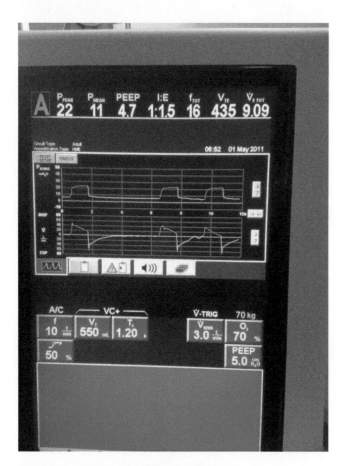

Fig. 45.7 Ventilator waveform before apnea test

45.5 Pearls and Pitfalls

- Pearls
  - The clinical examination should be performed by someone with experience or training in brain death examinations. Local regulations as well as hospital policies should be reviewed in order to determine the requirements for brain death. Some locales require a repeat examination by a different practitioner.
  - A patient with a cervical spine injury causing quadriplegia may not feel nail bed pressure and may be unable to respond to pain with more than facial movements.
- Pitfalls
  - Pupillary constriction less than 3 mm is not consistent with brain death.
  - Do not test oculocephalic reflex (doll's eyes) on patients who may have a cervical spinal cord injury from trauma.
  - Do not test the oculovestibular reflex with cold caloric testing in patients with a ruptured tympanic membrane.
  - A large number of patients may demonstrate spinal reflex movements during brain death. These reflexes may be triggered by touch, noxious stimuli, or removal of the ventilator. These movements can include plantar flexion, upper extremity posturing, eye opening, and the "Lazarus sign" (the arms raise off the bed and cross). Although these movements can be disconcerting to the health care team and family, they do not preclude a diagnosis of brain death.

45.6 Controversies

- Repeat examinations
  - The American Academy of Neurology guidelines recommend repeating the brain death examination at 6 h. The guidelines acknowledge that this is an arbitrary interval. Recent evidence suggests that the second examination may be unnecessary.

- Confirmatory Testing
  - Confirmatory testing is an option if specific elements of the clinical examination cannot be performed. For example, a trauma patient with suspected cervical spinal cord injuries precluding the oculocephalic reflex test would be a candidate for confirmatory testing.
  - Conventional cerebral angiography will demonstrate no filling beyond the carotid bifurcation or within the circle of Willis. Electroencephalography demonstrates no electrical activity. Transcranial Doppler ultrasonography will demonstrate vascular resistance associated with elevated intracranial pressure. Technetium-99m hexamethylpropylene-amine oxime brain scans demonstrate the "hollow skull" sign or no uptake of isotope in the brain (Fig. 45.9).
  - Newer modalities of confirmatory testing include computed tomography (CT) angiography and magnetic resonance imaging/magnetic resonance angiography (MRI/MRA). These tests are being used in some hospitals; however, the recent review by the American Academy of Neurology finds evidence insufficient to recommend using these newer modalities to confirm brain death.

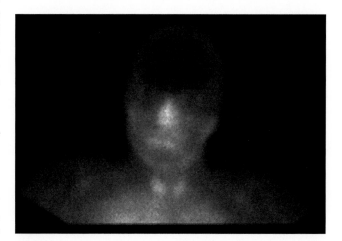

Fig. 45.9 "Empty skull sign" on nuclear medicine flow study confirms brain death

Selected Reading

A definition of irreversible coma: report of the Ad Hoc Committee of the Harvard Medical School to Examine the Definition of Brain Death. JAMA. 1968;205:337–40.

Lustbader D, O'Hara D, Wijdicks EF, et al. Second brain death examination may negatively affect organ donation. Neurology. 2011;76:119–24.

Practice parameters for determining brain death in adults (summary statement). The quality standards subcommittee of the American Academy of Neurology. Neurology. 1995;45:1012–4.

Saposnik G, Maurino J, Saizar R, Bueri JA. Spontaneous and reflex movements in 107 patients with brain death. Am J Med. 2005;118:311–4.

Wijdicks EF. Current concepts: the diagnosis of brain death. N Engl J Med. 2001;344:1215–21.

Wijdicks EF, Varelas PN, Gronseth GS, Greer DM, American Academy of Neurology. Evidence-based guideline update: determining brain death in adults: report of the Quality Standards Subcommittee of the American Academy of Neurology. Neurology. 2010;74:1911–8.

Part VII

Ophthalmic Procedures

Slit Lamp Examination

Bobby K. Desai

46.1 Indications

- A slit lamp magnifies structures of the eye (Fig. 46.1).
- Gives the operator a three-dimensional view of the area visualized.
- Used to delineate abnormalities that cannot be visualized by other means.
- Helpful in foreign body removal.

B.K. Desai, MD
Department of Emergency Medicine, University of Florida Health
Shands Hospital, Gainesville, FL, USA
e-mail: bdesai@ufl.edu

© Springer Science+Business Media New York 2016
L. Ganti (ed.), *Atlas of Emergency Medicine Procedures*, DOI 10.1007/978-1-4939-2507-0_46

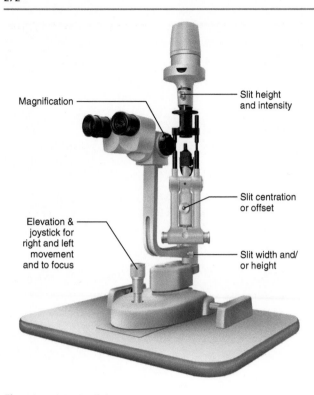

Fig. 46.1 A basic slit lamp

Magnification

Slit height
and intensity

Slit centration
or offset

Elevation &
joystick for
right and left
movement
and to focus

Slit width and/
or height

46.2 Contraindications

- Not to be used in patients who cannot tolerate an upright posture (e.g., trauma patients).
  - In these cases if a slit lamp examination is required, a portable slit lamp may be beneficial (Fig. 46.2).

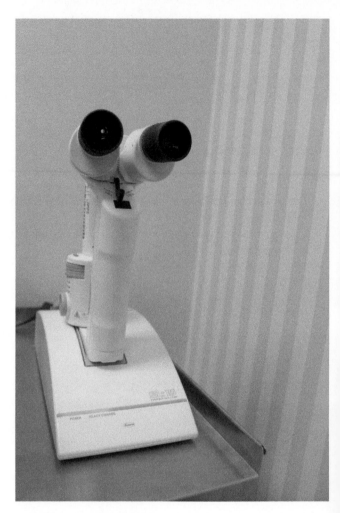

Fig. 46.2 A portable slit lamp

46.3   Materials

- The slit lamp is an eye-specific binocular stereoscope specifically designed to examine the eye and its structures and gives the practitioner a three-dimensional assessment of the eye.
- The operator has full movement of the microscope in all directions and the apparatus can be locked in place if required.
- Its light source can be manipulated to change the characteristics of the beam from its intensity to the angle at which it projects (Fig. 46.3).
  - A low-power setting is typically used for normal examination.
  - A higher-intensity beam is used when evaluating the anterior chamber with a narrow slit beam.
- It has colored filters typically built within the slit lamp.
  - Cobalt blue: Used with fluorescein dye to evaluate for corneal abrasions (Fig. 46.4) and avulsions; the dye will collect where the corneal epithelium is absent. It results in a yellow glow or hue visible through the microscope.
  - Green filter: Used to increase contrast of blood vessels. They appear black and the filter is useful for the assessment of hemorrhage.
- The operator is able to adjust the magnification of the microscopic typically through dial controls.
  - Low magnifications are most helpful for general examination.
  - Higher magnifications are used for examination of a particular area in fine detail.

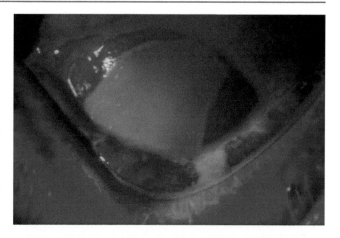

Fig. 46.4 Example of a corneal abrasion seen with a cobalt blue filter (With kind permission from Springer Science + Business Media: Das S, Chohan A, Snibson GR, Taylor HR. Capsicum spray injury of the eye. *International Ophthalmology*. 2005;26(4–5):171–3)

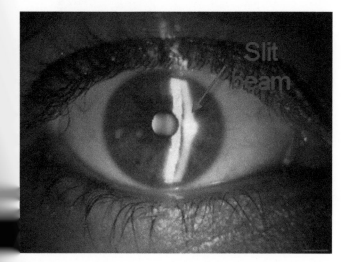

Fig. 46.3 The slit lamp beam and the reflection of the beam

46.4 Procedure

1. As part of a complete eye examination, informed consent is not generally required.
2. An explanation of the procedure and reassurance are helpful.
3. Lock the slit lamp before positioning the patient because unintended movement may inadvertently damage the equipment or cause injury to the operator or patient.
4. The apparatus has a chin and a head rest. Ask the patient to place the chin and forehead in the respective areas (Fig. 46.5).
5. Adjust the height of the apparatus and the patient's chair for optimum comfort (Figs. 46.6 and 46.7). It may be necessary for children to stand during the examination.
6. The patient may place his or her hands on the sides of the table that the lamp is mounted on; this ensures stability of both the lamp and the patient.
7. Adjust the eyepieces of the microscope to fit the operator.
8. Turn on the slit lamp at its lowest setting to avoid a sudden power surge that could potentially damage the bulb.
9. Move the stage forward and narrow the beam and angle it at 45° to the patient. Aim the beam laterally so as not to cause the patient discomfort.
10. Focus the beam by manipulating the joystick to move the apparatus forward and backward so that the beam is clearly visible and its lines are sharp.
11. For each area of the eye to be examined, inspect the area thoroughly using the joystick to slowly manipulate the slit lamp across the eye in all directions, using the height adjustment of the joystick to slightly raise and lower the slit lamp as needed.
    - The operator may find that the slit lamp may move too freely; in that case she or he may find slightly tightening the locking nut of the C-arm may provide better and more precise control.

Fig. 46.5 Appropriate positioning for a slit lamp examination

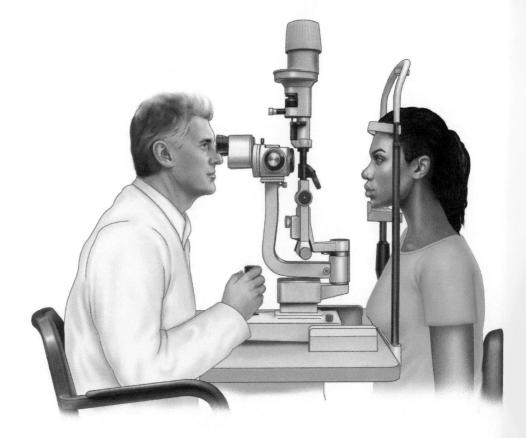

Fig. 46.6 The slit lamp is too high

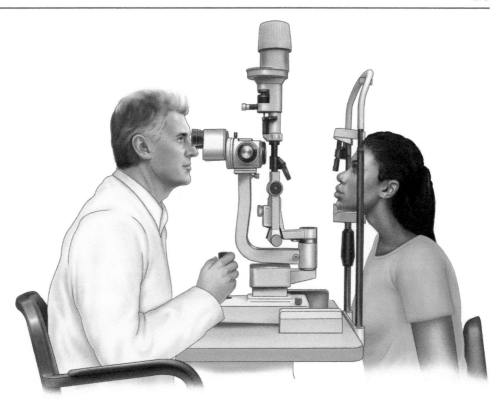

Fig. 46.7 The slit lamp is too low

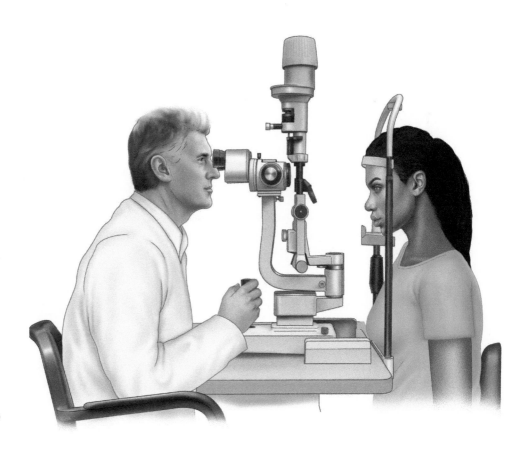

46.5 Complications

There are no complications following routine slit lamp examination.

46.6 Pitfalls

- Ensure a working bulb.
- Appropriately set the microscope's oculars for the operator's pupillary distance.
- Ensure all dials and knobs are firmly set.
- Inadequate focusing
- Patient noncompliance

46.7 Fluorescein Testing

46.7.1 Indications and Uses

- Examination of the cornea under a cobalt blue filter on a slit lamp or Wood's lamp: The chemical fluoresces under blue light and appears green under these circumstances.
- Useful for detecting corneal abrasions, corneal foreign bodies, and infections of the eye.

46.7.2 Procedure

- Fluorescein is typically used after installation of a topical anesthetic, which provides patient comfort especially for those with significant pathology.
- The fluorescein strip comes packaged in single-use wrappers (Fig. 46.8).
- Hold the strip by the white end and wet the orange end *lightly* because heavily moistening the strip may cause a significant amount of dye to be present, obscuring the examination.
  - A dry strip may be used, but it may irritate the patient's eye especially if already sensitive.
- If this occurs, the clinician may use tissue paper to gently blot the excess solution away.
  - The exception to this is the performance of the *Seidel test*, which is used to assess the eye for potential perforation (Fig. 46.9).
  - The clinician will instill a large amount of dye into the eye by wetting the orange strip copiously.
  - The clinician will next examine the eye for a stream of fluid leaking from the ruptured globe.

- This stream will fluoresce green or blue in distinction to the rest of the globe, which appears orange.
- The choice of solution to wet fluorescein strip is up to the clinician because saline, tap water, or the recently used anesthetic solution may be used safely.
- Place the now-wet orange end on the lower lid of the patient's eye.
- Ask the patient to blink several times to allow the solution to spread evenly.
- The clinician may use a Wood's lamp, penlight, or the cobalt blue filter on the slit lamp to examine the now-stained eye.
  - The slit lamp is preferable owing to the potential for missing small abrasions.

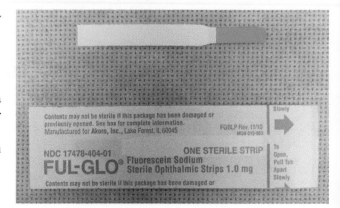

Fig. 46.8 A typical fluorescein strip package

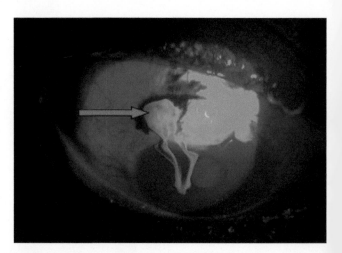

Fig. 46.9 A positive Seidel test (Reproduced with permission from: Lingam V, Panday M, George R, Shantha B. Management of complications in glaucoma surgery. *Indian J Ophthalmol.* 2011;59(Suppl1): S131–40)

46.7.3 Complications

- There is a theoretical risk of the development of superficial punctate keratitis from instillation of topical anesthetic before fluorescein testing.
- Discoloration of soft contact lenses.
- Potential for infection using premixed fluorescein solution.

46.7.4 Pitfalls

- Contact lens wearers should remove their lenses because the fluorescein will permanently stain the lens.
  - The wearer should not put the contacts back in for several hours.

Selected Reading

DuBois L. The slit lamp examination. In: DuBois L, Ledford JK, Daniels K, Campbell R, editors. Clinical skills for the ophthalmic examination: basic procedures. 2nd ed. Thorofare: Slack; 2006. p. 61–70.

Galor A, Jeng BH. Red eye for the internist: when to treat, when to refer. Cleve Clin J Med. 2008;75:137–44.

Lang GK. Ophthalmology: a short textbook. Stuttgart: Thieme; 2000.

Ledford JK, Sanders VN. The slit lamp primer. 2nd ed. Thorofare: Slack; 2006.

Eye Irrigation

Bobby K. Desai

47.1 Indications

Chemical burns to the eye
Removal of superficial foreign bodies

47.2 Contraindications

For suspected globe perforation, extreme care must be taken to not exacerbate the injury.

47.3 Materials and Medications

- Irrigating device—the Morgan lens (Fig. 47.1)
- Saline solution or lactated Ringer's (preferably warmed)
- Topical anesthetic drops (Fig. 47.2)
- Basin to secure the extruded solution
- Intravenous (IV) tubing to attach the IV bag to the Morgan lens
- pH paper (Fig. 47.3)

B.K. Desai, MD
Department of Emergency Medicine, University of Florida Health
Shands Hospital, Gainesville, FL, USA
e-mail: bdesai@ufl.edu

© Springer Science+Business Media New York 2016
B. Ganti (ed.), *Atlas of Emergency Medicine Procedures*, DOI 10.1007/978-1-4939-2507-0_47

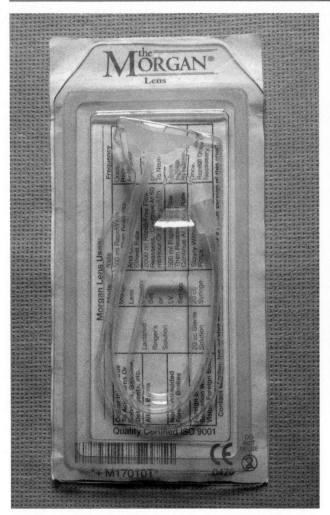

Fig. 47.1 The Morgan lens and packaging

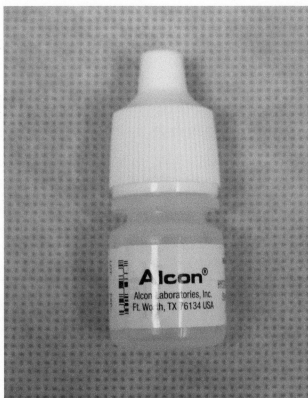

Fig. 47.2 Examples of topical anesthetics

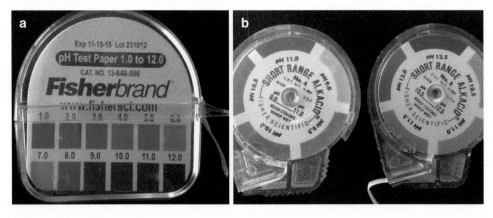

Fig. 47.3 (**a**, **b**) Examples of pH paper

47.4 Procedure

1. Informed consent is generally not required, although a thorough explanation to the patient is warranted.
2. Obtain pH of the eye *before* instilling anesthetic drops.
3. Anesthetize the eye(s) with topical anesthetic of choice by instilling drops within the lower lid and then asking the patient to blink several times in order to evenly distribute the solution.
4. Ensure there are no foreign bodies on the inside of the upper lids by inverting the upper lid.
   • Particulate foreign bodies may be removed with moistened cotton tip applicators.
5. After adequate anesthesia is ensured, place one end of the Morgan lens within the fornix of the upper lid (Fig. 47.4).

6. Next, gently retracting the lower lid will ensure smooth placement of the remaining portion of the Morgan lens (Fig. 47.5).
7. Using the end of the Morgan lens, screw in the prepared IV tubing (Fig. 47.6).
8. Attach the end of the IV tubing to the saline bag and place at height to allow for gravity to ensure a smooth flow of solution.
   • Continue to irrigate the eye until desired pH is obtained.
9. To remove the Morgan lens, use the opposite technique for insertion.

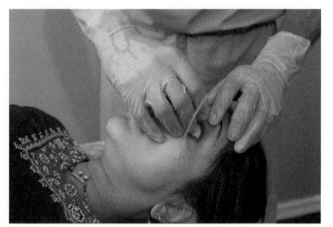

Fig. 47.4 Inserting the Morgan lens under the upper lid

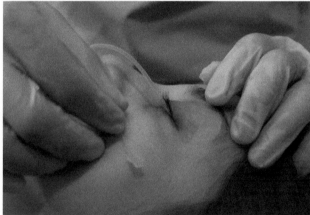

Fig. 47.6 The Morgan lens in place, ready to be attached to IV tubing for saline irrigation

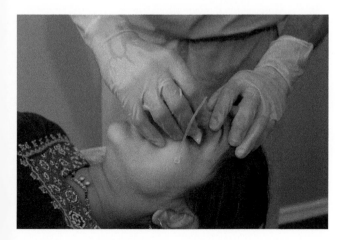

Fig. 47.5 Inserting the Morgan lens under lower lid

47.5 Complications

- Corneal abrasions may be caused by the Morgan lens and are treated in the usual fashion.
- Deep corneal injury may occur with inadequate irrigation.

47.6 Pearls and Pitfalls

- Note that alkali burns will require significant irrigation and more topical anesthesia may be required.

- Ophthalmological consultation may be required, especially for alkaline and hydrofluoric acid burns.

Selected Reading

Lang GK. Ophthalmology: a short textbook. Stuttgart: Thieme; 2000.

Rhee DJ, Pyfer MF, Rhee DM, editors. The Wills Eye manual: office and emergency room diagnosis and treatment of eye disease. 3rd ed. Philadelphia: Lippincott Williams & Wilkins; 1999.

Corneal Foreign Body Removal

Bobby K. Desai

48.1 Indications

- Presence of a corneal foreign body (Fig. 48.1)

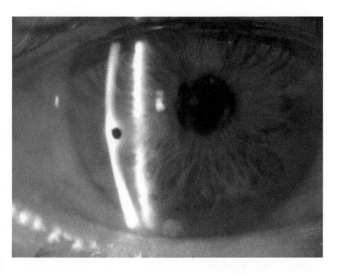

Fig. 48.1 Corneal foreign body (With kind permission from Springer Science+Business Media: Zuberbuhler B, Tuft S, Gartry D, Spokes D. Ocular Surface and Reconstructive Surgery. In: *Corneal Surgery*. 2013. 29–48)

48.2 Contraindications

- An uncooperative patient may require ophthalmological consultation as well as sedation.
- Suspected foreign bodies from high-velocity injuries must be referred to an ophthalmologist subsequent to initial evaluation.
- Any signs of globe penetration (e.g., hyphema) require emergent ophthalmological consultation.
- Overt globe rupture.
- Evidence of an inflammatory process such as iritis requires emergent ophthalmological consultation.
- Foreign bodies associated with corneal burns secondary to chemical exposure such as alkaline corneal burns will require emergent ophthalmological consultation.

B.K. Desai, MD
Department of Emergency Medicine, University of Florida Health
Shands Hospital, Gainesville, FL, USA
e-mail: bdesai@ufl.edu

© Springer Science+Business Media New York 2016
L. Ganti (ed.), *Atlas of Emergency Medicine Procedures*, DOI 10.1007/978-1-4939-2507-0_48

48.3   Materials and Medications

- Eye chart for visual assessment
- Cotton tip applicator
- Slit lamp or other source of magnification
- 27-Gauge needle or ophthalmic foreign body needle (Fig. 48.2)
- Topical ophthalmic anesthetic
- Ophthalmic burr (Fig. 48.3)

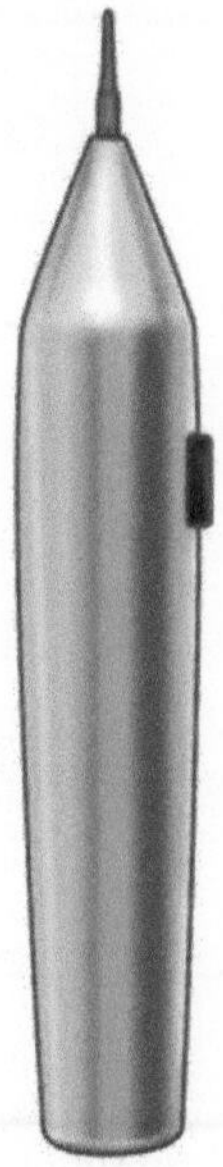

Fig. 48.3   Ophthalmic burr drill

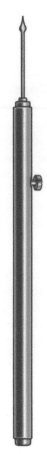

Fig. 48.2   Foreign body needle

48.4 Procedure

1. Informed consent may be required.
2. Visual acuity and a formal assessment of the eye should be done and documented.
3. Consider intraocular foreign body.
   - Computed tomography (CT) scan may be used to assess for the presence of an intraocular foreign body.
4. Eversion of the upper lid should be performed to evaluate for retained foreign body under the lid.
   - These usually can be removed by:
     - A moistened cotton tip applicator
     - Irrigation
5. Magnification is preferable, but some foreign bodies may be large enough to see with the naked eye.
6. Anesthetize the eye with topical anesthetic.
7. For multiple loose foreign bodies, removal may be attempted with irrigation after appropriate anesthesia.
8. Removal of the foreign body may be attempted with a moistened cotton swab.
   - Metallic foreign bodies recently embedded within the cornea may be difficult to remove in this fashion.
   - However, during the healing process, some metallic foreign bodies may be pushed closer to the surface during reepithelialization of the cornea. These potentially can be removed with this technique.
     - Care must be taken to avoid leaving a rust ring that could permanently stain the cornea.
9. A 27-gauge needle bent at a 90° angle may be used to remove foreign bodies by gently prying it out.
   - An advantage of using a needle is that any rust ring as well as any metallic foreign body can potentially be removed.
10. Technique: A slit lamp may be used to magnify the area.
    - See slit lamp chapter (Chap. 46) for details.
    - The patient should be informed about the procedure; formal informed consent may not be required.
    - Proper positioning is critical for success.
    - The patient's head should be fully forward and firmly placed against the head rest.
    - The patient's hands may be placed on the sides of the slit lamp stage for stabilization.
    - Apply topical anesthesia to the cornea.
11. Using the patient's cheek as a bolster potentially avoids significant movement of the needle if the patient unexpectedly moves.
    - Other modalities for stabilization include supporting the elbow by placing on a box or using towels.
12. Have the patient gaze at one point in the far distance.
    - Using the needle or burr as a scoop, gently manipulate the foreign body out.
      - Using a burr can allow for the total removal of any rust ring.
13. Once the foreign body is removed, patching is not required.
14. Consider application of topical antibiotics.
15. Tetanus prophylaxis should be given as for open other wounds.
16. Arrange follow-up with a primary care physician or preferably an ophthalmologist.

48.5 Complications

- Forceful attempts to dislodge a foreign body may result in corneal perforation.
- Incomplete removal of a foreign body.

Selected Reading

Lang GK. Ophthalmology: a short textbook. Stuttgart: Thieme; 2000.

Rhee DJ, Pyfer MF, Rhee DM, editors. The Wills eye manual: office and emergency room diagnosis and treatment of eye disease. 3rd ed. Philadelphia: Lippincott Williams & Wilkins; 1999.

Thomas SH, White BA. Foreign bodies. In: Marx J, Hockberger R, Walls R, editors. Rosen's emergency medicine: concepts and clinical practice. 7th ed. Philadelphia: Mosby; 2010. p. 715–32.

Ultrasound Evaluation of Retinal Detachment

49

Shalu S. Patel, L. Connor Nickels, and Rohit Pravin Patel

49.1 Indications

- To aid in the evaluation of vision loss or change in vision

49.2 Contraindications

- Relative: Suspicion of increased intraocular pressure
- Relative: Suspicion of globe rupture (see Chap. 50)

49.3 Materials and Medications

- Bedside ultrasound machine with high-frequency (7.5- to 10-MHz) linear transducer
- Transparent adhesive such as Tegaderm (optional)
- Sterile ultrasound gel
- Sterile gauze

49.4 Procedure

1. Position the patient supine with his or her eyes closed. The eyelid may be taped closed with a transparent adhesive if desired (Fig. 49.1).
2. Place a liberal amount of ultrasound gel over the eyelid.
3. Place the ultrasound probe over the eye in a transverse position.
4. Adjust the depth of the ultrasound so that the whole eye fills the screen.
5. Scan through the eye fully in the transverse and sagittal planes.
6. When viewing the ultrasound image, the normal eye is a circular hypoechoic structure (Fig. 49.2). The structures should be evaluated from anterior to posterior.
7. Identify the cornea. This is the first thin hypoechoic line in the anterior eye.
8. Continuing posteriorly, identify the anterior chamber, which is an anechoic area bordered by the cornea, iris, and lens. The iris is an echogenic linear structure, and the normal lens is anechoic.
9. Identify the vitreous chamber, the large anechoic region posterior to the lens.
10. Carefully evaluate the posterior globe. The normal retina cannot be distinguished from the other choroidal layers on ultrasound.
11. A detached retina will appear as a hyperechoic linear floating membrane in the posterior vitreous chamber (Fig. 49.3).
12. In the retrobulbar region, the optic nerve can be identified as a hypoechoic linear structure perpendicular to the globe (Fig. 49.3).

S.S. Patel, MD
Department of Emergency Medicine, Florida Hospital Tampa,
Florida Hospital Carrollwood, Tampa, FL, USA
e-mail: shalu314@gmail.com

L.C. Nickels, MD, RDMS (✉) • R.P. Patel, MD
Department of Emergency Medicine, University of Florida Health
Shands Hospital, Gainesville, FL, USA
e-mail: cnickels@ufl.edu; rohitpatel@ufl.edu

© Springer Science+Business Media New York 2016
L. Ganti (ed.), *Atlas of Emergency Medicine Procedures*, DOI 10.1007/978-1-4939-2507-0_49

Fig. 49.1 Probe positioning with Tegaderm applied to orbit: (**a**) sagittal view, (**b**) axial view

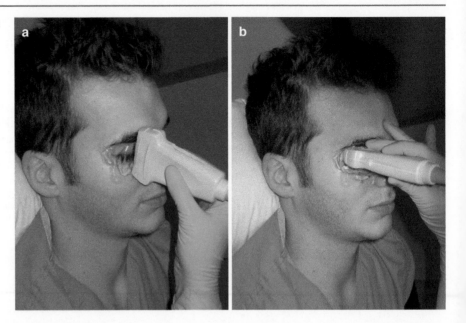

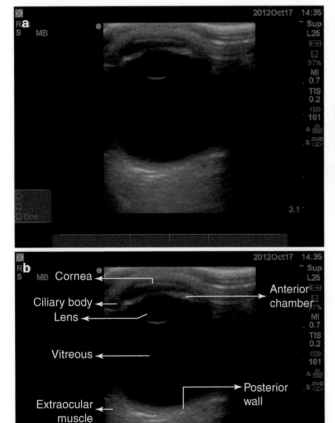

Fig. 49.2 Ocular ultrasound with normal anatomy findings ((**a**) without labels, (**b**) with anatomy labeled)

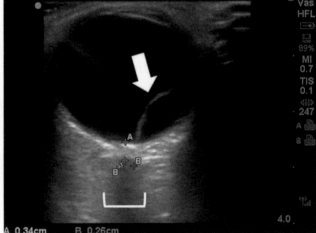

Fig. 49.3 Retinal detachment appears as a hyperechoic linear structure (*white arrow*). *White* bracket shows the optic nerve sheath shadow (see Chap. 50 for more information)

49.5   Complications

- Conjunctival infection
- Increased intraocular pressure (if too much pressure is applied)

49.6   Pearls and Pitfalls

- Pearls
  - Use a transparent adhesive such as Tegaderm to decrease the risk of conjunctival infection.
  - Use a liberal amount of gel to obtain the best images.
  - Use minimal pressure to obtain the best images.
  - False positives on ocular ultrasound may occur with disk edema or vitreous hemorrhage.

- Pitfalls
  - Subacute retinal detachments may be missed on ocular ultrasound.

Selected Reading

Blaivas M. Bedside emergency department ultrasonography in the evaluation of ocular pathology. Acad Emerg Med. 2000;7:947–50.

Blaivas M, Theodoro D, Sierzenski PR. Elevated intracranial pressure detected by bedside emergency ultrasonography of the optic nerve sheath. Acad Emerg Med. 2003;4:376–81.

Shinar Z, Chan L, Orlinksy M. Use of ocular ultrasound for the evaluation of retinal detachment. J Emerg Med. 2011;4:53–7.

Whitcomb MB. How to diagnose ocular abnormalities with ultrasound. AAEP Proc. 2002;48:272–5.

Ultrasonography in the Evaluation of Intraocular Pathology

Benjamin M. Mahon, Marie-Carmelle Elie,
L. Connor Nickels, and Rohit Pravin Patel

50.1 Indications

- Eye trauma
- Loss of vision or decreased vision
- Head injury
- Ocular pain
- Suspected foreign body

50.2 Contraindications

- None

50.3 Materials

- Linear probe (7.5–10 MHz)
- Tegaderm or other protective eye covering
- Copious amounts of water-soluble transmission gel

50.4 Procedure

1. Begin by asking the patient to close her or his eye, and then apply the Tegaderm or other suitable eye cover over both eyes.
2. Apply a copious amount of transmission jelly over both eyes.
3. Gently apply the ultrasound probe to the outer eyelid. If the operator has used a sufficient enough amount of jelly, the probe itself should not need to be in actual contact with the eyelid. This becomes of critical importance in suspected globe trauma or intraocular foreign body, when excess manipulation of the intraocular contents could precipitate further damage or worsening of present damage. Ensure the pressure is gentle enough to prevent this, but sufficient to obtain good imaging (see Chap. 49).
4. Image the normal eye first, to become familiar with the patient's anatomy (see Chap. 49), before proceeding to the suspected abnormal eye.
5. Start with low gain.
6. Ask the patient to move the eye slowly from the left to the right. This is called kinetic echography and will provide information elaborated upon later. Have the patient keep her or his eye straight ahead, as the operator phases up and down and side to side, between the transverse and the sagittal planes.
7. Increase gain slowly while the patient is moving the eye. Shifting from low gain to higher gain during the examination will help to prevent overlooking certain disease processes. As a fluid-filled structure, the eye provides its own acoustic window, and imaging is generally easy.

50.5 Complications

- Through excessive pressure applied to the eye, as described previously, further disruption of the intraocular contents and worsening of preexisting injury can occur.

50.6 Pearls and Pitfalls

- Pitfalls
  - Applying too much pressure to the globe and disrupting already damaged intraocular contents
  - Failing to image with full spectrum of gain
  - Using an insufficient amount of gel

B.M. Mahon, MD
Ponciana Medical Center, Kissimmee, FL, USA
e-mail: faust2k9@ufl.edu

M.-C. Elie, MD, RDMS (✉) • L.C. Nickels, MD, RDMS
R.P. Patel, MD
Department of Emergency Medicine, University of Florida Health
Shands Hospital, Gainesville, FL, USA
e-mail: elie@ufl.edu; cnickels@ufl.edu; rohitpatel@ufl.edu

© Springer Science+Business Media New York 2016
L. Ganti (ed.), *Atlas of Emergency Medicine Procedures*, DOI 10.1007/978-1-4939-2507-0_50

50.7 Specific Disease Processes/ Pathology [1]

50.7.1 Vitreous Hemorrhage (Fig. 50.1)

- Best seen in high gain.
- Clinical: Very common pathology. Seen as "floaters" on the visual field. Can cause blindness if large.
- Ultrasound: Appearance may vary. Early on in the evolution of a hemorrhage, these can be seen as small dots or mobile linear opacities that float freely in the back of the posterior chamber with eye movement. Has been described as a "snow-storm appearance." As hemorrhage ages, the blood organizes and membranes form, sometimes layering inferiorly owing to gravity.

50.7.2 Vitreous Detachment

- Best seen with higher gain.
- Clinical: Common in older patients. Presents as "flashers." Vitreous gel loses its attachment from the internal membrane lining.
- Ultrasound: Seen as "swaying seaweed." There are layering opacifications. Also seen as "snow-globe appearance." Concurrent vitreous hemorrhage is also common.
- Note: A small percentage of patients also have a retinal tear, so ophthalmology follow-up is necessary.

50.7.3 Retinal Detachment (Figs. 50.2 and 50.3)

- Best seen with lower gain.
- Clinical: Acute loss of vision, usually painless, often preceded by "flashers" and/or "floaters" as the neurosensory component of the retina pulls away from the retinal pigment epithelium. *An ophthalmological emergency.* Can be caused by ocular trauma or no known precipitant at all.
- Ultrasound: Seen as a taut, hyperechoic, linear opacity that moves with the eye, attached to the optic disc, in the posterior region of the globe.

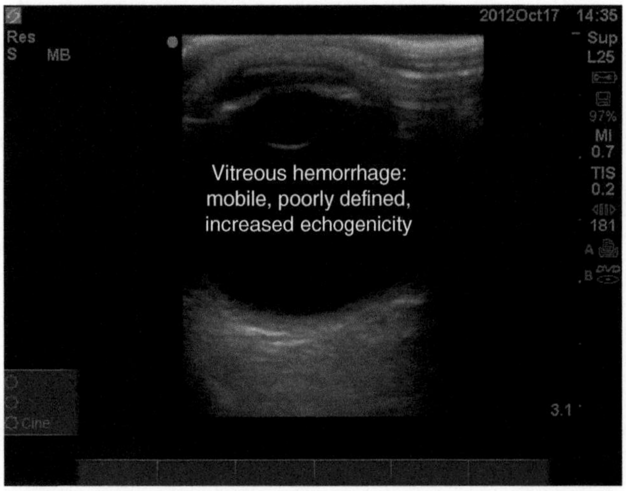

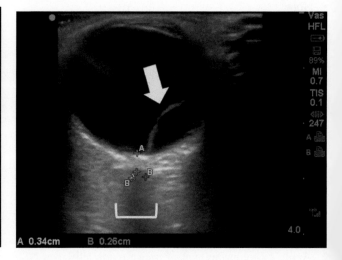

Fig. 50.1 Vitreous hemorrhage

Fig. 50.2 Retinal detachment ultrasound image

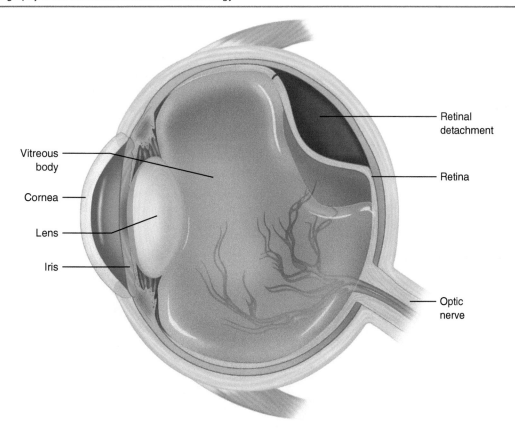

Fig. 50.3   Retinal detachment graphical representation

50.7.4 Intraocular Foreign Body (Fig. 50.4)

- Clinical: Usually a preceding episode of trauma, often from metalworking or landscaping.
- Ultrasound: Foreign bodies are seen as hyperechoic substances in the eye often with distal shadowing. Certain shadow patterns distal to the foreign body, as well as comet tails, can help to differentiate the type of foreign body material.

50.7.5 Globe Rupture (Fig. 50.5)

- Clinical: Usually the result of trauma. Frequently, the mechanism causing the injury has subsequently made the eye examination itself impossible, if edema, blepharospasm, hyphema, or distorted anatomy makes visualization of the posterior chamber too difficult. In these circumstances ultrasound can be immeasurably helpful.
- Ultrasound: Findings include decreased size of the anterior chamber, posterior chamber, or both, often with buckled sclera. Globe rupture should be suspected when the injury mechanism is present and any major distortion of the ocular anatomy is appreciated.

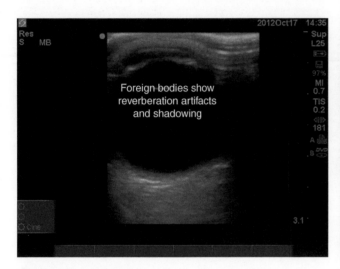

Fig. 50.4 Foreign bodies

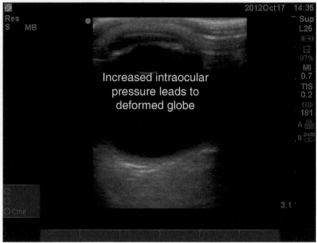

Fig. 50.5 Globe rupture

50.7.6 Increased ICP

- Clinical: Increased ICP is encountered in a number of pathological processes, such as closed head injury from trauma, altered mental status, pseudotumor cerebri, space-occupying lesion, or any other process causing intracranial injury. Physical examination may be suggestive of an intracranial process, but often key examination findings such as papilledema are not appreciated, owing to both limitations from the patient and their mental status, as well as limitations in the skill of the ED doctor, or the ability to dilate the eyes sufficiently, to appreciate the finding.

- Ultrasound: The size of the *optic nerve sheath diameter* is an indirect measurement of ICP. It is visualized as a hypoechoic linear strip radiating posteriorly from the edge of the back of the globe. A normal diameter is 5.0 mm or less. This measurement is taken at 3 mm back from the posterior edge of the globe (Fig. 50.6). Take measurements bilaterally to compare. Two or more measurements should be taken and then averaged on each side.

- A diameter greater than 5.0 mm, at 3.0 mm distal from the posterior globe border, is strongly suggestive of increased ICP and warrants further evaluation and imaging [2].

References

1. Blaivas M, Theodoro D, Sierzenski P. A study of bedside ocular ultrasonography in the emergency department. Acad Emerg Med. 2002;9:791–9.
2. Blaivas M, Theodoro D, Sierzenski P. Elevated intracranial pressure detected by bedside emergency ultrasonography of the optic nerve sheath. Acad Emerg Med. 2003;10:376–81.

Selected Reading

Mustafa M, Montgomery J, Atta H. A novel educational tool for teaching ocular ultrasound. Clin Ophthalmol. 2011;5:857–60.

Qureshi MA, Laghari K. Role of B-scan ultrasonography in preoperative cataract patients. Int J Health Sci (Qassim). 2010;4:31–7.

Shinar Z, Chan IL, Orlinsky M. Use of ocular ultrasound for the evaluation of retinal detachment. J Emerg Med. 2011;40:53–7.

Vodapalli H, Murthy SI, Jalali S, Ali MJ, Rani PK. Comparison of immersion ultrasonography, ultrasound biomicroscopy and anterior segment optical coherence tomography in the evaluation of traumatic phacoceles. Indian J Ophthalmol. 2012;60:63–5.

Whitcomb MB. How to diagnose ocular abnormalities with ultrasound. AAEP Proc. 2002;48:272–5.

Yoonessi R, Hussain A, Jang TB. Bedside ocular ultrasound for the detection of retinal detachment in the emergency department. Acad Emerg Med. 2010;17:913–7.

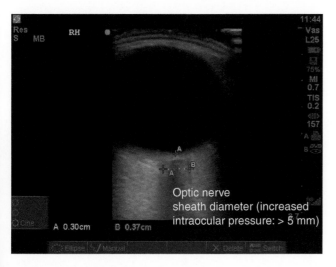

Fig. 50.6 Optic nerve sheath measurement

Tonometry

51

Bobby K. Desai

1.1 Indications

To measure intraocular pressure (IOP)

1.2 Contraindications

A relative contraindication is the presence of an active or indolent infection about the cornea or conjunctiva, unless a one-time-use device is used (e.g., a Tono-Pen XL).
Recent trauma to the eye.
Uncooperative patients because improper technique may cause damage to the eye.

1.3 Overview

Tonometry is the measurement of IOP obtained by evaluating the resistance of the eye to indentation by a force applied to it.

- Can be obtained by several methods.
- Two methods are routinely used in an emergency department setting:
  - *Impression tonometry*: measures the indentation made by a plunger carrying a known amount of weight.
  - More weight can be added to the apparatus.
  - The more weight needed to indent the cornea results in a higher IOP reading.
    - The Schiøtz tonometer is the most commonly used apparatus to utilize this method (Fig. 51.1).
- *Electronic indentation tonometry*: does not exert pressure on the eye (Fig. 51.2).

.K. Desai, MD
epartment of Emergency Medicine, University of Florida Health
ands Hospital, Gainesville, FL, USA
mail: bdesai@ufl.edu

Springer Science+Business Media New York 2016

Ganti (ed.), *Atlas of Emergency Medicine Procedures*, DOI 10.1007/978-1-4939-2507-0_51

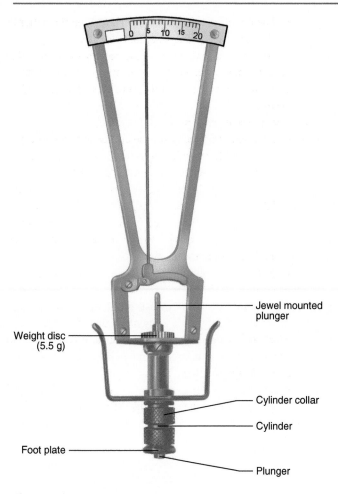

Fig. 51.1 Schiøtz tonometer

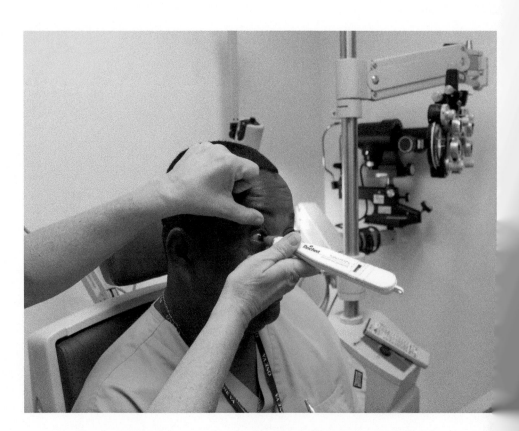

Fig. 51.2 Tono-Pen

51.4   Schiøtz Tonometry

51.4.1 Procedure: Schiøtz Tonometry (Fig. 51.3)

1. Carefully clean the apparatus between each patient.
   - Rubbing alcohol may be used.
   - Because it is metal, it can be autoclaved.
2. Calibrate the Schiøtz tonometer with the metal test block provided.
   - Test by placing the apparatus directly on the metal block.
   - The needle should be at "0" at the far end of the scale.
     - If not, loosen the screw at the base of the needle to rezero it.
     - Ensure that the needle is completely straight because any bend will produce an erroneous reading.
3. An explanation of the procedure is helpful because patient cooperation is critical for accurate results.
4. Anesthetize the eye with topical ophthalmic anesthetic of choice.
5. The patient should be in a recumbent position.
   - Have the patient focus on an area of the ceiling.
6. Hold the instrument with the aid of the curved arms at the side of the tonometer.

- The operator can rest her or his hand on the patient's cheek or forehead to maintain stability.
7. Gently rest the tonometer on the patient's eye such that the instrument is centered on the eye and the instrument is completely vertical; no pressure should be exerted on the eye.
8. Note the scale reading.
9. Lift the Schiøtz directly off the cornea to avoid injury.
10. Using the table provided with the Schiøtz, the operator may convert the scale reading into the IOP.
    - The scale is inversely proportional to the actual IOP.
    - If the scale is low (i.e., high IOP), the additional weights provided with the instrument may be used and the patient retested.

51.4.2 Pitfalls

- Ensure the plunger is clean because it can transmit infection.
- False readings may be obtained without proper calibration.
- Placing pressure on the instrument will cause false readings.

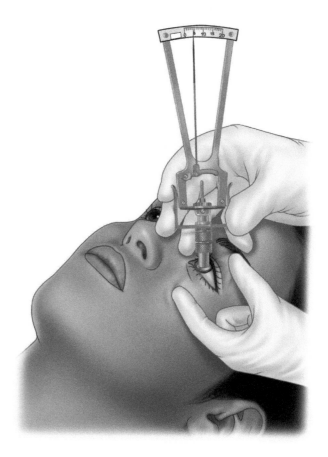

Fig. 51.3 Correct use of Schiøtz tonometer

51.5 Tono-Pen Tonometry

51.5.1 Overview

- Electronically measures IOP
  - Combines applanation and indentation tonometry
- Uses pressure-sensitive electronics to average four successive readings and displays the reading and a reliability factor digitally

51.5.2 Calibration of the Tono-Pen

- Should be performed once daily
- Hold the instrument with the tip down (Fig. 51.4).

- Press the black button twice.
  - The letters "CAL" will appear in the display.
- Press the black button again.
  - After a few seconds the word "UP" will appear.
- Rotate the instrument so that the tip points upward.
  - If "GOOD" appears, the Tono-Pen is ready for use.
  - If "BAD" appears, repeat the process until "GOOD" appears.
    - If "GOOD" does not appear, the device cannot be used.

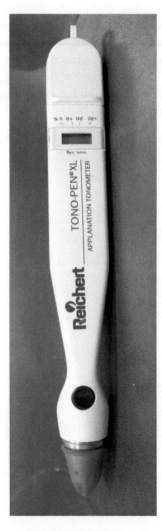

Fig. 51.4 Tono-Pen calibration position

51.5.3 Procedure: Tono-Pen Tonometry

1. An explanation of the procedure is helpful because patient cooperation is critical for accurate results.
2. Anesthetize the eye with the topical ophthalmic anesthetic of choice.
3. Place a probe cover on the unit.
4. The patient should be in a comfortable position because the unit can be used in any position.
   - Have the patient focus on a specific area.
5. The best way to hold the instrument is similar to that of a pen.
   - Ensure that the digital readout is visible.
6. The operator can rest his or her hand on the patient's cheek or forehead to maintain stability.
7. Hold the unit perpendicular to the patient's cornea.
8. Press the black button only once.
   - If "ICALI" is seen, followed immediately by a single row of dashes [– – – –], it indicates that the Tono-Pen requires calibration before it will measure.
   - If "====" is seen and a "beep" is heard, the unit is ready.
   - Proceed with measurement.
9. Gently touch the Tono-Pen to the cornea and withdraw (Fig. 51.5). Repeat several times.
   - Indentation is not required.
10. The unit will "chirp" and a digital reading will be displayed if a valid reading is obtained.
11. After four valid readings are obtained, the average of these measurements as well as a single bar that signifies statistical reliability will appear on the readout.
    - After the final beep if the liquid crystal display (LCD) readout shows "----," not enough valid readings were obtained.
    - In this case, the measurement must be repeated.

51.5.4 Pitfalls

- Unsuccessful calibration mandates a repeat attempt at calibration.
- Loosen the Ocu-Film tip cover and repeat for multiple failed attempts.
- Press the reset button and reattempt calibration.
- Replace the battery if necessary.
- If all else fails, use another device or Schiøtz tonometer.

Fig. 51.5 Proper use of
Tono-Pen

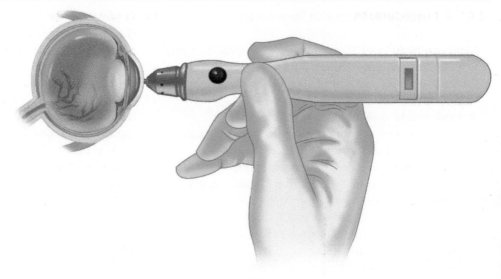

Correct

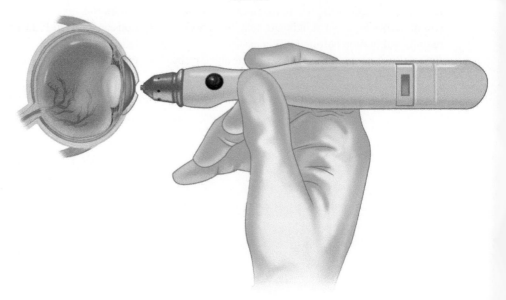

Incorrect

51.6 Complications

- Unusual if proper technique is used.
- If too much force is applied, a corneal abrasion may result.
- Infection when using an improperly sterilized Schiøtz tonometer.

Selected Reading

Lang GK. Ophthalmology: a short textbook. Stuttgart: Thieme; 2000.

Rhee DJ, Pyfer MF, Rhee DM, editors. The Wills eye manual: office and emergency room diagnosis and treatment of eye disease. 3rd ed. Philadelphia: Lippincott Williams & Wilkins; 1999.

Lateral Canthotomy

Benjamin M. Mahon and Bobby K. Desai

52.1 Indications

- Absolute indications: In the presence of presumed or confirmed retrobulbar hemorrhage
  - Acute visual loss
  - Intraocular pressure (IOP) greater than 40 mmHg (normal IOP is 10–20 mmHg)
  - Proptosis not amenable to retropulsion
- Relative indications: In the context of presumed or confirmed retrobulbar hemorrhage (Fig. 52.1)
  - Ophthalmoplegia
  - Cherry red macula
  - Profound eye pain
  - Afferent pupillary defect (Marcus Gunn pupil)
    - This defect is seen with the *swinging flashlight test.*

- Shine a light into both eyes; a normal response is equal constriction of both pupils.
- In those patients with an afferent papillary defect, when light is swung from an unaffected pupil to an affected pupil, the pupil will seem to paradoxically dilate, rather than constrict. The pupil on the nonaffected side will similarly dilate as light is shown into the affected eye. This results from injury to the afferent fibers of cranial nerve (CN) II on the affected side, while the efferent fibers, innervated by CN III, remain intact.
- This procedure is most effective if performed as soon as possible because irreversible vision loss can occur secondary to ischemia in as little as 90 min.

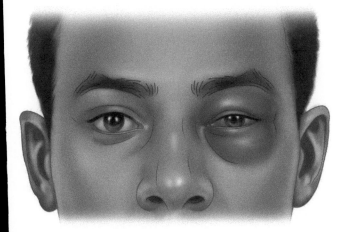

Fig. 52.1 Retrobulbar hemorrhage

B.M. Mahon, MD
Ponciana Medical Center, Kissimmee, FL, USA

B.K. Desai, MD (✉)
Department of Emergency Medicine, University of Florida Health
Shands Hospital, Gainesville, FL, USA
e-mail: bdesai@ufl.edu

© Springer Science+Business Media New York 2016
L. Ganti (ed.), *Atlas of Emergency Medicine Procedures*, DOI 10.1007/978-1-4939-2507-0_52

52.2 Contraindications

- Absolute
  - Globe rupture
- Relative
  - Suspected globe rupture: Heralded by a number of signs including hyphema, irregularly shaped pupil, exposed uveal tissue, or profound restriction of extra-ocular movement

52.3 Materials and Medications

- Straight hemostat
- Suture or iris scissors
- Forceps
- 1–2 % lidocaine with epinephrine
- Sterile gloves
- Sterile towels/drapes
- 4×4 gauze
- Face shield/mask
- Large-bore needle to withdraw anesthetic, 25-gauge needle to infiltrate
- 10-cc syringe
- Normal saline

52.4 Procedure

1. Position the patient
   - While waiting for the procedure to begin, the patient should initially be upright to produce any decrease in IOP that can be provided.
   - At the start of the procedure, lay the patient supine.
   - A cooperative patient is absolutely necessary because even slight movements can cause devastating iatrogenic injury.
   - If the patient is anxious or conscious, sedation may be required.
   - In extreme cases of altered mental status or combative trauma patients, endotracheal intubation and mechanical ventilation may be required.
2. Gently irrigate the affected eye to remove any debris.
3. Inject approximately 1–2 mL of 1–2 % lidocaine with epinephrine into the lateral canthus of the affected eye (Fig. 52.2).
4. Using a curved hemostat, gently crimp the skin over the lateral corner of the patient's eye down to the orbital rim for 3 min to establish hemostasis and set the boundaries for the incision.
   - Using forceps, use the hemostats to pick up the skin just crushed.
   - Raise the skin with forceps and then use scissors to make a 1- to 2-cm incision from the lateral corner of the eye extending laterally outward (Fig. 52.3).
     - This incision can often sufficiently decrease IOP.
     - It is feasible to remeasure the IOP at this point, and if it is still greater than 40 mmHg, proceed to the next step.
   - Visualize the lateral canthal tendon by retracting the inferior orbital lid inferiorly.
   - Direct the scissors along the lateral side of the orbital rim away from the globe, and cut the lateral canthal tendon inferiorly (Fig. 52.4).
   - At this point, again measure IOP, and if greater than 40 mmHg, proceed to the next step.
   - Direct the scissors along the lateral side of the orbital rim away from the globe, this time directed superiorly, and cut the superior crux of the lateral canthal tendon.

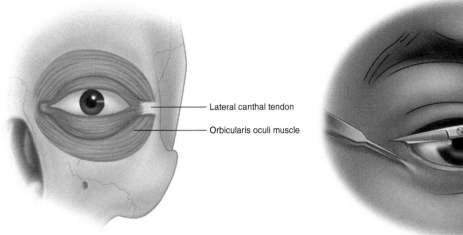

Fig. 52.2 Lateral canthal tendon

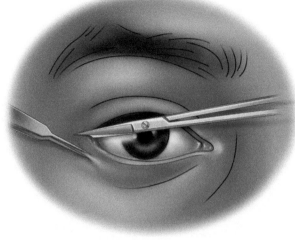

Fig. 52.4 Further cut to reduce intraocular pressure

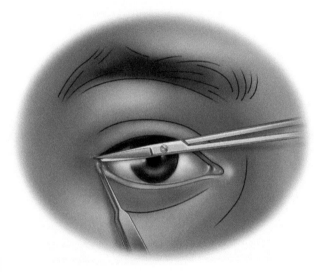

Fig. 52.3 Initial cut

52.5 Complications

- If one is making a superior incision, caution must be taken during this procedure to avoid injury to the lacrimal gland or artery.
- An additional complication of the procedure is ptosis due to iatrogenic injury to the levator aponeurosis, either partially or completely.
- The most obvious complication involves direct injury to the globe itself due to either operator error or poor patient control and immobility.
- Hemorrhage from inadequate hemostasis.
- Infection.

52.6 Pearls and Pitfalls

- Abrupt decrease in pain, decrease in IOP, and resolution of afferent pupillary defect will herald a successful procedure, assuming it was performed within an early enough time frame.
- Having an assistant present is beneficial.
  - In this case, the role of the assistant is to provide lateral retraction of the tissues to decrease likelihood of globe rupture.

- After cantholysis of the inferior component of the lateral canthal tendon, the lower lid will become lax as its attachment to the lateral wall is separated. This signifies a successful incision.
- Incisions made during this procedure generally heal without the need for suturing.
- Emergent ophthalmological consultation should ideally be sought before beginning this procedure.
- Emergent ophthalmological consultation is mandatory subsequent to the procedure.

Selected Reading

Goodall KL, Brahma A, Bates A, Leatherbarrow B. Lateral canthotomy and inferior cantholysis: an effective method of urgent orbital decompression for sight threatening acute retrobulbar haemorrhage. Injury. 1999;30:485–90.

McInnes G, Howes DW. Lateral canthotomy and cantholysis: a simple vision-saving procedure. CJEM. 2002;4:49–52.

Roberts JR, Hedges JR, editors. Clinical procedures in emergency medicine. 5th ed. Philadelphia: WB Saunders; 2009: Chap. 63.

Vassallo S, Hartstein M, Howard D, Stetz J. Traumatic retrobulbar hemorrhage: emergent decompression by lateral canthotomy and cantholysis. J Emerg Med. 2002;22:251–6.

Part VIII

Otorhinolaryngologic Procedures

Epistaxis Control

53

Benjamin M. Mahon and Bobby K. Desai

53.1 Etiology

- Anterior source: approximately 90 % of nosebleeds, usually Kiesselbach's plexus (Fig. 53.1)
  - Nose picking ("epistaxis digitorum")
  - Trauma
  - Infection
  - Nasal foreign body
  - Dry air
  - Atmospheric pressure alterations (e.g., increased altitude, lower arterial partial pressure of oxygen [PaO_2])
  - Allergies

- Blood dyscrasias
- Malignancy (e.g., leukemia, lymphoma)
- Posterior source: approximately 10 % of nosebleeds, usually sphenopalatine artery (Fig. 53.2)
  - Iatrogenic coagulopathy (e.g., warfarin, heparin, high-dose aspirin)
  - Blood dyscrasia
  - Liver failure
  - Renal failure
  - Malignancy
  - Older age

B.M. Mahon, MD
Ponciana Medical Center, Kissimmee, FL, USA

B.K. Desai, MD (✉)
Department of Emergency Medicine, University of Florida Health
Shands Hospital, Gainesville, FL, USA
e-mail: bdesai@ufl.edu

© Springer Science+Business Media New York 2016
L. Ganti (ed.), *Atlas of Emergency Medicine Procedures*, DOI 10.1007/978-1-4939-2507-0_53

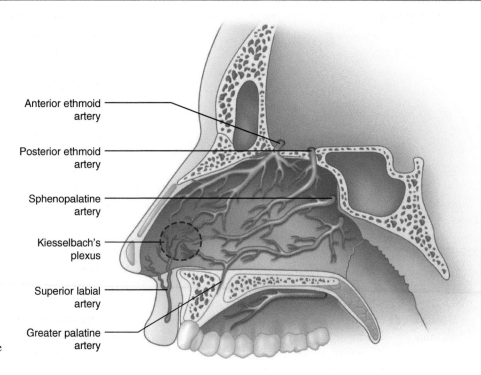

Fig. 53.1 Vascular supply to the nasal septum

Fig. 53.2 Vascular supply of the lateral wall of the nose

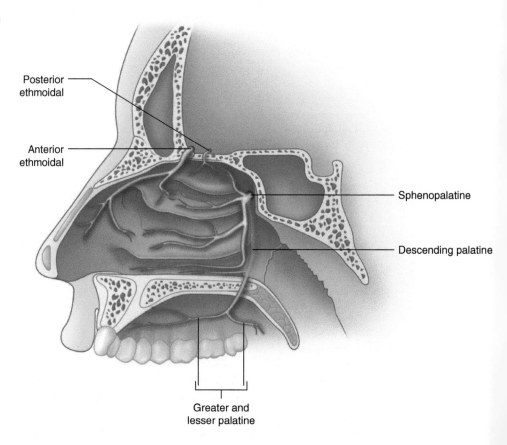

53.2 Indications

- Acute/recurrent epistaxis

53.3 Contraindications

- Resolution of epistaxis episode before arrival
- Massive facial trauma

53.4 Materials and Medications

- Headlight with focused beam
- Gown
- Gloves
- Mask with visor
- Full-body drape or sterile towels
- Nasal packing material (any or all of the following, as needed [see later]): several cotton pledgets, 3–5 feet of ½-inch ribbon gauze (preferably enriched with petroleum jelly and bacitracin), anterior epistaxis balloon nasal pack
- Topical vasoconstrictor (e.g., 1 % pseudoephedrine or 1:1000 epinephrine)
- Topical anesthetic (e.g., 4 % lidocaine solution or 2 % tetracaine)
- Nasal speculum
- Bayonet forceps
- Anterior epistaxis balloon (e.g., Rhino Rocket)
- Any of the following commercial products, as needed (see later): Gelfoam, Surgicel, Crosseal, and FloSeal
- Foley catheter

53.5 Procedure: Anterior Epistaxis

- Initial preparation
  1. Assemble necessary equipment at the bedside.
  2. Have the patient seated upright, with head and neck in the sniffing position.
  3. Universal precautions are mandatory: gown, glove, and mask.
  4. Drape the patient with towels or a large body drape.
  5. If initial evaluation using the headlamp and nasal speculum with gentle spreading in a vertical fashion or a simple visual examination reveals the source (anterior vs posterior), proceed with the appropriate management pathway as determined later.
     - If clot obstructs visualization, it is recommended for the patient to gently blow her or his nose once to remove any easily friable clots, and then proceed with immediate inspection. If anterior nose bleeds, go to the next step.
- Management of anterior epistaxis:
  1. Initial step in the management of anterior nosebleeds involves pinching the patient's nostrils firmly for at least 10–15 min.
     - This can be done by the patient.
     - Simple pressure is very often enough to provide appropriate hemostasis in anterior nosebleeds. If it fails, proceed to the next step.
  2. A topical vasoconstrictor of choice (e.g., cocaine, oxymetazoline, 1 % pseudoephedrine) can be applied to the septum and lateral walls of the nose either topically with cotton-tipped applicators or by using soaked pledgets.
  3. Continue to apply firm pressure to the nares for 10–15 min, and recheck the nose for evidence of bleeding.
  4. If the bleeding site can be easily visualized, chemical cautery may be attempted with silver nitrate (Fig. 53.3).
     - This can be accomplished with the help of a nasal speculum and a headlight.
     - It is advised to cauterize both the site itself and 0.5 cm around the site, by holding the silver nitrate stick to the site for at least 20 s until the bleeding stops.
     - If bleeding then stops, cover the site with an absorbable gelatin foam or an oxidized cellulose such as Gelfoam or Surgicel or simply apply topical antibiotic to the site.
  5. If there is continued bleeding, the clinician may apply either two elongated cotton pledgets or a commercially available substitute (e.g., a Rhino Rocket or similar device [Fig. 53.4]) presoaked in a few milliliters or a 1:1 mixture of a topical vasoconstrictor and an anesthetic. Combinations can include the previously cited two agents, plus 2 % tetracaine or 4 % lidocaine.
  6. Universal instructions for the insertion of a commercially available anterior nasal pack include (Fig. 53.5):
     - Soak the fabric via the manufacturer's recommended solution if required.
     - Insert antibiotic ointment in the nares to facilitate insertion.
     - Insert the entire length of the balloon along the inferior surface of the nasal cavity.
     - The fluid within the nasal cavity should cause it to expand spontaneously while in the nares, after which the remaining exposed string can be taped to the check.
     - For those devices that require air instillation, read the manufacturer's instructions on how much air to instill within the device.

7. Another option is to provide an anterior nasal packing using a few feet of ½-inch ribbon gauze (Fig. 53.6).
8. It is preferable if this gauze is impregnated with petroleum jelly and is enriched with bacitracin ointment.
   - If it is not, bacitracin can be applied to the strip before its insertion into the nasal cavity.
9. To facilitate the insertion, bayonet forceps can be used to gently lay each successive strip on top of the one before it.
10. Begin inferiorly, laying each strip on top of the other, about three or four layers at a time, with the end points protruding from the opening of the nasal cavity.
11. Pack the strands firmly.
12. It may take several feet to pack the entire nasal cavity.
13. This may be both uncomfortable for the patient and time consuming for the provider, so ensure adequate time and copious topical anesthetic.
14. Parenteral analgesic or anxiolytics may be required for any of these techniques.
15. If none of these resources is available, another technique requires the use of two cotton pledgets gently inserted into the nostrils after vasoconstrictor/anesthetic topical solution has been sprayed into the nose either manually or with the addition of bayonet forceps, where they will remain for 20 min, supplemented by firm pressure to the nares as described previously.
    - If the bleeding has then stopped, they can be removed at this time. If it does not, it is advised to repeat the previous step a second time, this time with a longer period of pressure, before proceeding to the next step.
16. If all of these techniques fail to control bleeding, the clinician may apply a sealant spray or foam enriched with thrombin to enhance clotting.
    - Commercially available options include Crosseal or FloSeal.
17. Finally, if none of these techniques manage to halt what one is sure is only an anterior, albeit persistent, nosebleed, consult the otolaryngologist for further guidance.
    - Another consideration at this point may be that the uncontrollable anterior nosebleed is really a posterior nosebleed from an undetermined location.
    - It may be prudent to proceed to the algorithm for treatment of posterior epistaxis, even if a posterior bleed is not specifically confirmed.

53.5.1 Complications

- Using an inadequate amount of packing when inserting the ribbon gauze, the entire product may serve as a plug with potential aspiration risk, rather than as a tool for hemostasis.
- Otitis, sinusitis, and toxic shock syndrome.

53.5.2 Pearls and Pitfalls

- Pearls
  - Be sure to perform a reevaluation of both the posterior oropharynx and the posterior nasopharynx after insertion of any of the previously discussed devices, and inspect for continued bleeding/oozing to ensure hemostasis has been accomplished.
  - For those patients with nasal packs in place, consider the use of oral antibiotics to avoid subsequent sinusitis, otitis, or toxic shock syndrome.
    - Appropriate antibiotic choices include cephalexin, clindamycin, or amoxicillin–clavulanic acid.
    - The use of antibiotics for short-term packing has not been proven.
  - Consider admission for elderly patients or for those patients with potential airway complications such as those patients with chronic obstructive pulmonary disease (COPD) and for those at risk for aspiration.
  - Have the patient follow up with otolaryngology within 2–3 days for reevaluation and packing removal.
  - Provide adequate discharge instructions warning the patient against nose blowing, sneezing with the mouth closed, or any movements or actions that cause a Valsalva maneuver.
  - The patient should try to keep his or her head elevated for the next 24–48 h even while sleeping to prevent potential aspiration.
- Pitfalls
  - Discharging a patient without an adequate period of observation.
  - Failing to ensure appropriate follow-up.
  - Providing inadequate discharge instructions.
  - Mistaking an anterior nosebleed for a posterior nosebleed.
  - Leaving silver nitrite on exposed nasal mucosa can lead to iatrogenic nasal septal perforation.
  - Not informing the patient that minimal oozing of blood from the nose can be expected.

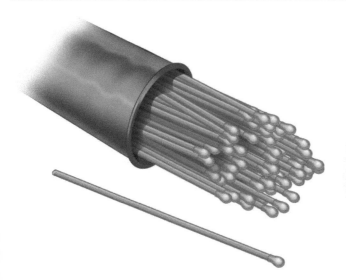

Fig. 53.3 Example of silver nitrate stick and packaging

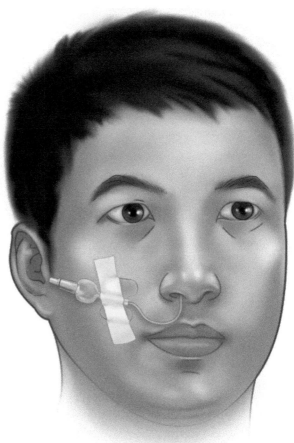

Fig. 53.5 Proper taping of a commercial anterior nasal pack

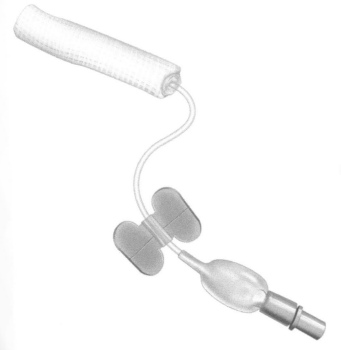

Fig. 53.4 Example of commercial nasal pack

Fig. 53.6 Gauze method

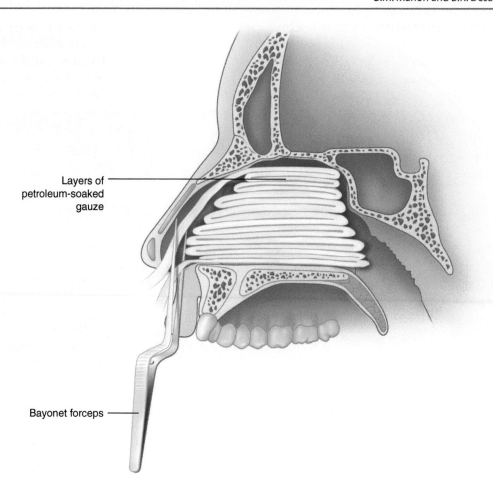

Layers of
petroleum-soaked
gauze

Bayonet forceps

53.6 Procedure: Posterior Epistaxis

- Preliminary Steps
  1. Owing to the possibility of extreme exsanguination from a posterior source of epistaxis or airway obstruction from a large clot dislodgment or large volume of blood aspiration, the stability of the patient's airway, breathing, and circulation must be ensured first.
     - Appropriate interventions entirely depend on the presentation of the patient and therefore are not described in this chapter.
     - Patients with posterior epistaxis can lose a large volume of blood quickly, so this needs to be an initial consideration.
  2. Consider establishing intravenous access and placing the patient on a cardiac monitor.
  3. Because patients with posterior epistaxis tend to be either older, on various blood thinners, or to potentially have some type of coagulopathy, consider obtaining a complete blood count, prothrombin time, and partial thromboplastin time as part of the preliminary workup.
  4. Consider a blood type and screen.
- Management of posterior epistaxis:
  1. Inspect the nares as described in the previous section on anterior nosebleeds.
  2. Several of the techniques discussed may be attempted but may not be successful.
  3. Assemble necessary equipment at the bedside.
  4. Have the patient seated upright, with the head and neck in the sniffing position.
  5. Universal precautions including a gown, glove, and mask should be employed.
  6. Drape the patient with towels or a large body drape.
  7. Apply a combination of a topical vasoconstrictor and anesthetic to the nose.
     - An appropriate choice (e.g., 1 % pseudoephedrine or 1:1000 epinephrine in a 1:1 ratio with 4 % lidocaine or 2 % tetracaine)
     - Be aware, however, that there are situations in which the bleeding may be too brisk, and this step may need to be avoided owing to time constraints and the volume of bleeding. So it is not unheard of to be required to intervene in posterior epistaxis without this initial step.
  8. Otolaryngology should be consulted as early as possible in the workup of this condition, both for admission and in case the following techniques fail.
  9. An advised initial step for the treatment of posterior epistaxis is to proceed directly to insertion of a unilateral or, preferably, bilateral posterior nasal pack or balloon.
     - An example of these is the elongated version of the Rhino Rocket as described previously.
     - Insertion and securing of the product proceed essentially the same way, except that it is inserted deeper into the posterior oropharynx.
  10. Consider the use of a dedicated posterior balloon, such as a Nasostat or Epistat (Fig. 53.7).
      - These devices are double-balloon systems that are lubricated preferably with bacitracin (sterile jelly is also appropriate) and inserted into the posterior nasopharynx.
      - The posterior balloon is then inflated with the product-specific quantity of air.
      - The product is then withdrawn slightly to ensure that the posterior balloon is situated firmly in its desired location of the posterior nasal cavity.
      - The anterior balloon is then inflated with the device-specific quantity of normal saline, and the device is secured.
- If the previously discussed resources are not available, a clinician can insert an adult-caliber Foley catheter into the posterior nasopharynx, with inflation of the balloon, and gentle traction anteriorly to ensure the bulb is situated similarly to the Nasostat or Epistat, firmly in the posterior nasal cavity to tamponade off the bleeding (Fig. 53.8).
- If all of these techniques still fail to control bleeding, an otolaryngologist will likely need to intervene, performing techniques outside the scope of practice of the emergency physician, including electrocautery, submucosal lidocaine/epinephrine injections, or other surgical interventions.
- The final step in the management of this patient includes admission to a monitored bed.

53.6.1 Pearls and Pitfalls

- Pearls
  - Consult otolaryngology early in the workup as soon as a posterior bleed is identified.
  - Patients receiving packing will still need to be placed on antibiotics, such as a first-generation cephalosporin, clindamycin, or amoxicillin–clavulanic acid.
  - Perform a good physical examination concomitantly with the management of the bleed specifically geared toward assessing the patient's volume status (orthostatics, capillary refill, heart rate), because the patient may have significant volume loss depending on the duration and quantity of the bleed.
  - Take a good history including prior bleed, prior admission requirements owing to epistaxis, any anticoagulant use, blood dyscrasias, and so on.

- Pitfalls
  - Misidentifying a posterior bleed as an anterior bleed. This can be catastrophic if the patient is discharged. Reference the "Etiology" section earlier.
  - Discharging the patient.
  - Consulting otolaryngology too late.
  - Underestimating the volume of blood loss. It may be helpful to think of these patients as trauma patients in their initial management and to proceed down the standard primary survey/intervention/secondary survey/ intervention approach, ensuring that the volume needs are identified early.
  - Infection.
  - Pressure necrosis of the septum.
  - Hypoxia.
  - Aspiration.
  - Arrhythmias.
  - Dysphagia.
  - Dislodgment of the pack.

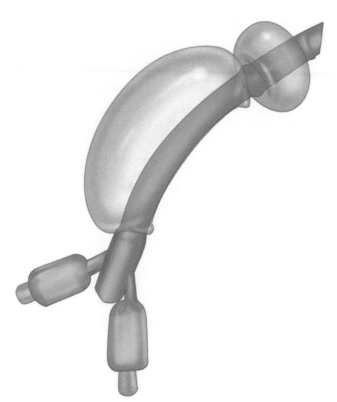

Fig. 53.7 Example of posterior balloon

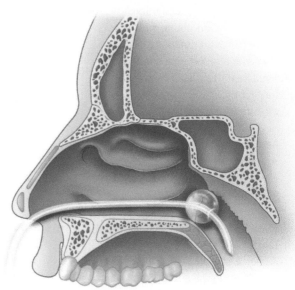

Fig. 53.8 Foley catheter in the posterior nasopharynx

Selected Reading

Buttaravoli P. Minor emergencies, splinters to fractures. 2nd ed. Philadelphia: Mosby; 2007.

Kucik CJ, Clenney T. Management of epistaxis. Am Fam Physician. 2005;71(2):305–11.

Marx JA, Hockberger RS, Walls RM, editors. Rosen's emergency medicine: concepts and clinical practice. 6th ed. Philadelphia: Mosby; 2006.

Pope LE, Hobbs CG. Epistaxis: an update on current management. Postgrad Med J. 2005;81(955):309–14.

Singer AJ, Blanda M, Cronin K, et al. Comparison of nasal tampons for the treatment of epistaxis in the emergency department: a randomized controlled trial. Ann Emerg Med. 2005;45:134–9.

Summers SM, Bey T. Chapter 239. Epistaxis, Nasal Fractures, and Rhinosinusitis. In: Tintinalli's Emergency Medicine, 7th ed. New York, NY: McGraw Hill; 2011.

Treatment of Septal Hematoma

Bobby K. Desai

54.1 Indications

- Septal hematomas occur after force applied to the nasal cartilage results in leakage of blood from the perichondrium (Figs. 54.1 and 54.2). They may be unilateral or bilateral.
- Untreated, this hematoma can expand and mechanically obstruct the blood vessels that supply the nasal cartilage.

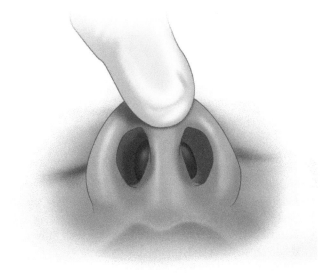

Fig. 54.1 Example of a septal hematoma

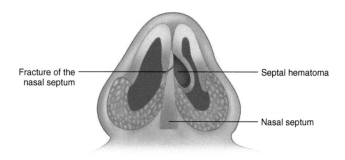

Fig. 54.2 Diagram of a septal hematoma

B.K. Desai, MD
Department of Emergency Medicine, University of Florida Health
Shands Hospital, Gainesville, FL, USA
e-mail: bdesai@ufl.edu

© Springer Science+Business Media New York 2016
L. Ganti (ed.), *Atlas of Emergency Medicine Procedures*, DOI 10.1007/978-1-4939-2507-0_54

54.2 Contraindications

- In the setting of massive facial trauma, airway protection and consultation with otolaryngology or oral surgery may be required.

54.3 Materials and Medications

- 5-cc syringe
- 20-gauge needle (may use larger-gauge needle, but smaller ones may not allow for adequate suctioning).
- Topical antiseptic
- Sterile drapes, gown, eye protection, and gloves
- Light source—preferably a head lamp
- If using procedural sedation, specific medications of choice are needed as well as monitoring and resuscitation equipment
- Nasal speculum
- 4 % liquid cocaine or 4 % liquid lidocaine for anesthesia
- Topical vasoconstrictor of choice (oxymetazoline or phenylephrine)
- Scalpel (#15 blade)
- Suction setup
- Saline for irrigation
- Sterile gauze
- Iodoform packing or sterile rubber band
- Anterior nasal pack (Rhino Rocket)
- Intravenous antibiotics to cover *Staphylococcus aureus*, group A β-hemolytic streptococci, *Streptococcus pneumonia,* and *Haemophilus influenzae*

54.4 Procedure

- Preprocedure
  - Explain the procedure to the patient.
  - Informed consent may be required.
- Procedure—unilateral (Fig. 54.3):
1. Place the patient in a seated position if the procedure is to be done without procedural sedation.
   - If performing the procedure under procedural sedation, the patient may be placed in the supine position with appropriate monitoring and resuscitation equipment on standby.

2. Provide local anesthesia by applying the topical anesthetic of choice to cotton pledgets, wringing out the excess before insertion.
   - Remove after 10 min.
   - If using lidocaine, a topical vasoconstrictor may be required that may be mixed with the lidocaine or applied directly on the nasal mucosa before the procedure.
3. Using a nasal speculum, open the affected nares vertically as wide as possible. Horizontal use may obscure the hematoma.
4. Using a #15 blade, make a vertical incision at the hematoma extending the incision posteriorly at its base.
   - Take care not to make too deep an incision because septal perforation may occur.
5. Suction and gauze should be at the ready to remove as much blood as possible.
6. Pack the incision site with iodoform gauze or a sterile rubber band in order to keep the incision open to prevent accumulation of blood.
7. This packing can be held in place with an anterior nasal pack.
   - The pack should be placed in both nares to prevent deformity of the nasal septum.
8. Consider administration of a dose of intravenous antibiotics.
9. Send the patient home with a prescription for oral antibiotics.
10. Arrange follow-up for 24 h.
- Procedure—bilateral (Fig. 54.4):
1. If bilateral hematomas are present, otolaryngology consultation should be sought.
2. One method involves the incision of one side only through the nasal septum so that both may drain through one side.
   - Care must be taken NOT to penetrate the overlying mucosa of the other side.
3. The second option is to repeat the unilateral drainage procedure on the contralateral side.
4. Care must be taken to not have the incision exactly in the same location as the contralateral side owing to the risk of permanent septal perforation.

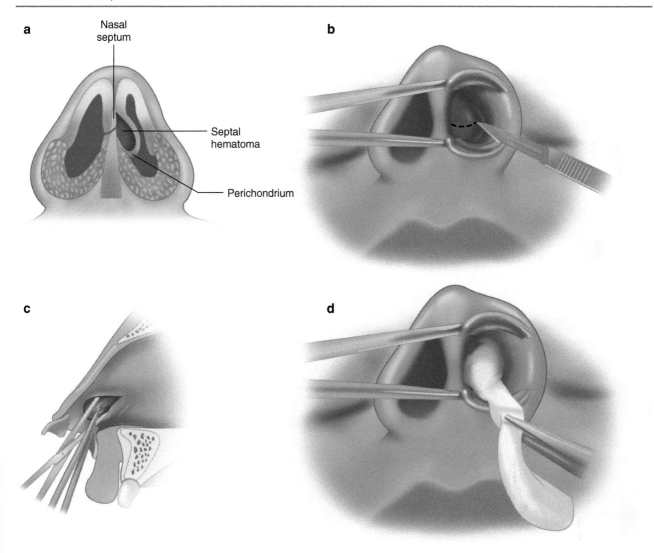

Fig. 54.3 (**a–d**) Technique for drainage of a unilateral septal hematoma

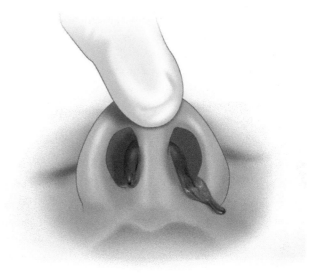

Fig. 54.4 Technique for drainage of a bilateral septal hematoma

54.5　Pitfalls and Complications

- Bleeding
- Infection: toxic shock syndrome
- Deformity of the nose
- Permanent septal perforation
- Inadequate drainage
- Reaccumulation of blood
- Development of septal abscess

Selected Reading

Ginsburg CG. Consultation with the specialist: nasal septal hematoma. Pediatr Rev. 1998;19:142–3.

Savage RR, Valvich C. Hematoma of the nasal septum. Pediatr Rev. 2006;27:478–9.

Nasal Foreign Body Removal

Bobby K. Desai

55.1 Indications

- Visualized foreign body (FB) on inspection
- Continued unilateral nasal discharge of unknown etiology
- Recurrent epistaxis

55.2 Contraindications: Need Urgent Referral

- Those cases in which the emergency physician is not confident of success.

- Combative patients who are not candidates for conscious sedation.
- Embedded FBs.
- Penetrating injuries with an FB.
- Button batteries that cannot be removed.
- Patients with bleeding diathesis.
- Respiratory distress.
- FBs superior and medial to the middle turbinate owing to risk of puncture to the cribriform plate.
- Chronic FBs may be difficult to visualize and these should be referred.

B.K. Desai, MD
Department of Emergency Medicine, University of Florida Health
Shands Hospital, Gainesville, FL, USA
e-mail: bdesai@ufl.edu

© Springer Science+Business Media New York 2016
L. Ganti (ed.), *Atlas of Emergency Medicine Procedures*, DOI 10.1007/978-1-4939-2507-0_55

55.3 Materials and Medications

- 1 % lidocaine without epinephrine (solution) for anesthesia
- 2 % lidocaine jelly
- 0.5 % phenylephrine to vasoconstrict vessels
- Nasal speculum (Fig. 55.1)
- Headlamp or other direct lighting instrument

- Ambu bag (Fig. 55.2)
- Alligator forceps (Fig. 55.3)
- Curved hook (Fig. 55.4)
- Foley catheter
- Suction: schuknecht catheter (Fig. 55.5)
- Eye and biohazard protection for the clinician

Fig. 55.1 (**a–c**) Example of nasal speculum

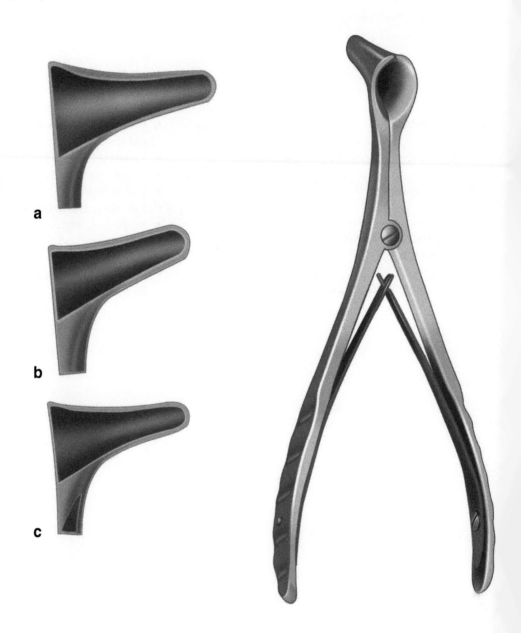

a

b

c

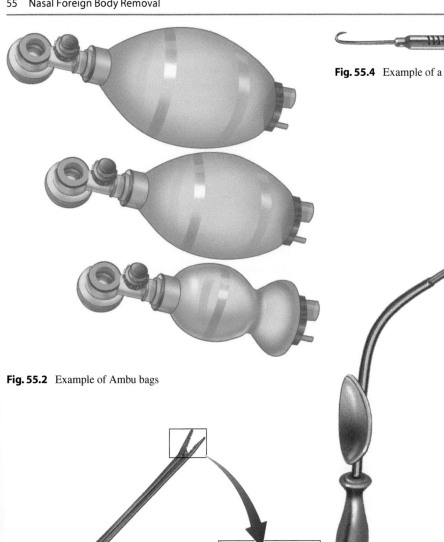

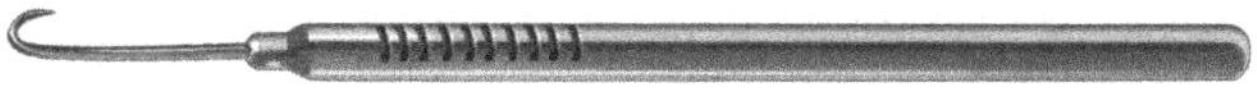

Fig. 55.4 Example of a curved hook

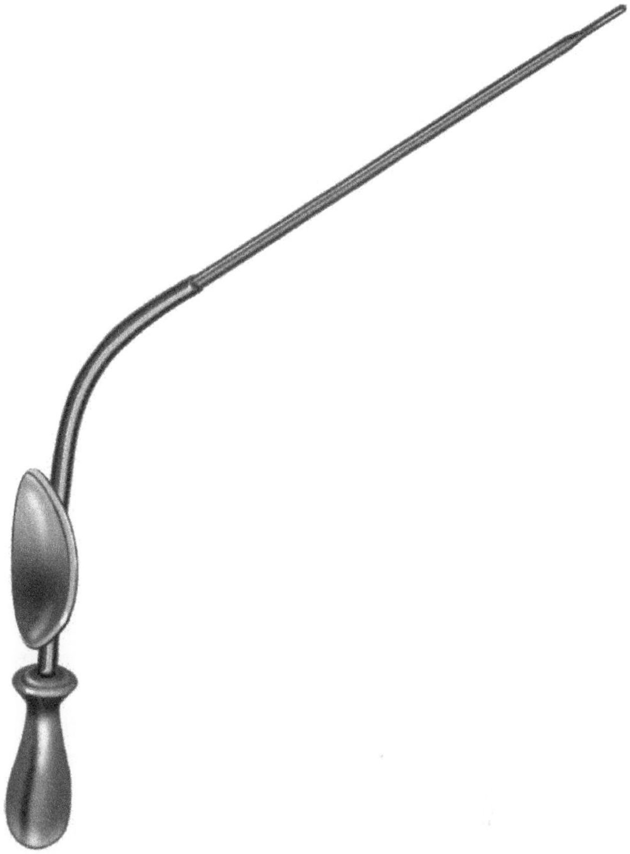

Fig. 55.2 Example of Ambu bags

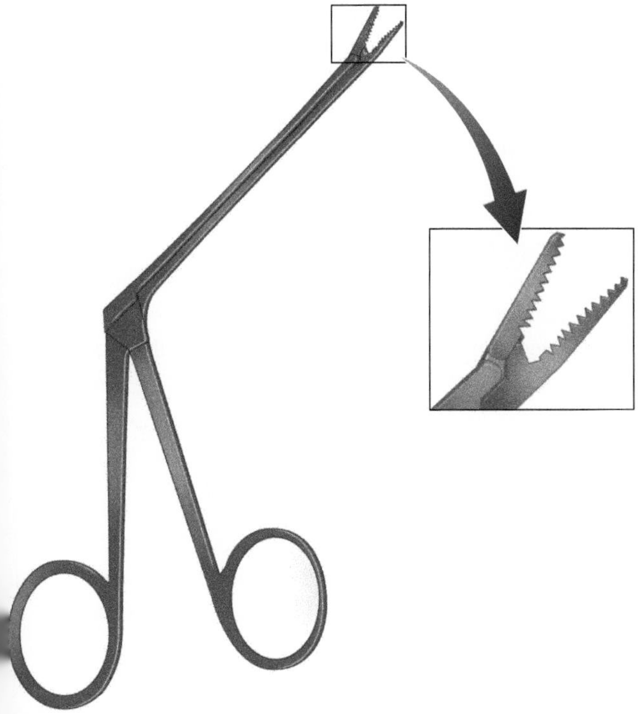

Fig. 55.5 Example of a schuknecht suction tube

Fig. 55.3 Example of alligator forceps

55.4 Procedures (Based on the Method Chosen)

55.4.1 Alligator Forceps

- Perhaps the easiest method to use for easily visualized FBs.
- Care must be taken for those FBs that are easily broken apart (e.g., peas) to ensure that all of the matter has been removed.
- Using a nasal speculum, spread the nares as much as possible to maximize visualization.
- Stabilize the head with the nondominant hand, or for children, consider a papoose board to secure the patient.
- Attempt to grasp the FB with the forceps.
- After removal, ensure the complete removal of the object and ensure that no other FBs are present.

55.4.1.1 Pitfalls and Complications

- Pushing the object deeper into the nares.
- Inability to totally remove the FB.
- Attempted removal of an embedded FB may cause significant bleeding.

55.4.2 Curved Hook

- Used for nongraspable objects especially in the anterior nares.
- Using a nasal speculum, spread the nares as much as possible to maximize visualization.
- Stabilize the head with the nondominant hand, or for children, consider a papoose board to secure the patient.
- Pass the hook behind the object, or if the object has holes, the hook may be placed inside the hole to facilitate removal.
- Slowly withdraw the hook, thereby removing the FB.
- After removal, ensure the complete removal of the object and ensure that no other FBs are present.

55.4.2.1 Pitfalls and Complications

- This technique cannot be used if the object cannot be directly visualized because significant trauma may arise owing to the misplacement of the hook.
- Attempted removal of an embedded FB may cause significant bleeding.

55.4.3 Foley Catheter Removal

- Use a 5 or 6 French catheter.
- Anesthetize the nares with lidocaine with or without epinephrine and vasoconstrict the nasal vessels with phenylephrine.
- Ensure that the Foley balloon has no leaks.
- Place the patient in a supine position.
  - Consider procedural sedation for children and/or a papoose board.
- Lubricate the Foley tip and balloon with lidocaine jelly.
- Advance the tip past the object.
- Blow up the balloon with 2–3 mL of air and gently withdraw the catheter.
  - The amount of air may need to be adjusted depending on the size of the object to be withdrawn.
  - Pulling too quickly may cause a soft FB to break apart.

55.4.3.1 Pitfalls and Complications

- This technique may be used if the FB is not visible.
- In order for this technique to work, the catheter must be able to slide posterior to the object in order for the balloon to pull out the object.

55.4.4 Suction

- A small metal suction catheter—the schuknecht catheter—may be used.
- The suction is placed against the FB and slowly withdrawn.
- This technique works best for round smooth objects visualized in the anterior nares.

55.4.4.1 Pitfalls and Complications

- May not work for posteriorly displaced FBs.
- May not work for objects too tightly entrenched in the nares.

55.4.5 Nasal Positive Pressure

- This technique works best for round FBs occluding the nares.
- Place the patient in a supine position.
  - Consider a papoose board to secure the patient.
- Apply pressure to the contralateral nares to occlude it.
- Connect an Ambu bag to high-flow oxygen.
  - Use a facemask that covers only the mouth.
- Place the mask on the patient's mouth and allow it to expand by covering the thumbhole.
- If this pressure is insufficient to expel the object, the Ambu bag may be compressed to add pressure to the attempt.
- This may allow the object to be seen and grasped in the anterior nares.

55.4.5.1 Pitfalls and Complications

- Too much pressure could theoretically rupture the tympanic membranes.

Selected Reading

Backlin SA. Positive-pressure technique for nasal foreign body removal in children. Ann Emerg Med. 1995;25:554–5.

Chan TC, Ufberg J, Harrigan RA, et al. Nasal foreign body removal. J Emerg Med. 2004;26:441–5.

Kadish H. Ear and nose foreign bodies: it is all about the tools. Clin Pediatr. 2005;44:665–70.

Cerumen Removal

56

Bobby K. Desai

56.1 Indications

- Hearing loss
- Profound dizziness
- Pain

56.2 Contraindications

- Uncooperative patient
- Potential for foreign bodies
- Prior surgery to ear or mastoid
- History of middle or outer ear disease

56.3 Materials and Medications

- Ear speculum (Fig. 56.1).
- Eye and biohazard protection for the clinician
- Headlamp or other direct lighting instrument
- Cerumen-softening solutions
  - Carbamide peroxide
  - Mineral oil or other oil-based agents including almond or olive oil
  - Liquid docusate sodium
  - Acetic acid
  - Sodium bicarbonate
- Alligator forceps (Fig. 56.2)
- Curved hook or cerumen spoon (Figs. 56.3 and 56.4)
- Suction—Schuknecht catheter
- Irrigation setup
  - Ear syringe (Figs. 56.5 and 56.6)
- 20- to 60-mL syringe with an 18-gauge angiocath attached
  - Commercial ear irrigation setup
  - Water (tap water may be used)
  - Basin or other collection device
  - Towels

B.K. Desai, MD
Department of Emergency Medicine, University of Florida Health
Shands Hospital, Gainesville, FL, USA
e-mail: bdesai@ufl.edu

© Springer Science+Business Media New York 2016
L. Ganti (ed.), *Atlas of Emergency Medicine Procedures*, DOI 10.1007/978-1-4939-2507-0_56

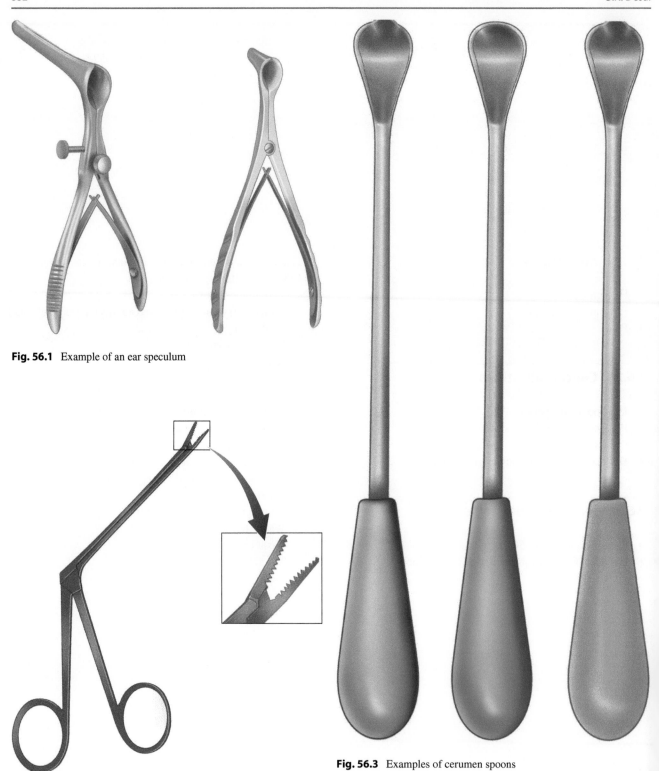

Fig. 56.1 Example of an ear speculum

Fig. 56.2 Example of alligator forceps

Fig. 56.3 Examples of cerumen spoons

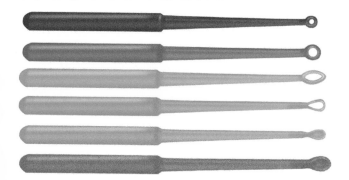

Fig. 56.4 Examples of ear curettes

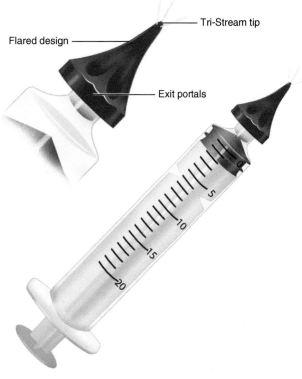

Tri-Stream tip

Flared design

Exit portals

Fig. 56.6 Example of a specialized ear syringe

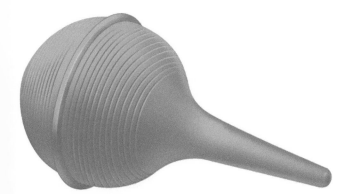

Fig. 56.5 Example of a typical bulb syringe used in irrigation

56.4 Procedure

1. Explain the procedure to the patient to facilitate cooperation.
    - Some discomfort may be involved, including a sensation of pressure and the cold, wet feeling from the water used.
    - Nausea, vomiting, or a sensation of vertigo may also be experienced.
        - Consider pretreatment of vertigo with agent of choice.
2. The patient may be seated or supine with the head slightly turned to the affected side to facilitate the collection of fluid.
3. Stabilize the head with the nondominant hand, or for children, consider a papoose board to secure the patient.
4. Pull the ear up and out to straighten the ear canal.
5. Before irrigation, if the cerumen is hard, alligator forceps or a cerumen spoon may be used under direct visualization to remove as much cerumen as possible.
6. Use a cerumen-softening agent before irrigation by instilling and leaving in for 30 min to maximize softening.
7. Place a collection device next to the patient's ear, or alternatively, have the patient hold a basin near the ear to collect any liquid.
8. Attach an angiocath to a 20- or 60-mL syringe, place the tip of the catheter within the ear canal, and aim toward the tympanic membrane.
9. Slowly inject the solution into the ear canal.
    - Care must be taken to limit the force used owing to the potential for tympanic membrane rupture.
    - The fluid can be injected in short bursts or all at once.
10. Direct the stream as much as possible toward the rear of the cerumen to be removed.

11. Continually reassess the ear canal to ensure that all cerumen has been removed.
    - If one large piece remains, use a cerumen hook to facilitate removal.
12. If the patient complains of severe sharp pain, stop the procedure and assess the tympanic membrane for rupture.
    - Consider referral or otolaryngological consultation at this point.
13. After successful removal, dry the ear canal with cotton-tipped applicators to prevent otitis externa.

56.5 Pitfalls and Complications

- Owing to instillation of room temperature water, a caloric response may occur including vertigo, nausea, and vomiting.
- Rupture of the tympanic membrane.
- Unsuccessful irrigation secondary to inadequate time given to softening agents before attempting removal.
- Bleeding of the external auditory canal.
- Otitis externa.
- Hearing loss.

Selected Reading

Blake P, Matthews R, Hornibrook J. When not to syringe an ear. N Z Med J. 1998;111:422.

McCarter D, Courtney AU, Pollart SM. Cerumen impaction. Am Fam Physician. 2007;75:1523–8.

Roland PS, Smith TL, Schwartz SR, et al. Clinical practice guideline: cerumen impaction. Otolaryngol Head Neck Surg. 2008;139:S1–21.

Ear Foreign Body Removal

57

Bobby K. Desai

57.1 Indications

- Visualized foreign body (FB) on inspection.
- Continued unilateral otorrhea of unknown etiology mandates a search.
- Recurrent bleeding.
- History of FB placement by patient.

57.2 Contraindications: Need Urgent Referral

- Those cases in which the emergency physician is not confident of success.
- Combative patients are not candidates for conscious sedation.
- Embedded FBs.
- Penetrating injuries with an FB.
- FBs close to the tympanic membrane.
- Consider referral of spherical FBs because these may be difficult to grasp.

- Chronic FBs may be difficult to visualize; these should be referred.
- Consider referral for those patients who have attempts made at other institutions.

57.3 Materials and Medications

- Ear speculum (Fig. 56.1)
- Eye and biohazard protection for the clinician
- Headlamp or other direct lighting instrument
- Alligator forceps (Fig. 56.2)
- Curved hook (Fig. 57.1) or cerumen spoon (Fig. 56.3)
- Suction—Schuknecht catheter (Fig. 57.2)
- Irrigation setup
  - Ear syringe (Fig. 57.3)
  - 20- to 60-mL syringe with an 18-gauge angiocath attached
  - Water (tap water may be used)
  - Basin or other collection device
  - Towels
- Cyanoacrylate (Fig. 57.4)

B.K. Desai, MD
Department of Emergency Medicine, University of Florida Health
Shands Hospital, Gainesville, FL, USA
e-mail: bdesai@ufl.edu

© Springer Science+Business Media New York 2016
L. Ganti (ed.), *Atlas of Emergency Medicine Procedures*, DOI 10.1007/978-1-4939-2507-0_57

Fig. 57.1 Example of a curved hook

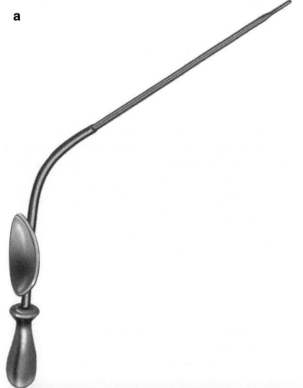

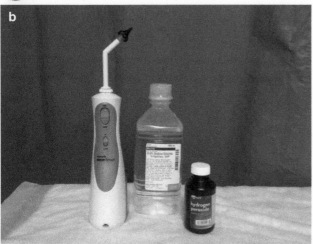

Fig. 57.2 (**a**) Example of a Schuknecht suction tube, (**b**) example of ear irrigation setup using a Waterpik system

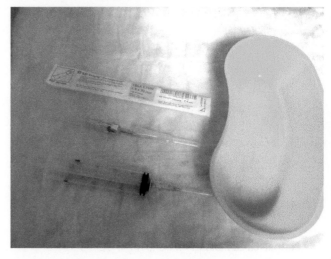

Fig. 57.3 Example of a typical syringe used in irrigation

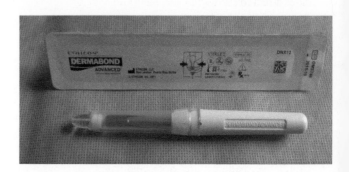

Fig. 57.4 Example of cyanoacrylate

57.4 Procedures (Based on the Method Chosen)

57.4.1 Alligator Forceps

- Ideal for easily visualized FBs, especially graspable FBs in the lateral third of the ear canal.
  - May have limited success with rounded objects.
- Care must be taken for those FBs that are easily broken apart (e.g., peas) to ensure that all of the matter has been removed.
  - May need irrigation subsequent to the attempt.
- Explain the procedure to the patient to facilitate cooperation.
- Pull the ear up and out to straighten the ear canal.
- Consider using a specialized otoscope with magnification (an operating otoscope) to maximize visualization.
- The patient may be seated or supine with the unaffected side turned to the gurney or examining chair.
- Stabilize the head with the nondominant hand, or for children, consider a papoose board to secure the patient.
- Attempt to grasp the FB with the forceps.
  - If using an ear speculum, attempt to bring the object as close as possible to the speculum in order to stabilize it and slowly remove both.
- After removal, ensure the complete removal of the object and ensure that no other FBs are present.

57.4.1.1 Pitfalls and Complications

- Pushing the object deeper into the auditory canal.
- Inability to totally remove the FB.
- Attempted removal of an embedded FB may cause significant bleeding.

57.4.2 Curved Hook

- Ideal for spherical objects in the lateral third of the auditory canal.
- Can be used for non-graspable objects especially in the lateral third of the auditory canal.
- Direct visualization is necessary to avoid trauma to the ear canal.
- Consider using a specialized otoscope with magnification (an operating otoscope) to maximize visualization.
- Explain the procedure to the patient to facilitate cooperation.
- The patient may be seated or supine with the unaffected side turned to the gurney or examining chair.

- Stabilize the head with the nondominant hand, or for children, consider a papoose board to secure the patient.
- Pull the ear up and out to straighten the ear canal.
- Pass the hook behind the object, or if the object has holes, place the hook inside the hole to facilitate removal.
  - In order for this technique to succeed, there must be sufficient area near the object to facilitate the hook going behind it.
- Slowly withdraw the hook, thereby removing the FB.
- After removal, ensure the complete removal of the object and ensure that no other FBs are present.

57.4.2.1 Pitfalls and Complications

- Pushing the object deeper into the auditory canal.
- This technique cannot be used if the object cannot be directly visualized because significant trauma may arise owing to the misplacement of the hook.
- Attempted removal of an embedded FB may cause significant bleeding.
- Do not use this technique if the object is close to the tympanic membrane owing to risk of rupture.

57.4.3 Suction

- A small metal suction catheter—the Schuknecht catheter—may be used.
- Ideal for hard rounded objects in the lateral third of the ear canal.
  - Does not work as well for those objects closer to the tympanic membrane owing to lack of suction and the narrow ear canal
- Direct visualization of the object is mandatory.
  - The catheter must be placed directly on the object for this technique to succeed.
- Explain the procedure to the patient to facilitate cooperation.
- The patient may be seated or supine with the unaffected side turned to the gurney or examining chair.
- Stabilize the head with the nondominant hand, or for children, consider a papoose board to secure the patient.
- Pull the ear up and out to straighten the ear canal.
- Place the suction against the FB and slowly withdraw.

57.4.3.1 Pitfalls and Complications
- Pushing the object deeper into the auditory canal
- May not work for objects too tightly entrenched in the ear canal

57.4.4 Irrigation

- Useful for small particulate matter unable to be grasped by forceps or too small for a hook to pull out.
  - Cannot be used for button batteries or vegetable matter.
    - Irrigation may cause an alkaline necrosis with the button battery.
    - Vegetable matter may expand, increasing the difficulty of removal.
- Explain the procedure to the patient to facilitate cooperation.
  - Some discomfort may be involved, including a sensation of pressure and a feeling cold wetness from the water used.
- The patient may be seated or supine with the head slightly turned to the affected side to facilitate collection of fluid.
- Stabilize the head with the nondominant hand, or for children, consider a papoose board to secure the patient.
- Pull the ear up and out to straighten the ear canal.
- Place a collection device next to the patient's ear, or alternatively, have the patient hold a basin.
- Attach an angiocath to a 20- or 60-mL syringe and place the tip of the catheter within the ear canal, or use a Waterpik system.
- Slowly inject the solution into the ear canal.
  - Care must be taken to limit the force used owing to the potential for tympanic membrane rupture.
- Direct the stream as much as possible toward the rear of the object(s) to be removed.
- Continually assess the ear canal to ensure that all foreign matter has been removed.
- If the patient complains of severe sharp pain, stop the procedure and assess the tympanic membrane for rupture.
  - Consider referral or otolaryngological consultation at this point.

57.4.4.1 Pitfalls and Complications
- Owing to instillation of room temperature water, a caloric response may occur including vertigo, nausea, and vomiting.
- Rupture of the tympanic membrane.

57.4.5 Cyanoacrylate

- Useful for objects that can be directly visualized.
- Ideal for hard rounded objects in the lateral third of the ear canal.
  - Does not work as well for those objects closer to the tympanic membrane owing to lack of visualization
- Direct visualization of the object is mandatory.
  - The stick with the cyanoacrylate must be placed directly on the object for this technique to succeed.
- Consider using a specialized otoscope with magnification (an operating otoscope) to maximize visualization.
- Explain the procedure to the patient to facilitate cooperation.
- The patient may be seated or supine with the unaffected side turned to the gurney or examining chair.
- Stabilize the head with the nondominant hand, or for children, consider a papoose board to secure the patient.
- Pull the ear up and out to straighten the ear canal.
- Place a small amount of cyanoacrylate on the end of a cerumen spoon or wooden end of a cotton-tipped swab.
- Using direct visualization, place the stick in the ear canal and touch the FB.
- Leave the stick on the object for approximately 30–60 s to facilitate drying of the glue.
- Remove the stick and the FB.

57.4.5.1 Pitfalls and Complications
- This technique cannot be used if the object cannot be seen.
- The object must be relatively smooth to facilitate placement of the glue.

Selected Reading

Hanson RM, Stephens M. Cyanoacrylate-assisted foreign body removal from the ear and nose in children. J Paediatr Child Health. 1994;30:77–8.

Kadish H. Ear and nose foreign bodies: it is all about the tools. Clin Pediatr. 2005;44:665–70.

Treatment of Auricular Hematoma

58

Bobby K. Desai

58.1 Indications

- Presence of auricular hematoma
  - These occur after significant force is applied to the ear.
  - This type of hematoma will separate the perichondrium from the cartilage.
    - Untreated, this hematoma prevents the development of new cartilage, subsequently deforming the auricle, causing *cauliflower ear* (Figs. 58.1 and 58.2).

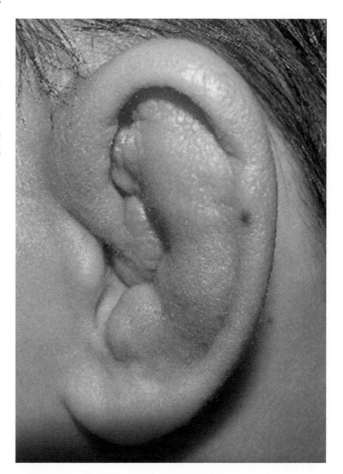

Fig. 58.1 Example of a cauliflower ear

B.K. Desai, MD
Department of Emergency Medicine, University of Florida Health
Shands Hospital, Gainesville, FL, USA
e-mail: bdesai@ufl.edu

© Springer Science+Business Media New York 2016
. Ganti (ed.), *Atlas of Emergency Medicine Procedures*, DOI 10.1007/978-1-4939-2507-0_58

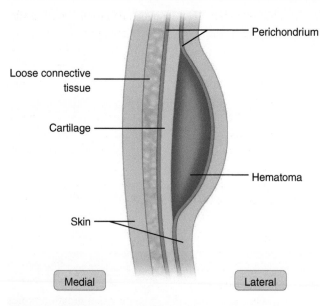

Fig. 58.2 Schematic of auricular hematoma

58.2 Contraindications

- Uncooperative patient.
- Evidence of infection mandates plastic surgery or otolaryngology consultation.
- Significant trauma to area around the ear.

58.3 Materials and Medications

- 5-cc syringe
- 20-gauge needle (may use larger-gauge needle, but smaller ones may not allow for adequate suctioning)
- Topical antiseptic
- Sterile drapes, gown, eye protection, and gloves
- 1 % lidocaine for anesthesia
- Scalpel (#11 or #15 blade)
- Suction setup
- Saline for irrigation
- Hemostat and forceps
- Penrose drain or plain gauze packing
- Xeroform gauze
- Laceration tray setup
    - Needle driver
    - 4–0 Nonabsorbable suture
- Antibiotic ointment
- Gauze bandages

58.4 Procedure (Needle Aspiration)

1. Explain the procedure to the patient.
2. Informed consent may be required.
3. The patient may be seated or supine with the unaffected side turned to the gurney or examining chair.
4. Stabilize the head with the nondominant hand, or for children, consider a papoose board to secure the patient.
    - Consider procedural sedation for children.
5. Carefully clean the area with an antiseptic solution of choice (povidone-iodine [Betadine] or chlorhexidine solution) and allow to dry.
6. Anesthetize the area where the hematoma is of greatest diameter with 1 % lidocaine.
7. Inject the hematoma itself to promote increased anesthesia.
8. The clinician should prepare for the procedure by practicing universal precautions.
9. Drape the patient's ear.
10. Attach a 20-gauge needle to a syringe.
    - A 5-cc syringe should be sufficient.
11. Attempt to aspirate the hematoma contents with the prepared syringe (Fig. 58.3).

12. "Milking" the hematoma may be required to fully remove the clot.
    • If the hematoma has been present for sufficient time for the blood to completely clot, needle aspiration will fail, and an alternative technique, described later, may be necessary to completely evacuate the hematoma.
13. Place antibiotic ointment around the injection site.
14. Loosely dress the area.
15. Refer to an otolaryngologist or a plastic surgeon for follow-up care.

If needle aspiration fails, a larger incision may be required using the following procedure:

1. Perform the previously discussed steps.
2. Consider a local field block of the greater auricular nerve.
3. Make an incision over the hematoma, following the anatomy of the helix (Fig. 58.4).
    • The incision should be 5–6 mm in length and curvilinear, following the concavity of the helix.
    • More than one incision may be required.
4. Remove the hematoma with hemostats or forceps.
    • Suctioning may be used as well.
5. Copiously irrigate the cavity with saline to make certain of complete removal of the hematoma.
6. Insert the Penrose drain or plain packing into the incision.

7. Antibiotic ointment may be applied to the incision site.
8. Place the Xeroform gauze over the incision site.
9. Apply a compression dressing to the ear (Fig. 58.5).
    • Place dry cotton into the ear canal to protect from possible drainage and subsequent infection (Fig. 58.6).
    • Mold Xeroform gauze in and around the contours of the helix (Fig. 58.7).
    • With the aid of an assistant, place gauze behind the pinna and over the Xeroform gauze already molded to the anterior portion of the ear (Fig. 58.8).
    • Place more fluffed gauze over the ear (Fig. 58.9).
    • While the assistant holds the anterior and posterior gauze in place, use a web roll (Kerlix) around the head to keep the gauze in place. Then wrap the head with an ACE wrap or stretchy bandage (Figs. 58.10 and 58.11).
    • These steps are critical to maintain equal compression of the ear, which will help prevent future deformity.
    • Alternatively, dental rolls can be secured with suture to the anterior and posterior site of the drained hematoma (Fig. 58.12).
10. Place the patient on prophylactic antibiotics.
11. Refer to an otolaryngologist or a plastic surgeon for follow-up care.

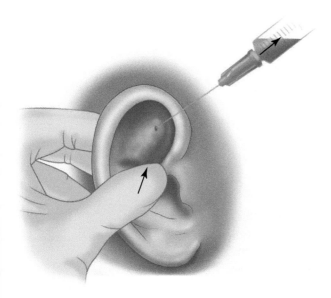

Fig. 58.3 Aspiration of a hematoma

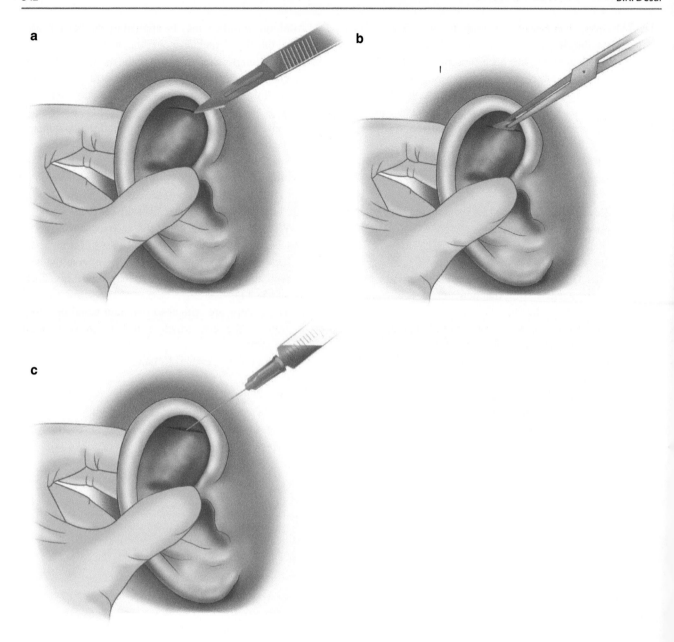

Fig. 58.4 Incision of an auricular hematoma. (**a**) Incision; (**b**) removal of clot with forceps; (**c**) aspiration of blood with syringe

Fig. 58.5 Materials needed for compression dressing

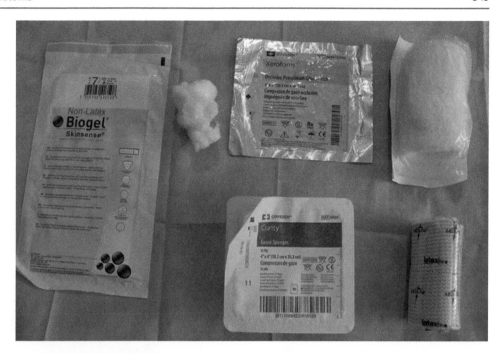

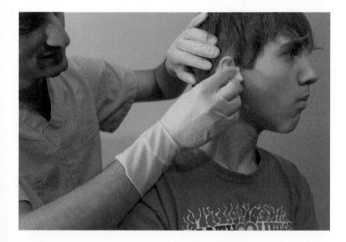

Fig. 58.6 Place cotton in the ear to prevent drainage into ear

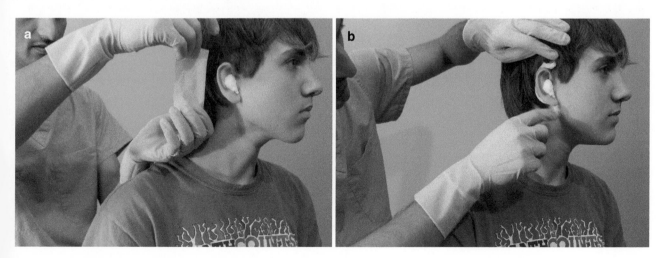

Fig. 58.7 (**a, b**) Mold Xeroform gauze around ear helix

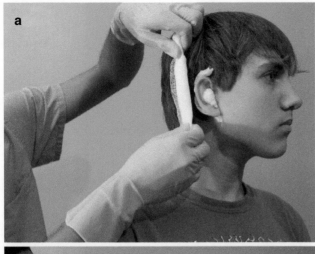

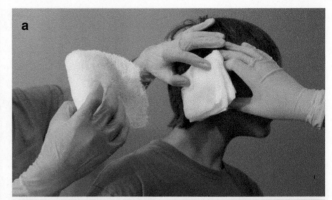

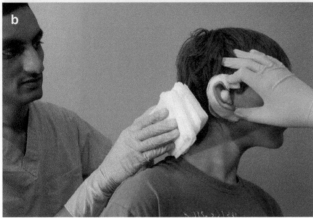

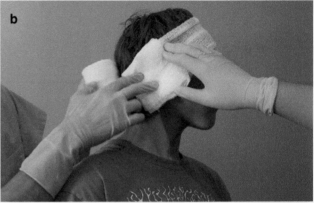

Fig. 58.8 (**a, b**) Mold sterile gauze on top of Xeroform gauze around ear helix

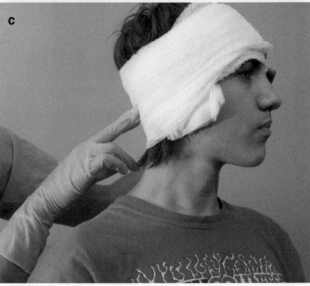

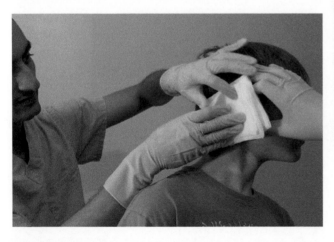

Fig. 58.10 (**a–c**) Wrap head with Kerlix (sterile gauze roll)

Fig. 58.9 Pad outside of ear with 4×4 gauze pads

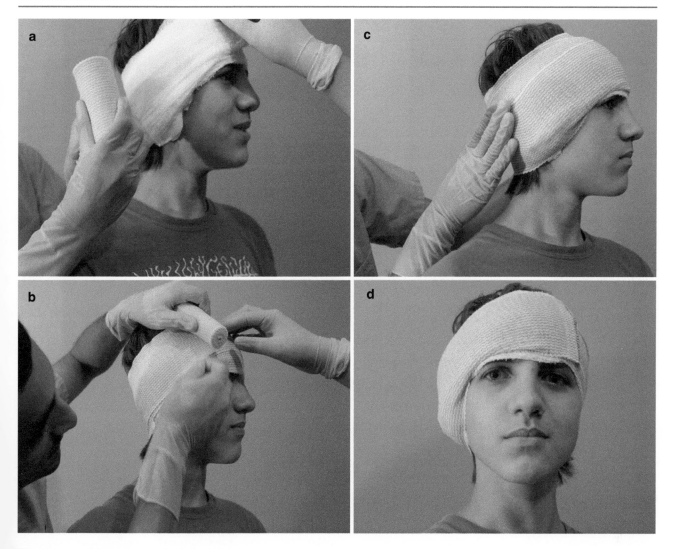

Fig. 58.11 (**a**–**d**) Wrap head with elastic bandage

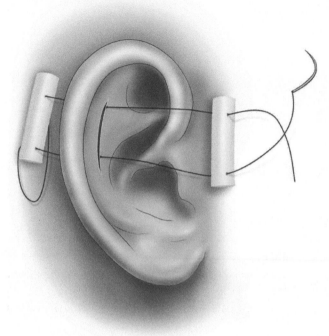

Fig. 58.12 Dental rolls secured to the ear

58.5   Pitfalls and Complications

- Bleeding
- Infection—perichondritis
- Deformity of the auricle
- Inadequate clot removal
- Hematomas present for several days warrant a plastic surgery or an otolaryngology consultation

Acknowledgement The authors would like to thank Thor Shiva Stead for serving as the subject in many of the photographs in this chapter.

Selected Reading

O'Donnell BP, Eliezri YD. The surgical treatment of traumatic hematoma of the auricle. Dermatol Surg. 1999;25:803–5.

Starck WJ, Kaltman AI. Current concepts in the surgical management of traumatic auricular hematoma. J Oral Maxillofac Surg. 1992;50:800–2.

Incision and Drainage of Peritonsillar Abscess

Melinda W. Fernandez and Bobby K. Desai

59.1 Indications

- Peritonsillar abscess

59.2 Contraindications

- Absolute
  - Malignancy
  - Vascular malformations
- Relative
  - Pediatric patient
  - Severe trismus
  - Uncooperative patient

59.3 Materials and Medications

- #11 or #15 scalpel
- 27-gauge 1.5-inch needle, 18- to 20-gauge 1.5-inch or longer needle
- 5-mL syringe, 10- to 20-mL syringe
- Tape
- Trauma shears
- Viscous lidocaine
- Lidocaine 1 % with epinephrine
- Laryngoscope with MAC 3 or 4 *or* tongue blade(s) and headlamp or other light source
- Suction setup with Frazier or tonsil suction tip

M.W. Fernandez, MD
Department of Emergency Medicine, University of Florida Health, Gainesville, FL, USA
e-mail: mindyfernandez@ufl.edu

B.K. Desai, MD (✉)
Department of Emergency Medicine, University of Florida Health Shands Hospital, Gainesville, FL, USA
e-mail: bdesai@ufl.edu

59.4 Procedure: Aspiration

1. Informed consent may be required.
2. Raise head of bed to at least 60° and place a pillow or other support behind the patient's head.
3. Prepare an 18- to 20-gauge 1.5-inch needle on a 10- to 20-mL syringe with a needle guard.
   - This can be accomplished by using trauma shears to cut 1–1.5 cm off the distal plastic needle cover and replacing the cover over the needle.
   - This now creates a guard to prevent deep penetration into vascular structures (Fig. 59.1).
4. Topically anesthetize area with viscous lidocaine (alternatively, can use Cetacaine [benzocaine, tetracaine hydrochloride, and butamben] spray)
5. Using lidocaine 1 % with epinephrine and a 27-gauge 1.5-inch needle on a 5-mL syringe, infiltrate 1–2 mL into the area. Blanching should be apparent.
6. Palpate the oropharynx with the gloved finger to evaluate for fluctuance.
7. Assemble a MAC 3 or 4 intubation blade on a laryngoscope handle and open into the light-on position. Insert the blade into the patient's mouth, and advance the blade as far posteriorly as possible without inducing gagging. Have the patient hold the laryngoscope handle. Alternatively, use a tongue blade and head lamp or other light source, but the laryngoscope technique allows for an unobstructed view of the area and the weight of the handle helps hold the patient's mouth open.
8. Using the previously prepared needle guard on the long 18- to 20-gauge needle on a 12-mL syringe, insert the needle into the most fluctuant area (as determined from the previous examination), aspirating as the needle advances (Fig. 59.2). The most fluctuant area will usually be located in the superior pole of the tonsil.
   - It is very important to be careful not to angle the needle laterally toward the carotid artery. Also remember, this is a peritonsillar abscess so do not aspirate the tonsil itself.

© Springer Science+Business Media New York 2016
L. Ganti (ed.), *Atlas of Emergency Medicine Procedures*, DOI 10.1007/978-1-4939-2507-0_59

9. After aspiration, if there is a pus return, remove as much purulent drainage as possible. Typical drainage is between 2 and 6 mL. If a large amount of pus is obtained (>6 mL), incision and drainage (I&D) may be indicated. (See later for details on I&D.)

10. If the aspirate did not return pus, attempt aspiration again by moving the insertion site 1 cm inferiorly to the middle pole of the peritonsillar space. If there is still no pus aspirated, make a final attempt by moving again 1 cm inferiorly to the lower pole of the peritonsillar space.

11. Suction should be set up, readily available, and turned on. Use suction to prevent the patient from aspirating or swallowing any purulent drainage.

12. Expect a small amount of bleeding when the procedure is complete and the needle is removed.

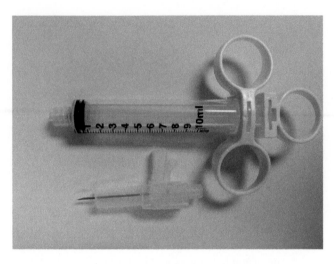

Fig. 59.1 Guard to prevent deep penetration of vascular structures

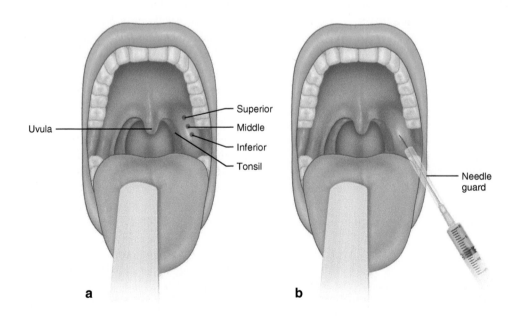

Fig. 59.2 Aspiration of a peritonsillar abscess: (**a**) Aspirate superior pole first. If no pus aspirated, move 1 cm inferior to the middle pole. If still no pus, make final attempt by moving 1 more cm inferiorly to the inferior pole. (**b**) Demonstrates use of needle guard

59.5   Procedure: Incision and Drainage

1. Raise the head of the bed and anesthetize the area as described previously.
2. Have suction set up with a Fraser or tonsil tip, available, and turned on.
3. Have the patient hold the laryngoscope handle after the blade has been inserted orally as described previously.
4. Fashion a blade guard on a #11 or #15 blade scalpel by taping over the blade with only 0.5 cm of the blade

exposed at the tip. Incise the area that was previously aspirated with a small stab incision. Suction the area.
5. Insert a curved Kelly clamp into the incision and open gently to enter the abscess cavity and break up loculations (Fig. 59.3). Suction as necessary.
6. Have the patient gargle with a saline solution and expectorate.
7. Do not pack the abscess cavity.
8. Observe for 2–4 h for bleeding.

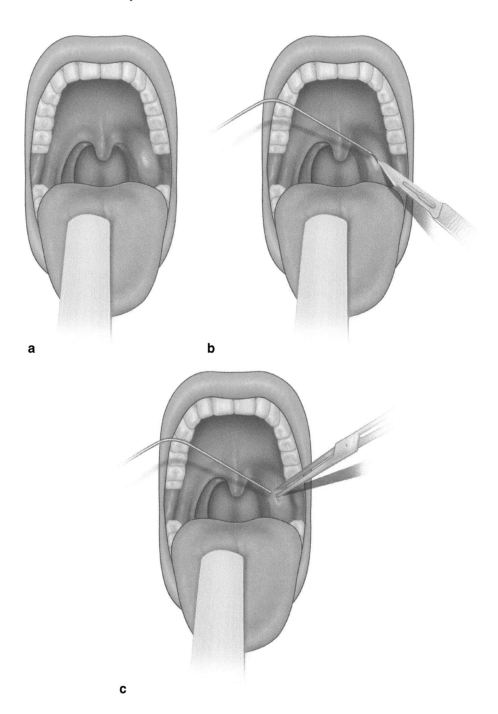

a   b

c

Fig. 59.3 Incision and drainage of peritonsillar abscess: (**a**) Gain access with appropriate lighting. (**b**) Fashion a blade guard on a #11 or #15 blade scalpel by taping over the blade with only 0.5 cm of the blade exposed at the tip. Incise the area that was previously aspirated with a small stab incision. (**c**) Insert a curved Kelly clamp into the incision and open gently to enter the abscess cavity and break up loculations. Do not pack!

59.6 Complications

- Aspiration or incision of the carotid artery
- Excessive bleeding
- Aspiration of purulent material
- Pain

59.7 Pearls and Pitfalls

- Pearls
    - Airway protection should always be considered. Intubation may be necessary for very large abscesses with airway compromise.
    - Bedsides ultrasound is a valuable tool in confirming the diagnosis of peritonsillar abscess. Perform using the intracavitary probe covered with a sterile glove or other appropriate probe cover and insert into the oropharynx. The abscess will appear as any other abscess: an encapsulated, hypoechoic structure. Doppler flow can also be used to locate the carotid artery relative to the abscess.
    - Empirical oral antibiotics after aspiration or I&D are considered usual care and should cover for group A streptococcus and oral anaerobes.
        - Amoxicillin/clavulanate or clindamycin is the most commonly used.
    - A single dose of high-dose steroids may be helpful in relieving symptoms.
    - Patients who cannot tolerate oral fluids, cannot take oral antibiotics, or who appear to have a toxic response should be admitted. Others may be discharged with 24-h follow-up.
- Pitfalls
    - The carotid artery is located approximately 2.5 cm posterolaterally to the tonsils. Take care that the needle is not inserted too far laterally or the risk of aspirating the carotid artery is increased.
    - Incision into the tonsil itself may cause excessive bleeding. Aspiration or incision into the tonsil will likely miss the abscess altogether and may result in misdiagnosis.
    - There is a 1–15 % failure and recurrence rate.

Selected Reading

Afarian H, Lin M. Tricks of the trade—say "ah!"—needle aspiration of peritonsillar abscess. ACEP News. 2008;27(5):38.

Braude DA, Shalit M. A novel approach to enhance visualization during drainage of peritonsillar abscess. J Emerg Med. 2008;35:297–8.

Galioto NJ. Peritonsillar abscess. Am Fam Physician. 2008;77:199–202.

Ozbek C, Aygenc E, Tuna EU, Selcuk A, Ozdem C. Use of steroids in the treatment of peritonsillar abscess. J Laryngol Otol. 2004;118:439–42.

Roberts J, Hedges J, editors. Clinical procedures in emergency medicine. 5th ed. Philadelphia: Saunders; 2009. p. 1184–9.

Vieira F, Allen SM, Stocks RM, Thompson JW. Deep neck infection. Otolaryngol Clin North Am. 2008;41:459–83.

Incision and Drainage of Sublingual Abscess

60

Melinda W. Fernandez and Bobby K. Desai

60.1 Indications

- Sublingual abscess (Fig. 60.1)

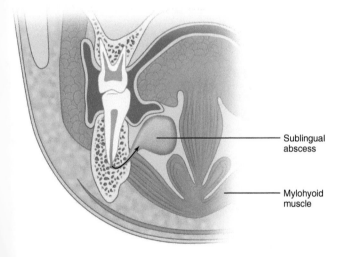

Fig. 60.1 Sublingual abscess

M.W. Fernandez, MD
Department of Emergency Medicine, University of Florida
Health, Gainesville, FL, USA
e-mail: mindyfernandez@ufl.edu

B.K. Desai, MD (✉)
Department of Emergency Medicine, University of Florida Health
Shands Hospital, Gainesville, FL, USA
e-mail: bdesai@ufl.edu

© Springer Science+Business Media New York 2016
, Ganti (ed.), *Atlas of Emergency Medicine Procedures*, DOI 10.1007/978-1-4939-2507-0_60

60.2 Contraindications

- Relative
  - Pediatric patient
  - Severe trismus—may need sedation or drainage in the operating room
  - Uncooperative patient—may need sedation or drainage in the operating room
  - Coagulopathy, patients taking anticoagulants, or patients with a known bleeding disorder

60.3 Materials and Medications (Fig. 60.2)

- #11 scalpel
- Hemostats
- Penrose drain
- 4-0 silk suture
- 25- to 27-gauge 1.5-inch needle for injecting anesthetic
- 18- to 20-gauge needle for drawing up anesthetic
- 5- to 10-mL syringe or control syringe
- Viscous lidocaine (or other topical anesthetic)
- Lidocaine 1 % with epinephrine
- Light source
- Suction setup with tonsil suction tip
- Culture swab

Fig. 60.2 Materials needed: #11 scalpel, hemostats, Penrose drain, 4-0 silk suture, 25–27-gauge 1.5-inch needle for injecting anesthetic, 18- to 20-gauge needle for drawing up anesthetic, 5- to 10-mL syringe or control syringe, viscous lidocaine (or other topical anesthetic), lidocaine 1 % with epinephrine, light source, suction setup with tonsil suction tip, culture swab (optional)

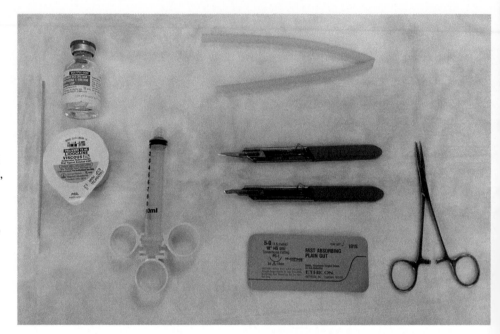

60.4   Procedure: Incision and Drainage

1. After explaining the procedure, risks, and benefits to the patient, put the head of the bed in the most comfortable working position for the clinician and the patient. Alternatively, the clinician may also elect to position the patient in an upright procedure chair that has multiple positions.
2. Apply viscous lidocaine topically with a cotton-tipped swab to the area to be injected with anesthetic. Leave in place for a minute or 2. Alternatively, spray the area with a topical anesthetic spray.
3. Have suction set up with a tonsil tip, available, and turned on.
4. Draw up the appropriate amount of lidocaine with epinephrine into a 5-mL syringe (control syringe if available).
5. Direct light source to area to be worked on. *Adequate lighting is essential.* Options include a headlamp or an overhead adjustable light.
6. Change needle to the 27-gauge needle and inject 1–2 mL of lidocaine with epinephrine using an inferior alveolar block. Alternatively, anesthetize the floor of the mouth around the most fluctuant area. Avoid injecting through infected tissue to avoid possible spread into deeper spaces.
7. Using the scalpel, make an intraoral stab incision superficially at the lowest point of the pus accumulation (Fig. 60.3). This will facilitate evacuation of pus under gravity. Have the suction catheter in the mouth and allow the purulent material to drain into the suction.
8. Obtain a specimen of the purulent fluid for culture and sensitivity.

9. Insert a hemostat into the incision to facilitate drainage, but do not open it up to avoid injury to neurovascular structures. Gently massage the soft tissue surrounding the abscess to assist drainage. Suction as necessary to avoid swallowing or aspirating the pus.
10. Once adequate drainage has been achieved, place a small Penrose drain (or other rubber-type drain) into the cavity, and stabilize on one side with a silk suture that goes through the drain and the mucosa (Fig. 60.4).
11. Have the patient rinse and spit with a half-strength peroxide solution followed by either water or saline.
12. Watch for signs of bleeding or upper airway symptoms.
13. Ensure that the patient can tolerate oral fluids before discharge.

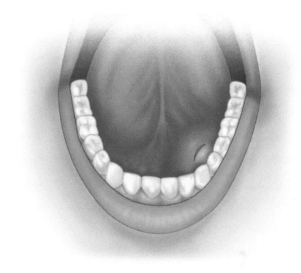

Fig. 60.3 Incise lowest portion of abscess

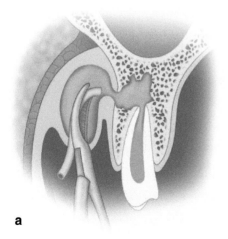
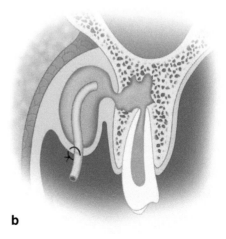

a   b

Fig. 60.4 (**a**) Using hemostats, place small Penrose drain into the abscess cavity. (**b**) Suture Penrose in place with a silk suture that goes through the drain and the mucosa

60.5 Complications (Generally Minimal)

- Excessive bleeding (apply pressure—to avoid potential nerve injury, do not cauterize or ligate unless absolutely necessary)
- Aspiration of purulent material (have the patient sit upright and use suction as the abscess is incised)
- Pain

60.6 Pearls and Pitfalls

- Pearls
  - Airway protection is paramount. Infections in this space can quickly spread to the submandibular region and can compromise the airway owing to swelling (Ludwig's angina).
    - Assess for elevation of the floor of the mouth and tongue, ability to lie supine, drooling, stridor, and restlessness.
    - If these signs are present, emergent surgical airway will be necessary before incision and drainage (I&D).
  - The sublingual space is bounded superiorly by the oral mucosa and inferiorly by the mylohyoid muscle.
  - Infected premolars and first molars drain into this space because the apices of their roots are located superior to the mylohyoid muscle.
  - The source molar should be extracted as soon as possible after I&D.
  - Empirical oral antibiotics after I&D should cover for group A streptococcus and oral anaerobes. Penicillin remains the drug of choice, but clindamycin or amoxicillin–clavulanic acid can be substituted.
- Pitfalls
  - The lingual artery, vein, and nerve are contained in the posterolateral area of the floor of the mouth, and the hypoglossal nerve is nearby. These must be avoided when performing I&D for sublingual abscesses.

Selected Reading

Flynn TR, Shanti RM, Levi MH, Adamo AK, Kraut RA, Trieger N. Severe odontogenic infections, part 1: prospective report. J Oral Maxillofac Surg. 2006;64:1093–103.

Reichman E, Simon R, editors. Emergency medicine procedures. New York: McGraw-Hill Education; 2003. p. 1342–5.

Roberts J, Hedges J, editors. Clinical procedures in emergency medicine. 5th ed. Philadelphia: Saunders; 2009. p. 1184–9.

Vieira F, Allen SM, Stocks RM, Thompson JW. Deep neck infection. Otolaryngol Clin North Am. 2008;41:459–83.

Incision and Drainage of Parotid Duct Abscess

61

Melinda W. Fernandez and Bobby K. Desai

61.1 Indications

- Parotid duct abscess

61.2 Contraindications

- Absolute
  - None
- Relative
  - Pediatric patient
  - Severe trismus—may need sedation or drainage in the operating room
  - Uncooperative patient—may need sedation or drainage in the operating room
  - Coagulopathy, patients taking anticoagulants, or patients with a known bleeding disorder

61.3 Materials and Medications (Fig. 61.1)

- #11 scalpel
- 4×4 gauze
- Hemostat
- Penrose drain or ¼-inch packing gauze
- Light source (headlamp or overhead light)
- Culture swab
- 4-0 silk suture
- 25- to 27-gauge needle, 1.5–2 inches long
- 18-gauge needle to withdraw anesthetic from vial
- 5-mL syringe
- Viscous lidocaine or other topical anesthetic
- Lidocaine with epinephrine
- Suction setup with Frazier or tonsil suction tip

M.W. Fernandez, MD
Department of Emergency Medicine,
University of Florida Health, Gainesville, FL, USA
e-mail: mindyfernandez@ufl.edu

B.K. Desai, MD (✉)
Department of Emergency Medicine, University of Florida Health
Shands Hospital, Gainesville, FL, USA
e-mail: bdesai@ufl.edu

© Springer Science+Business Media New York 2016
L. Ganti (ed.), *Atlas of Emergency Medicine Procedures*, DOI 10.1007/978-1-4939-2507-0_61

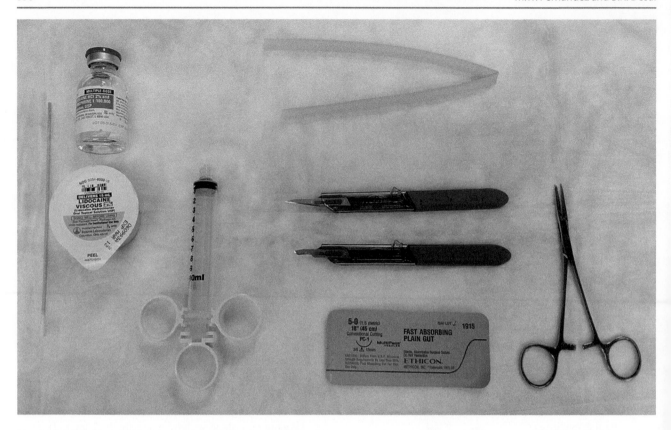

Fig. 61.1 Materials needed: #11 scalpel, hemostats, Penrose drain, 4-0 silk suture, 25- to 27-gauge 1.5-inch needle for injecting anesthetic, 18- to 20-gauge needle for drawing up anesthetic, 5- to 10-mL syringe or control syringe, viscous lidocaine (or other topical anesthetic), lidocaine 1 % with epinephrine, light source, suction setup with tonsil suction tip, culture swab (optional)

61.4   Procedure (Figs. 61.2 and 61.3)

1. After explaining the procedure, risks, and benefits to the patient, put the head of the bed in the most comfortable working position for the operator and the patient. Alternatively, position the patient in an upright procedure chair that has multiple positions.
2. Find the most fluctuant area. Apply viscous lidocaine topically with a cotton-tipped swab to the area to be injected with anesthetic. Leave in place for a minute or 2. Alternatively, spray the area with a topical anesthetic spray.
3. Have suction setup with a tonsil tip, available, and turned on.
4. Draw up the appropriate amount of lidocaine with epinephrine into a 5-mL syringe (control syringe if available).
5. Direct light source to area to be worked on. *Adequate lighting is essential.* Options include a headlamp or an overhead adjustable light.
6. Change needle to a 25- or 27-gauge needle. Inject 1–2 mL of lidocaine with epinephrine just beneath the mucosal surface. Avoid injecting through infected tissue to avoid possible spread into deeper spaces.

7. Using the scalpel, make an intraoral stab incision superficially into the area of greatest fluctuance (Fig. 61.4). Have the suction catheter in the patient's mouth and allow the purulent material to drain into the suction.
8. Obtain a specimen of the purulent fluid for culture and sensitivity.
9. Insert a hemostat into the incision to facilitate drainage, but do not open it up in order to avoid injury to neurovascular structures. Gently massage the soft tissue surrounding the abscess to assist drainage. Suction as necessary to avoid swallowing or aspirating the pus.
10. Have the patient rinse and spit with a half-strength peroxide solution.
11. Place a small Penrose drain (or other rubber-type drain) into the cavity, and stabilize on one side with a silk suture that goes through the drain and the mucosa. Alternatively, cut a strip of ¼- inch packing gauze and insert into the abscess cavity.
12. Have the patient rinse and spit with a half-strength peroxide solution followed by either water or saline.
13. Watch for signs of bleeding or upper airway symptoms.
14. Ensure that the patient can tolerate oral fluids before discharge.

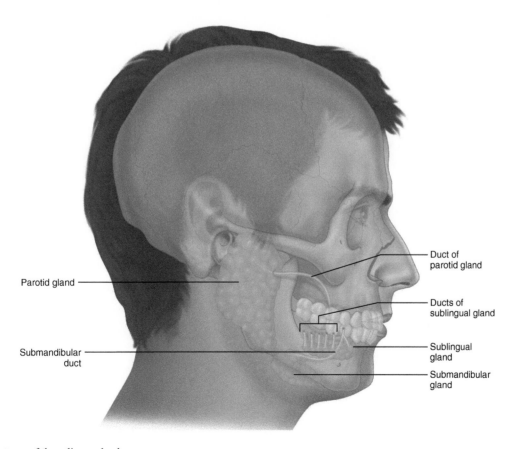

Fig. 61.2 Anatomy of the salivary glands

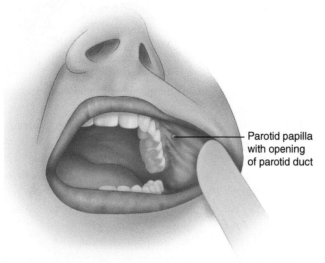

Fig. 61.3 Parotid papilla: opening of the parotid gland located adjacent to third upper molar

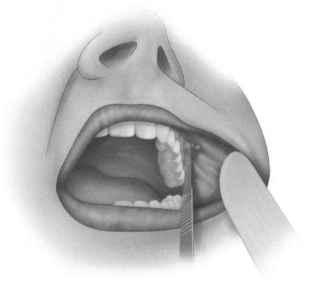

Fig. 61.4 Parotid abscess; make a superficial stab into most fluctuant area

61.5 Complications

- Complications are generally minimal but may include:
  - Excessive bleeding (apply pressure; to avoid potential nerve injury, do not cauterize or ligate unless absolutely necessary)
  - Aspiration of purulent material (have the patient sit upright and use suction as the abscess is incised)
  - Pain

61.6 Pearls and Pitfalls

- Airway protection should always be considered.
- Empirical oral antibiotics after incision and drainage are considered usual care and should cover for group A streptococcal and oral anaerobes. Penicillin remains the drug of choice, but clindamycin or amoxicillin–clavulanic acid can be substituted.
- Patients who cannot tolerate oral medications, cannot take oral antibiotics, or who appear to have a toxic response should be admitted. Pediatric patients should be admitted. Others may be discharged with 24-h follow-up.

Selected Reading

Reichman E, Simon R, editors. Emergency medicine procedures. New York: McGraw-Hill Education; 2003. p. 1346–9.

Roberts J, Hedges J, editors. Clinical procedures in emergency medicine. 5th ed. Philadelphia: Saunders; 2009. p. 1184–9.

Parotid papilla with opening of parotid duct

Techniques of Mandibular Anesthesia

Susana Perry, Joshua Perry, and Rosalia Rey

62.1 Inferior Alveolar Nerve Block

62.1.1 Nerves Anesthetized

- Inferior alveolar, branch of the posterior division of the mandibular nerve (V3, branch of the trigeminal nerve)
- Incisive
- Mental
- Lingual (usually)

62.1.2 Areas Anesthetized (Fig. 62.1)

- Mandibular teeth to midline
- Body of the mandible
- Buccal mucoperiosteum, mucous membrane anterior to the mandibular first molar
- Anterior two thirds of the tongue and floor of the mouth (via the lingual nerve)
- Lingual soft tissues and periosteum (via the lingual nerve)

S. Perry, DMD (✉)
Department of Pediatric Dentistry, University of Florida College of Dentistry, University of Florida Health Shands Hospital, Gainesville, FL, USA
e-mail: sperry@dental.ufl.edu

J. Perry, DMD
Department of Prosthodontics, University of Florida College of Dentistry, University of Florida Health Shands Hospital, Gainesville, FL, USA
e-mail: jperry@dental.ufl.edu

R. Rey, DDS
Department of Restorative Dental Sciences, University of Florida College of Dentistry, University of Florida Health Shands Hospital, Gainesville, FL, USA
e-mail: RREY@dental.ufl.edu

Fig. 62.1 Areas anesthetized with inferior mandibular nerve block

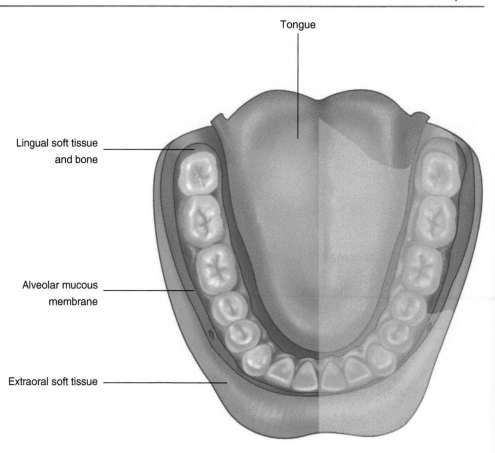

Tongue

Lingual soft tissue and bone

Alveolar mucous membrane

Extraoral soft tissue

62.1.3 Indications

- When buccal soft tissue anesthesia is necessary
- When lingual soft tissue anesthesia is needed
- When performing procedures on multiple mandibular teeth in one quadrant

62.1.4 Contraindications

- Infection or acute inflammation in the area of injection
- Patients who might bite their lip or tongue (e.g., very young child or physically or mentally handicapped adult or child)
- In relation to local anesthetic use

Absolute
- Local anesthetic allergy
  - Avoid all local anesthetics in the same chemical class (e.g., esters).

- Bisulfite allergy
  - Avoid vasoconstrictor-containing local anesthetics.

Relative
- Atypical plasma cholinesterase
- Methemoglobinemia (idiopathic or congenital)
- Significant liver dysfunction (American Society of Anesthesiologists [ASA] III–IV)
- Significant kidney dysfunction (ASA III–IV)
- Significant cardiovascular disease (ASA III–IV)
  - Avoid high concentrations of vasoconstrictors.
  - Use local anesthetics with epinephrine concentrations of 1:200,000 or 1:100,000 or 3 % mepivacaine or 4 % prilocaine.
- Clinical hyperthyroidism (ASA III–IV)
  - Avoid high concentrations of vasoconstrictors.
  - Use local anesthetics with epinephrine concentrations of 1:200,000 or 1:100,000 or 3 % mepivacaine or 4 % prilocaine.

62.1.5 Materials and Medications

- Local anesthetic carpule (1.7–1.8 mL)
  - Mepivacaine 3 % (+epinephrine 1:100,000)
  - Articaine HCl 4 % (+epinephrine 1:100,000 or 1:200,000)
  - Lidocaine HCl 2 % (+ epinephrine 1:50,000 or 1:100,000) (Fig. 62.2)
  - Bupivacaine HCl 0.5 % +epinephrine 1:200,000
- Aspirating syringe (Fig. 62.3)

- Needle (Fig. 62.4)
  - Gauge refers to the lumen of the needle: The smaller the number, the greater the diameter of the lumen.
  - Needles are color coded by gauge: red = 25 gauge, yellow = 27 gauge, and blue = 30 gauge.
  - *Recommendations: For inferior alveolar nerve (IAN) block, it is best to use a 25-gauge long needle.*
- Mouth props
- Retractors

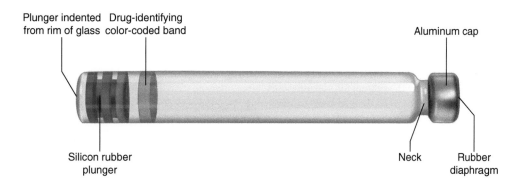

Plunger indented from rim of glass   Drug-identifying color-coded band   Aluminum cap

Silicon rubber plunger   Neck   Rubber diaphragm

Fig. 62.2 Local anesthetic carpule (1.7–1.8 mL)

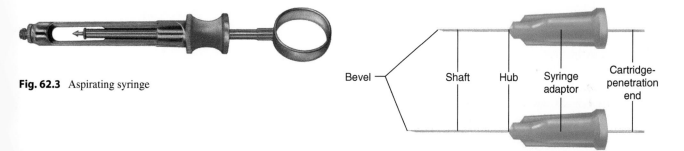

Fig. 62.3 Aspirating syringe

Bevel   Shaft   Hub   Syringe adaptor   Cartridge-penetration end

Fig. 62.4 Needle

62.1.6 Procedure

1. Target area: IAN as it passes downward toward the mandibular foramen.
2. Landmarks.
   (a) Coronoid notch
   (b) Pterygomandibular raphe
   (c) Occlusal plane of mandibular posterior teeth
3. Procedure.
   (a) Correct position for operator.
      (i) For a right IAN block, a right-handed administrator should sit at the 8 o'clock position facing the patient.
      (ii) For a left IAN block, a right-handed administrator should sit at the 10 o'clock position facing in the same direction as the patient.
   (b) Recommended to position the patient supine and with the mouth wide open.
   (c) Place thumb on the coronoid notch and index finger extraorally on the posterior border of the ramus in order to estimate the distance between these two points (Fig. 62.5).
      (i) The needle insertion should be three fourths of the anteroposterior distance from the coronoid notch to the deepest part of the pterygomandibular raphe.
   (d) Place the barrel of the syringe in the corner of the mouth on the contralateral side, usually corresponding to the premolars.
   (e) Slowly advance the needle until bony resistance is met.
      (i) For anxious or sensitive patients, a small volume of anesthetic may be deposited as the soft tissue is penetrated.
      (ii) Average depth of penetration to bony contact will be 20–25 mm, approximately two thirds to three fourths the length of a long needle.
      (iii) If the bone is contacted too soon (less than half the length of a long needle), the needle tip is usually located too far anteriorly (laterally) on the ramus. To correct:

• Withdraw it slightly from the tissues and bring the syringe barrel anteriorly toward the lateral incisor or canine; reinsert to the proper depth.
      (iv) If the bone is not contacted, the needle tip is usually located too far posterior (medial). To correct:
• Withdraw it slightly in tissue (leaving approximately one fourth its length in tissue), and reposition the syringe barrel more posteriorly (over the mandibular molars).
• Continue the insertion until contact with the bone is made at an appropriate depth (20–25 mm).
   (f) Aspirate. If negative, slowly deposit 1.5 mL of anesthesia over 60 s.
   (g) Wait 3–5 min before commencing the dental procedure.
4. Precaution: *Do not deposit anesthesia if the bone is not contacted.* The needle tip may be resting within the parotid gland near the facial nerve (cranial nerve VII), and a transient paralysis of the facial never may occur if solution is deposited.

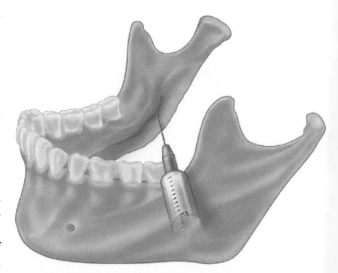

Fig. 62.5 Needle orientation for inferior alveolar nerve block

62.2   Buccal Nerve Block

62.2.1 Nerve Anesthetized

- Buccal nerve, a branch of the anterior division of the mandibular nerve

62.2.2 Area Anesthetized (Fig. 62.6)

- Soft tissues and periosteum buccal to the mandibular molars

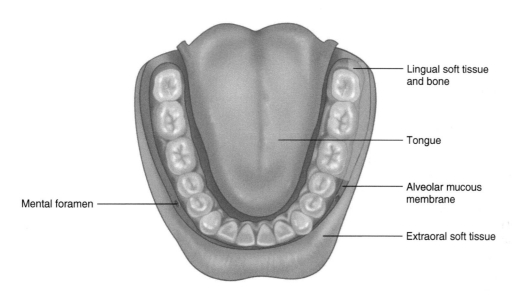

Fig. 62.6 Areas anesthetized with buccal nerve block

62.2.3 Procedure

1. A 25-gauge long needle is recommended.
2. Landmarks: mandibular molars and mucobuccal fold.
3. Orient the bevel of the needle *toward* the bone during injection.
4. Correct positioning.
   (a) For a right buccal nerve block, a right-handed administrator should sit at the 8 o'clock position directly facing the patient.
   (b) For a left buccal nerve block, a right-handed administrator should sit at the 10 o'clock facing in the same direction as the patient.
5. Procedure.
   (a) With the index finger, pull the buccal soft tissues in the area of injection laterally to allow for better visualization.
   (b) Align the syringe parallel to the occlusal plane of the teeth.
   (c) Penetrate the mucous membrane at the injection site, distal and buccal to the last molar (Fig. 62.7).
6. If tissue at the injection site becomes swollen, stop depositing solution.

62.3 Mental Nerve Block

62.3.1 Nerve Anesthetized

• Mental nerve, a terminal branch of the inferior alveolar nerve

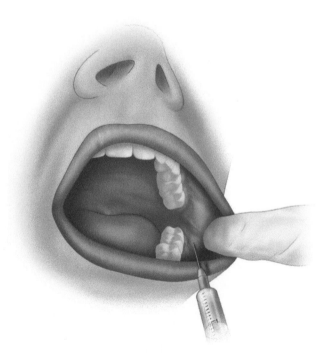

Fig. 62.7 Needle orientation for buccal nerve block

62.3.2 Area Anesthetized (Fig. 62.8)

- Buccal mucous membranes anterior to the foramen (around the second premolar) to the midline and skin of the lower lip

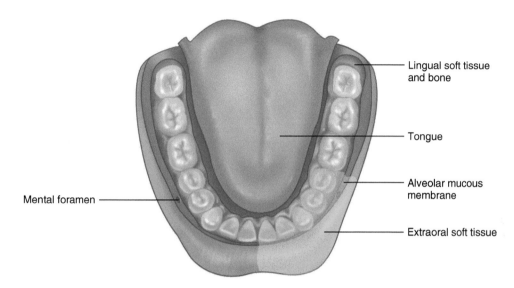

Fig. 62.8 Areas anesthetized with mental nerve block

62.3.3 Indications

- For buccal soft tissue anesthesia in procedures such as:
  - Soft tissue biopsies
  - Suturing of soft tissues

62.3.4 Procedure

1. Area of insertion: mucobuccal fold at or just anterior to the mental foramen.
2. Orientation of bevel should be *toward* the bone during injection.
3. Operator should sit in front of the patient so that the syringe is below the patient's line of sight.
4. Locate the mental foramen.
   (a) Place the index finger in the mucobuccal fold and press against the body of the mandible in the area of the first molar.
   (b) Move the finger anteriorly until the bone beneath the finger feels somewhat concave.

(c) Mental foramen is usually found around the apex of the second premolar.
(d) Orient the needle with the bevel directed toward the bone.
(e) Penetrate the mucous membrane and advance needle slowly; penetration depth is usually 5–6 mm.
(f) If aspiration is negative, deposit approximately one third of the cartridge over 20 s.
   (i) If the site balloons, stop the deposition of anesthetic and remove the syringe.

Selected Reading

Bennett CR. Monheim's local anesthesia and pain control in dental practice. 6th ed. St. Louis: Mosby; 1978.

Gow-Gates GAE. Mandibular conduction anesthesia: a new technique using extraoral landmarks. Oral Surg. 1973;36:321–8.

Jastak JT, Yagiela JA, Donaldson D. Local anesthesia of the oral cavity. Philadelphia: WB Saunders; 1995.

Malamed SF. The Gow-Gates mandibular block: evaluation after 4275 cases. Oral Surg. 1981;51:463.

Malamed SF. Handbook of local anesthesia. 5th ed. St. Louis: Mosby; 2004.

Reduction of Dislocated Temporomandibular Joint

63

Christopher J. Spencer and Geraldine Weinstein

63.1 Indications

- Open lock: associated with yawning, vomiting, or opening the mouth wide
- Open lock: associated with a dental procedure
- Open lock: associated with endoscopy
- Open lock: associated with oral intubation
- Time duration: acute to 3 weeks or less duration

63.2 Contraindications for Closed Reduction

- Absolute
  - Head trauma with fracture of the skull, maxilla, mandible, or mandibular Condyles

- Relative
  - Dislocation of 30 days or longer (will likely be unable to accomplish reduction without general anesthesia and/or open surgical approach)

63.3 Materials and Medications

- Local anesthetic syringe.
- Lidocaine 2 % 1–2 mL.
- 25- to 27-gauge needle (long or approximately 2 inches long).
- Betadine (povidone-iodine) or other skin antiseptic preparation.
- Gauze padding for thumbs.
- Consider a muscle relaxant.
- Consider conscious sedation.

.J. Spencer, DDS • G. Weinstein, DDS (✉)
Department of Restorative Dental Sciences, University of Florida
ollege of Dentistry, Gainesville, FL, USA
-mail: cspencer@dental.ufl.edu; gweinstein@dental.ufl.edu

## 63.4	Procedure

63.4.1 Manual Closed Reduction *without* Local Anesthesia (Figs. 63.1)

1. Position the patient in an upright posture with the mandible at the physician's flexed elbow height (physician's comfortable position).

2. Place the thumbs on the mandibular molars with wrapping around the thumbs to protect from possible biting force once the mandible reduces.
3. Apply bilateral firm force in an inferior direction.
4. The mandible will move rapidly in an inferior and then a posterior direction as the condyles slide back over the height of their respective articular eminences.

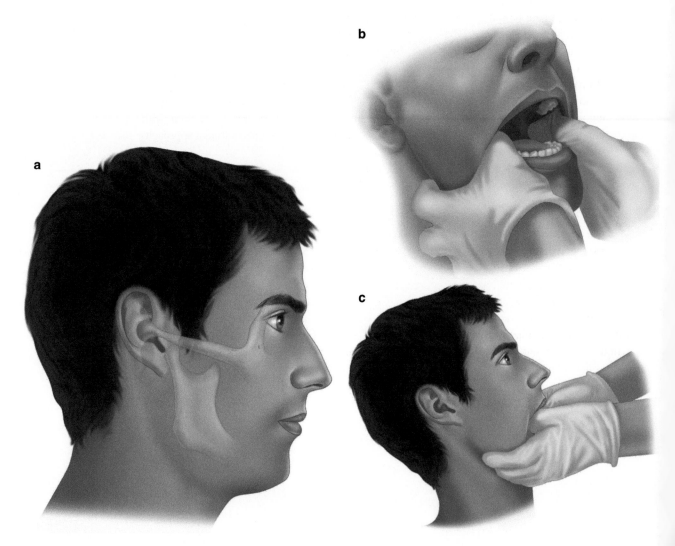

Fig. 63.1 Reduction in progress: (**a**) In a mandibular dislocation, the condyle will be anterior and superior to the articular eminence. (**b**) Position the thumbs on mandibular molars, and apply firm pressure in an inferior direction to distract the TM joint condyles so that they can reposition themselves into the glenoid fossa so that the TM joint can be reduced. (**c**) Lateral view of the distraction force with direction in an inferior direction to distract the condyle of the TM joint

63.4.2 Manual Closed Reduction *with* Local Anesthesia

- If the mandible will not respond to closed reduction with just thumb pressure, likely the masticatory muscles are contracting with sufficient force to prohibit the condyles from being sufficiently distracted owing to pain.

1. Reduction of pain in the temporomandibular joint (TMJ) with local anesthesia.
2. *Auriculotemporal block of V3:*
    - The auriculotemporal nerve that innervates the TMJ may be anesthetized inferior to the TMJ capsule. It can be accessed through the skin just anterior to the tragus.
    - With the patient's mouth wide open (it already is in this case), a triangular-shaped hollow will be evident inferior and posterior to the mandibular condyle. Insert the needle at a 20-degree anterior inclination, in the horizontal plane, at the level of the inferior border of the tragus of the ear (Fig. 63.2). The bevel of the needle should be anterior.
    - The needle should be inserted behind the (posterior) ramus and approximately 2 cm deep (aiming for the medial aspect of the posterior border of the ramus). If the posterior border of the ramus is contacted, the needle will need to be directed in a more posterior direction. Then deposit 1–2 mL of lidocaine 2 %.
3. Then, as before, place the thumbs in a bilateral position on the patient's mandibular molars, and depress the mandible to distract the condyles in an inferior direction.
4. Conscious sedation may be utilized if the reduction procedure has been arduous and stressful for the patient.

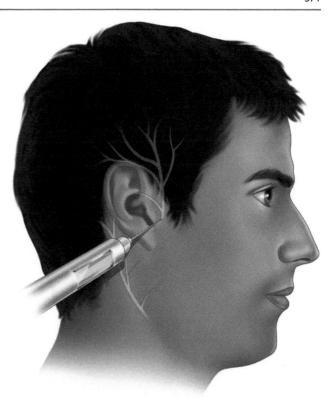

Fig. 63.2 Infiltration of cranial nerve V, the auriculotemporal branch (V3)

63.5   Complications

- Inability to reduce the condyles manually which may lead to more invasive procedures.
- If the condition is acute (≤24 h) and not associated with trauma, there are few if any significant complications or risks for this procedure.

63.6   Pearls

- The manual pressure required on the mandibular molars needs to be sustained and very firm.
- If both condyles are dislocated, it is likely beneficial to attempt one side at a time.
- The clinician needs to protect the thumbs from the impact of the patient's molars during the sudden successful reduction because the biting forces are significant in the molar region.

Selected Reading

Chan TC, Harrigan RA, Ufberg J, Vilke GM. Mandibular reduction. J Emerg Med. 2008;34:435.

Donlon WC, Truta MP, Eversole LR. A modified auriculotemporal nerve block for regional anesthesia of the temporomandibular joint. J Oral Maxillofac Surg. 1984;42:544.

Huang IY, Chen CM, Kao YH, Chen CM, Wu CW. Management of long-standing mandibular dislocation. Int J Oral Maxillofac Surg. 2011;40:810–4.

Prabhakar V, Singla S. Bilateral antersuperior dislocation of the intact mandibular condyles in the temporal fossa. Int J Oral Maxillofac Surg. 2011;40:640–3.

Thagarajah T, Mcculloch N, Thangarajah S, Stocker J. Bilateral temporomandibular joint dislocation in a 29-year-old man: a case report. J Med Case Rep. 2010;4:263.

Dry Socket (Alveolar Osteitis, Fibrinolytic Osteitis)

64

Michael A. Abraham, Amir Azari, Jennifer Westcott, and Franci Stavropoulos

64.1 Indications (Fig. 64.1)

- Definition: severe pain occurring 2–3 days after tooth extraction
- Recent tooth extraction, especially of a mandibular tooth or an impacted third molar
- Partially or completely visible bone socket
- Intense radiating pain (often to the ear)
- Fetid odor without suppuration
- Absence of swelling, lymphadenitis, or bacteremia
- Foreign bodies present in the extraction socket

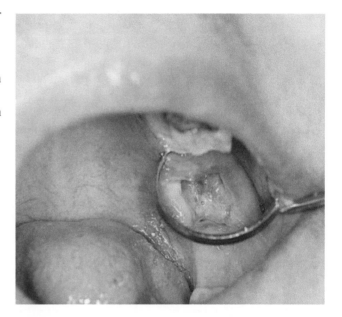

Fig. 64.1 Clinical photograph suggestive of a dry socket. Clinical correlation is necessary

M.A. Abraham, DMD (✉)
United States Air Force, Dental Corps, Minot, ND, USA
e-mail: mikeabrahamdmd@gmail.com

A. Azari, DMD
Department of Oral and Maxillofacial Surgery, Oregon Health and Science University, Portland, OR, USA
e-mail: Azari@OHSU.edu

J. Westcott, DMD
Private Practice, Palm Beach Gardens, FL, USA
e-mail: Jwestcott561@gmail.com

F. Stavropoulos, DDS
Department of Dental Specialties – Oral and Maxillofacial Surgery, Gundersen Health System, La Crosse, WI, USA
e-mail: Mfstavro@gundersenhealth.org

© Springer Science+Business Media New York 2016
L. Ganti (ed.), *Atlas of Emergency Medicine Procedures*, DOI 10.1007/978-1-4939-2507-0_64

64.2 Contraindications

- Absolute
  - Osteomyelitis
  - Jaw fracture
- Relative
  - Retained roots
  - Infection

64.3 Materials and Medications

- Warm saline or 0.12 % aqueous chlorhexidine solution
- 12-mL syringe with curved tip (Monoject® syringe)
- 25-gauge needle, syringe
- Local anesthetic, 2 % lidocaine 1:100,000 epinephrine
- Suction with small tip or gauze
- Socket dressing
  - Gelfoam or small gauze strips
- Socket medicament
  - Sultan dry socket paste® (guaiacol, balsam of Peru, eugenol, 1.6 % chlorobutanol), iodoform, or eugenol® (zinc oxide eugenol dental cement)
- Curved forceps

64.4 Procedure

1. Administer local anesthesia as necessary.
2. Remove any sutures closing the extraction site.
3. Irrigate the wound gently with warm saline or 0.12 % aqueous chlorhexidine.
4. Carefully suction or gently dry any excess saline; the socket area should be isolated from saliva by using gauze or cotton rolls.
5. Gently place iodoform-soaked gauze, Gelfoam soaked in eugenol, or Sultan dry socket paste in the extraction socket with forceps/Monoject syringe.
6. Rinse with saline and replace the dressing as needed for the first 2–3 days and every 2–3 days thereafter.
7. Remove the dressing, if it does not dissolve, without replacement once the pain has resolved.
8. Pain medication (nonsteroidal anti-inflammatory drugs [NSAIDS] or narcotics) should be prescribed if necessary.
9. Follow-up with dentist.

64.5 Complications

- Delayed healing
- Wound dehiscence

64.6 Pearls and Pitfalls

- *Pearls*
  - Wound irrigation may be so painful at the first visit that administration of a local anesthetic without a vasoconstrictor should be considered.
  - The patient should experience profound pain relief within minutes of placement of the soaked medicated dressing.
  - If a medicated dressing is necessary for more than 2 weeks, reevaluate for development of osteomyelitis.
  - "Dry socket" is not a progressive disease but may persist for 10–14 days whether treated or not; therapy is palliative.
  - Instruct the patient to avoid the following, which can cause changes of pressure in the mouth:
    - Smoking
    - Using a straw
    - Spitting
    - Drinking carbonated beverages (e.g., soda, seltzer water, beer)
- *Pitfalls*
  - Avoid over manipulating the socket because this will increase the amount of exposed bone and pain.

Selected Reading

Bloomquist D, Hooley J, Whitacre R. A self-instructional guide: surgical complications. 3rd ed. Seattle: Stroma; 1983.

Matocha DL. Postsurgical complications. Emerg Med Clin North Am. 2000;18:549–64.

Roberts G, Scully C, Shotts R. Dental emergencies. West J Med. 2001;175:51.

Postextraction Hemorrhage

Michael A. Abraham, Amir Azari, Jennifer Westcott, and Franci Stavropoulos

65.1 Indications

- Recent tooth extraction site, presenting with more than a slight oozing of blood
- Full evaluation indicating amount of blood loss, present physical condition, and reason for hemorrhage including coagulopathy or medication use

65.2 Contraindications

- Absolute
  - None
- Relative
  - None

65.3 Materials and Medications

- 2×2 gauze pad
- Saline
- 25-gauge needle, syringe
- Local anesthetic without vasoconstrictor—2 % lidocaine plain

M.A. Abraham, DMD (✉)
United States Air Force, Dental Corps, Minot, ND, USA
e-mail: mikeabrahamdmd@gmail.com

A. Azari, DMD
Department of Oral and Maxillofacial Surgery, Oregon Health and Science University, Portland, OR, USA
e-mail: Azari@OHSU.edu

J. Westcott, DMD
Private Practice, Palm Beach Gardens, FL, USA
e-mail: Jwestcott561@gmail.com

F. Stavropoulos, DDS
Department of Dental Specialties – Oral and Maxillofacial Surgery, Gundersen Health System, La Crosse, WI, USA
e-mail: Mfstavro@gundersenhealth.org

- Gelfoam® (absorbable gelatin-compressed sponge) or oxidized cellulose
- Topical thrombin
- Suture kit with 3-0 chromic gut suture or 3-0 Vicryl® suture (synthetic absorbable sterile surgical suture composed of a copolymer made from 90 % glycolide and 10 % L-lactide)
- Hemostat

65.4 Procedure

1. Use suction and saline irrigation to gently rinse the affected area. If a "liver" clot is present, irrigate and remove it with suction.
2. Determine the source of hemorrhage without local anesthesia, if possible, because the use of local anesthetic with an added vasoconstrictor may obscure bleeding sites.
3. Moisten a folded 2×2 gauze pad with saline and place it directly onto the extraction site.
4. Instruct the patient to apply firm biting pressure, and observe for 1 h, changing gauze as necessary.
5. If bleeding persists, an intraoral nerve block should be performed.
   - Blocks are preferred to infiltrations; anesthetic with epinephrine infiltrated near the bleeding site will produce only temporary local hemostasis from vasoconstriction.
6. Gently curette the tooth extraction socket and remove areas of old blood clot or granulation tissue.
7. Check soft tissue for associated arterial bleeding.
   - If hemorrhage is localized to soft tissue, use pressure or tie off vessels.
8. Fold Gelfoam® into a small cylinder to fit into the extraction socket.
9. Place Gelfoam® with topical thrombin or Surgicel® (absorbable hemostat) into the socket and hold in

Springer Science+Business Media New York 2016
Ganti (ed.), *Atlas of Emergency Medicine Procedures*, DOI 10.1007/978-1-4939-2507-0_65

375

position with a figure-of-eight stitch using 3-0 chromic gut suture or 3-0 Vicryl suture (Figs. 65.1 and 65.2).

10. Fold 2×2 gauze, moisten it with saline, and place it over the suture.
11. Instruct the patient to bite down with firm pressure for 30 min; repeat as necessary.
12. Follow-up with dentist.

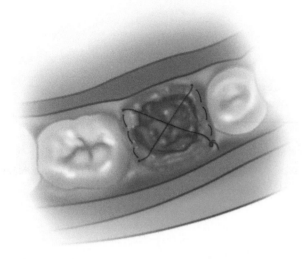

Fig. 65.1 A resorbable figure-of-eight suture placed over an extraction socket

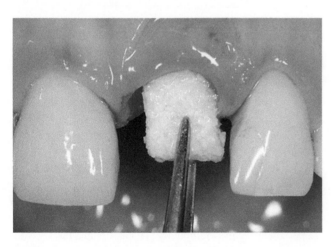

Fig. 65.2 Gelfoam® (absorbable gelatin-compressed sponge) being placed into the extraction socket (Photograph courtesy of Dr. Michael Abraham)

65.5 Complications

- Continued bleeding due to lack of patient compliance.
- Continued bleeding due to coagulopathy or medication use.
- If bleeding persists and coagulopathy is identified, the administration of intravenous blood replacement products may be necessary.

65.6 Pearls and Pitfalls

- Pearls
  - Minor bleeding concerns may be addressed at home by instructing the patient to bite on the affected area with a tea bag for 30 min (tannic acid in tea is a vasoconstrictor).
  - It is normal for an extraction socket to ooze slight amounts of blood for 12–24 h; it is normal for patients to see some blood on their pillow after waking.
  - The patient should be instructed to avoid the following, which can cause changes of pressure in the mouth:
    - Smoking
    - Using a straw
    - Spitting
    - Drinking carbonated beverages (e.g., soda, seltzer water, beer)
- Pitfalls
  - Small amounts of blood mixed with saliva may deceptively appear as large amounts of blood.

Selected Reading

Bloomquist D, Hooley J, Whitacre R. A self-instructional guide: surgical complications. Seattle: Stroma; 1983. pp. 50–5.

Hupp JR, Ellis III E, Tucker MR, editors. Contemporary oral and maxillofacial surgery. 5th ed. St. Louis: Mosby Elsevier; 2008. p. 195–7.

Fractured Tooth

Geraldine Weinstein

66.1 Indications (Fig. 66.1)

- Temporary repair of an acute dental fracture until follow-up by a dentist can be secured.

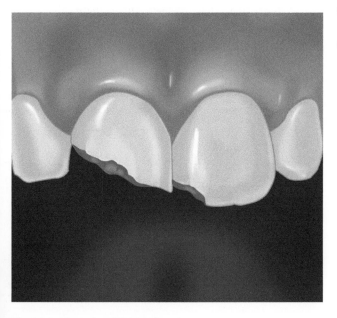

Fig. 66.1 Examples of fractured teeth

66.2 Methods of Sustaining Dental Fracture

- Traumatic injury to the head/facial area
- Falling down
- Extensive tooth decay that has undermined the integrity of the tooth structure
- Biting down on something hard

G. Weinstein, DDS
Department of Restorative Dental Sciences,
University of Florida College of Dentistry,
Gainesville, FL, USA
e-mail: gweinstein@dental.ufl.edu

© Springer Science+Business Media New York 2016
L. Ganti (ed.), *Atlas of Emergency Medicine Procedures*, DOI 10.1007/978-1-4939-2507-0_66

66.3   Four Types of Fractured Tooth
(Fig. 66.2)

- *Type 1*: contained to the enamel of the tooth, asymptomatic, and can be treated easily with a composite filling by a dentist.
- *Type 2*: involves a fracture through the dentin layer of the tooth. The patient may experience some sensitivity to

temperature changes and chewing. Depending on the severity, treatment may include a root canal and a restoration by a dentist.

- *Type 3*: involves the pulp of the tooth and will require endodontic treatment by a dentist.
- *Type 4*: a root fracture in the tooth that makes it nonrestorable and requiring extraction. It is diagnosed by means of a periapical radiograph taken in a dental office.

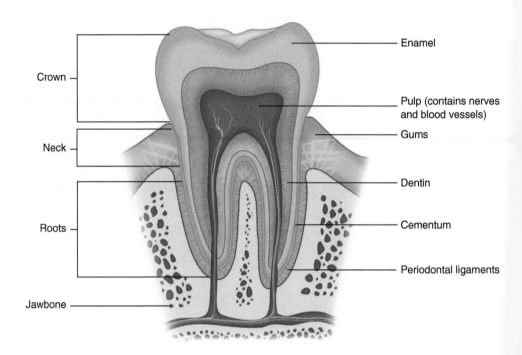

Crown

Neck

Roots

Jawbone

Enamel

Pulp (contains nerves and blood vessels)

Gums

Dentin

Cementum

Periodontal ligaments

Fig. 66.2 Anatomy of a tooth

66.4 Contraindications

- *Relative*
  - Patients at high risk of aspiration owing to intoxication and altered mental status

66.5 Materials and Medications

- Warm saline or 0.12 % aqueous chlorhexidine solution for irrigation of tissues and tooth
- Irrigating syringe
- Suction with a small tip
- Gauze to control hemorrhage
- Resorbable sutures and local anesthetic as needed for soft tissue lacerations
- Temporary tooth restoration material like intermediate restorative material (IRM) and glass ionomer (like Fuji)

66.6 Procedure

1. Have the patient rinse the mouth out with warm water to clean out any debris. Apply an ice pack to the affected cheek to reduce swelling.
2. Anesthetize the area, either locally at the tooth apex or with a nerve block (mental or inferior alveolar).
3. Irrigate the area; assess the fracture intraorally and check for soft tissue lacerations. Use the gauze with finger pressure to control bleeding in the soft tissue or the tooth.
4. Check if the tooth or bony segment is mobile. If so, a referral to a dentist or oral surgeon is necessary as soon as possible for proper assessment.
5. Type II fractures (fracture limited to dentin layer): cover the exposed surface with a temporary dental cement. In a pinch, 2-octyl cyanoacrylate (Dermabond) is an acceptable secondary alternative (Fig. 66.3).
6. Type III (pulp involved)
   - Provide immediate dental follow-up and analgesics.
   - Initiate antibiotic coverage with penicillin or clindamycin.

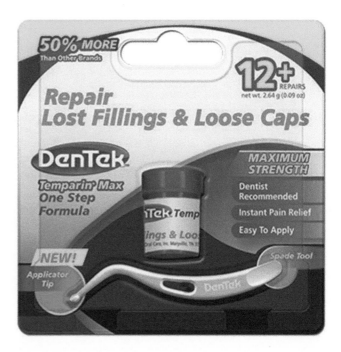

Fig. 66.3 Example of temporary dental cement (Reproduced with permission from DenTek Oral Care, Inc.)

66.7 Complications

- Loss of a tooth
- Infection or abscess
- Aspiration of a segment or a whole tooth
- Cosmetic deformity

66.8 Pearls

- Be certain to perform a thorough intraoral examination, looking for tooth fragments or lacerations that may be hiding fragments.
- Dental blocks are very useful for pain control.
- If a tooth is not mobile and the *pulp is exposed*, immediate referral (within a few hours) to a dentist is necessary for extraction or endodontic (root canal) treatment of the tooth. Placement of a temporary-type restoration on this tooth is *not* recommended at this time because it may exacerbate symptoms. Prescribe pain medication and possibly antibiotics when the tooth's pulp is exposed and the patient is unable to see the dentist within 24 h.
- If the tooth is not mobile and *the pulp is not exposed*, a temporary restoration can be placed on the tooth and the patient referred to a dentist for treatment. The fractured part of the tooth should be saved in the event that it can be used. If temporary tooth restoration is unavailable in the emergency department, advise the patient that it is readily available at local pharmacies.
- ALL DENTAL FRACTURES, EXCEPT TYPE I, REQUIRE DENTAL FOLLOW-UP WITHIN 24 h.

Dental Avulsion Management

Laura Tucker and Abimbola O. Adewumi

67.1 Indications

- The tooth is completely displaced *out* of its socket, leading to severance of the neurovascular pulp supply and separation of the periodontal ligament (Fig. 67.1).
- Diagnosis
  - Clinically, the socket is found empty or filled with coagulum.
  - Imaging (occlusal, periapical, and lateral views of the affected tooth and surrounding area) (Fig. 67.2):
- Confirm vacuous socket.
- Ensure that the missing tooth is not intruded.
- Diagnose root fracture or alveolar fracture.

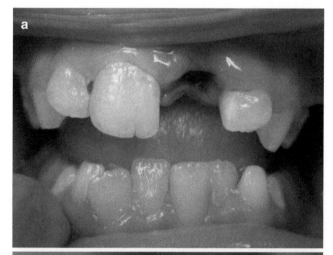

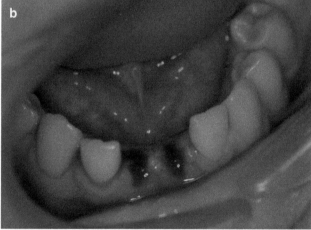

Fig. 67.1 (**a**, **b**) Empty socket following traumatic dental avulsion

. Tucker, DDS • A.O. Adewumi, BDS, FDSR (✉)
epartment of Pediatric Dentistry, University of Florida Health
hands Hospital, Gainesville, FL, USA
-mail: lauragracesullivan@gmail.com; aadewumi@dental.ufl.edu

Springer Science+Business Media New York 2016
Ganti (ed.), *Atlas of Emergency Medicine Procedures*, DOI 10.1007/978-1-4939-2507-0_67

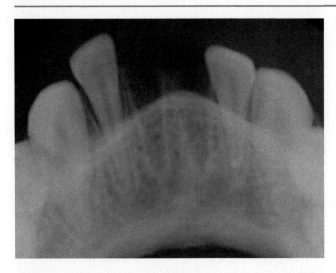

Fig. 67.2 Lower occlusal radiograph shows a complete avulsion of the mandibular right and left central incisors

67.2 Contraindications

- Absolute
  - Avulsed tooth is a primary tooth.
    - DO NOT REPLANT OR REPOSITION AVULSED PRIMARY TEETH.
    - Replantation of primary teeth increases the potential for damage to the developing permanent tooth owing to the increased frequency of pulpal necrosis.
- Relative
  - Fractured root (further intervention required before replantation)
  - Alveolar fracture (further intervention required before replantation)
  - Prolonged extraoral dry time and out of compatible solution (>1 h)
  - Immunocompromised host or congenital heart disease
  - Severe seizure disorder that may put tooth at risk for coming out while the airway is compromised
  - Patient with potential to lose airway reflexes

67.3 Materials and Medications

- Hank's Balanced Salt (Save-A-Tooth) solution or milk in which to preserve tooth until it can be replanted
  - Normal saline if neither of those is available
- Normal saline rinse
- 20- or 18-gauge cannula for gentle irrigation of the socket
- Absorbable suture for gingival lacerations, if present
- Flexible splint materials
  - Round dental wire
  - A flat pliable metal long enough to cover the affected tooth and the two teeth on other side (e.g., the metal nasal bridge from a respirator mask)
- Fixative
  - Dental adhesive
  - Dermabond or some other brand of cyanoacrylate for adhesive skin closures

67.4   Procedure

1. Be certain the tooth is a permanent one and not a primary tooth.
2. If not done by the patient, gently wash the tooth under water for approximately 10 s.
   - Be certain to hold the tooth by the crown, not the root (Fig. 67.3)
3. If the tooth cannot be replanted immediately, place the tooth in Hank's solution or milk.
4. If no such media is available, instruct the patient to hold the tooth inside his or her mouth between the cheek and the gums.
5. Gently replant the tooth, using digital pressure only into as anatomical a position as possible (Fig. 67.4).
   - Assess clinically for alignment.
   - Radiograph for confirmation.
6. Suture any gingival lacerations if present.
7. Apply a flexible splint, securing the affected tooth to the teeth on either side.
   - Consider using skin adhesive both to secure the tooth to its neighbors and, perhaps, to apply a makeshift splint until the patient can be seen by her or his dentist.
     - Towel dry the teeth as best as possible.
     - Apply skin adhesive (using the standard applicator) to the lateral edges of the avulsed tooth where it will make contact with its adjacent teeth.
     - If dental wire is available, apply adhesive to the buccal surfaces of the three teeth (the avulsed tooth central to the other two) and apply length of metal to the Fixodent (Fig. 67.5).
8. Systemic antibiotics with anaerobic coverage is empirical.
9. Ascertain tetanus status for the patient; update if uncertain.

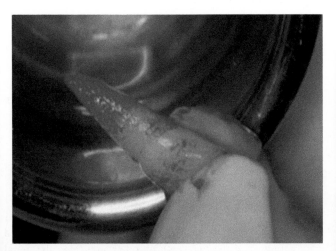

Fig. 67.3   Proper way to hold an avulsed tooth

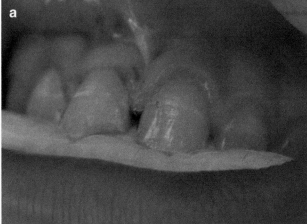

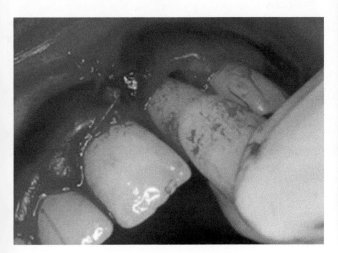

Fig. 67.4   Gentle replantation using digital pressure

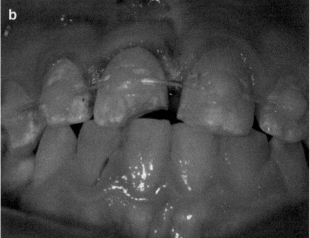

Fig. 67.5   (**a, b**) Splint stabilization

67.5 Complications

- Primary teeth
  - Dilaceration (bend) in the permanent tooth crown
  - Enamel defect of the lower permanent incisors as a result of avulsion of the preceding primary tooth
- Permanent teeth
  - Discoloration as a result of loss of vitality of the avulsed tooth.
  - Ankylosis of the alveolar ridge, leading to functional and aesthetic changes.
  - Replacement resorption occurs when the replanted tooth is slowly replaced with bone.
  - External inflammatory resorption is a progressive loss of tooth associated with destruction of adjacent alveolar bone.
  - Infection
  - Aspiration of an inadequately secured replanted tooth.

67.6 Pearls and Pitfalls

- Pearls
  - At the initial examination, make sure that all avulsed teeth are accounted for.
    - If not, a radiographic examination is necessary to ensure that the missing tooth is not completely intruded (pushed into the gum) or has sustained a root fracture with loss of the coronal fragment.
  - In children, always consider the likelihood of nonaccidental trauma (abuse).
  - Short-term and long-term dental follow-up cannot be emphasized enough.
- Pitfalls
  - If the avulsed tooth cannot be accounted for, aspiration is a possibility.
- Prognosis
  - Depends on extraoral dry time (length of time the tooth has been out of the mouth and not stored in an appropriate medium):
    - Ideally, tooth should be implanted within 5 min.
    - Extraoral dry time greater than 60 min has a poor prognosis for periodontal healing.
  - Depends on stage of root development of the avulsed tooth (Fig. 67.6)
- The more advanced the root development, the lower the probability of pulp healing and survival.

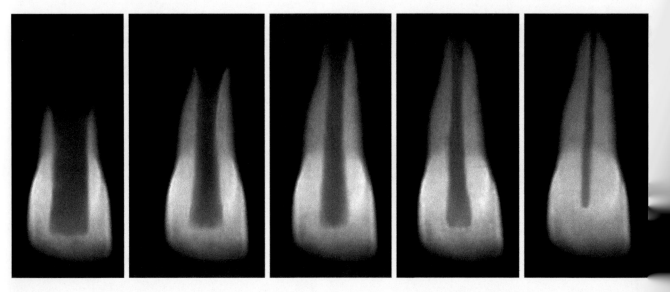

Fig. 67.6 The various stages of root development, from the less advanced (*open apex, left*) to the more advanced (*closed apex, right*)

Selected Reading

AAPD Council on Clinical Affairs. Guideline on management of acute dental trauma. AAPD reference manual. Chicago: American Academy of Pediatric Dentistry; 2010–2011. pp. 202–12.

Andreasen FM, Andreasen JO. Avulsions. In: Andreasen JO, Andreasen FM, Andersson L, editors. Textbook and color atlas of traumatic injuries to the teeth. 4th ed. Oxford: Blackwell; 2007. p. 444–88.

Andreasen JO, Jensen SS, Sae-Lim V. The role of antibiotics in preventing healing complications after traumatic dental injuries: a literature review. Endod Topic. 2006;14:80–92.

Finucane D, Kinirons MJ. External inflammatory and replacement resorption of luxated, and avulsed replanted permanent incisors: a review and case presentation. Dent Traumatol. 2003;19: 170–4.

Flores MT, Andersson L, Andreasen JO, et al. Guidelines for the management of traumatic dental injuries. II. Avulsion of permanent teeth. Dent Traumatol. 2007;23:130–6.

Hile LM, Linklater DR. Use of 2-octyl cyanoacrylate for the repair of a fractured tooth. Ann Emerg Med. 2006;47:424–6.

The dental trauma guide. Available at: www.dentaltraumaguide.org.

Excision of Thrombosed External Hemorrhoid

68

Latha Ganti

68.1 Indications

- Acute pain within 72 h of thrombosis onset
- The thrombosis will be visible as a bluish-purplish painful mass in perianal area (Fig. 68.1).

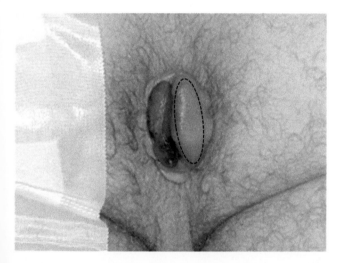

Fig. 68.1 Bluish-purplish appearance of an external thrombosed hemorrhoid. The *ellipse* denotes the area of the elliptical incision to be made (Reproduced with permission from: Fargo and Latimer [3])

68.2 Contraindications

- Absolute
  - Severe coagulopathy
  - Hemodynamic instability
  - Concurrent internal hemorrhoid with rectal prolapse
  - Painless rectal mass (external hemorrhoids are almost always painful, so a painless mass is not a thrombosed external hemorrhoid; also, the whole point of doing this procedure is to provide pain relief).
- Relative
  - Allergy to local anesthetics
  - Perianal infection
  - Inflammatory bowel disease
  - Serious systemic illness or comorbidity that could increase risk of procedure

68.3 Materials and Medications

- Sterile gloves and drape
- Alcohol swabs or pads
- 10 % povidone-iodine or chlorhexidine prep
- 2 % lidocaine with epinephrine
- 5 ml syringe with 25 or 27 gauge and 18 gauge needles
- #11 or #15 scalpel blade and handle
- Direct light source
- Forceps
- Iris scissors
- 4×4 gauze pads
- Adhesive tape
- 3-0 absorbable suture
- 1/4 inch iodoform packing
- Silver nitrate sticks
- Sterile dressing

L. Ganti, MD, MS, MBA
Professor of Emergency Medicine, University of Central Florida, Orlando, FL, USA

Director, SE Specialty Care Centers of Innovation, Orlando Veterans Affairs Medical Center, Orlando, FL, USA
e-mail: lathagantimd@gmail.com

© Springer Science+Business Media New York 2016
L. Ganti (ed.), *Atlas of Emergency Medicine Procedures*, DOI 10.1007/978-1-4939-2507-0_68

68.4   Procedure

1. Patient should be in either prone, left lateral decubitus, or jackknife position (Fig. 68.2).
2. Place 2 vertically oriented pieces of tape down each buttock from lower back to upper thigh. Next, place a perpendicular (horizontal) strip spreading buttocks to either side, securing gurney (Fig. 68.3).
3. Place sterile drape over field and center direct lighting over field (Fig. 68.4).
4. Wipe area with alcohol.
5. Inject 1–2 cc of anesthetic into base of hemorrhoid.
6. Clean area with povidone-iodine or chlorhexidine prep.
7. Make an elliptical incision in the roof of the hemorrhoid, being careful to avoid anal sphincter muscle.
8. Remove blood clot(s); multiple clots are often present.
9. If profuse bleeding is a problem, consider cauterization with silver nitrate sticks.
10. Wound can be closed with figure-of-8 absorbable suture OR can be loosely packed with1/4 inch iodoform gauze if not suturing (do not suture wound closed with packing inside).
11. Cover wound with 4×4 gauze folded in half and taped into place (Fig. 68.5).

- Discharge medicines:
  - Antibiotics generally not necessary.
  - Prescribe ibuprofen and/or acetaminophen for analgesia. Avoid opiates, which are constipating.
  - Prescribe stool softeners, to be taken two to three times daily.
- Discharge instructions to patient:
  - Sitz baths 3–4 times daily, for 20 min, warm not hot water.
  - Packing should fall out spontaneously in 2 days.
  - Keep well hydrated.
  - Use gauze to protect underclothing from soilage/blood stains.
  - Return to ED if pain persists beyond 48 h.

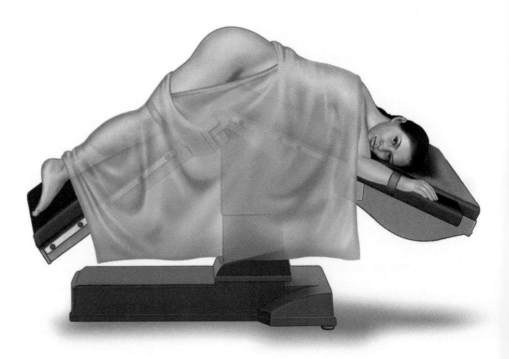

Fig. 68.2 Jackknife position

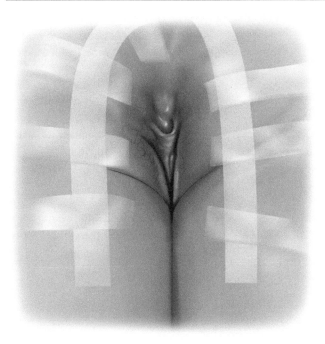

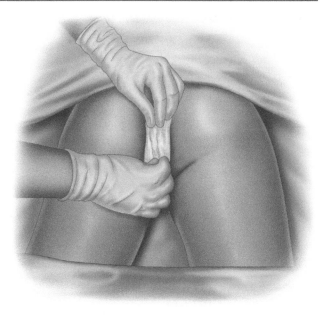

Fig. 68.5 Dress wound with sterile gauze

Fig. 68.3 Taping of buttocks to maximize visualization of hemorrhoid

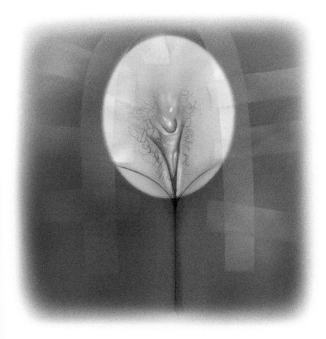

Fig. 68.4 Direct lighting over field

68.5   Complications

- Common
  - Bleeding: usually self-limited. Can apply cautery or figure-of-8 suture if not previously done
  - Pain: usually controlled with ibuprofen or acetaminophen
  - Perianal skin tag: benign
- Rare
  - Infection rate is 5 % [1].
  - Recurrence rate is 5–19 %, vs. 30 % for simple lancing [2].
  - Stricture and/or incontinence: prevented by avoiding underlying external anal sphincter muscle

68.6   Pearls and Pitfalls

- Pearls
  - Elliptical excision of the hemorrhoid results in much lower recurrence rate than simple lancing.
  - Risk factors for thrombosed external hemorrhoids include constipation, 2nd or 3rd trimester pregnancy, and traumatic vaginal delivery.

- Pitfalls
  - Excision of multiple hemorrhoids in circumferential fashion on all sides of the anal canal can cause anal stenosis.
  - Excision of a painless mass: if it is *painless*, it is *not* a thrombosed external hemorrhoid.

References

1. Lorber BW. Thrombosed external hemorrhoid excision. Medscape. com. www.emedicine.medscape.com/article/81039. Accessed 27 July 2014.
2. Rivadeneira DE. Outpatient and surgical procedures for hemorrhoids. UpToDate.com. http://www.uptodate.com/contents/outpatient-and-surgical-procedures-for-hemorrhoids. Accessed 27 July 2014.
3. Fargo MV, Latimer KM. Evaluation and management of common anorectal conditions. Am Fam Physician. 2012;85(6):624–30.

Selected Reading

Fargo MV, Latimer KM. Evaluation and management of common ano-rectal conditions. Am Fam Physician. 2012;85(6):624–30.
Jongen J, Bach S, Stübinger SH, Bock JU. Excision of thrombosed external hemorrhoid under local anesthesia: a retrospective evaluation of 340 patients. Dis Colon Rectum. 2003;46(9):1226–31.

Diagnostic Peritoneal Lavage

Latha Ganti

69.1 Indications (Table 69.1)

- Inability to perform FAST exam due to lack of equipment or operator
- Hemodynamically unstable patient in whom FAST exam is negative or equivocal

Table 69.1 Comparison parameters for DPL, FAST, and CT [1]

	DPL	FAST	CT
Speed	10–15 min	Fastest: <5 min	Variable
Repeatable	Yes, but rarely done	Yes, and frequently done	Yes, but not done often
Cost	$	$$	$$$
Invasive	Yes	No	No
Mobile	Yes	Yes	No
Advantages	Most sensitive for mesenteric and hollow viscus injuries	Highest specificity	Highly accurate but can be hampered by patient movement
Disadvantages	Misses retroperitoneal and diaphragm injuries	Hampered by subcutaneous or intra-abdominal air, obesity, and pelvic fractures. Significant false-negative rate	Misses diaphragm, small bowel, and pancreatic injuries. Small but significant risk of radiation-associated malignancy. Cannot be done at bedside

. Ganti, MD, MS, MBA
rofessor of Emergency Medicine, University of Central Florida,)rlando, FL, USA

irector, SE Specialty Care Centers of Innovation, Orlando
eterans Affairs Medical Center, Orlando, FL, USA
mail: lathagantimd@gmail.com

Springer Science+Business Media New York 2016

. Ganti (ed.), *Atlas of Emergency Medicine Procedures*, DOI 10.1007/978-1-4939-2507-0_69

69.2   Contraindications

- Absolute
  - Indication for laparotomy already exists.
- Relative
  - 2nd or 3rd trimester pregnancy
  - Previous lower abdominal surgery
  - Inexperienced operator
  - Abdominal wall infection
  - Coagulopathy
  - Cirrhosis
  - Morbid obesity

69.3   Materials and Medications

- 10 % povidone iodine prep
- 1 % lidocaine with epinephrine
- Fenestrated drape
- #10 scalpel blade and scalpel holder
- Skin retractors
- Hemostats
- Diagnostic peritoneal lavage (DPL) catheter (standard peritoneal dialysis catheter)
- 10 cc syringe
- Warmed lactated Ringer's or normal saline solution
- Skin stapler
- Simple suture tray with suture material

69.4   Procedure

69.4.1 Patient Preparation

- Place patient in supine position.
- Ensure nasogastric and urethral catheter (Foley) are in place.
- Prep and drape the area from the umbilicus to the symphysis pubis.
- Anesthetize the skin using 1 % lidocaine with epinephrine in the midline where incision will be made (Fig. 69.1).

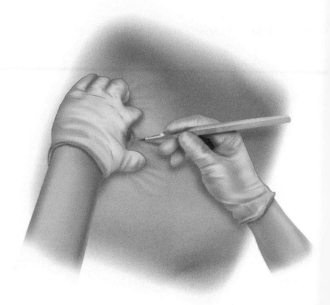

Fig. 69.1 Anesthetize skin where incision will be made (supraumbilical incision shown here, can also make infraumbilical incision)

69.4.2 Three DPL Techniques

- Semiopen (Seldinger) technique
    1. Using a #10 scalpel blade, make a 2 cm incision either superior or inferior to the umbilicus.
    2. Dissect subcutaneous fat until linea alba is exposed.
    3. Hold incision open with skin retractors (Fig. 69.2).
    4. Grasp fascia with hemostats on either side of midline.
    5. Insert 18 gauge needle at 45° angle toward pelvis (Fig. 69.3).
    6. First "pop" will be heard once fascia is penetrated.
    7. Second "pop" will be heard once peritoneum is traversed.
    8. Pass guidewire through needle into pelvis (should pass easily without resistance).
    9. Remove needle while keeping wire stable.
    10. Pass dilator over the wire through fascia, and remove (Fig. 69.4).
    11. Slip DPL catheter over guidewire aiming toward pelvis.
    12. Aspirate peritoneal contents with syringe; aspiration of blood is a positive DPL and means immediate laparotomy (can stop DPL procedure here).
    13. If no blood is immediately obvious, then connect the DPL catheter to a liter of warmed lactated Ringer's (LR) or normal saline (NS) solution for lavage (ensure setup has no one-way valves as solution and peritoneal fluid need to be able to freely mix).
    14. Place LR or NS bag on floor once it is almost empty (minimum 300–350 ml for adults or 10–15 ml/kg for children) and allow intra-abdominal fluid to return (Fig. 69.5).
    15. Send fluid for analysis (Table 69.2).
    16. Irrigate wound, and close skin only with staples or sutures.
- Open technique
    1. Make a 5 cm incision inferior to the umbilicus over linea alba and directly visualize peritoneal cavity.
    2. Both fascia (absorbable suture) and skin (nonabsorbable suture) need to be closed.
- Closed technique
    1. Access peritoneal cavity via percutaneous needle access.
    2. No surgical closure required.

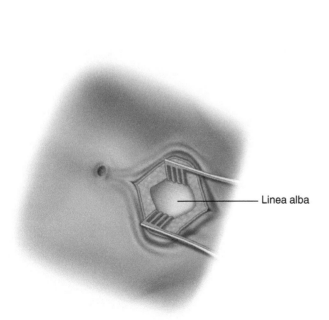

Fig. 69.2 Hold incision open with skin retractors

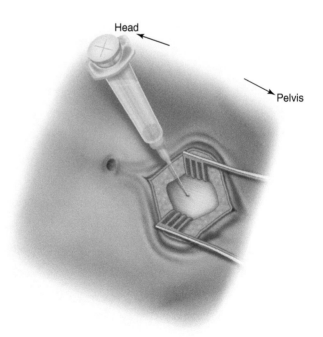

Fig. 69.3 Insert 18 gauge needle at 45° angle toward the pelvis

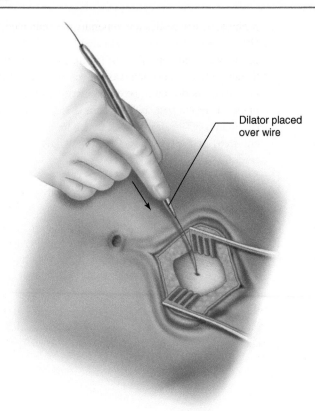

Fig. 69.4 Pass dilator over the wire through fascia and remove

Table 69.2 Diagnostic peritoneal lavage red blood cell criteria (per mm³) [2]

	Positive	Indeterminate
Immediate gross return of blood via catheter	Any amount	
Immediate return of food particles/intestinal contents	Any amount	
Aspiration of blood	10 cc	
RBC in blunt trauma	100,000	20,000–100,000
RBC in penetrating trauma	10,000	5000–10,000
RBC in gunshot wound	5000	1000–5000
Amylase level (IU/L)	≥175	
Alkaline phosphatase level (IU/L)	≥3	
WBCs (per mm³)	>500	250–500

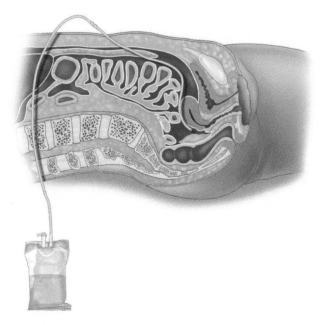

Fig. 69.5 Lavage

69.5 Complications

- Wound infection or dehiscence
- Intraperitoneal injury to organs or vessels (iatrogenic hemoperitoneum)
- Unnecessary laparotomy due to false-positive result from bleeding within rectus sheath or from site of incision
- Potential failure to recover lavage fluid due to:
  - Inadvertent placement of the catheter into the preperitoneal space
  - Compartmentalization of fluid by adhesions
  - Obstruction of fluid outflow (e.g., by omentum)
  - Fluid pooling in the intrathoracic cavity due to diaphragmatic injury
- Incisional hernia

69.6 Pearls and Pitfalls

- Pearls
  - When properly done, complication rate for DPL is low.
- Prophylactic antibiotics are generally not indicated.
- Pitfalls
  - Inadequate decompression of stomach and urinary bladder increases the chance of injury to these organs; thus, nasogastric and Foley decompression is an important step in patient preparation.

References

1. Jagminas L. Diagnostic peritoneal lavage. Medscape.com. http://emedicine.medscape.com/article/82888-overview#a17. Accessed 28 Aug 2014.
2. Marx JA. Diagnostic peritoneal lavage. In: Ivatury RR, Cayten CG, editors. The textbook of penetrating trauma. Baltimore: Williams & Wilkins; 1996. p. 337.

Selected Reading

Whitehouse JS, Weigelt JA. Diagnostic peritoneal lavage: a review of indications, technique, and interpretation. Scand J Trauma Resusc Emerg Med. 2009;17:13.

Latha Ganti

An abdominal wall hernia is a protrusion of the intestine through an opening or area of weakness in the abdominal wall. See Table 70.1 for types of abdominal hernias and Fig. 70.1 for locations along the abdominal anatomy.

Table 70.1 Types of abdominal hernias

Type	Defect	Most commonly seen in	Notes
Inguinal	Intestine or bladder protrudes through abdominal wall or into inguinal canal in the groin	Men because of a natural weakness in this area	96 % of all groin hernias are inguinal; 4 % are femoral
Femoral	Intestine enters canal carrying femoral artery into the upper thigh	Women, especially those who are pregnant or obese	
Incisional	Intestine pushes through abdominal wall at the site of previous abdominal surgery	Elderly or overweight people who are inactive after abdominal surgery	
Umbilical	Part of the small intestine passes through abdominal wall near the navel	Newborns and obese women or those who have had many children	In children, not repaired until age five because often resolve on their own
Hiatal	Upper stomach squeezes through hiatus, an opening in the diaphragm through which the esophagus passes		

. Ganti, MD, MS, MBA
rofessor of Emergency Medicine, University of Central Florida,
rlando, FL, USA

irector, SE Specialty Care Centers of Innovation, Orlando
eterans Affairs Medical Center, Orlando, FL, USA
mail: lathagantimd@gmail.com

Springer Science+Business Media New York 2016
Ganti (ed.), *Atlas of Emergency Medicine Procedures*, DOI 10.1007/978-1-4939-2507-0_70

Fig. 70.1 Types of abdominal wall hernias

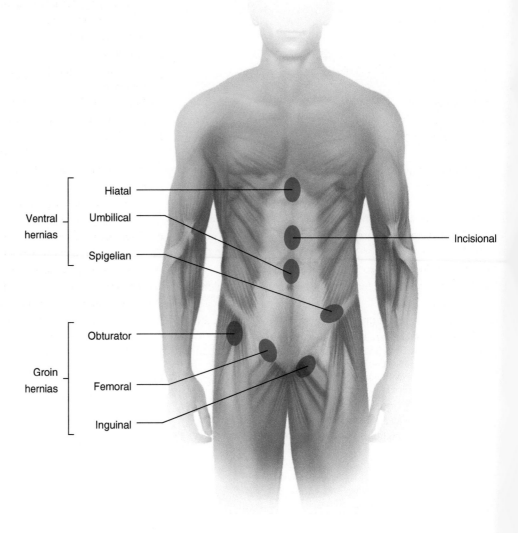

70.1   Indications

- Incarcerated hernia

70.2   Contraindications

- Absolute
  - Strangulated hernia (could result in placing dead bowel into abdominal cavity)
- Relative
  - Inability to get patient relaxed enough
  - Previous unsuccessful attempts

70.3   Materials and Medications

- Ice or cold compress
- Stretcher or gurney that can tilt to provide Trendelenburg position
- Moderate sedation drugs if providing moderate sedation
- Truss for post-procedure

70.4   Procedure

1. Patient positioning:
   - For abdominal hernia: place patient supine.
   - For groin hernia in adult: place in 20 ° of Trendelenburg.
   - For groin hernias in children: place in unilateral frog leg position (Fig. 70.2).
2. Apply ice or cold compress directly over hernia site to reduce swelling.
3. Administer opiate analgesia or moderate/procedural sedation.
4. Wait up to 30 min as hernia may reduce spontaneously after swelling has gone down and patient is relaxed.
5. Gently apply steady pressure distally on the tissue at the neck of the hernia with one hand and with other hand, guide hernia proximally through fascial defect. Too much pressure distally can cause hernia to balloon further, making manual reduction difficult. Takes up to 15–20 min. Do not rush procedure.
6. Once hernia is reduced, pain will improve.
7. An external support garment or truss (Fig. 70.3) can be helpful to hold reduced hernia in place and serve as a temporizing measure until surgical repair can be done.
8. Advise patient to schedule elective surgical repair.
9. If unable to reduce the hernia, obtain surgical consultation. Do not force repeated attempts.

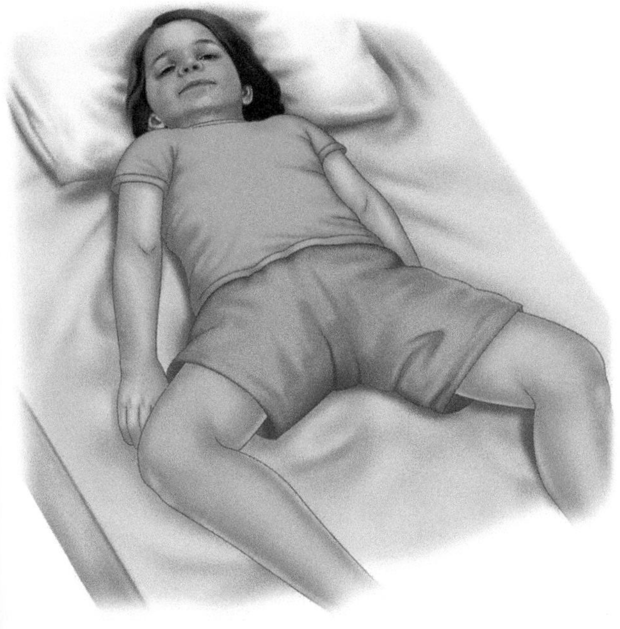

Fig. 70.2 Frog leg position in child

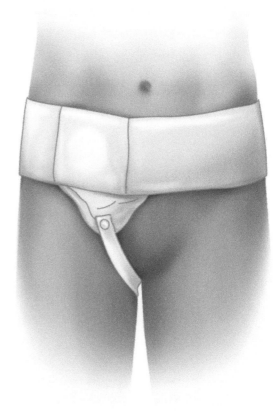

Fig. 70.3 An example of a truss, or external support, that can be useful as a temporizing measure until definitive hernia repair can be done

70.5 Complications

- Pain.
- Inability to achieve manual reduction, leading to strangulation of the hernia.
- Strangulation can result in peritonitis and sepsis.
- Recurrence.
- Hydrocele.

70.6 Pearls and Pitfalls

- Pearls
  - Definitive treatment for a hernia is surgery (herniorrhaphy). Without surgery, hernias grow larger over time; they do not disappear. Small hernias are easier to fix and result in fewer complications.
  - The only hernia that can resolve on its own is an umbilical hernia in a child.
  - Trusses, bandages, and tape may provide some comfort but do not reduce risk of incarceration or strangulation.
  - Note that if a truss is worn, it should be in place after reduction of the hernia. Also, it can be impractical in hot climates.
- Pitfalls
  - When the constricting neck and the protrusion are both reduced into the abdomen together (known as a reduction *en masse*), without actually reducing the hernia itself, strangulation ensues even though it appears one has reduced the hernia.
  - If there is still considerable pain after the reduction, it is likely the reduction was not successful or that dead bowel has been reduced into the abdominal cavity.
  - Not recognizing strangulation leads to gangrenous bowel, peritonitis, and sepsis.

Selected Reading

Campanelli G, Canziani M, Frattini F, et al. Inguinal hernia: state of the art. Int J Surg. 2008;6 Suppl 1:S26–8.

Jenkins JT, O'Dwyer PJ. Inguinal hernias. BMJ. 2008;336(7638):269–72.

Moses S. Hernia reduction. 2014. http://www.fpnotebook.com/mobile/Surgery/GI/HrnRdctn.htm. Accessed Sept 15, 2014.

Extended Focused Assessment with Sonography for Trauma

71

Coben Thorn and L. Connor Nickels

71.1 Indications

- Blunt abdominal or chest trauma
- Penetrating abdominal or chest trauma
- Undifferentiated hypotension
- The "E" in EFAST refers to the "extended" ability to detect lung pathology such as a pneumothorax or hemothorax during the otherwise standard trauma FAST exam using the same equipment with or without an additional transducer probe.
- Specific findings that can be detected on extended focused assessment with sonography for trauma (EFAST):
    - Pericardial fluid
    - Pleural fluid
    - Free intraperitoneal fluid
    - Pneumothorax
- Free fluid appears as anechoic or black.

71.2 Contraindications

- Need for immediate operative intervention

C. Thorn, MD
Department of Emergency Medicine, Bon Secours St. Francis
Health System, Greenville, SC, USA
e-mail: cobenthorn@gmail.com

L.C. Nickels, MD, RDMS (✉)
Department of Emergency Medicine,
University of Florida Health Shands Hospital, Gainesville, FL, USA
e-mail: cnickels@ufl.edu

71.3 Materials and Medications

- Ultrasound machine
- Probe(s): phased array probe (5 to 1 MHz) or curved array probe (5 to 2 MHz)
    - Phased array has a smaller footprint, allowing easier access between intercostal spaces (Fig. 71.1); however, curved array provides better resolution of images

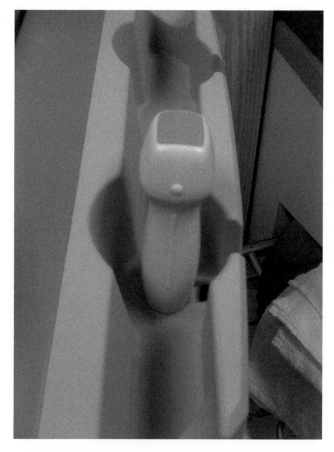

Fig. 71.1 Phased array transducer (P17) with a small footprint that is helpful to fit between the ribs and can be used for focused assessment with sonography for trauma (FAST) examination

© Springer Science+Business Media New York 2016
L. Ganti (ed.), *Atlas of Emergency Medicine Procedures*, DOI 10.1007/978-1-4939-2507-0_71

(Fig. 71.2). The linear array transducer (L38, 10–5 MHz) is good for lung images.

- Gel
- Skilled ultrasound operator
- ± Laboratory work, cardiac monitor, and two large-bore intravenous (IV) needles
  - All trauma alerts and unstable patients must have all of these.

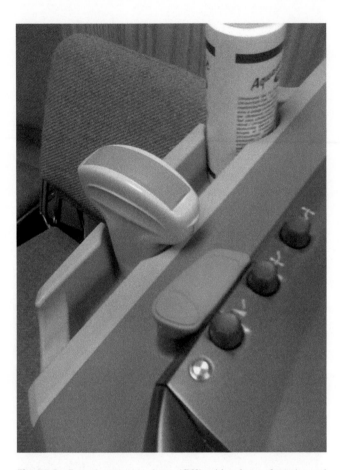

Fig. 71.2 Curved array transducer (C60) with a larger footprint and better resolution for deeper imaging that can be used for FAST examination as well as lung examination

71.4 Procedure

1. Ultrasound machine in the abdominal preset.
2. Patient in the supine position.
3. Phased array or curved array probe for focused assessment with sonography for trauma (FAST) and linear array for lung.
4. Begin scanning the patient in a systematic fashion.
   - All the views should be scanned by thoroughly sweeping through the area in question in order to maximize the information obtained.
   - All views should be obtained in the same order every time.
   - Obtain all four views, five views if pneumothorax is included.

71.4.1 Subxiphoid Four-Chamber View
(Fig. 71.3)

1. Examine for free pericardial fluid.
   - Anechoic (black) stripe seen between the myocardium and the pericardium
2. Probe is placed in the subxiphoid area.
3. Indicator is to the patient's right.
4. Probe is directed toward the patient's left shoulder.
5. Use a shallow angle in the head to feet direction.
6. Should adequately visualize the following:
   - Liver edge superficially
   - Right ventricle
   - Left ventricle
   - Right atrium
   - Left atrium
7. If unable to obtain this view, proceed to *parasternal long-axis view*:
   - Probe is placed perpendicular at the left parasternal border.
   - Third to fourth intercostal space.
   - Indicator is to the patient's right shoulder.
   - Coronal section through the heart's long axis should adequately visualize the following:
     - Right ventricle most superficially
     - Left ventricle
     - Mitral valve
     - Left atrium
     - Aortic valve
     - Aortic outflow tract

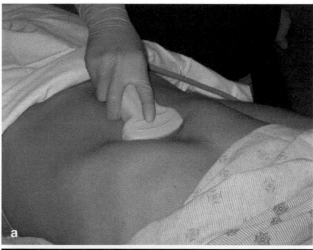

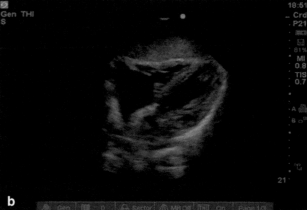

Fig. 71.3 (**a**) Image shows how to obtain the subxiphoid four-chamber view of the heart using the curved array transducer (C60) (Photograph courtesy of F. Eike Flach, MD).(**b**) Ultrasound image of four-chamber view of the heart (Used with permission from First aid for the emergency medicine clerkship 3rd Ed, McGraw Hill, 2011.) *RV* right ventricle, *LV* left ventricle, *RA* right atrium, *LA* left atrium

71.4.2 Right Upper Quadrant View (Fig. 71.4)

1. Examine for free fluid in all of the following areas:
   - Right intrathoracic space
     - Anechoic area above the diaphragm
   - Morison's pouch: hepatorenal space
     - Anechoic stripe between the liver and the kidney
   - Right paracolic gutter
     - Anechoic collection surrounding the inferior tip of the kidney
2. Probe is placed in the midaxillary line on the right.
3. Indicator is directed toward the patient's head.
4. Probe is in the coronal plane, angle can be aimed obliquely while scanning anterior to posterior.

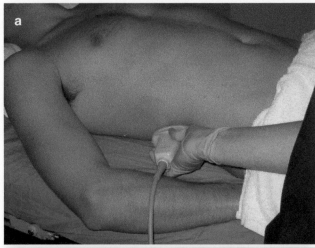

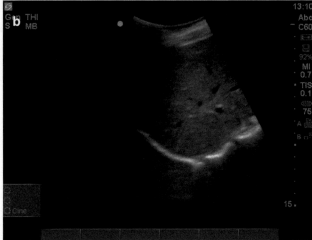

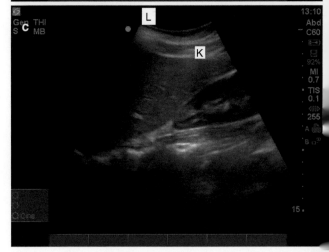

Fig. 71.4 (**a**) Image shows how to obtain the right upper quadrant view of the FAST exam using the curved array transducer (C60). The probe is aimed slightly obliquely in the coronal plane to get a better view between the ribs (Photograph courtesy of F. Eike Flach, MD). (**b**) Ultrasonographic view of the liver. (**c**) Ultrasonographic view of the liver–kidney interface (Morison's pouch). *L* liver, *K* kidney

71.4.3 Left Upper Quadrant View (Fig. 71.5)

1. Examine for free fluid in all of the following areas:
   - Left intrathoracic space
     - Anechoic area above the diaphragm
   - Subphrenic space
     - Anechoic stripe below the diaphragm and above the spleen
   - Splenorenal space
     - Anechoic stripe between the spleen and kidney
   - Left paracolic gutter
     - Anechoic collection surrounding the inferior tip of the kidney
2. Probe is placed in the midaxillary line on the left.
3. Indicator is directed toward the patient's head.
4. Probe in the coronal plane, angle can be aimed obliquely while scanning anterior to posterior.

71.4.4 Pelvic View (Figs. 71.6 and 71.7)

1. Examine for intraperitoneal free fluid in the pelvis:
   - Anterior pelvis, above the bladder
     - Anechoic fluid above the bladder
   - Posterior cul-de-sac (pouch of Douglas)
     - Anechoic fluid posterior to the bladder or uterus
2. Probe is placed above the pubic symphysis over the bladder.
3. Scan through in both planes:
   - Transverse plane (Fig. 71.6)
     - Indicator is to the patient's right.
     - Scan through the bladder in the head to feet direction.
   - Sagittal plane (Fig. 71.7)
     - Indicator is aimed to the patient's head.
     - Scan through the bladder in a right to left direction.

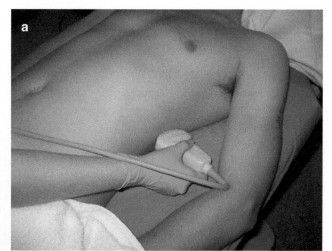

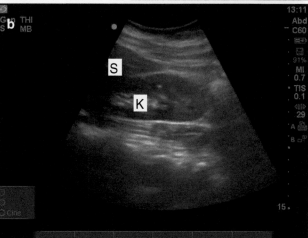

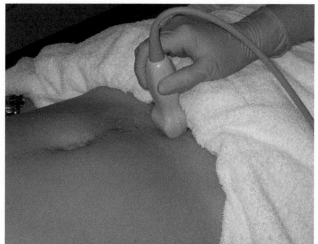

Fig. 71.6 Transverse pelvic view of the FAST examination using the phased array transducer (P17). With gentle force, the probe is pressed downward in order to look back behind the pubic symphysis and view the bladder (Photograph courtesy of F. Eike Flach, MD)

Fig. 71.5 (a) Image shows how to obtain the left upper quadrant view of the FAST examination using the curved array transducer (C60). Again, the probe is aimed slightly obliquely and is placed more superiorly in the midaxillary line (Photograph courtesy of F. Eike Flach, MD). (b) Ultrasonographic view of spleen–kidney interface. *S* spleen, *K* kidney

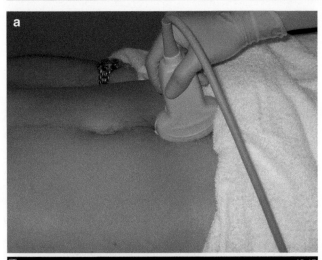

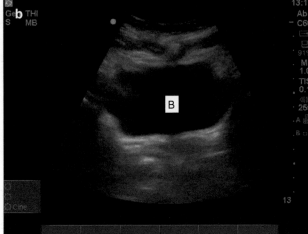

71.4.5 EFAST with Lung Views
(Figs. 71.8 and 71.9)

1. Examine for pneumothorax:
   - Lung sliding
     - Absence: pneumothorax
     - Presence: normal lung
   - M mode tracing
     - Stratosphere sign: pneumothorax
     - Seashore sign: normal lung
2. Probe is placed on the anterior chest in the midaxillary line.
3. Level of the second to fourth intercostal spaces.
4. Sagittal position.
5. Center the probe over the pleural line between the ribs.
   - Find the rib and then slide the probe toward the head or feet to center the pleural line.
6. Observe for lung sliding.
7. Press M mode and move the line over the pleural line and press M mode again to get the tracing.
8. Examine multiple other areas anteriorly, moving distally, and in midaxillary line laterally, moving from superior to inferior.

Fig. 71.7 (a) Sagittal pelvic view of the FAST exam using the curved array transducer (C60). With gentle force, the probe is pressed downward in order to look back behind the pubic symphysis and view the bladder (Photograph courtesy of F. Eike Flach, MD). (b) Ultrasonographic view of the bladder. *B* bladder

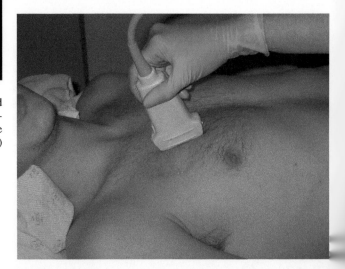

Fig. 71.8 Right lung view of the extended focused assessment with sonography for trauma (EFAST) examination using the linear array transducer (L38). The probe is placed in the sagittal plane on the anterior chest in the midaxillary line approximately at the second intercostal space and centered over the pleural line (Photograph courtesy of F. Eike Flach, MD)

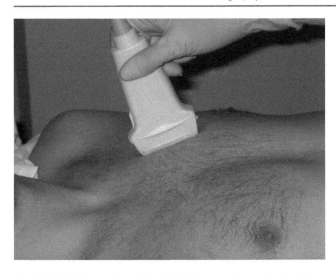

Fig. 71.9 Left lung view of the EFAST examination using the linear array transducer (L38) (Photograph courtesy of F. Eike Flach, MD)

71.5 Complications

- Overreliance on ultrasound to rule out abdominal injury:
  - FAST examinations do not detect retroperitoneal bleeding, solid organ injury, contained subcapsular hematomas, and bowel injuries.
- Not scanning through the object in question could lead to false-negative results.

71.6 Pearls and Pitfalls

- Always follow the ABCs (airway, breathing, circulation) first in any unstable patient.
- Always make sure the depth is set adequately.
  - Recommend starting deeper to make sure positive findings are not missed and then adjustments can be made from there.
- The curved array probe may be used throughout the entire EFAST for convenience if necessary.

71.6.1 Subxiphoid Four-Chamber View

- For larger body habitus, need to parallel the probe with the body in the subxiphoid area and use firm pressure to press the entire probe downward so as to look up under the xiphoid process at the heart.
- Moving the entire probe more to the patient's right in the subxiphoid area while still looking toward the left shoulder may improve visualization by using the liver as a window.
- Fat pad:
  - May be mistaken for pericardial fluid
  - Contains echoes and, therefore, is hypoechoic rather than anechoic
  - Should only be present anteriorly
    - Fluid should be gravity dependent, completely encircling the heart, and seen in multiple views.

71.6.2 Right Upper Quadrant View

- Normal artifacts of mirroring and loss of the spine are obscured when pleural fluid is present and, instead, the anechoic fluid is seen and there is loss of mirroring and continuation of the spine.

71.6.3 Left Upper Quadrant View

- Same as right upper quadrant view
- May be more difficult view to find than in right upper quadrant view for all of the following:
  - Spleen and kidney are more posterior and superior than in right upper quadrant view.
  - Spleen is smaller and less of a window for viewing.

71.6.4 Pelvic View

- Bowel can be mista0ken for free fluid or vice versa, but holding the probe still and observing can sometimes help distinguish the two.
  - Peristalsis will occur with bowel.
  - Internal echoes may be present in bowel.

71.6.5 Lung Views

- Ultrasound is more sensitive than a supine portable chest x-ray.
  - Apex anteriorly in midaxillary line.
- Rib
  - Hyperechoic horizontal line with a dense shadow posteriorly
  - Evenly spaced along the chest

- Pleural line
  - First hyperechoic line deep to the rib.
  - Actually includes the visceral and parietal pleura, but appears as one line.
  - Lung sliding is present in normal lung.
  - Comet tail artifact.
  - M mode tracing will be the same in normal lung and pneumothorax above the pleural line and different below the pleural line.
    - Seashore sign (Fig. 27.5a):
      - Appears as waves washing up on the shore.
      - Granular appearance represents movement.
    - Stratosphere sign (Fig. 27.5b):
      - Appears as straight lines
      - Bar code appearance

Selected Reading

Brunett P, Cameron P. Trauma in adults. In: Tintinalli J, Stapczynski J, Ma OJ, Cline D, Cydulka R, Meckler G, editors. Emergency medicine: a comprehensive study guide. 7th ed. New York: McGraw Hill; 2012. p. 1671–5.

Ma JO, Mateer JR, Blaivas M. Trauma. In: Emergency ultrasound. Course Materials; New York, NY: McGraw Hill; 2008. pp. 7–109.

Saul T, Rivera M, Lewiss R. Ultrasound image quality. ACEP News. 2011;4:24–5.

Nasogastric Tube Placement

72

David P. Nguyen, L. Connor Nickels,
and Giuliano De Portu

72.1 Indications

- Evaluation of upper gastrointestinal (GI) bleeding (history of melena, bright red blood per rectum, or coffee-ground emesis)
  - Only in the cases in which frank blood is obtained, the sensitivity/specificity in detecting upper GI bleeding is poor.
  - It should not be used for diagnostic purposes. It is used to remove blood that is irritating the stomach and to determine whether bleeding is still occurring (lavage does not clear).
- Commonly used in decompression of the GI tract (partial/complete small bowel obstruction)
- Prevents aspiration and gastric dilation in intubated patients
- Used during gastric lavage and/or removal of toxins (activated charcoal) for acute overdose or poisonings

72.2 Contraindications

- Absolute
  - Facial trauma with possible cribriform plate fracture
- Relative
  - Severe coagulopathy (consider orogastric tube placement)
  - Esophageal strictures and alkali ingestions (possible esophageal perforation)
  - Esophageal varices (studies show that it is actually safe)

72.3 Materials and Medications

- For awake patients, consider pretreatment: lidocaine gel (2 % viscous)/nebulized lidocaine (4 or 10 %), vasoconstrictors (e.g., phenylephrine 0.5 %), and antiemetic (e.g., ondansetron 4 mg).
- 16- or 18-French sump tube lubricating jelly
- 50- or 60-mL syringe stethoscope

D.P. Nguyen, DO
Department of Emergency Medicine, Rush-Copley Medical
Center, Aurora, IL, USA
e-mail: davidpnguyen@yahoo.com

L.C. Nickels, MD, RDMS (✉) • G. De Portu, MD
Department of Emergency Medicine,
University of Florida Health Shands Hospital, Gainesville, FL, USA
e-mail: cnickels@ufl.edu; gdeportu@ufl.edu

Springer Science+Business Media New York 2016
Ganti (ed.), *Atlas of Emergency Medicine Procedures*, DOI 10.1007/978-1-4939-2507-0_72

72.4   Procedure

- Preparation
  1. Awake patients, should receive antiemetics 15 min before procedure.
  2. Anesthetize both nares at least 5 min before placement.
     - Spray vasoconstrictor into both nares.
     - Inject about 5 mL of lidocaine gel along the floor of the nose.
     - Nebulized lidocaine via facemask also reduces both nasal and pharyngeal discomfort.
  3. Elevate the head of the bed to an upright position (when possible).
  4. Estimate tube insertion distance by measuring the tube from the xiphoid to the earlobe and then to the tip of the nose. Add 6 in. to this estimate and note the total distance. This helps with placement in the stomach and prevents esophageal placement or coiling in stomach. Mark the tube with markers or tape at the desired length.
  5. Lubricate the nasogastric (NG) tube.
- Insertion (Fig. 72.1)
  1. Always insert the tube gently into the nares along the floor of the nose under direct visualization. Always point inferiorly (do not point upward).
  2. If resistance is encountered, try to apply a small amount of pressure. STOP if unable to advance. Try the other side. It is necessary to prevent bleeding or dissecting the tissues.
  3. Have the patient flex his or her head forward when the tube is in the nasopharynx. This helps direct the tube toward the correct placement in the esophagus and not the trachea. Have the awake and cooperative patient sip water from a straw and swallow as the tube enters the oropharynx.
  4. Making the tube more rigid by placing it in cold water will help advance it because the "warmer" tube will tend to coil.
  5. Once the tube is in the esophagus, rapidly advance the tube into the stomach, taking into consideration the previously marked depth.
- Confirmation of tube placement
  1. Insufflate air into the end of the NG tube, via a 50- or 60-mL syringe, while auscultating for a rush of air (borborygmi) over the stomach.
  2. Aspiration of gastric contents (pH<4, there is >90 % gastric placement).
  3. The awake and cooperative patient should be able to talk, and if coughing or severe discomfort occurs, consider that esophageal or bronchial placement might have occurred.
  4. Radiographic evaluation:
     - "Gold standard" is to evaluate simple radiograph for position.
     - Consider in comatose patients.
- Secure the tube
  1. Tape the NG tube in place by taping both the tube and the nose. A butterfly bandage is typically used. Some companies produce a specific fixation for the tube.
  2. Secure the tube to where it does not press on the medial or lateral nostril (can lead to bleeding/necrosis).

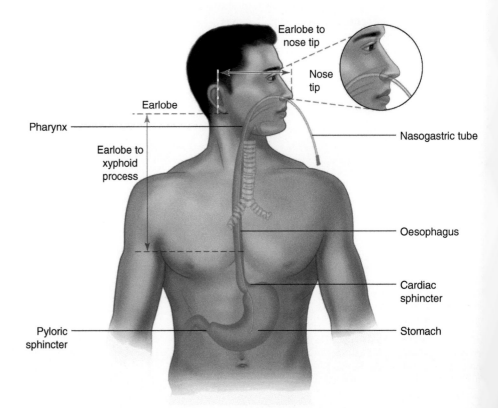

Fig. 72.1   NG tube placement

72.5   Complications

- Inability to pass the tube
- Bleeding
- Curling of the NG tube in the patient's mouth
- Pulmonary placement
- Nasal necrosis

72.6   Pearls

- Pearls
    - NG tube placement was ranked #1 as the most painful procedure in the emergency department so it is imperative to maintain patient's comfort by using anesthetics and even maybe intravenous anxiolytics.
    - Estimate the proper length of the tube before passage to avoid placing the tip of the tube in the esophagus or excessively coiling it in the stomach.

- If leaving the tube for a prolonged period of time, make sure that the suction is set "intermittent" or "off" to prevent irritation to the gastric mucosa owing to direct pressure.

Selected Reading

Chun DH, Kim NY, Shin YS, Kim SH. A randomized, clinical trial of frozen versus standard nasogastric tube placement. World J Surg. 2009;33:1789–92.

Goff JS. Gastroesophageal varices: pathogenesis and therapy of acute bleeding. Gastroenterol Clin North Am. 1993;22:779.

Henneman PL. Gastrointestinal bleeding. In: Marx J, Hockberger R, Walls R, editors. Rosen's emergency medicine: concepts and clinical practice. 7th ed. Philadelphia: Mosby; 2010.

Tho PC, Mordiffi S, Ang E, Chen H. Implementation of the evidence review on best practice for confirming correct placement of nasogastric tube in patients in an acute care hospital. Int J Evid Based Healthc. 2011;9:51–60.

Esophageal Foreign Body Removal

David P. Nguyen, L. Connor Nickels,
and Rohit Pravin Patel

73.1 Indications

- Patient presenting with any one or combination of the following:
  - Foreign body sensation in throat, neck, substernal chest, or epigastric area
  - Clear history of ingestion
  - Dysphagia
  - Airway compromise
  - Drooling
  - Inability to tolerate fluids
  - Inability to tolerate solids
  - Evidence of perforation
  - Active bleeding
- All unstable patients should have immediate airway management and urgent endoscopy.
- FBs lodged superior to the epiglottis may be retrieved by emergency physicians in an emergent situation, but generally, a consultant should be present, whether ear, nose, and throat, gastroenterology, or general surgery.

73.2 Contraindications

- Absolute
  - None
- Relative
  - Performing rapid sequence intubation (RSI) in a patient with an FB that could compromise the airway.
  - Generally, if the patient is breathing on their own, collaborate with a consultant on the best method to secure the airway (emergency department, intensive care unit, operating room).
  - Treating with glucagon repeatedly if it is inducing vomiting and/or not working.
  - Conservatively managing a patient who should otherwise undergo a procedure for removal.

73.3 Materials

- Esophagoscopy/endoscopy is the definitive diagnostic and therapeutic procedure for impacted esophageal FBs.
  - Generally, should not be performed by an emergency physician.
  - Devices used include forceps, baskets, polypectomy snares, and nets.
  - Endoscopic techniques include push into stomach, push plus fragmentation, pull with retrieval forceps, and pull with various items (basket, snare, nets).
- Foley catheter removal
  - Widely used technique for recently ingested single, smooth, blunt, and radiopaque objects
  - #12 to #16 French Foley catheter
  - Forceps (bayonet and Magill) of various sizes
  - Often done under fluoroscopic guidance
- Bougienage
  - A single, smooth object, such as a coin, lodged less than 24 h in a patient with no respiratory distress or esophageal disease can be advanced successfully into the stomach by using bougienage.
  - Dilator size is selected based on age:
    - 1–2 years: 28 French
    - 2–3 years: 32 French
    - 3–4 years: 36 French
    - 4–5 years: 38 French
    - Longer than 5 years: 40 French
- Relaxation of the lower esophageal sphincter (LES)
  - Some FBs lodged at the LES can be medically managed by relaxation of the LES.

D.P. Nguyen, DO
Department of Emergency Medicine, Rush-Copley Medical
Center, Aurora, IL, USA
e-mail: davidpnguyen@yahoo.com

L.C. Nickels, MD, RDMS (✉) • R.P. Patel, MD
Department of Emergency Medicine,
University of Florida Health Shands Hospital, Gainesville, FL, USA
e-mail: cnickels@ufl.edu; rohitpatel@ufl.edu

© Springer Science+Business Media New York 2016
L. Ganti (ed.), *Atlas of Emergency Medicine Procedures*, DOI 10.1007/978-1-4939-2507-0_73

– Most ingested FBs and impacted food boluses eventually pass spontaneously.
  - 1–2 mg of glucagon intravenously
  - 0.4–0.8 mg of nitroglycerin sublingually
  - 5–10 mg of nifedipine sublingually
  - Carbonated beverage

73.4   Procedure

- Push technique and push with fragmentation technique (generally performed by specialists)
  1. First accepted endoscopic method.
  2. Gentle pressure is applied with the tip of the endoscope on the esophageal food bolus after air insufflation.
  3. If pressure does not disimpact the bolus, fragmentation can be attempted but is generally avoided owing to unknown pathology behind the food bolus.
- Foley catheter removal
  1. Moderate sedation and nasopharyngeal topical anesthesia may be used.
  2. Place the patient in a head-down Trendelenburg position.
  3. Check for symmetrical balloon inflation of the Foley catheter.
  4. Under fluoroscopy, visually pass the catheter distal to the FB.
  5. Fill the balloon slowly with 3–5 mL of saline or contrast agent.
  6. Using steady, gentle traction, withdraw the catheter with the balloon inflated distal to the FB.
  7. Grasp the object with fingers, forceps, or clamp once it is visualized in the oropharynx.
- Bougienage
  1. Topical anesthesia is recommended.
  2. Blind esophageal bougienage resembles placement of an orogastric tube.
  3. Place the patient in a sitting position.
  4. Pass a well-lubricated, appropriately sized bougie posteriorly along the roof of the mouth, following the natural curve of the soft palate caudally to the hypopharynx.
  5. Encourage the patient to swallow (to help pass the dilator through the cricopharyngeus muscle).
  6. Ask the patient to phonate to help exclude accidental laryngeal intubation.
  7. Once past the cricopharyngeus muscle, extend the head to aid the bougie in passing distally to the stomach.
  8. Post-procedure radiograph is used to confirm passage into the stomach.
- Relaxation of the LES
  1. Premedicate with an antiemetic, such as ondansetron.
  2. Administer 1–2 mg of glucagon intravenously (0.02–0.03 mg/kg in children, not to exceed 0.5 mg) with the patient in a sitting position over 1–2 min.
  3. Carbonated beverages given after glucagon ingestion have shown to have higher success rates.
  4. An alternative is to use either sublingual nitroglycerin (1–2 0.4 mg tabs) or 5–10 mg of nifedipine to relieve LES tone.
  5. This procedure does not work in patients with structural abnormalities.

73.5   Complications

- Esophageal FBs may cause esophageal pressure leading to edema, necrosis, infection, laceration, and/or perforation.
- Be cognizant of time (risk of complications is higher the longer the FB is left in place) and treatment side effects (i.e., do not continue to give patient water or glucagon if these induce vomiting).
- Aspiration and perforation during procedures listed previously.
- Late complications: esophageal stricture, abscess, mediastinitis, tracheoesophageal fistula, vascular injuries, pneumothorax, pericarditis, aspiration pneumonia, and vocal cord paralysis.

73.6   Pearls

- Esophageal foreign bodies can be lodged in the upper (proximal), middle, or lower (distal) one third:
  - Proximal: cervical web, Zenker's diverticulum
  - Middle: eosinophilic esophagitis, cancer, radiation structure, spastic dysmotility
  - Distal: peptic stricture, eosinophilic esophagitis, cancer, achalasia, esophageal diverticula, spastic dysmotility
- Because food bolus impactions are generally associated with pathology, follow-up evaluation for these abnormalities should be considered.
- Esophagus foreign bodies should not be allowed to remain in the esophagus beyond 24 h from presentation.
- Button/disc batteries in esophagus (emergent removal)
  - Considered an emergency, because liquefaction necrosis and perforation can occur rapidly.
  - Most common ingestions are hearing aid batteries.
  - If in stomach, and patient is a symptomatic, can wait up to 24 h.
- Sharp objects (emergent removal)

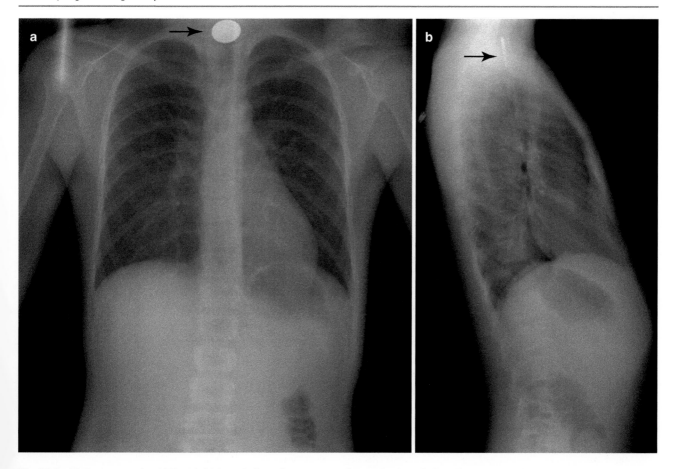

Fig. 73.1 (**a**) Anteroposterior (AP) and (**b**) lateral views demonstrating a coin in the esophagus. A coin in the trachea would present in the opposite manner—the coin would be seen on edge in the AP view and flat on the lateral view (Reproduced with permission from McGraw-Hill: Stead LG, et al. *First Aid for the Pediatrics Clerkship*. New York: McGraw-Hill, 2010)

- – Cause the majority of complications (~35 %) with esophageal FBs.
- – Direct visualization with endoscopy is the only appropriate removal technique.
- Magnets (urgent removal)
- – Can cause necrosis and fistula formation due to the way they adhere to the mucosa
- Esophageal coins (remove within 24 h) (Fig. 73.1)
- – Up to 80 % of coins at the LES will pass spontaneously within 24 h without interventions. The watchful waiting approach is used only in patients with single coins and who are asymptomatic.
- – Common complications of these procedures include mild bleeding, lip laceration, bradycardia with Foley catheter insertion, and teeth injuries.
- – Some protocols include RSI as part of the management process and should be considered if lifesaving.

Selected Reading

ASGE Standards of Practice Committee. Management of ingested foreign bodies and food impactions. Gastrointest Endosc. 2011; 73:1085.

Bhargava R, Brown L. Esophageal coin removal by emergency physicians: a continuous quality improvement project incorporating rapid sequence intubation. CJEM. 2011;13:28–33.

Conway WC, Sugawa C, Ono H, Lucas CE. Upper GI foreign body: an adult emergency hospital experience. Surg Endosc. 2007; 21:455–60.

Katsinelos P, Kountouras J, Paroutoglou G, et al. Endoscopic techniques and management of foreign body ingestion and food bolus impaction in the upper gastrointestinal tract: a retrospective analysis of 139 cases. J Clin Gastroenterol. 2006;40:784–9.

Activated Charcoal

74

Deylin I. Negron Smida and Judith K. Lucas

74.1 Indications

- Single-dose activated charcoal (AC) (Fig. 74.1)
  - Does not meet criteria for gastric emptying.
  - Gastric emptying may be too harmful.
  - Ingestion of toxic xenobiotic is known to be adsorbed by AC.
  - Ingestion occurred with a time frame amenable to adsorption by AC, or clinical factors are present that suggest that not all of the xenobiotic had already been systemically absorbed.
  - Ingestion of extended- or sustained-release formulations.
- Multiple-dose activated charcoal therapy (MDAC)
  - Life-threatening ingestion of:
    - Carbamazepine
    - Phenobarbital
    - Quinine
    - Theophylline
    - Dapsone

- Life-threatening ingestion of another xenobiotic that undergoes enterohepatic recirculation and is adsorbed to AC
- Ingestion of a significant amount of a slowly released xenobiotic
- Ingestion of a xenobiotic known to form concretions or bezoars, such as aspirin

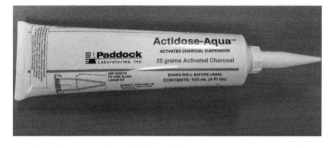

Fig. 74.1 Activated charcoal (AC)

D.I.N. Smida, MD
Department of Emergency Medicine, University of Pittsburgh
Medical Center, Saint Margaret Hospital, Pittsburgh, PA, USA
e-mail: Deylin.negron@gmail.com

J.K. Lucas, MD (✉)
Department of Emergency Medicine,
University of Florida Health Shands Hospital,
Gainesville, FL, USA
e-mail: judithklucas@ufl.edu

74.2 Contraindications

- Absolute
  - Gastric perforation
  - Gastrointestinal ileus, obstruction, or diminished peristalsis
  - Nonintubated patients with the potential of losing protective airway reflexes
  - Intestinal obstruction
  - Ingestion of:
    - Corrosives
    - Petroleum distillates
- Relative
  - Altered or decreased level of consciousness unless intubated.
  - Vomiting.
  - Xenobiotic has limited toxicity at almost any dose.
  - Dose ingested is less than the dose expected to produce significant illness.
  - Presentation many hours after ingestion.
  - Minimal signs or symptoms of poisoning.
  - Ingested xenobiotic has a highly efficient antidote.
  - Administration of charcoal may increase the risk of aspiration (i.e., hydrocarbons).

74.3 Materials and Medications

- Nasogastric (NG) tube/orogastric (OG) tube (Fig. 74.2)
- Baby bottle with split nipple (designed for drinking of slurry solutions, such as thickened formulas) or sippy cup without the valve
- Absorbent pad
- Basin
- Water-soluble lubricant
- Tubing connected to suction device
- Flavored syrup

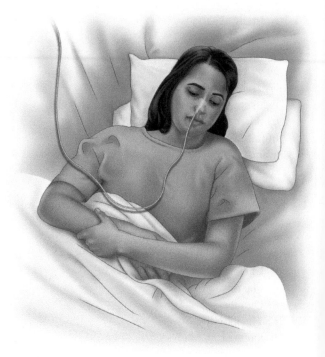

Fig. 74.2 Drinking AC (by cup, sippy cup, or bottle) is effective, but it may also be infused via nasogastric or orogastric tube

74.4   Procedure

- Single-dose administration
  - Adult
    - Can be taken via a cup and straw (drunk) if the patient is cooperative.
    - The optimal dose of AC is unknown.
    - 50–100 g/dose (1 g/kg), administered at a rate no less than 12.5 g/h or its equivalent.
    - If vomiting is anticipated, an intravenous antiemetic is recommended.
  - Children
    - 1 g/kg or 10:1 ratio of AC to drug ingested.
    - After massive ingestion, give 2 g/kg.
    - Many children will drink the suspension from a bottle or sippy cup, especially if it is mixed with juice or flavored syrup (e.g., chocolate or strawberry).
- MDAC
  - Adults: 0.5–1 g/kg every 2–4 h for 24–48 h
  - Children (<12 y old): 0.25–0.5 g/kg every 2–4 h or rate of 0.2 g/kg/h for 24–48 h
- Mixtures
  - Ready to drink
  - Powder form
    - Add eight parts water to the selected powdered form.
    - Gatorade or juices can also be used to help hide the flavor and texture.
    - In children, the AC can be mixed with cold chocolate or some other flavored syrup, which also hides the flavor.
  - Shake liquid suspension well for 1 min.
  - If the patient vomits, the dose should be repeated. Smaller, more frequent, dosing may be better tolerated, and an antiemetic may be needed.

74.5   Complications

- Aspiration pneumonitis
- Transient constipation
- Intestinal bezoars
- Bowel obstruction
- Diarrhea, dehydration, hypermagnesemia, and hypernatremia with coadministered cathartics or MDAC
- Vomiting
- Corneal abrasion if spilled in the eyes

74.6   Pearls and Pitfalls

- Pearls
  - If an OG or NG tube is used, time should be allowed for the last dose to pass through the stomach before the tube is removed. Suctioning the tube before removal may prevent subsequent AC aspiration.
  - With children, the colder and sweeter the solution and if the color is camouflaged (cup with a lid or a sippy cup), there will be increased success at oral administration (vs NG/OG).
- Pitfalls
  - No evidence-based literature supports the assertion that AC changes clinical outcome.
  - Xenobiotics and AC adsorption (Table 74.1).
  - Incorrect application (e.g., into the lungs) results in pulmonary aspiration, which can be fatal if unrecognized.
    - Incorrect placement of NG/OG tube into trachea.
    - Administration of AC to a patient with an ileus (e.g., in anticholinergic overdoses).
  - No specific contraindication for AC in pregnant women; however, diarrhea or hypernatremia in the mother may adversely affect the fetus.

Table 74.1 Absorption of xenobiotics by AC

Good absorption	Poor absorption
Acetaminophen	Alkali
Bupropion	Chlorpropamide
Caffeine	Doxepin
Carbamazepine	Ethanol or other alcohols
Chlordecone	Ethylene glycol
Dapsone	Fluoride
Digitoxin	Heavy metals
Nadolol	Imipramine
Phenobarbital	Inorganic salts
Phenylbutazone	Iron
Phenytoin	Lithium
Salicylate	Methotrexate
Theophylline	Mineral acids
	Potassium
	Tobramycin
	Valproate sodium
	Vancomycin

Selected Reading

American Academy of Clinical Toxicology; European Association of Poisons Centres and Clinical Toxicologists. Position statement and practice guidelines on the use of multi-dose activated charcoal in the treatment of acute poisoning. J Toxicol Clin Toxicol. 1999;37:731–51.

Chyka PA, Seger D. American Academy of Clinical Toxicology; European Association of Poisons Centres and Clinical Toxicologists. Position statement: single-dose activated charcoal. J Toxicol Clin Toxicol. 1997;35:721–41.

Gude A, Hoegberg LCG. Techniques to prevent gastrointestinal absorption. In: Nelson LS, Lewin NA, Howland MA, et al., editors. Goldfrank's toxicologic emergencies. 9th ed. New York: McGraw-Hill; 2011. p. 93–7,431.

Lie D. Use of activated charcoal in drug overdose. Medscape family medicine. 25 Mar 2004. www.medscape.com/viewarticle/471331

Olson KR. Emergency evaluation and treatment. In: Olson KR, Anderson IB, Benowitz NL, et al., editors. Poisoning and drug overdose. 5th ed. New York: McGraw-Hill; 2007. p. 1–56.

Gastric Lavage

75

Deylin I. Negron Smida and Judith K. Lucas

75.1 Indications

- Recent ingestion (<30–60 min).
- Life-threatening exposure where there is a high suspicion that a xenobiotic is still present in the stomach and evacuation is expected to contribute to an improved outcome (e.g., iron, tricyclic antidepressants).
- Ingested agent is not absorbed with activated charcoal (e.g., pesticides, hydrocarbons, iron, alcohols, lithium, and solvents).
- Activated charcoal is unavailable.
- Ingestion exceeds adsorptive capacity of initial activated charcoal dosing (e.g., >100 mg/kg of pills).
- Ingestion of an agent likely to form a durable mass or bezoars after overdose.

75.2 Contraindications

- Vomiting
- Unintubated patients with potential to lose airway protective reflexes
- Ingestion of a xenobiotic with aspiration potential (e.g., hydrocarbon) without intubation
- Ingestion of caustic substances (alkali or acidic)
- Ingestion of sharp metals
- Ingestion of a foreign body (e.g., drug packet)
- Risk for hemorrhagic gastrointestinal perforation
- Ingestion of xenobiotic in a form known to be too large to fit into the lumen of the orogastric tube
- Nontoxic ingestions

75.3 Materials and Medications

- Orogastric tube (Ewald tube or the Tum-E-Vac) (Fig. 75.1)
  - Adults and adolescents: 36–40 French
  - Children: 22–28 French
- Pen or tape to mark the length of the tube
- Water-soluble lubricant
- Suction
- Emesis basin
- Absorbent pad
- Catheter-tip syringe with 2 mL water/saline to check position of the tube
- Room temperature irrigation fluid
- Bite block or oral airway to prevent patients from biting down on the tube

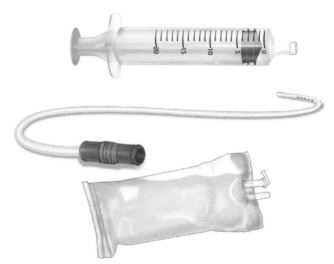

Fig. 75.1 Materials needed for gastric lavage include a large-bore nasogastric tube, a 60-cc non-Luer-Lok syringe, and a solution, typically normal saline, for lavage

D.I.N. Smida, MD
Department of Emergency Medicine, University of Pittsburgh Medical Center, Saint Margaret Hospital, Pittsburgh, PA, USA
e-mail: Deylin.negron@gmail.com

J.K. Lucas, MD (✉)
Department of Emergency Medicine,
University of Florida Health Shands Hospital,
Gainesville, FL, USA
e-mail: judithklucas@ufl.edu

Springer Science+Business Media New York 2016
Ganti (ed.), *Atlas of Emergency Medicine Procedures*, DOI 10.1007/978-1-4939-2507-0_75

423

75.4 Procedure

1. If there is potential airway compromise, endotracheal or nasotracheal intubation should precede orogastric lavage.
2. Place an oral airway or a bite block to prevent biting of the endotracheal tube if the patient recovers consciousness or has convulsions during the procedure.
3. Ensure suction apparatus is available and functioning.
4. Place the patient in an upright-seated position if awake and alert.
5. Place patient in the left lateral decubitus position if obtunded.
6. Before insertion, the proper length of tubing to be passed should be measured from the mouth, back to the ear, and down anterior to the chest and abdomen, beyond the point where any side ports on the tube would be beyond the level of the estimated lower esophageal sphincter (Figs. 75.2 and 75.3).
7. If the patient is still awake, insert the gastric tube to the level of the glottis, and encourage the patient to swallow.
8. Pass the tube to the stomach.
    (a) Coughing, airflow, or fog from the tube raises the concern for inadvertent tracheal positioning.
9. After the tube is inserted, it is essential to confirm that the distal end of the tube is in the stomach, by "popping" 5–10 mL of air into the tube while someone is listening with a stethoscope over the stomach.

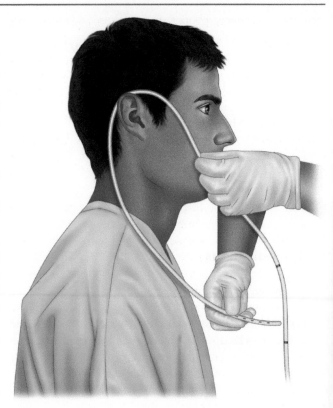

Fig. 75.3 Measuring correct placement of the tube. Place the distal tip over the stomach and wrap the tube up behind the ear (usually the right ear because the tubes generally pass easier through the right nares) and around the nares. The black line or centimeter mark at the level of the nares is the point of insertion when passage stops

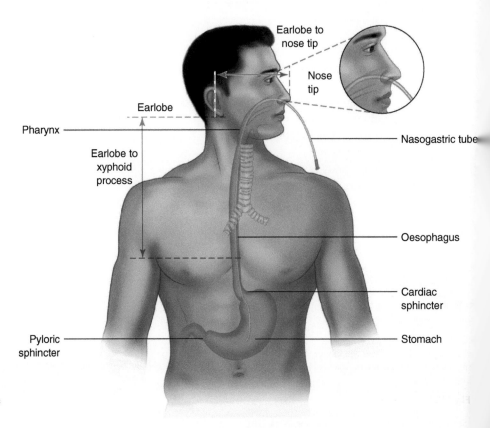

Fig. 75.2 Diagram illustrates appropriate placement of the lavage tube

10. In adults, 250-mL aliquots of a room temperature saline lavage solution are instilled via a funnel or lavage syringe. In children, aliquots should be 10–15 mL/kg to a maximum of 250 mL and suctioned back out of the tube attached to low to moderate continuous wall suction. Instillation of lavage solution and suction is repeated (Fig. 75.4).

11. Orogastric lavage should continue for at least several liters in an adult and/or at least 0.5–1 L in a child if the return is free of debris or until no particulate matter returns and the effluent lavage solution is clear.

12. Those caring for the patient must remain protected at all times, using goggles, mask, gown, and gloves. If the ingested poison is toxic via pulmonary or skin absorption, isolate the ingestant immediately in a self-contained wall suction unit.

13. Any material still in the stomach should be withdrawn, and immediate instillation of the activated charcoal should be considered for large ingestions of xenobiotics known to be adsorbed by activated charcoal.

75.5 Complications

- Vomiting
- Esophageal tears or perforation after orogastric tube insertion
- Inadvertent tracheal intubation and/or airway trauma
- Aspiration pneumonitis

75.6 Pearls and Pitfalls

- Pearls
  - You must use a large-bore orogastric tube for maximal efficacy.
  - The left lateral decubitus position is recommended because the pylorus points upward in this orientation. This position theoretically helps prevent the xenobiotic from passing through the pylorus during the procedure.
- Pitfalls
  - Large drug packets, adherent masses of pills, and plant and mushroom fragments will not pass through a 40-French lavage tube.

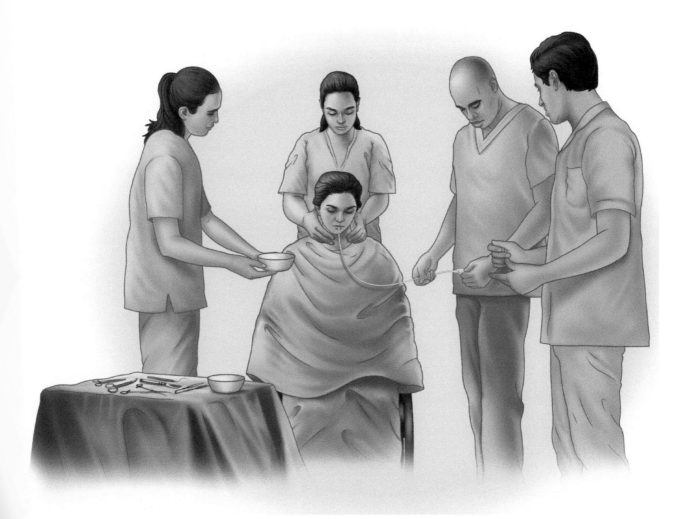

Fig. 75.4 Lavage in progress

Selected Reading

Gude A, Hoegberg LCG. Techniques to prevent gastrointestinal absorption. In: Nelson LS, Lewin NA, Howland MA, et al., editors. Goldfrank's toxicologic emergencies. 8th ed. New York: McGraw-Hill; 2006. p. 91–3.

Olson KR. Poisoning & drug overdose. In: Olson KR, Anderson IB, Benowitz NL, et al., editors. Emergency evaluation and treatment. 6th ed. New York: McGraw-Hill; 2012.

Smilktein MJ. Techniques used to prevent gastrointestinal absorption of toxic compounds. In: Nelson LS, Lewin NA, Howland MA, et al., editors. Goldfrank's toxicologic emergencies. 7th ed. New York: McGraw-Hill; 2002. p. 46–8.

Whole-Bowel Irrigation

76

Judith K. Lucas

76.1 Indications

- Whole-bowel irrigation (WBI) should not be used routinely in the management of the poisoned patient (because there is no clinical proof it will change clinical outcome).
- Ingestion of significant amount of medications.
  - Not adsorbed by activated charcoal
    - Lead, lithium, arsenic, and zinc
    - Substantial amounts of iron (high morbidity and no other effective method to gastrointestinal decontamination)
  - Sustained-release medications or enteric-coated drugs
  - Disk batteries distal to the pylorus
  - Whole transdermal patches (fentanyl, clonidine, nicotine)
  - Drug concretions
  - Ingested packets of illicit drugs

76.2 Contraindications

- Absolute
  - Bowel obstruction
  - Bowel perforation
  - Ileus
  - Hemodynamic instability
  - Compromised or unprotected airway
  - Intractable vomiting

- Relative
  - Concurrent or recent administration of activated charcoal (may decrease the effectiveness of activated charcoal)

76.3 Materials and Medications

- Topical anesthesia, although not mandatory, will reduce the pain of nasogastric (NG) tube placement.
  - 10 % lidocaine spray
  - Lidocaine gel
- Small-bore (12-French) NG tube (Fig. 76.1).
- Tape for securing the NG tube.
- Reservoir or feeding bag used for NG tube feedings (Fig. 76.2).
- Intravenous pole.
- Bedside commode or toilet (Fig. 76.3).
- Polyethylene glycol-electrolyte solution (PEG-ES) (Fig. 76.4).
- Antiemetic.
  - No absolute indication for prophylactic use
  - May be helpful if vomiting ensues during infusion
    - Metoclopramide
      - Antiemetic
      - *Increases gastric motility*

J.K. Lucas, MD
Department of Emergency Medicine,
University of Florida Health Shands Hospital,
Gainesville, FL, USA
e-mail: judithklucas@ufl.edu

© Springer Science+Business Media New York 2016
L. Ganti (ed.), *Atlas of Emergency Medicine Procedures*, DOI 10.1007/978-1-4939-2507-0_76

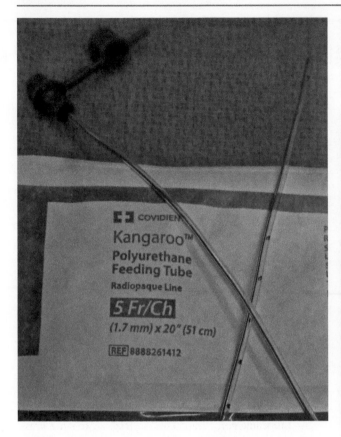

Fig. 76.1 Nasogastric (NG) tube. Typically, the infusion of the lavage solution is too rapid to be taken orally, so an NG tube can be placed. Since the irrigation solution is of low viscosity, a small-bore NG tube should be used for comfort

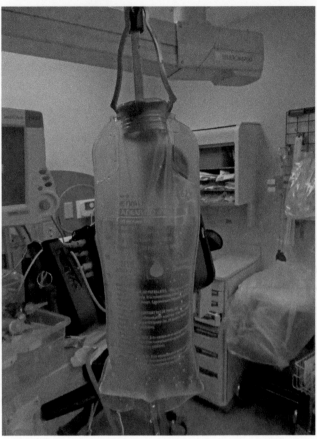

Fig. 76.2 Bag from which the lavage solution will drain; it is similar to the bags used for gastrostomy tube feeding

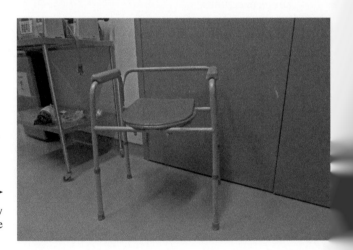

Fig. 76.3 Almost always, the patient will need to be seated on or very near a portable commode, as once the irrigation solution starts to move through the bowels, defecation will occur rapidly

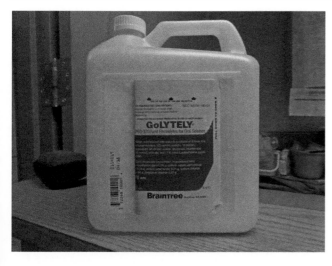

Fig. 76.4 Example brands of intestinal irrigation electrolyte solutions

76.4 Procedure

1. An NG tube is required because most patients will not drink the PEG-ES at the necessary rate.
2. Place a small-bore (12-French) NG tube to a sufficient distance that the tip lies in the central portion of the stomach.
3. Confirm NG placement with a radiograph.
4. Attach the tube to the reservoir bag of PEG-ES and hang from an elevated site (an extended intravenous pole).
5. The patient should be seated in an upright position.
   - Promotes settling of the intoxicant in the distal portion of the stomach
   - Decreases the likelihood of vomiting
6. Dosing:
   - Children 9 months to 6 years: 500 mL/h
   - Children 6–12 years: 1,000 mL/h
   - Adolescents/adults: 1,500–2,000 mL/h
7. Collect effluent.
8. Continue infusion.
   - Until the rectal effluent is the same color as the influent (i.e., clear), usually between 4 and 6 h.
   - You may continue beyond clear effluent if clinical evidence indicates ongoing effectiveness:
     - Continued pill fragments or drug packets are present in the effluent.
     - Radiographic evidence that pills, pharmacobezoars, or packets are still present.

76.5 Complications

- Nausea, vomiting, and bloating
- Misplacement of the NG tube
- Esophageal perforation owing to NG tube placement
- Aspiration pneumonitis in the unprotected airway

76.6 Pearls

- Overall, WBI is probably more effective than gastric lavage, but probably less effective than activated charcoal in preventing poison absorption (when the intoxicant can be adsorbed to charcoal).
- Vomiting.
  - Usually secondary to the ingestant (i.e., emetogenic toxins, such as iron)
  - May be due to rate of infusion
    - Slow rate by 50 % for 30–60 min.
    - Then return to original rate.
- If resistance is encountered during NG tube placement, do not force passage. Remove and redirect.

Selected Reading

Bailey B. To decontaminate or not to decontaminate? the balance between potential risks and foreseeable benefits. Clin Pediatr Emerg Med. 2008;9:17–23.

Hanhan UA. The poisoned child in the pediatric intensive care unit. Pediatr Clin North Am. 2008;55:669–86. xi.

Lheureux P, Tenenbein M. Position paper: whole bowel irrigation. American Academy of Clinical Toxicology/European Association of Poison Centres and Clinical Toxicologists. J Toxicol Clin Toxicol. 2004;42:843–54.

Othong R. Whole-bowel irrigation. MedScape Reference: drugs, diseases, and procedures. Updated: Aug 2011

Postuma R. Whole bowel irrigation in pediatric patients. J Pediatr Surg. 1982;17:350–2.

Sengstaken-Blakemore Tube

77

Thomas T. Nguyen, Etan Eitches,
and Stephanie Wetmore-Nguyen

77.1 Indications

- Life-threatening esophageal variceal bleed refractory to endoscopy and medical therapy
- Life-threatening esophageal variceal bleed refractory to medical therapy in the absence of possible endoscopy

77.2 Contraindications

- Absolute
  - Known esophageal rupture
  - Unable to intubate or maintain airway
- Relative
  - History of prior esophageal trauma or strictures
  - Recent surgery of the gastroesophageal junction
  - Resolved or resolving variceal bleeding

77.3 Materials and Medications

- Sengstaken-Blakemore (SB) tube (Fig. 77.1)
- 60-mL syringe with catheter tip (Fig. 77.2)
- Sphygmomanometer (Fig. 77.3) or cuffalator (Fig. 77.4)
- Y-Tube connector (Fig. 77.5) or 3-way stop-valve connector (Fig. 77.6)
- Vacuum suction device and tubing (Fig. 77.7)
- Tube clamps (4) (Fig. 77.8)
- Lubricant (water soluble)
- Lidocaine (Xylocaine) spray or gel
- Anchoring device such as a football helmet or catcher's mask (Fig. 77.9)
- Cup of water and straw if the patient is awake
- Scissors (Fig. 77.10)
- Intubation equipment
- Sterile water

T.T. Nguyen, MD (✉)
Department of Emergency Medicine,
Mount Sinai Beth Israel, New York, NY, USA
e-mail: tnguyen@chpnet.org

E. Eitches, MD
Department of Emergency Medicine,
Beth Israel Medical Center, New York, NY, USA
e-mail: eeitches@gmail.com

S. Wetmore-Nguyen, MD
Department of Emergency Medicine,
New York-Presbyterian Hospital/Columbia University Medical Center,
New York, NY, USA
e-mail: slw9004@nyp.org

© Springer Science+Business Media New York 2016
L. Ganti (ed.), *Atlas of Emergency Medicine Procedures*, DOI 10.1007/978-1-4939-2507-0_77

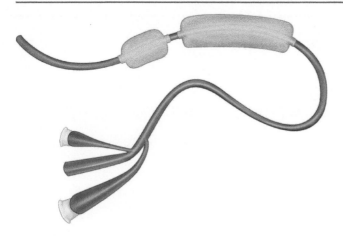

Fig. 77.1 Sengstaken-Blakemore (SB) tube

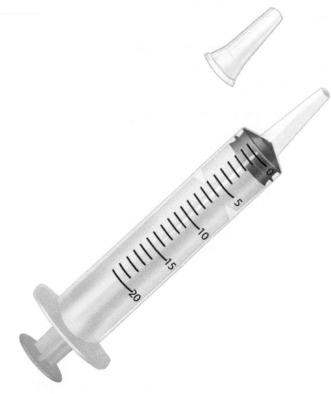

Fig. 77.2 Syringe

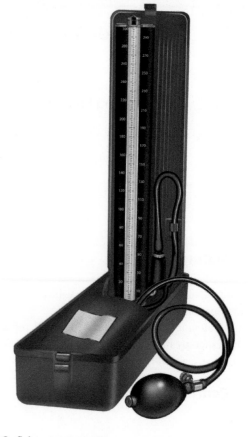

Fig. 77.3 Sphygmomanometer

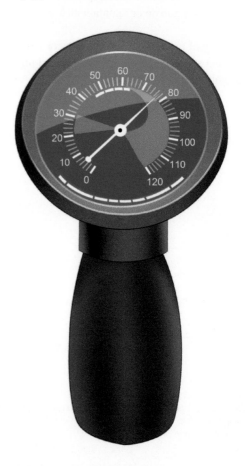

Fig. 77.4 Cuffalator

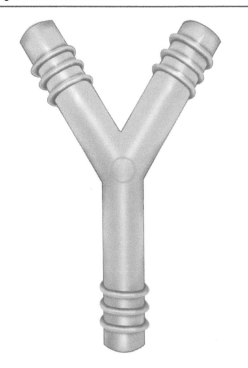

Fig. 77.5   Y-Tube connector

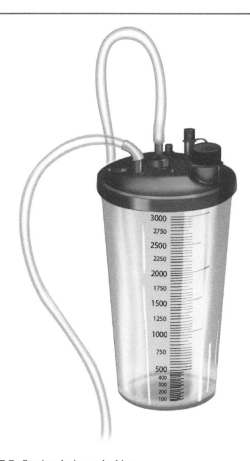

Fig. 77.7   Suction device and tubing

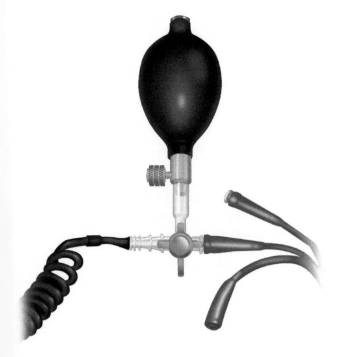

Fig. 77.6   3-way stop-valve tube connector

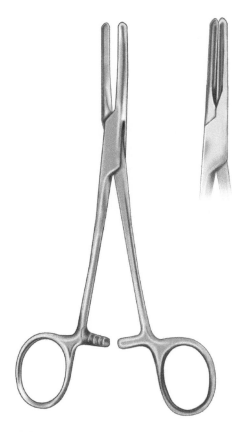

Fig. 77.8   Tube clamps

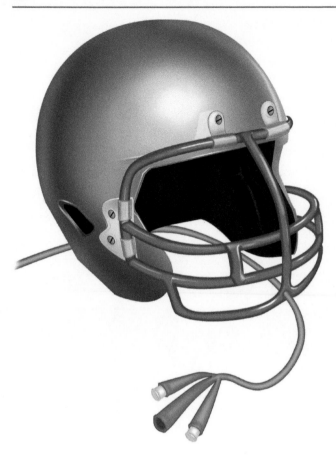

Fig. 77.9 Helmet traction setup

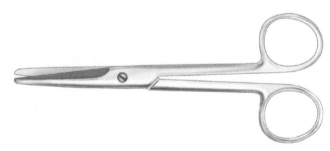

Fig. 77.10 Scissors

77.4   Procedure

1. Sedate and/or intubate the patient for adequate control of the patient during the procedure.
2. Ensure that the SB tube balloons are functional by inflating and deflating the balloons to ensure the absence of leaks.
3. Perform gastric lavage and irrigate the stomach with copious amount of sterile water.
4. Coat the distal and proximal portions of the SB tube with a thin layer of lubricating jelly or lidocaine gel. Spray the nasal passage with lidocaine spray.
5. Pass the SB tube via the nasogastric (NG) or the orogastric route (in intubated patients) to the 50-cm line. You may confirm placement with x-ray.
6. Inflate the gastric balloon to 200 mL of air and clamp the tube.
7. Apply gentle traction of 1–2 lb (0.4–2 kg) of force until it is felt that the gastric balloon has lodged at the gastroesophageal junction (Fig. 77.11).
8. Secure the tube to an anchor (e.g., football helmet or catcher's mask) placed on the patient's head.
9. Aspirate and lavage the gastric aspiration port. If it is clear of blood, do not inflate the esophageal balloon.
10. If it is not clear of blood, connect the esophageal tube of the SB tube to the sphygmomanometer/cuffalator using the 3-way stop-valve device (Fig. 77.12). You may use the Y-Tube connector instead.
11. Inflate the esophageal balloon to the lowest pressure determined to stop bleeding, typically 20–45 mmHg. Clamp the balloon.
12. Place an NG tube until it is felt overlying the top of the esophageal balloon of the SB tube. Check for further proximal esophageal bleed through aspiration and gentle lavage. Attach this NG tube to intermittent section to aid in the clearance of secretions.
13. Obtain a portable radiograph to confirm the position of the SB tube.
14. The esophageal tube should be at the lowest pressure that prevents bleeding and kept inflated for 24 h or until other definitive treatment is obtained.

Fig. 77.11 Proper placement
of the balloons

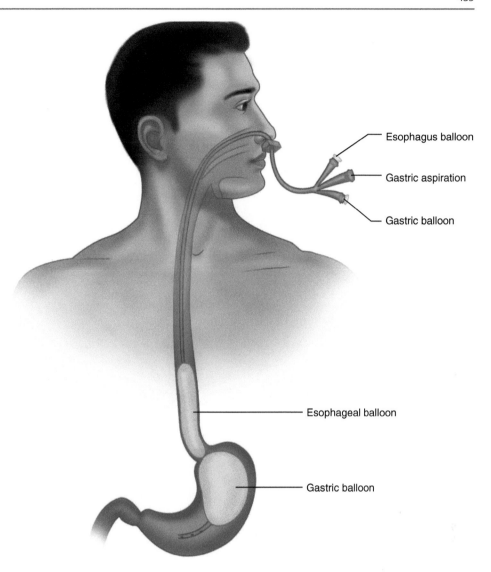

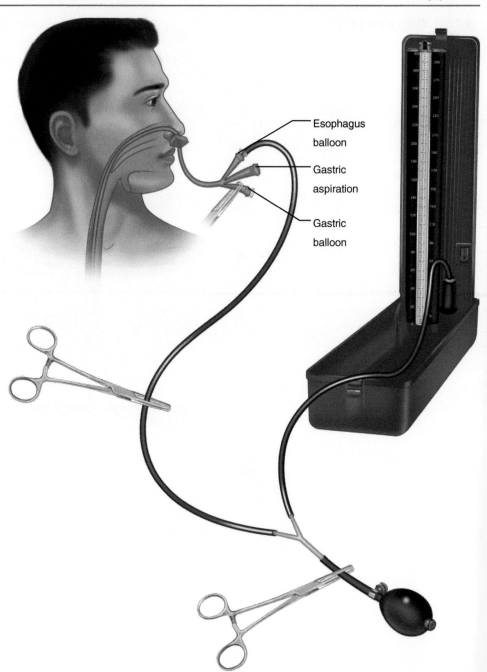

Fig. 77.12 Connection of the sphygmomanometer to the esophagus balloon port

Esophagus balloon

Gastric aspiration

Gastric balloon

77.5   Complications

- Esophageal rupture occurs owing to esophageal erosion and necrosis owing to a balloon tamponade effect on tissue perfusion or overzealous balloon inflation.
- Airway obstruction owing to gastric tube deflation or failure, allowing esophageal tube to move up and occlude airway. Keep scissors near the patient to cut the SB tube lumens and remove the tube as necessary.
- Regurgitation and aspiration pneumonia from failure to adequately suction oropharyngeal secretions.

77.6   Pearls and Pitfalls

- Pearls
  - The esophageal balloon should not be inflated if the gastric balloon alone stops the bleeding.
  - Never inflate the esophageal balloon without the inflating the gastric balloon first. This will prevent it from slipping proximally into the oropharynx and obstructing the airway.
  - Nausea, vomiting, or aspiration is highly likely to occur. Use antiemetics and lavage the stomach before the procedure.
  - Intubate if there is airway compromise or risk of aspiration into the lungs.
  - Inflate the esophageal balloon only to the minimum pressure necessary to stop the variceal bleeding.
  - Using a catcher's mask may be more practical and comfortable for the recumbent patient.
- Pitfalls
  - The SB tube may induce hiccups.

Selected Reading

Bauer J, Kreel I, Kark A. The use of the Sengstaken-Blakemore tube for immediate control of bleeding esophageal varices. Ann Surg. 1974;179:273–7.

Henneman PL. Gastrointestinal bleeding. In: Rosen P, Barkin RM, editors. Emergency medicine. 6th ed. St. Louis: Mosby; 1998.

Remonda G, Morachioli N, Petruzzelli C. The use of the Sengstaken-Blakemore tube for immediate control of bleeding esophageal varices. Ann Osp Maria Vittoria Torino. 1981;24:115–20.

Sengstaken RW, Blakemore AH. Balloon tamponage for the control of hemorrhage from esophageal varices. Ann Surg. 1950;131:781–9.

Treger R, Graham T, Dea S. Sengstaken-Blakemore tube. Available at http://emedicine.medscape.com/article/81020-overview#a01. Accessed 18 May 2014.

Gastrostomy Tube Placement

78

Nathaniel Lisenbee and Latha Ganti

There are several types of gastrostomy tubes and related procedure variations:

- Procedure variations:
  - Open gastrostomy tube (G tube)
  - Percutaneous endoscopic gastrostomy (PEG) tube
  - Laparoscopic G tube

- Tube types:
  - PEG tube (Fig. 78.1)
  - Malecot tube (Fig. 78.2)
  - Balloon G tube (Fig. 78.3)
  - Low-profile G tube (nonobturated, button) (Fig. 78.4)
  - Low-profile G tube (obturated, button) (Fig. 78.5)

N. Lisenbee, MD
U. S. Air Force Medical Center Keesler, Biloxi, MI, USA
e-mail: nate4085@ufl.edu

L. Ganti, MD (✉)
Professor of Emergency Medicine, University of Central Florida, Orlando, FL, USA

Director, SE Specialty Care Centers of Innovation, Orlando Veterans Affairs Medical Center, Orlando, FL, USA
e-mail: lathagantimd@gmail.com

© Springer Science+Business Media New York 2016
L. Ganti (ed.), *Atlas of Emergency Medicine Procedures*, DOI 10.1007/978-1-4939-2507-0_78

Fig. 78.1 Percutaneous endoscopic gastrostomy (PEG) tube

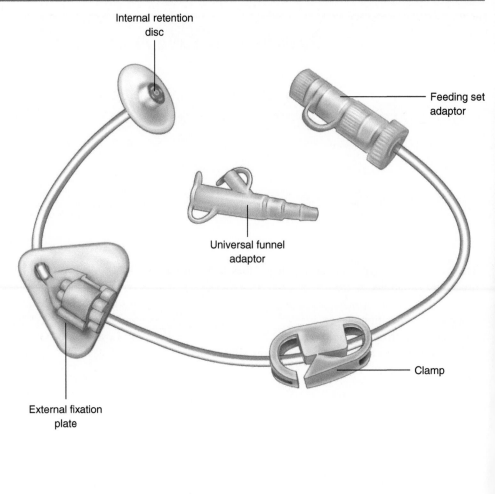

Internal retention disc

Feeding set adaptor

Universal funnel adaptor

External fixation plate

Clamp

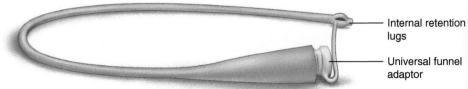

Internal retention lugs

Universal funnel adaptor

Fig. 78.2 Malecot tube

Fig. 78.3 Balloon gastrostomy tube

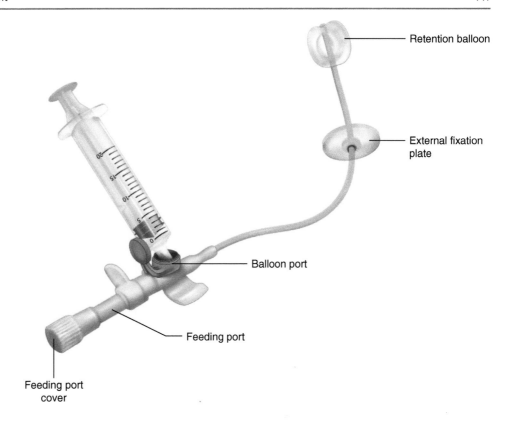

Retention balloon

External fixation plate

Balloon port

Feeding port

Feeding port cover

Feeding port

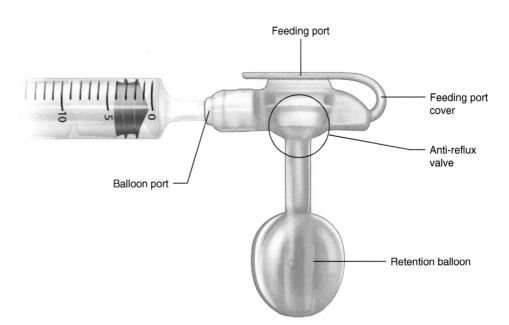

Feeding port cover

Anti-reflux valve

Balloon port

Retention balloon

Fig. 78.4 Low-profile gastrostomy tube (nonobturated, button)

Fig. 78.5 Low-profile gastrostomy tube (obturated, button)

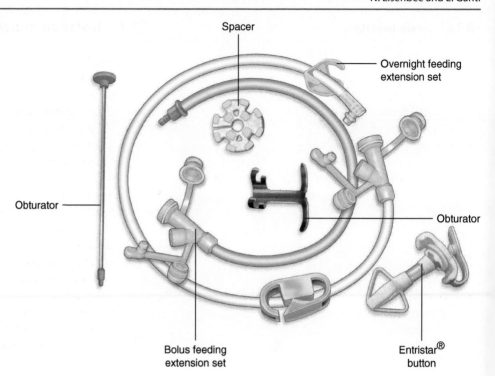

Spacer

Overnight feeding extension set

Obturator

Obturator

Bolus feeding extension set

Entristar® button

78.1   Indications

- Inability to swallow
  - Neurological deficit
  - Head trauma
  - Facial burns
  - Decreased mental status
- Need for gastric decompression
  - Gastric outflow obstruction
  - Small bowel obstruction (SBO), ileus, or volvulus
  - Intra-abdominal malignancy

78.2   Contraindications

- Absolute
  - Peritonitis
  - Ascites
- Relative
  - Hemodynamic instability
  - Coagulopathy
  - Abdominal wall infection at surgical site
  - History of gastric resection
  - Portal hypertension
  - Gastric varices

78.3   Materials and Medications

- Materials
  - Gloves
  - Lubricant
  - G tube (commercial kit) or Foley catheter
  - Sterile saline
  - External bolster
  - Multiple syringes
  - Suture material
  - Needle driver
  - Scissors
  - Stethoscope
- Medications
  - PEG tube placement
    - Moderate sedation (e.g., propofol, midazolam, fentanyl)
    - Local anesthesia (e.g., lidocaine, bupivacaine)
  - Open or laparoscopic G tube placement (not an emergency department procedure)
    - General anesthesia

78.4 Procedure (PEG Tube Replacement)

1. If the G tube is only partially removed upon patient presentation, the tube must first be removed.
2. Remove the G tube by deflating the balloon and pull gently on the tube while applying pressure to the abdominal wall at the surgical site.
3. The G tube should slide out easily with gentle traction, and the procedure should be discontinued if it does not.
4. Initially, it is important to assess the tract to determine the size and potential need for dilation.
5. If necessary for tube passage, the tract can be dilated with a cotton-tipped applicator or hemostat; however, be sure to dilate gently because it is possible to create a false tract.
6. Once the tract has been assessed, obtain the appropriate tube for replacement.
7. Initially, attempt replacement of the patient's G tube with an identical tube.
8. If an identical tube is not available, attempt placing a small Foley catheter in the tract to ensure that it stays open.
9. To initiate placement, place lubricant on the tube and carefully advance the tube into the tract.
10. Once the tube is in place, secure an air-filled syringe to the tip of the tube and insufflate a small amount of air into the stomach while auscultating to confirm passage of air into the stomach.
11. Secondary procedural confirmation can be performed by aspirating gastric contents from the tube.
12. Once placement is verified, do not forget to inflate the balloon with saline and then pull the tube backward until it abuts the inside of the stomach wall (Fig. 78.6).
13. Finally, it is very important to secure the external portion of the tube to prevent the tube from being lost into the stomach.
14. Commercial G tubes are accompanied by a bolster made specifically for the specific type of G tube in order to provide security of tube placement.

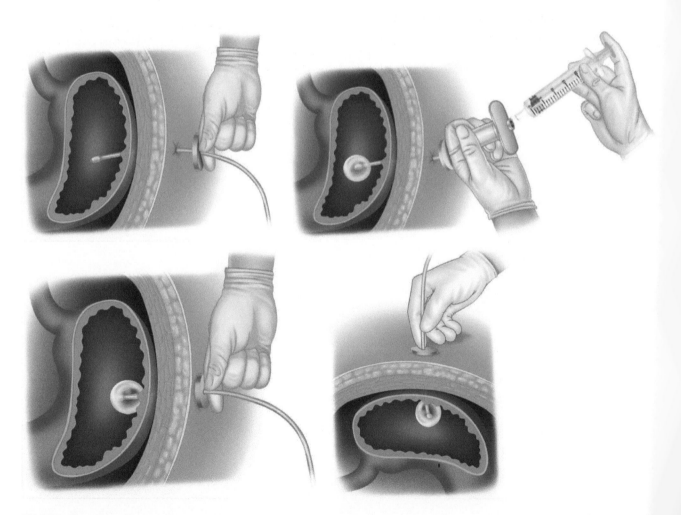

Fig. 78.6 Placement of low-profile gastrostomy tube

15. If a Foley catheter is used to maintain tract patency, an external bolster must be created using the following steps:
    • Trim a 2- to 3-in. portion from the tip of the catheter.
    • Cut two small holes just above each other on the 2- to 3-in. trimmed catheter portion.
    • Slide the external portion of the Foley catheter through both holes of the bolster.
    • Slide the bolster down the Foley catheter to the abdominal wall.
    • Secure the two ends of the bolster to the skin in order to maintain patency of the Foley catheter.
    • An interventional radiologist may also be contacted to advance the tube over a wire under fluoroscopic guidance.
16. Radiographic confirmation.
    • Typically, G tube placement is confirmed by injecting approximately 20 mL of Gastrografin® (diatrizoate meglumine, diatrizoate sodium) water-soluble contrast into the G tube, followed shortly by an abdominal x-ray.
    • Proper placement will result in an abdominal radiograph showing contrast outlining the stomach (Fig. 78.7).

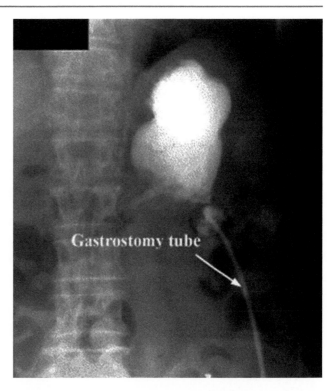

Gastrostomy tube

Fig. 78.7 An anteroposterior abdominal radiograph after PEG tube placement and injection of 25 mL of gastrografin. The tube can be seen projecting up the left side of the abdomen, and contrast medium appears to enter the stomach lumen. The balloon is not visualized in the stomach (Reproduced with permission from: Burke DT, El Shami A, Heinle E, and Pina BD. Comparison of gastrostomy tube replacement verification using air insufflation versus gastrografin. Archives of physical medicine and rehabilitation. 2006;87(11): 1530–3.)

78.5 Pearls and Pitfalls

- Pearls
  - Even if a patient's G tube is only partially removed upon presentation to the emergency department, the tube likely needs complete removal and replacement.
  - Most G tubes are easily removed at the bedside; however, some are not able to be safely removed in the emergency department setting. Thus, if the tube does not withdraw easily, attempt to contact the proceduralist who placed the tube in order to inquire about the best method for removal.
- Pitfalls
  - Never use barium contrast when confirming G tube placement radiographically because barium can cause significant intra-abdominal damage if accidentally injected in the intraperitoneal cavity.

78.6 Complications

- Aspiration
- Surgical site infection
- Bleeding
- Pneumoperitoneum
- Accidental perforation of the colon or small bowel
- Tube dislodgment
- Peritonitis

Selected Reading

Arora G. Medscape: percutaneous endoscopic gastrostomy tube placement. Retrieved 3 Jan 2013, from http://emedicine.medscape.com/article/149665-overview#a09.

Gauderer MW, Ponsky JL, Izant Jr RJ. Gastrostomy without laparotomy: a percutaneous endoscopic technique. J Pediatr Surg. 1980; 15:872–5.

Great Ormand street hospital for children website. Retrieved 3 Jan 2013, from www.gosh.nhs.uk/EasySiteWeb/GatewayLink.aspx?alId=102263.

Sarani B. Percutaneous endoscopic gastrostomy tube placement. In: Falter F, editor. Bedside procedures in the ICU. Philadelphia: Springer; 2012. p. 113–22.

Tawa Jr NE, Fischer JE. Metabolism in surgical patients. In: Townsend Jr CM, Beauchamp RD, Evers BM, Mattox KL, editors. Sabiston textbook of surgery. 18th ed. Philadelphia: Elsevier; 2007.

Paracentesis

79

Shalu S. Patel and Bobby K. Desai

79.1 Indications

- Diagnosis of infection in ascites
- Diagnosis of malignant ascites
- Diagnosis of hemoperitoneum in traumas
- Relief of abdominal pressure/pain or respiratory compromise secondary to ascites

79.2 Contraindications

- Severe coagulopathy
  - Prothrombin time (PT)>21 s
  - International normalized ratio (INR)>1.6
  - Platelets <50,000/mm^3
- Skin infection over the needle insertion site
- Acute abdomen that requires surgery
- Pregnancy
- Distended bowel
- Intra-abdominal adhesions

79.3 Materials and Medications

- 18- to 22-gauge 1.5- to 3.5-in. needle or angiocatheter, 25-gauge needle
  Lidocaine 1 or 2 % (10 mL)
  Syringes

- 10 mL (1), 50 mL (2)
- 1-L vacuum bottle (4) (if therapeutic tap)
- Thoracentesis kit tubing or any high-pressure connection tubing (if therapeutic tap)
- Sterile gloves
- Surgical pen (recommended)
- Povidone-iodine (Betadine) or other skin antiseptic
- Sterile drape
- Sterile gauze (4×4)
- Band-Aid
- Bedside ultrasound (recommended)

79.4 Procedure (Fig. 79.1)

1. Position the patient supine. If possible, adjust the head of the bed to make a 45° angle to help the fluid accumulate in the pocket. Sometimes, it may also be beneficial to have the patient lie recumbent toward the site of drainage.
2. Scan the abdomen with an ultrasound to determine whether there is a pocket of fluid that can be drained. This also allows the physician to see how far the needle needs to be inserted and how deep it can be placed without risking injury to the bowel (Fig. 79.2).
3. Mark the optimal needle insertion site with a surgical pen.
4. Prepare the skin and drape in a sterile fashion.
5. Using lidocaine, anesthetize the appropriate area subcutaneously and then continue to insert the needle, and inject anesthetic through the deeper tissues until ascitic fluid can be drawn back.
6. Withdraw the needle.
7. When ready for the paracentesis, stretch the skin caudad and insert the needle or angiocatheter (connected to a syringe) while aspirating. Then, release the skin and continue to insert the needle or angiocatheter through the peritoneal wall until fluid is retrieved. This will create a "Z-track" that will decrease leakage of peritoneal fluid through the skin.

S. Patel, MD
Department of Emergency Medicine, Florida Hospital Tampa,
Florida Hospital Carrollwood, Tampa, FL, USA
e-mail: shalu314@gmail.com

K. Desai, MD (✉)
Department of Emergency Medicine,
University of Florida Health Shands Hospital,
Gainesville, FL, USA
e-mail: bdesai@ufl.edu

Springer Science+Business Media New York 2016
Ganti (ed.), *Atlas of Emergency Medicine Procedures*, DOI 10.1007/978-1-4939-2507-0_79

447

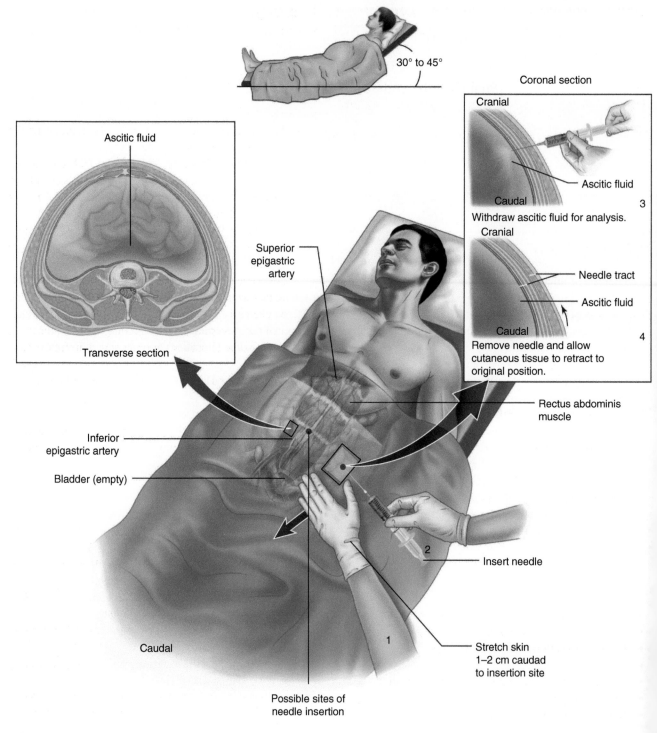

Fig. 79.1 Paracentesis procedure

8. Once fluid is retrieved, push in the catheter and remove the needle portion (if used) or hold the needle steady.

9. Aspirate from the catheter to ensure that it is in the appropriate location.

10. If fluid easily is aspirated, unscrew the syringe and connect a 50-mL syringe to the needle or catheter and fill it with fluid. This may be done twice. Alternatively, if the

procedure is done for therapeutic purposes, attach th[e] tubing that is already connected to the vacuum bottle t[o] the catheter and allow the vacuum to withdraw fluid int[o] the collection bottles.

11. If fluid cannot be aspirated easily, the catheter can b[e] repositioned further in the pocket or turned by 4[5°] sequentially as needed.

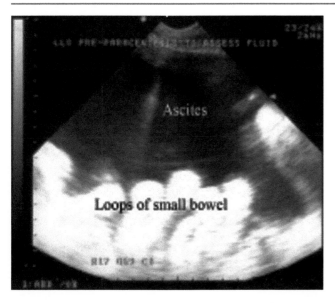

Fig. 79.2 Ultrasound to determine whether there is a pocket of fluid that can be drained

12. Once the fluid is aspirated, pull out the needle or angio-catheter and hold pressure with gauze. Bleeding should be minimal.
13. Place a Band-Aid or other dressing over the site.
14. Send the fluid to the laboratory. Generally, laboratory analyses include protein, albumin, specific gravity, glucose, bilirubin, amylase, lipase, triglyceride, lactate dehydrogenase (LDH), cell count and differential, culture and sensitivity (C&S), Gram stain, acid-fast bacillus (AFB), fungal culture, cytology, and pH.

79.5 Complications

- Persistent leakage from the needle insertion site
- Abdominal wall hematoma
- Bowel perforation
- Introduction of infection
- Hypotension (after a large-volume paracentesis)
- Dilutional hyponatremia
- Hepatorenal syndrome
- Bleeding
- Postparacentesis circulatory dysfunction

79.6 Pearls and Pitfalls

- Pearls
  - The preferred site of entry is in the midline of the abdomen, below the umbilicus.
  - The serum-ascites albumin gradient (SAAG) can be used to identify the cause of the ascites. It is calculated by subtracting the albumin concentration in the ascites from the albumin concentration in the serum. A high gradient (>1.1 g/dL) suggests portal hypertension, whereas a low gradient (<1.1 g/dL) suggests other causes.
  - Postparacentesis circulatory dysfunction (PPCD) occurs secondary to hypovolemia after large-volume paracentesis (>4 L) in cirrhotic patients. It is associated with worsening hyponatremia, renal dysfunction, shorter time to ascites recurrence, and increased mortality. Prevention of PPCD has been demonstrated with the administration of 6–8 g of albumin per liter of ascites removed.
- Pitfalls
  - Polymorphonuclear lymphocyte (PMN) count greater than 250/mm^3 is diagnostic of spontaneous bacterial peritonitis.

Selected Reading

Ginès P, Cárdenas A, Arroyo V, Rodés J. Management of cirrhosis and ascites. N Engl J Med. 2004;350:1646–54.

Ginès P, Tito L, Arroyo V, et al. Randomized comparative study of therapeutic paracentesis with and without intravenous albumin in cirrhosis. Gastroenterology. 1988;94:1493–502.

Ruiz del Arbol L, Monescillo A, Jimenéz W, et al. Paracentesis-induced circulatory dysfunction: mechanism and effect on hepatic hemodynamics in cirrhosis. Gastroenterology. 1997;113:579–86.

Runyon BA. Paracentesis of ascitic fluid. A safe procedure. Arch Intern Med. 1986;146:2259–61.

Wong CL, Holroyd-Leduc J, Thorpe KE, Straus SE. Does this patient have bacterial peritonitis or portal hypertension? How do I perform a paracentesis and analyze the results? JAMA. 2008;299:1166–78.

Anal Fissure Management

David P. Nguyen, L. Connor Nickels, and
Giuliano De Portu

80.1   Indications

- An anal fissure is a small ulcer of the mucosa at the anal verge (Fig. 80.1).
- It is the most common cause of intense sudden rectal bleeding.
- Posterior midline anal fissures are the most common type (90 %).
  - Mostly found in young adults (30–50 y) but can occur at any age.
  - Usually associated with constipation (firm, large-caliber, painful bowel movements) or chronic diarrhea.
  - Most uncomplicated fissures resolve in 3–4 weeks.
- Can be extremely painful, during and after defecation.
- Classified as acute or chronic.
- Now believed to be caused by reduced anal blood flow in the posterior midline, anal sphincter hypertonia, and thus mucosal ischemia.

D.P. Nguyen, DO
Department of Emergency Medicine, Rush-Copley Medical
Center, Aurora, IL, USA
e-mail: davidpnguyen@yahoo.com

L.C. Nickels, MD, RDMS (✉) • G. De Portu, MD
Department of Emergency Medicine, University of Florida Health
Shands Hospital, Gainesville, FL, USA
e-mail: cnickels@ufl.edu; gdeportu@ufl.edu

© Springer Science+Business Media New York 2016
L. Ganti (ed.), *Atlas of Emergency Medicine Procedures*, DOI 10.1007/978-1-4939-2507-0_80

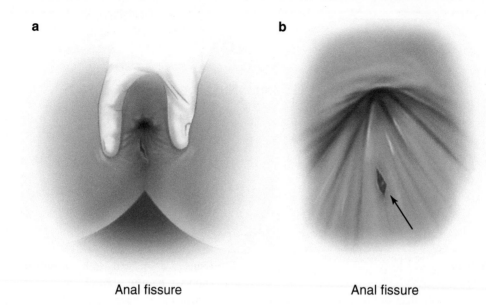

Anal fissure   Anal fissure

Fig. 80.1 (**a, b**) Anal fissures

80.2 Contraindications

- Digital rectal examination should be avoided unless the diagnosis is in doubt.
- Surgical procedures are generally reserved for when medical management has failed after 1–3 months of treatment.

80.3 Materials and Medications

- Standard precautions barrier protection for the provider.
- Good light source.
- Optional emergency department treatments:
  - Topical anesthetic/preparation (Anusol [pramoxine hydrochloride; zinc oxide] with cortisone).
  - Nitroglycerin (0.2 %) or nifedipine gel (2 %) is second-line therapy (relaxes muscles and promotes blood flow).

80.4 Procedure

1. In a private, calm environment, gently spread the buttocks for complete visual inspection.
   - This may cause an increase in the patient's pain and spasming.
   - If a fissure is clearly identified, stop here.
2. Apply topical anesthetic/preparation for symptomatic relief (optional, as the physician may want to just start with the treatments that follow).
3. Discharge the patient with conservative therapy management.
4. In acute anal fissures (onset of 3–6 weeks), medical management is indicated along with dietary modifications (WASH regimen [warm baths, analgesia, stool softeners, high-fiber diet]):
   - Warm sitz baths.
     - Usually 20 min soaking each time
     - Recommended after every bowel movement
     - At least twice per day if not having regular bowel movements
   - High-fiber diet with fiber supplements.
   - Increase fluid intake.
   - May add stool softeners, if needed.
   - If chronic or the previous regimen has been exhausted, one of the following may be considered:
     - 0.2–0.4 % nitroglycerin cream applied to anal area
       - May cause headache
       - Recommend wearing a glove to prevent absorption through digital skin

- Calcium channel blockers:
  - Topical nifedipine
  - 2 % diltiazem cream
- Botulinum toxin A injection:
  - Controversial; may have poorer success rates than surgery

5. Provide surgical referral for nonhealing wounds.
   - Lateral internal sphincterotomy is the surgical procedure of choice.

80.5 Complications

- Infection
- Abscess
- Bleeding
- Chronic fissure formation
- Postsurgical fecal incontinence

80.6 Pearls and Pitfalls

- Pearls
  - Multiple or recurrent fissures are associated with Crohn's disease, tuberculosis, syphilis, human immunodeficiency virus (HIV), and malignancy.
- Pitfalls
  - Suspect child abuse if an anal fissure is found in a child.

Selected Reading

Feldman M, Friedman LS, Brandt LJ, editors. Sleisenger and Fordtran's gastrointestinal and liver disease. 9th ed. Philadelphia: Saunders; 2010.

Marx J, Hockberger R, Walls R, editors. Rosen's emergency medicine. 7th ed. Philadelphia: Mosby; 2010. Chapter 94: Disorders of the anorectum

Öztürk H, Onen A, Dokucu AI, Otçu S, Yağmur Y, Yucesan S. Management of anorectal injuries in children: an eighteen-year experience. Eur J Pediatr Surg. 2003;13:249–55.

Townsend CM Jr, Beauchamp RD, Evers BM, Mattox KL, editors. Sabiston textbook of surgery. 19th ed. Philadelphia: Saunders; 2012. Chapter 53: Anus

Bladder Catheterization

81

Maritza A. Plaza-Verduin and Judith K. Lucas

81.1 Indications

- Obtaining a sterile urine specimen
- Preventing or relieving urinary retention
- Close monitoring of urine output for fluid balance with an indwelling urinary catheter
- Urgent cystourethrography
- Child with contusion or burns to the perineum and at risk for meatal swelling and obstruction to urine outflow
- Temporary measure to relieve lower urinary tract obstruction
- Neurogenic bladder
- Anesthesia-induced and/or surgery-induced urinary retention has occurred.

81.2 Contraindications

- Absolute
  - Potential urethral injury from trauma
    - Pelvic fractures
    - Known trauma to the urethra
    - Blood at the meatus

- Relative
  - Recent genitourinary surgery (consult with a urologist before placing a catheter)

81.3 Materials and Medications

- Bladder catheterization kit:
  - Sterile gloves
  - Sterile drapes
  - Povidone-iodine (Betadine) solution
  - Cotton sponges or applicators for sterilizing solution
  - Lubricant
  - Specimen collection cup
  - Catheter
    - 5-French feeding tube for neonates
    - 8-French catheters for Infants
    - 10- to 12-French catheters in older children
- Local anesthetic (if desired—2 % lidocaine hydrochloride jelly)
- Absorbent pad

M.A. Plaza-Verduin, MD
Pediatric Division, Department of Emergency Medicine, Arnold Palmer Hospital for Children, Orlando, FL, USA
e-mail: mari.plazav@gmail.com

J.K. Lucas, MD (✉)
Department of Emergency Medicine,
University of Florida Health Shands Hospital,
Gainesville, FL, USA
e-mail: judithklucas@ufl.edu

© Springer Science+Business Media New York 2016
L. Ganti (ed.), *Atlas of Emergency Medicine Procedures*, DOI 10.1007/978-1-4939-2507-0_81

81.4 Procedure

1. Inspect the urinary catheterization tray for all the appropriate materials.
2. Place the patient supine with an absorbent pad under the buttocks.
   (a) Girls should be placed in the frog-leg position (Fig. 81.1).
3. Before sterilizing the field, locate the urethral opening.
4. Remove any powder, ointments, or medicated creams the child might have on the perineum.
5. If needed, apply anesthetic to the area.
   (a) Soak a cotton ball with anesthetic (2 % lidocaine hydrochloride jelly) and hold over the urethra opening for 2 min.
   (b) 0.5–2.0 mL of anesthetic can also be injected into the urethra.
6. Sterilize the area and place drapes appropriately, exposing the genitalia.
7. Catheterization of males
   (a) If uncircumcised, gently retract foreskin, *if possible*, for cleaning and visualization of the meatus.
   (b) Hold the penis using the nondominant hand at a 90° angle from the body (Fig. 81.2).
   (c) Lubricate the catheter tip.
   (d) Insert the lubricated catheter into the meatal opening and advance it while applying gentle traction to the penis from the base of the penis.
   (e) If resistance is met, maintain gentle pressure with the catheter.
      • *Do not attempt to force the catheter that could create a false tract or traumatic fistula.*
   (f) Advance the catheter until urine is obtained, approximately inserting the catheter to just beyond the penile length.
   (g) Once completed, gently withdraw the catheter.
   (h) Clean the area, wiping away the Betadine solution.
   (i) If uncircumcised, pull the foreskin over the glans to avoid paraphimosis.
8. Catheterization of females
   (a) Sterilization of the area should occur from anterior to posterior.
   (b) Have an assistant hold the labia majora apart.
      (i) If no assistant is available, use the nondominant hand to hold the labia apart.
         • Holding the labia majora with a gentle outward, lateral, and upward traction will help visualize the meatus (Fig. 81.3).

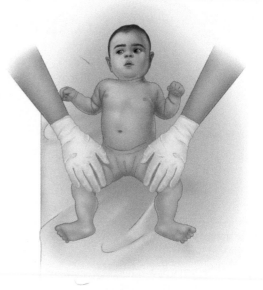

Fig. 81.1 Infant held in the frog-leg position for catheterization

Fig. 81.2 Bladder
catheterization of a male; penis
should be held perpendicular to
the body

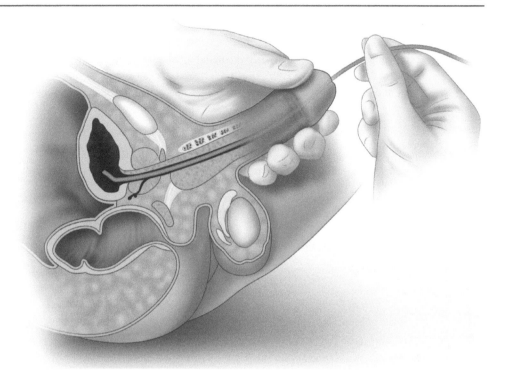

Gentle lateral and
outward traction
of labia majora

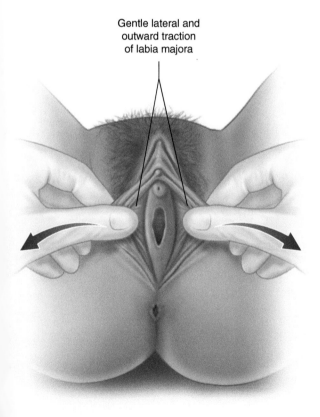

Fig. 81.3   Positioning of labia for better visualization of the meatus

- Downward displacement of the cephalad aspect of the vaginal introital fold with a cotton-tipped applicator can help visualize the urethral meatus (Fig. 81.4).

(c) Lubricate the catheter tip.

(d) Insert the lubricated catheter into the meatal opening. Advance slowly until urine is obtained (Fig. 81.5).

(e) Once completed, gently withdraw the catheter.

(f) Clean area, wiping away the Betadine solution.

Fig. 81.4 Better visualization of the meatus is achieved with downward displacement of the introital mucosa

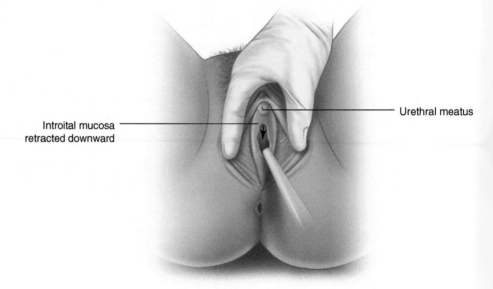

Introital mucosa retracted downward

Urethral meatus

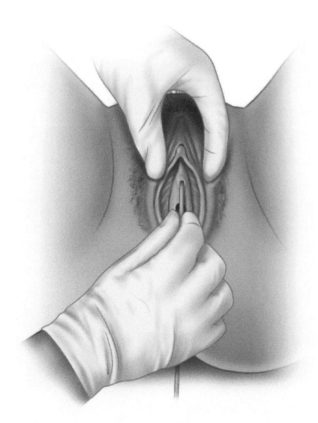

Fig. 81.5 Bladder catheterization of a female

81.5   Complications

- Urethral or bladder injury
- Infection if sterile field not maintained
- Paraphimosis owing to failure to restore a retracted fore-skin to its normal position

81.6   Pearls and Pitfalls

- Pearls
  - It is not necessary to fully retract a foreskin. This only causes trauma and increases the likelihood of paraphi-mosis. As the infant/boy ages, the foreskin will loosen and the naturally occurring adhesions will spontane-ously release.
  - The urethral meatus in an infant female is usually tucked just above the redundant hymen (as opposed to the more anteriorly located meatus in the adult woman) and often looks like a dimple or small blind pouch.
  - Using viscous lidocaine in lieu of, or blended with, lubricant anesthetizes the meatus and urethra as the catheter passes.
  - Have the specimen cup at the ready because, at times, once the (usually cold) Betadine or antiseptic solution is applied, the infant often releases the urine and it can be caught, literally, midstream.
  - In the uncircumcised male, be certain to return the foreskin over the glans to avoid paraphimoses.
- Pitfalls
  - If catheterizing a child in search of infection, send a urine culture regardless of the urinalysis results because the younger infants can have false-negative urinalysis and still have positive cultures.

Selected Reading

American Academy of Pediatrics, Subcommittee on urinary tract infection, steering committee on quality improvement and management. Urinary tract infection: clinical practice guideline for the diagnosis and management of the initial UTI in febrile infants and children 2 to 24 months. Pediatrics. 2011;128:595–609.

Beno S, Schwab S. Bladder catheterization. In: King C, Henretig FM, editors. Textbook of pediatric emergency procedures. 2nd ed. New York: Lippincott Williams & Wilkins; 2008.

Cheng YW, Wong SN. Diagnosing symptomatic urinary tract infection in infants by catheter urine culture. J Paediatr Child Health. 2005;41:437–40.

Gerard LL, Cooper CS, Duethman KS, et al. Effectiveness of lidocaine lubricant for discomfort during pediatric urethral catheterization. J Urol. 2003;170:564–7.

Kozer E, Rosenbloom E, Goldman D, et al. Pain in infants who are younger than 2 months during suprapubic aspiration and transure-thral bladder catheterization: a randomized, controlled study. Pediatrics. 2006;118:e51–6.

Pelvic Examination and Wet Preparation

82

Nauman W. Rashid, Elaine B. Josephson, and Muhammad Waseem

82.1 Indications

- Lower abdominal or pelvic pain
- Vaginal bleeding or discharge
- Cancer screening
- Pregnancy
- Exposure to sexually transmitted disease
- Sexual assault

82.2 Contraindications

- Physical or mental disability
- Recent gynecological surgery
- Third-trimester pregnancy with bleeding
- Premenstrual females (may not be indicated in adolescents, who are not sexually active, unless there is discharge, bleeding, suspicion for abuse, or a foreign body)
- If a speculum examination is necessary, examination under general anesthesia should be considered.

N.W. Rashid, MD
Department of Emergency Medicine, WellStar Kennestone Hospital, Marietta, GA, USA
e-mail: naumanrashid@hotmail.com

E.B. Josephson, MD
Department of Emergency Medicine, Lincoln Medical and Mental Health Center, Weill Cornell Medical College of Cornell University, Bronx, NY, New York
e-mail: elaine.Josephson@nychhc.org

M. Waseem, MD (✉)
Department of Emergency Medicine, Lincoln Medical and Mental Health Center, New York, NY, USA
e-mail: waseemm2001@hotmail.com

82.3 Materials and Medications

- Examination table with stirrups (Fig. 82.1)
- Reliable light source
- Appropriately sized speculum (Fig. 82.2)
- Endocervical brush or spatula
- Culture swab for gonorrhea and chlamydia
- Large cotton swabs for vaginal discharge or bleeding (Fig. 82.2)
- pH paper
- Saline and potassium hydroxide dropper bottles for wet preparations
- Lubricating gel
- Disposable gloves (Fig. 82.2)
- Small stool or chair for examiner

82.4 Procedure

1. Obtain permission from patient before beginning examination.
2. Chaperone should be present (medical staff member).
3. Make sure the examination table is clean and appropriately draped.
4. Have the patient in a loose-fitting gown.
5. Place the patient on the examination table in the lithotomy position with both feet in the stirrups and have the patient's pelvis as close to the edge of the table as possible.
6. Turn on the light source and adjust for optimum illumination. Put on the disposable gloves.
7. Communicate the procedure well to the patient.
8. Begin the examination with inspection and palpation of the abdomen.
9. Examine the external genitalia. Evaluate the skin, labia minora and majora, clitoris, urethral meatus, vaginal

L. Ganti (ed.), *Atlas of Emergency Medicine Procedures*, DOI 10.1007/978-1-4939-2507-0_82

Fig. 82.1 Examination table with stirrups

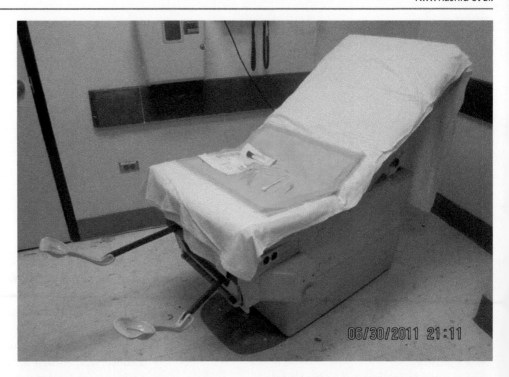

Fig. 82.2 Gloves, speculum, and swabs

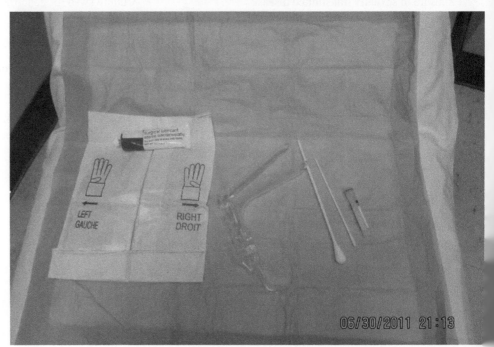

canal, and Bartholin glands (Fig. 82.3). Look for skin abnormalities, lesions, masses, rashes, excoriation, abscesses, discharge, bleeding, or trauma. Palpate for tenderness.

10. Lubricate the appropriate-size speculum (mostly medium size). Insert the speculum through the vaginal opening with gentle downward pressure. The speculum should advance without any resistance until the cervical os is visualized.

11. Inspect the vaginal walls for any lesions or masses (Fig. 82.4). The cervical os is inspected to see if it is open or closed. Cervical cultures for gonorrhea and chlamydia are obtained with a cotton swab and sent for microbiology.

12. A sample of the discharge or bleeding is taken with a large cotton swab. The color, odor, and amount should be noted. The pH of the vaginal discharge can be evaluated. Normal pH is less than 4.5. An elevated pH indicates an infection (Table 82.1).

Fig. 82.3 Female external genitalia

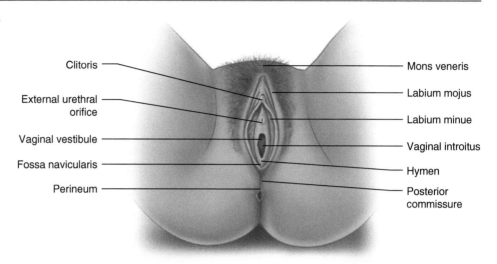

Clitoris

External urethral orifice

Vaginal vestibule

Fossa navicularis

Perineum

Mons veneris

Labium mojus

Labium minue

Vaginal introitus

Hymen

Posterior commissure

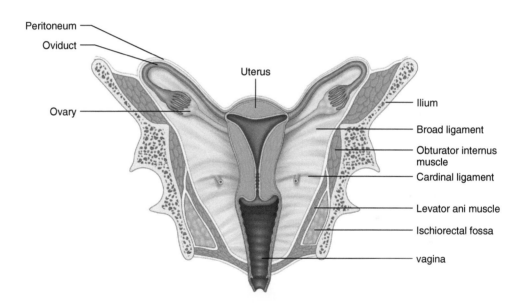

Peritoneum

Oviduct

Uterus

Ovary

Ilium

Broad ligament

Obturator internus muscle

Cardinal ligament

Levator ani muscle

Ischiorectal fossa

vagina

Fig. 82.4 Female internal genitalia

Table 82.1 Wet preparation interpretation

Organism	Preparation	pH	Microscope	Cervix	Appearance of discharge
Bacterial vaginosis	Saline	>4.5	Clue cells	Redness	Thin, milky, fishy odor
Trichomoniasis	Saline	>4.5	Motile flagella	Strawberry red	Yellow-green, foamy
Yeast	Potassium hydroxide	3.8–4.5	Budding yeast pseudohyphae	Normal	White, cottage cheese

3. Next, a bimanual examination should be performed (Fig. 82.5). Lubricating gel is applied to the nondominant gloved hand and the index and middle finger are inserted into the vagina until the cervix is felt. The other hand is placed on the abdomen to palpate the uterus and ovaries. Pressure is applied to the abdomen while the vaginal hand is elevated upward.

14. The cervix is palpated to elicit any cervical motion tenderness. The uterus is palpated and the size, position, and mobility are noted. The adnexa are examined for masses and tenderness. If a mass is palpated, the size, mobility, consistency, and tenderness are noted.

15. The final part of the pelvic examination is the rectovaginal examination. Lubricate the index and middle fingers

of the left hand. Place the index finger in the vagina and the middle finger in the rectum. Palpate for any fistulas or masses. With the finger, also palpate the uterosacral ligaments, the broad ligaments, and the pelvic side walls. The finger is then gently removed and any feces are inspected for mucous or occult blood.

16. A wet preparation is made by obtaining a sample of the vaginal discharge and placing it in a vial mixed with saline solution. A drop of the solution is placed on a microscopic slide and examined under high magnification for the presence of clue cells (Fig. 82.6) diagnostic for bacterial vaginosis and trichomonads (Fig. 82.7) diagnostic for trichomoniasis. For yeast, two drops of the solution is mixed with two drops of potassium hydroxide. Presence of hyphae is diagnostic of candida (yeast) species (Fig. 82.8)

82.5   Complications

- Urinary tract infection
- Vaginal bleeding
- Cramping

82.6   Pearls and Pitfalls

- Pearls
  - Good communication is essential to ensure the patient is comfortable and not anxious.
  - The chaperone should be a medical staff member.
  - Do not skip the pelvic examination if the patient is menstruating.
- Pitfalls
  - Do not forget to perform a complete abdominal exam along with the pelvic exam to rule out any GI etiology.
  - In older females (>50), perform the DRE for a stool occult sample as a possible source of bleeding.

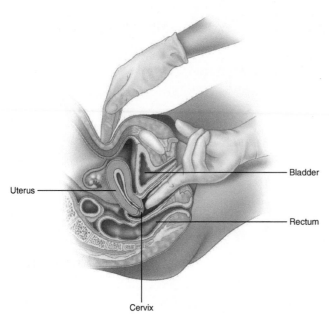

Fig. 82.5 Bimanual pelvic examination

Fig. 82.6 Photomicrograph of a vaginal smear specimen depicting two epithelial cells, a normal cell, and an epithelial cell with its exterior covered by bacteria giving the cell a roughened, stippled appearance known as a "clue cell" (From the CDC Public Health Image library)

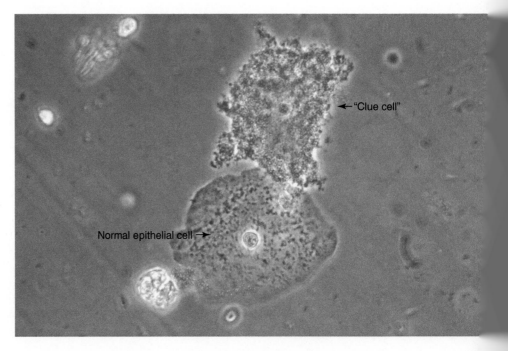

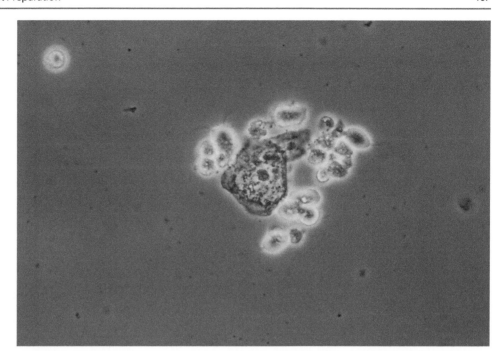

Fig. 82.7 Photomicrograph of trichomonads in wet mount prepared witvh physiological saline (From the CDC Public Health Image library)

Fig. 82.8 *Candida albicans* from vaginal wet prep (From the CDC Public Health Image library)

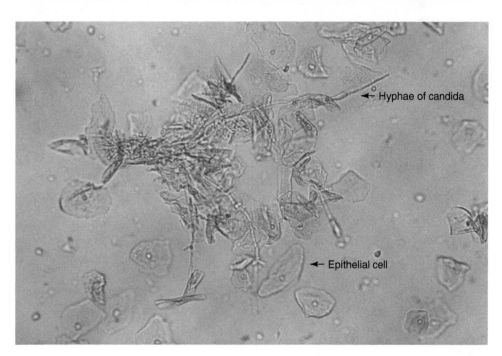

← Hyphae of candida

← Epithelial cell

Selected Reading

Brown J, Fleming R, Aristzabel J, Gishta R. Does pelvic exam in the emergency department add useful information? West J Emerg Med. 2011;12:208–12.

Butler J, Barton D, Shepherd J, Reynolds K, Kehoe S. Gynaecological examinations. Good not bad medicine. BMJ. 2011;342:d1760.

Carr SE, Carmody D. Outcomes of teaching medical students core skills for women's health: the pelvic examination educational program. Am J Obstet Gynecol. 2004;190:1382.

Katz VL, Lentz G, Lobo RA, Gershenson D, editors. Comprehensive gynecology. 5th ed. Philadelphia: Mosby; 2007.

Tiemstra J, Chico P, Pela E. Genitourinary infections after a routine pelvic exam. J Am Board Fam Med. 2011;24:296–303.

Bartholin Gland Abscess/Cysts Drainage

83

Holly H. Charleton, Marylin Otero, Diane F. Giorgi, and Joseph A. Tyndall

83.1 Indications

- Bartholin gland cysts larger than 1 cm or painful
- Bartholin gland abscess

83.2 Contraindications

- Absolute
  - None
- Relative
  - Recurrent/complex abscess requiring general anesthesia in operating room
  - Coagulopathy

83.3 Procedure Types

- Incision and drainage (I&D)
- Iodoform packing
- Word catheter
- Jacobi ring catheter
- Silver nitrate stick ablation (after I&D)

H.H. Charleton, MD
Emergency Department, The Brooklyn Hospital Center,
Brooklyn, NY, USA
e-mail: Hcmd08@gmail.com

M. Otero, MD
Department of Emergency Medicine, Franklin Hospital,
Valley Stream, NY, USA
e-mail: momd42@hotmail.com

D.F. Giorgi, MD
Department of Emergency Medicine, Mount Sinai Queens,
New York, NY, USA
e-mail: dgiorgi@earthlink.net

J.A. Tyndall, MD (✉)
Department of Emergency Medicine, University of Florida Health,
Gainesville, FL, USA
e-mail: tyndall@ufl.edu

© Springer Science+Business Media New York 2016
L. Ganti (ed.), *Atlas of Emergency Medicine Procedures*, DOI 10.1007/978-1-4939-2507-0_83

83.4   Materials

- Sterile gloves
- Sterile skin preparatory solution/swabs and drapes
- Lidocaine 1 % (local anesthesia); may give oral or intravenous sedatives or analgesics
- Needles 25 or 27 gauge with 3-mL syringe for lidocaine injection
- Scalpel #11 for incision
- Culture swab
- Hemostat or suture kit
- Word catheter (if choosing that method) (Fig. 83.1)
- Jacobi ring catheter (if choosing that method) (Fig. 83.2)
- 3-mL syringe with saline for inflation of Word catheter balloon
- Silver nitrate stick (if choosing that method)
- Gauze pads for bleeding and effluents
- Iodoform packing

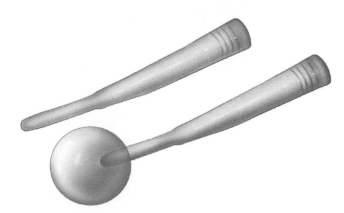

Fig. 83.1 Word catheter (inflated/deflated)

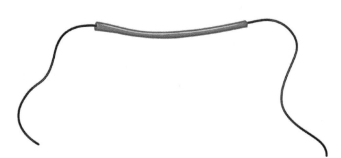

Fig. 83.2 Jacobi ring catheter

83.5   Procedures

83.5.1 Incision and Drainage

1. Obtain informed consent from the patient.
2. Place the patient in the lithotomy position.
3. Prepare the cyst/abscess and the surrounding area with sterilizing fluid/swabs and drape the area, leaving the cyst/abscess accessible for the procedure (Fig. 83.3)
4. May need to hold traction to the labia to fully expose the cyst/abscess (Fig. 83.4).
5. Inject 1–4 mL of lidocaine at the planned site of incision (Fig. 83.5).
6. Hold one side of the cyst/abscess with a forceps or hemostat to maintain traction while incising.
7. With a #11 scalpel, make an incision approximately 0.5–1 cm and 1.5 cm deep in the introitus or behind the hymnal ring to prevent vulvar scarring. The incision should be made through the fluctuant area of the abscess on the mucosal surface. The incision should be linear and large enough to fit the Word catheter (if using that method).
8. Drain the cyst/abscess completely, using the hemostat to break up the loculations.
9. Culture the abscess with a swab and send to microbiology.
10. All previous steps should be done regardless of the procedure type to follow.

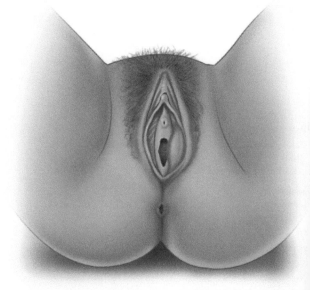

Fig. 83.3 Cyst/abscess accessible for the procedure

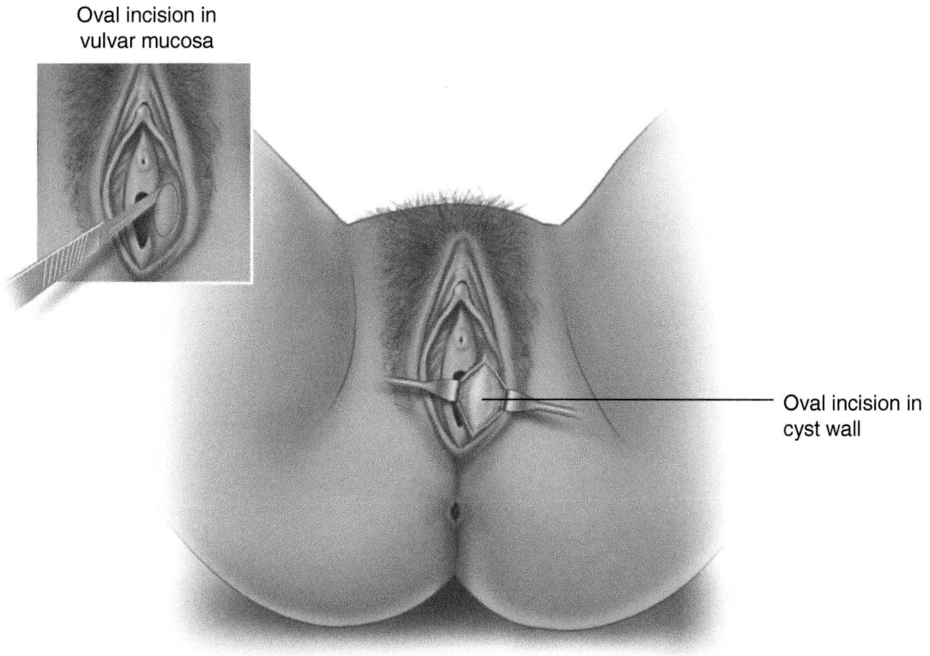

Fig. 83.4 May need to hold
traction to the labia to fully expose
the cyst/abscess

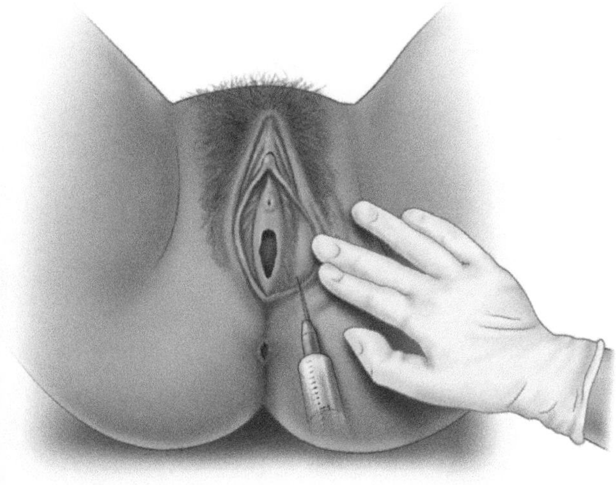

Oval incision in
vulvar mucosa

Oval incision in
cyst wall

Fig. 83.5 Inject 1–4 mL of lidocaine at the planned site of incision

83.6 Iodoform Packing

1. Pack with iodoform packing, grasping the end of the packing material with a hemostat and inserting deeply within the cavity.
2. The cavity should be filled with the packing material and a small piece left exposed (for ease of retrieval during follow-up).
3. Clean the site and cover with gauze.

83.6.1 Word Catheter

- After culturing the abscess
  1. Place the Word catheter into the incision site as deep as possible (if the incision is too large, the catheter will slip out) (Fig. 83.6).
  2. Inflate the balloon of the Word catheter with 2–3 mL of saline or water injected into the hub with a needle and syringe (Fig. 83.7).
  3. Tuck the end of the Word catheter into the vagina for comfort purposes.
  4. The catheter should remain in place for 4 weeks to allow for epithelialization of the tract.

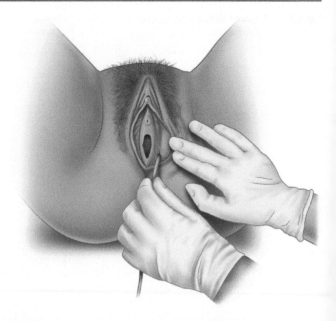

Fig. 83.6 Place the Word catheter into the incision site as deep as possible

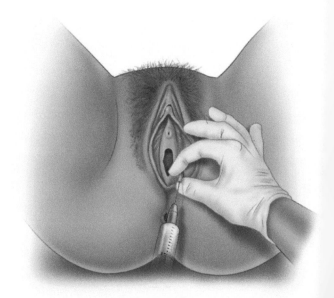

Fig. 83.7 Inflate the balloon of the Word catheter with 2–3 mL of saline or water injected into the hub with a needle and syringe

83.6.2 Jacobi Ring Catheter

1. Grasp one end of the Jacobi ring with a hemostat and pass it through the initial incision site.
2. At this time, use a hemostat to break loculations and culture the material for microbiology.
3. Pull the Jacobi ring through the abscess cavity (be careful not to pull the suture out of the catheter) and make a second incision to pull the catheter out through it.
4. The two ends of the catheter are then tied, forming a ring.

83.6.3 Nitrate Stick

- After sending the culture
  1. Take the silver nitrate stick and place it deep within the cyst/abscess cavity (Fig. 83.8).
  2. The patient is instructed to return in 48 h for removal of the remaining nitrate material and necrotic tissue and wound cleaning.
  3. The patient should be warned of side effects including pain, chemical burns of nearby tissue, edema, discharge, and scarring.

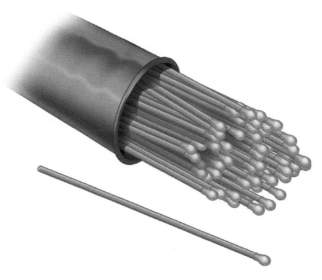

Fig. 83.8 Silver nitrate sticks

83.7 Aftercare

- Follow-up care is required after each of these procedures.
- A high-risk patient (e.g., diabetic) may need to be covered with broad-spectrum antibiotics.
- Pregnant women are also considered high risk and should be given antibiotics and followed closely.
- The patient should be instructed to remain on pelvic rest (nothing in vagina) while the catheter is in place, wear a pad owing to discharge, use sitz baths and analgesics for pain control, and follow up 1–2 days after the procedure.

Although a few other methods are available for draining Bartholin cyst/abscess including marsupialization, carbon dioxide laser vaporization, and excision, these methods are typically done by gynecologists and rarely, if ever, performed by an emergency department physician.

Selected Reading

Chen KT, Robert LB, Falk SJ. Disorders of Bartholin's gland. Available at: WWW.Uptodate.com.

Chen KT, Robert LB, Falk SJ. Word catheter placement for treatment of Bartholin's cysts and abscesses. Available at: WWW.Uptodate.com.

Gennis P, Li SF, Provataris J, et al. Jacobi ring catheter treatment of Bartholin's abscesses. Am J Emerg Med. 2005;23:414–5.

Vitaly KA, Mosquera C. Novel technique for management of Bartholin gland cysts and abscesses. J Emerg Med. 2008;36:388–90.

Wechter ME, Wu JM, Marzano D, Haefner H. Management of Bartholin duct cyst and abscesses: a systematic review. Obstet Gynecol Surv. 2009;64:395–404.

Sexual Assault Forensic Examination

Rajnish Jaiswal, Mary T. Ryan, and Muhammad Waseem

When the survivor of a sexual assault seeks medical care, in addition to addressing their medical needs, their forensic needs must also be addressed. This is best achieved by a specialist examiner, who is trained to conduct a Sexual Assault Forensic Examination (SAFE). When the examiner is a nurse, she or he is referred to as a Sexual Assault Nurse Examiner (SANE). In designated centers, the forensic examiner and the nurse, physician, law enforcement officials, social workers, and patient advocates work together as a Sexual Assault Response Team (SART).

The process of caring for survivors of sexual assault continues to evolve and reflects the advances in forensic science, judicial reform and our understanding of assault survivor psychology.

However, when an emergency medical condition exists, it should be addressed by the designated medical team. The role of the SAFE examiner becomes secondary in these situations. Life- or limb-threatening injuries always take priority over forensic evidence collection, although emergency medical care can often be rendered without compromising existing evidence.

84.1 Indications

- Survivors of sexual assault who seek and consent to forensic examination.
- The upper limit of time for evidence collection varies from state to state (e.g., 96 h in New York State [1]).

84.2 Contraindications

- Absolute
  - If the survivor does not consent to evidence collection
- Relative
  - If the upper time limit has been exceeded

84.3 Materials and Medications

- Ideally, a designated SAFE room should be available.
- Standardized sexual assault evidence collection kits.
- Gloves.
- Camera.
- Portable light source.
- Swab dryer.
- Wood's lamp.
- Anoscope.
- Colposcope, ideally with a camera.
- Support material for survivors: information pamphlets, clothing.
- Prophylactic medications: antibiotics, antiretrovirals, contraceptives.

R. Jaiswal, MD
Department of Emergency Medicine, New York Medical College, Metropolitan Hospital Center, New York, NY, USA
e-mail: Rajnish.Jaiswal@gmail.com

M.T. Ryan, MD • M. Waseem, MD (✉)
Department of Emergency Medicine, Lincoln Medical and Mental Health Center, New York, NY, USA
e-mail: maryryanmd@aol.com; waseemm2001@hotmail.com

© Springer Science+Business Media New York 2016
L. Ganti (ed.), *Atlas of Emergency Medicine Procedures*, DOI 10.1007/978-1-4939-2507-0_84

84.4 Procedure: "Prepare the Patient, Prepare the Room"

1. Informed Consent
   - A separate consent is required for the SAFE. Obtaining consent has important psychosocial implications for the survivor and returns "control" and "choice" to him or her at this critical time [2]. If the survivor chooses not to undergo a SAFE, the examiner must respect his or her decision. Consent is not an "all-or-none" phenomenon and survivors can chose to consent to some steps and decline others. The examiner should be respectful of their decision.
   - Consent for the SAFE should include consent for evidence collection, forensic photography, release of evidence to law enforcement, and permission to discuss the findings of the SAFE with investigators.
2. Law Enforcement Involvement
   - State laws vary in terms of reporting requirements for sexual assault. The examiner should be familiar with the requirements in the state in which she or he practices. All survivors should be offered law enforcement involvement and the benefits of doing so should be outlined to them.
3. Evidence Collection
   - Sexual assault evidence collection kits are specialized preassembled kits containing essential materials for collecting and preserving evidence (Fig. 84.1). The kit contains written instructions, swabs, envelopes, body diagrams, and an integrity seal for the examiner's use.
4. Forensic Interview and History Taking
   - The forensic interview is the first step in the SAFE process. It is a therapeutic as well as a forensic exercise, designed to establish rapport with the survivor, offer support, and gather information to help guide the medical care and direct evidence collection. Acquiring information is a continuous process that ends only when the survivor-SAFE interaction ends.
   - The survivor's exact words with quotation marks should be recorded. A simple factual account of events should be documented. Avoid biased or prejudicial language, such as "allegedly" or "claims." Relevant information includes the time of the assault, the type of contact involved (offender-survivor and survivor-offender), the number of people involved, and the survivor's activities since the assault. A basic medical and obstetrical-gynecological history is also relevant. The SAFE interview is not an investigative interview. Investigation of the sexual assault is the role of law enforcement.
5. General Physical Examination
   - The patient should be asked to undress over a paper sheet to allow any trace evidence to fall and be collected. She or he should be given a gown to wear. A

systematic head-to-toe examination should be undertaken. Identify any injuries, no matter how minor. Document them in writing, on a body diagram (Fig. 84.2), and, when possible, with photography. Pay attention to areas that can be easily overlooked: in the mouth, behind the ears, under the chin, and the soles of the feet, for example. Take time to palpate the scalp for areas of tenderness.

6. Injury Documentation
   - Always take time during documentation. Describe the type of injury—abrasion, contusion, laceration, or bite mark. Document the size and site of the injury, ideally include a measuring device in the photograph. A commonly used scale is the one provided by the American Board of Forensic Odontology (ABFO) (Fig. 84.3). If an injury appears to have a shape or pattern (e.g., linear, circular, curvilinear, petechial), describe it without drawing specific conclusions.
7. Bite Marks
   - Bite marks require additional evaluation because they may have salivary trace evidence associated with them. In addition to being described and photographed, they should be swabbed and the dried swabs included in the evidence collection kit.
8. Forensic Pelvic Examination
   - The purpose of the genital examination (external and speculum) is to identify injury and collect forensic evidence.
9. Inspection
   - Visually examine the external genitalia. Separate the labia and look in skin folds and at the posterior fourchette for injury. The TEARS mnemonic (T=tear, E=ecchymosis, A=abrasions, R=redness, S=swelling) is a useful tool while inspecting and documenting. External genital injury findings can be photographed using a standard camera (digital or conventional 35 mm) or a colposcope camera for additional magnification.
10. Speculum Examination
    - Insert a moistened speculum under a good light source and inspect the vault and cervix for any injuries or possible trace evidence for collection (pooled secretions, hair, retained condom, debris). A colposcope (Fig. 84.4) is a useful adjunct and allows for magnification and assists in injury identification and photodocumentation.
    - Bimanual pelvic examination may be a part of some protocols but is not mandatory.
11. Rectal Examination
    - Inspect the area looking for fissures, bleeding, or secretions. Anoscopy, if indicated by this history and permitted by the survivor, should be performed and the findings documented and photographed.

12. Evidence Collection
   - The evidence collection kit should be opened and the contents laid out in a systematic way. Once the evidence collection kit has been opened, it cannot be left unattended at any time. Each envelope should be labeled with the survivor's name and the time and date of collection. The required swabs and slides are included in the kit.

13. Collection of Biological Material
   - Evidence collection will include oral, anal, and vaginal swabs. Swabs should be allowed to air dry before being placed back in the envelopes. Trace evidence should be collected and may include nail scrapings, dried secretions, loose hair collection, and possible foreign bodies (e.g., soil, condom). A Wood's lamp may help the examiner to identify dried secretions on skin or clothing. When each step is completed, the envelope will be closed, sealed, and signed by the examiner and returned to the box.
   - When completed, the Sexual Assault Evidence Collection Kit (SAECK) is closed, the provided evidence seal placed on the box, and the seal signed and dated by the examiner. The evidence is then given to law enforcement (if the patient consents) or maintained in a predesignated, secure locked area if law enforcement is not yet involved in the case. Each time evidence is passed from person to person, the transfer must be documented in writing to ensure it is not compromised or tampered with in any way. This is the underlying principle of maintaining a "Chain of Custody." This chain must be maintained for evidence to be admissible in court.

14. Collection of Clothing
   - Clothing may be considered "evidence" and collected in some cases. Depending on the case, this may include underwear and any feminine hygiene products. These may fit in the evidence collection kit itself. Larger items of clothing and/or shoes will need to be collected separately. They should be placed in an appropriately sized paper bag and labeled with the patient's name. The bag should be sealed, signed, and dated by the examiner in the same way as all other evidence. Any additional evidence should remain with the SAECK. The survivor should be provided with replacement clothes and underwear.

5. Forensic Photography
   - Although the examiner is not expected to be a specialized forensic photographer, photodocumentation of injuries is an important part of the SAFE. A separate consent is required. Either a conventional 35-mm camera or a high-resolution digital camera is acceptable.
   - At least one image should include the survivor's face or some form of identifying marks. Near and far images should be taken. The camera should be held at 90° to the surface to avoid distortion of the image.

A tape measure should be included when an injury is being photographed. An identifier, like medical record number or case number, should be visible in the image if possible. The examiner should document in the records that photographs were taken.

16. Investigations
   - Baseline complete blood count (CBC), chemistry panel, and liver function tests are generally drawn before initiation of human immunodeficiency virus (HIV) prophylaxis. Serologic tests for syphilis, hepatitis B virus (HBV), hepatitis C virus, and HIV should be obtained. Urine should be sent for analysis and pregnancy testing. Urine for toxicology may be useful in selected cases. Testing for gonorrhea and chlamydia before starting prophylactic antibiotics may be undertaken, but this remains controversial.

17. Prophylaxis
   - Survivors should be offered prophylaxis against pregnancy, common sexually transmitted infections, HBV, and HIV. The current Centers for Disease Control and Prevention (CDC) guidelines recommend the following:
     (a) HBV vaccination should be offered to sexual assault victims at the time of the initial examination if they have not been previously vaccinated. Postexposure HBV vaccination, without hepatitis B immunoglobulin (HBIG), should adequately protect against HBV infection. Follow-up doses of vaccine should be administered 1–2 and 4–6 months after the first dose.
     (b) An empirical antimicrobial regimen for chlamydia, gonorrhea, and trichomonas should be offered.
        - Recommended regimens:
           – *Ceftriaxone* 125 mg intramuscularly in a single dose
           – *PLUS*
           – *Metronidazole* 2 g orally in a single dose
           – *PLUS*
           – *Azithromycin* 1 g orally in a single dose
           – *OR*
           – *Doxycycline* 100 mg orally twice a day for 7 days
     (c) Emergency contraception protocols are state and institution specific. A negative pregnancy test should be documented before evidence collection. Commonly prescribed regimens are "Plan B," "Ovral," and the recently approved "Ella."
     (d) Update tetanus profile if indicated.
     (e) HIV postexposure prophylaxis.
        - All patients with significant exposure should receive pretest counseling and postexposure prophylaxis as per CDC guidelines [3]. The regimens are complex (Table 84.1).

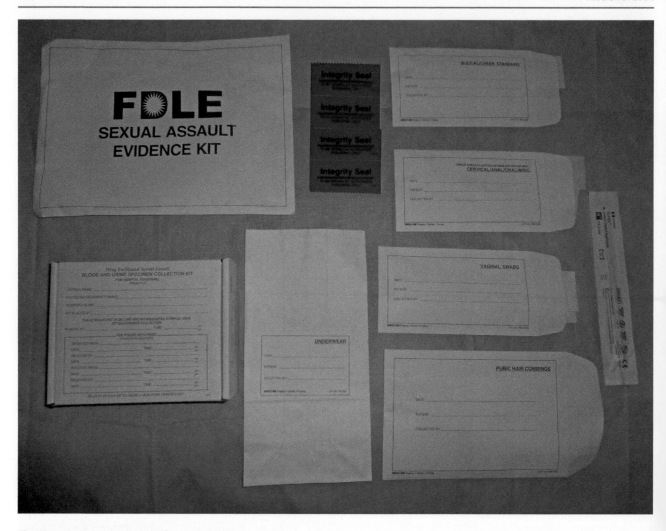

Fig. 84.1   Sexual assault evidence collection kit

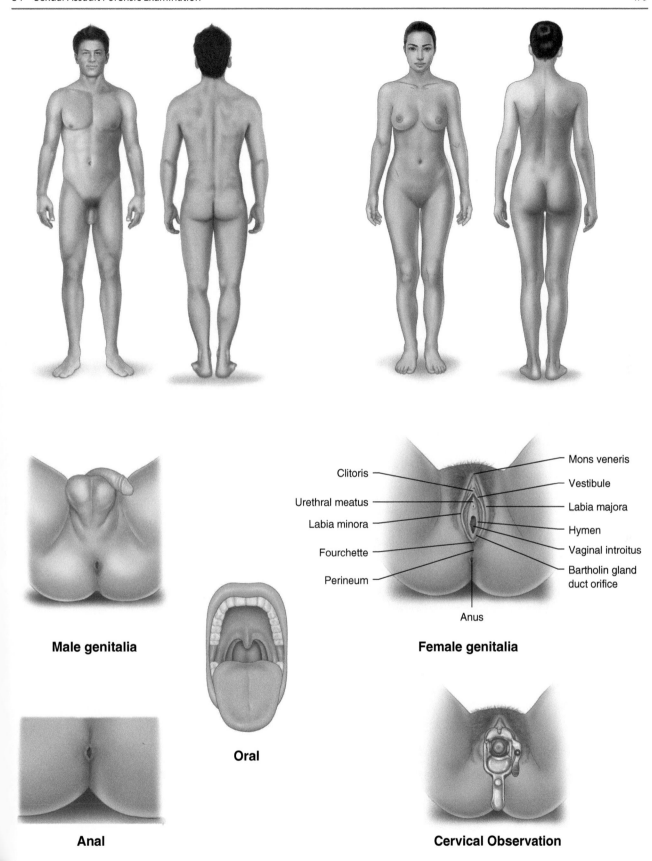

Male genitalia

Oral

Anal

Female genitalia

Clitoris

Urethral meatus

Labia minora

Fourchette

Perineum

Mons veneris

Vestibule

Labia majora

Hymen

Vaginal introitus

Bartholin gland
duct orifice

Anus

Cervical Observation

Fig. 84.2 Traumagram

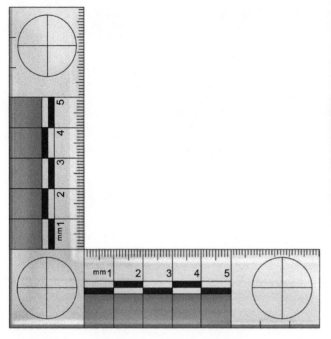

Fig. 84.3 American Board of Forensic Odontology (ABFO) scale (Courtesy Bronx SART Program)

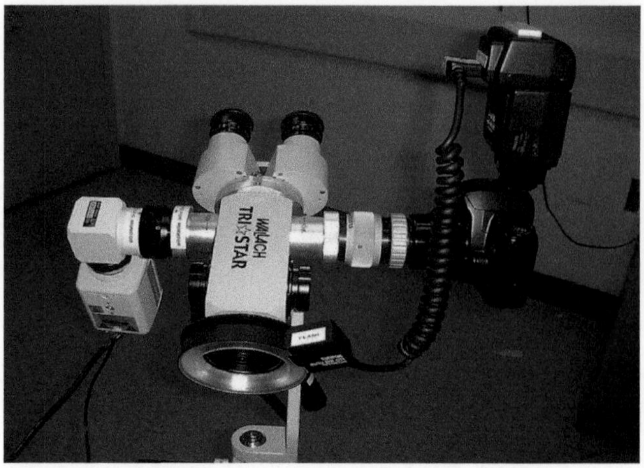

Fig. 84.4 Colposcope (Courtesy Bronx SART Program)

Table 84.1 Postexposure prophylaxis as per Centers for Disease Control and Prevention (CDC) guidelines [3]

Regimen	Dosage
Zidovudine (Retrovir, ZDV, AZT) + lamivudine (Epivir®, 3TC); *available as Combivir™*	ZDV: 300 mg twice daily or 200 mg three times daily, with food; total: 600 mg daily 3TC: 300 mg once daily or 150 mg twice daily Combivir: one tablet twice daily
Zidovudine (Retrovir, ZDV, AZT) + emtricitabine (Emtriva, FTC)	300 mg twice daily or 200 mg three times daily, with food; total: 600 mg/day, in 2 or 3 divided doses; FTC: 200 mg (one capsule) once daily
Tenofovir DF (Viread, TDF) + lamivudine (Epivir, 3TC)	300 mg once daily; 3TC: 300 mg once daily or 150 mg twice daily
Tenofovir DF (Viread, TDF) + emtricitabine (Emtriva, FTC)	TDF: 300 mg once daily; FTC: 200 mg once daily Truvada: one tablet daily

AZT azidothymidine, *FTC* emtricitabine, *3TC* lamivudine, *TDF* tenofovir disoproxil fumarate, *ZDV* zidovudine

84.5   Pearls and Pitfalls

- Pearls
  - Survivors will need to have both medical and psychosocial follow-up. Medical referrals should include gynecology and primary care for follow-up of their baseline serology, testing and completion of HBV vaccination regimen, and so on.
  - Referrals for counseling and information with 24-h hotlines should be provided. Recovery from a sexual assault is a process and is best achieved by a long-term support network [4].
- Pitfalls
  - It is estimated that survivors are men in fewer than 10 % of cases, although sexual assault in males appears to be greatly underreported. The same principles for evidence and prophylaxis apply for the SAFE.

References

1. Department of Health, State of New York. Acute care of the adult patient reporting sexual assault. 2004.
2. Criminal Victimization in the United States 2010. Washington, DC: US Department of Justice, Office of Justice Programs, Bureau of Justice Statistics; 2010.
3. Varghese B, Maher JE, Peterman TA, et al. Reducing the risk of sexual HIV transmission. Sex Transm Dis. 2002;29:38–43.
4. Parekh V, Brown CB. Follow up of patients who have been recently sexually assaulted. Sex Transm Infect. 2003;79:349.

Treatment of Priapism

Jeffrey Kile, Katrina John, and Amish Aghera

85.1 Indications

- Ischemic ("low-flow") priapism

85.2 Contraindications

- To cavernosal aspiration/irrigation
  - Nonischemic ("high-flow") priapism
  - Overlying cellulitis
  - Uncontrolled bleeding disorder
  - Skin infection at the site of injection
- To intracavernosal injection of vasoactive agents (α-adrenergic sympathomimetics)
  - Severe hypertension
  - Dysrhythmias
  - Monoamine oxidase inhibitor use

85.3 Materials and Medications (Fig. 85.1)

- Sterile gloves
- Antimicrobial solution and swabs
- 4×4 gauze sponges
- Local anesthetic (1 % lidocaine 5 mL and 0.5 % bupivacaine 5 mL, without epinephrine)
- 10-mL syringe
- 20-mL syringe
- 19- or 21-gauge butterfly or straight needles (2)
- Blunt needle
- 27-gauge needle
- Normal saline, 1000 mL
- Phenylephrine 1 % solution (10 mg/mL), 1 mL

Kile, MBBS, PhD, MPH (✉) • K. John, MBBS
epartment of Emergency Medicine, Eisenhower Medical Center,
ancho Mirage, CA, USA
mail: jeffrey.kile@gmail.com; trenjohn@me.com

. Aghera, MD
epartment of Emergency Medicine, Maimonides Medical Center,
ew York, NY, USA
mail: aaghera@maimonidesmed.org

Springer Science+Business Media New York 2016
Ganti (ed.), *Atlas of Emergency Medicine Procedures*, DOI 10.1007/978-1-4939-2507-0_85

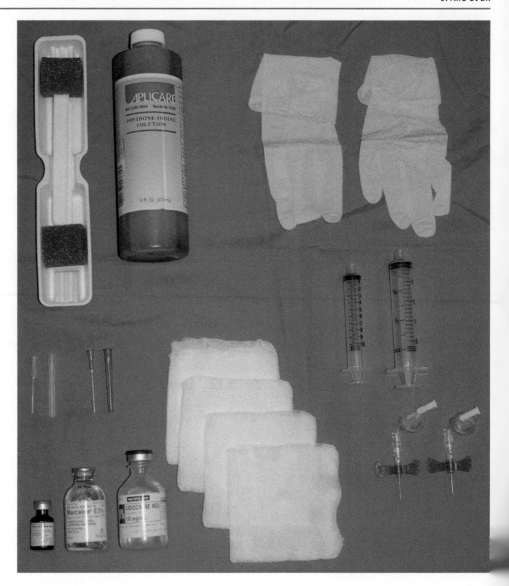

Fig. 85.1 Materials and medications

85.4   Noninvasive Therapy Preprocedure

1. Administer analgesia (e.g., parenteral opiates, benzodiazepines).
2. Administer subcutaneous terbutaline as soon as the diagnosis is suspected (0.25–0.5 mg subcutaneous in quadriceps, deltoid, or gluteus maximus) and repeat after 20 min if necessary.
    • If resolution of priapism does not occur with subcutaneous terbutaline, proceed to cavernosal aspiration.

85.5   Procedures

85.5.1   Dorsal Penile Nerve Block Procedure

1. Position the patient in the supine position.
2. Apply povidone-iodine solution liberally to the penis and scrotum using a 4×4 gauze pad.
3. Clean the glans and shaft of the penis in a circular motion.
4. Establish a sterile field by placing drapes between the scrotum and the shaft, above the shaft, and on either side (Fig. 85.2).
5. Draw up 5 mL 0.5 % bupivacaine and 5 mL 1 % lignocaine (both without epinephrine) into a single syringe.
6. Using a 27-gauge needle, inject local anesthetic superficially to raise skin wheals at the (dorsal) 2 and 10 o'clock positions as proximal to the base of the penis as possible.
7. Insert the needle through the wheal at the 2 o'clock position at the base of the penis until it contacts the pubic symphysis.
8. Withdraw the needle slightly and walk the needle in a caudal fashion down the pubis until the needle passes immediately below the symphysis and advance to a depth of 5 mm deeper than the depth of the pubic symphysis (Fig. 85.3).
    • A transmitted "pop" may be felt as the needle penetrates the superficial penile fascia beneath the symphysis.
9. Aspirate to confirm the tip of the needle is not within the lumen of a vessel.
10. Inject 4 mL of solution.
11. Repeat the injection of local anesthetic as outlined at the 10 o'clock position of the penile base to anesthetize the right dorsal penile nerve (Fig. 85.4).

Fig. 85.2 Priapism in sterile field

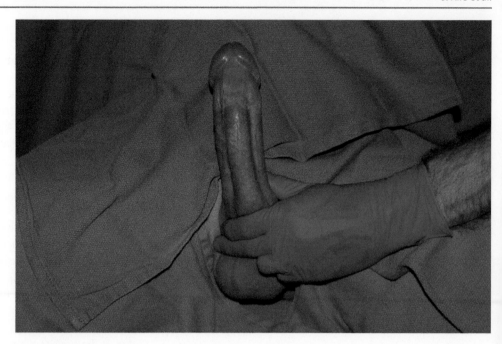

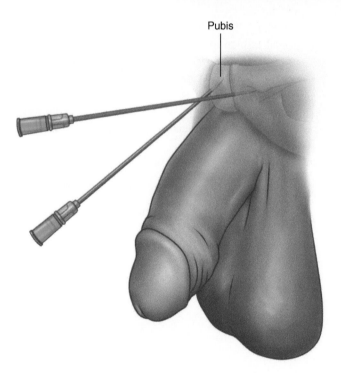

Pubis

Fig. 85.3 Schematic anatomy of dorsal penile nerve block

Fig. 85.4 Injection of local anesthetic

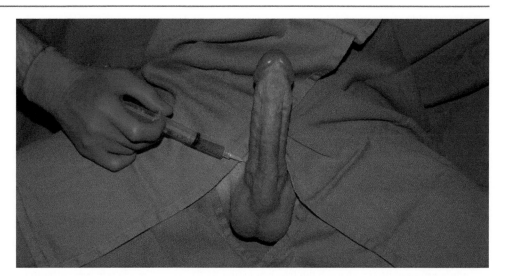

85.5.2 Cavernosal Aspiration Procedure

1. Attach a 19- or 21-gauge needle to a syringe.
2. Puncture the corpus cavernosa at the 2 o'clock or 10 o'clock position (~+60° or −60° from the midline) on the suprapubic aspect of the penis approximately 3 cm from the penile base, directing the needle straight toward the center of the ipsilateral cavernosum.
   - Never use the glans as a puncture site during this procedure.
3. Advance the needle slowly while drawing back on the plunger until blood is visible in the syringe (blood is usually easily aspirated).
4. Once blood is obtained, do not advance further, stabilize the needle, and use one hand to aspirate 20–30 mL of blood while milking the corpus with the free hand (Fig. 85.5).
   - The needle should not be advanced further once blood is visible in the syringe to minimize the risk of injury to the cavernosal artery.
   - Avoid excessive negative pressure on the plunger because this often halts aspiration.
   - If detumescence is not achieved using the above steps, proceed with the following steps.

5. Insert an irrigation needle by puncturing the corpus cavernosum on the same side of the penis punctured with the aspiration needle, approximately 1 cm from the penile base.
6. Irrigate the oxygen-depleted blood in the cavernosa by injecting 20–30 mL of 0.9 % normal saline via the proximal needle in exchange for the blood aspirated (Fig. 85.6).
7. Repeat the cycle of aspiration of 20- to 30-mL volumes of blood from the distal needle followed by irrigation with an equal volume of 0.9 % normal saline via the proximal needle until flow into the syringe of dark red (oxygen-depleted) blood ceases and bright red (oxygen-rich) blood is aspirated or until detumescence is achieved (Fig. 85.7).
   - When removing the needle after cavernosal aspiration, compress the puncture site for approximately 1 min to prevent hematoma formation.
8. Wrap the detumescent penis in gauze or an elastic bandage to prevent return of priapism and to compress the puncture site(s) (Fig. 85.8).

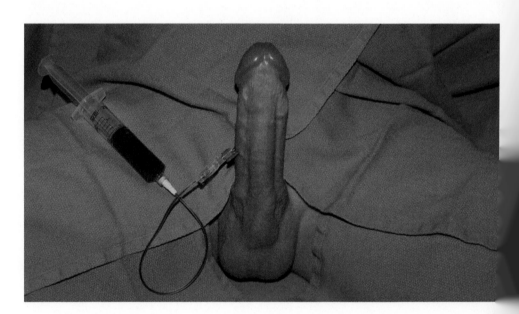

Fig. 85.5 Aspiration of cavernosal blood

Fig. 85.6 Aspiration and irrigation of cavernosal blood

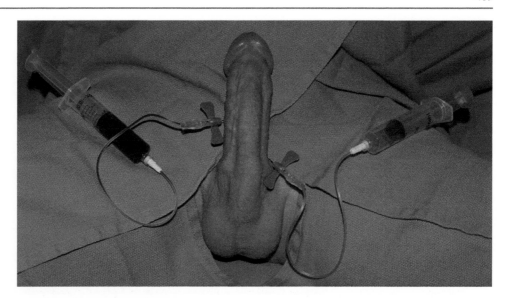

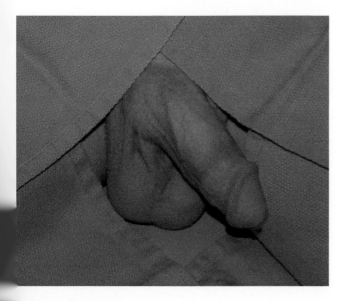

Fig. 85.7 Detumescence

Fig. 85.8 Detumescent penis wrapped in compression dressing

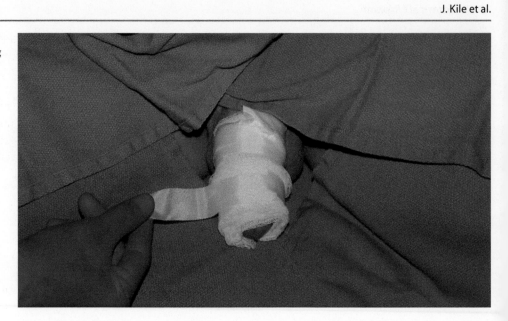

85.5.3 Intracorporeal Injection Procedure

1. Prepare a diluted concentration of 100 µg/mL (1 mg/10 mL) phenylephrine solution by aspirating 0.1 mL of standard 1 % (10 mg/mL) phenylephrine solution into a 10-mL syringe and then adding normal saline to a total volume of 10 mL
2. Attach a 25- or 27-gauge needle to the syringe.
3. Puncture the corpus cavernosum at the 2 o'clock *or* 10 o'clock position (~+60° or −60° from the midline) on the suprapubic aspect of the penis approximately 1 cm from the penile base.
   - Puncture only one side of the penis.
4. Confirm the position of the needle by drawing back on the plunger to aspirate blood from the corpus cavernosa.
5. Inject 1 mL of phenylephrine solution every 3–5 min.
   - Repeat injections of phenylephrine (up to the maximum dose of 1000 µg) should be continued until the erection resolves; only thereafter should this procedure be abandoned in favor of the more invasive approach of surgical shunt.
6. Wrap the detumescent penis in gauze or an elastic bandage to prevent the return of priapism and to compress the puncture site(s).

85.6 Complications

- Of cavernosal aspiration/irrigation
  - Hematoma (at puncture site)
  - Infection (at insertion site or systemic)
  - Thrombosis
  - Arteriovenous fistula
  - Pseudoaneurysm formation
  - Traumatic puncture of dorsal penile or urethra
  - Exsanguination (secondary to dislodgement of catheter)
  - Cerebrovascular accident (secondary to air embolism)
- Of intracavernosal injection of vasoactive agents (α-adrenergic sympathomimetics)
  - Fibrosis of the corpora, pain, penile necrosis, urinary retention
  - Phenylephrine toxicity
  - Acute hypertension, headache, reflex bradycardia, tachycardia, palpitations, cardiac arrhythmia

85.7 Pearls and Pitfalls

- Pearls
  - In ischemic priapism, the penis and corpora cavernosa are rigid and tender to palpation.
  - Ischemic priapism commonly results from an underlying hypercoagulable state, tumor, infection, neurological impairment ("spinal shock"), or vasoactive drug use.
  - During intracorporeal injection, the patient should be monitored for known side effects of sympathomimetics, including hypertension, headache, reflex bradycardia, tachycardia, palpitations, and cardiac arrhythmia. In addition, in patients with elevated cardiovascular risk profiles, blood pressure and electrocardiographic monitoring should be performed.
  - Seek a urological consult as soon as possible for any patient presenting with priapism.
  - Resolution of priapism can be verified by measurement of cavernous blood gases or measurement of blood flow by color duplex ultrasonography.
  - Phenylephrine is the sympathomimetic agent of choice for intracavernosal injection because it is has a lower likelihood of causing adverse cardiovascular side effects than other agents. If this is unavailable, alternatives include epinephrine, norepinephrine, ephedrine, metaraminol, and etilephrine.
  - Intracavernous aspiration/irrigation/injection therapy is unlikely to resolve ischemic priapism lasting for 48 h or longer. In such cases, immediate surgical shunting is first-line treatment.
  - Once detumescence is achieved, any unmetabolized drugs in the corpus cavernosa enter the venous circulation, and thus, dosages of any vasoactive drugs injected must be monitored carefully.
- Pitfalls
  - The most common complication of ischemic priapism is complete erectile dysfunction.

85.8 Considerations

85.8.1 Blood Gas Analysis

This investigation provides a rapid distinction between ischemic and nonischemic priapism. Blood aspirated from the corpus cavernosum in ischemic priapism is dark in color with partial pressure of oxygen (PO_2) less than 30 mmHg, partial pressure of carbon dioxide (PCO_2) greater than 60 mmHg, and pH less than 7.25. In nonischemic priapism, respective values will be PO_2 greater than 90 mmHg, PCO_2 less than 40 mmHg, and pH of 7.4 (Table 85.1).

Table 85.1 Summary of cavernosal blood gas findings

	pH	PO_2 (mm Hg)	PCO_2 (mm Hg)
Ischemic priapism	<7.25	<30	>60
Arterial blood	7.40	>90	<40
Mixed venous blood	7.35	40	50

PCO_2 partial pressure of carbon dioxide, $PO2$ partial pressure of oxygen

85.8.2 Sickle Cell Testing

The sickle-solubility test detects any sickle hemoglobin (therefore, it is positive in patients with either sickle cell train or sickle disease). Hemoglobin electrophoresis with 10 % or greater HbS suggests sickle cell disease. Anemia and increased reticulocyte count may also be present in sickle cell disease.

85.8.3 Hemoglobin Electrophoresis

Confirmatory test for sickle status after a positive sickle-solubility test.

85.8.4 Complete Blood Count

White blood cell (WBC) count may suggest infection or blood dyscrasia. Hemoglobin (Hb) and reticulocyte counts may suggest sickle cell disease.

85.8.5 Color Duplex Ultrasonography

Blood flow in cavernosal arteries is absent or minimal in ischemic priapism, whereas flow velocity is normal to high in nonischemic priapism.

85.8.6 Urine Toxicology and Psychoactive Drug Screen

The following drugs have been associated with priapism: antihypertensives, anticoagulants, antidepressants, alcohol, marijuana, cocaine, and other illegal substances. Intracavernous injection therapy using drugs such as alprostadil, papaverine, prostaglandin E1, phentolamine, and others may precipitate priapism.

Selected Reading

Burnett AL, Bivalacqua TJ. Priapism: new concepts in medical and surgical management. Urol Clin North Am. 2011;38:185–94.

Dubin J, Davis JE. Penile emergencies. Emerg Med Clin North Am. 2011;29:485–99.

Montague DK, Jarow J, Broderick GA, et al; Members of the Erectile Dysfunction Guideline Update Panel; American Urological Association. American Urological Association guideline on the management of priapism. J Urol. 2003;170:1318–24.

Shrewsberry A, Weiss A, Ritenour CW. Recent advances in the medical and surgical treatment of priapism. Curr Urol Rep. 2010;11: 405–13.

Vilke GM, Harrigan RA, Ufberg JW, Chan TC. Emergency evaluation and treatment of priapism. J Emerg Med. 2004;26:325–9.

Reduction of Phimosis/Paraphimosis

86

Justin Chen and Muhammad Waseem

Phimosis occurs when the distal aspect of the prepuce cannot be retracted over the glans.

Paraphimosis is a true urological emergency; it occurs when retracted paraphimotic foreskin cannot be replaced to its normal position past the coronal sulcus, resulting in venous and lymphatic congestion leading to arterial occlusion, ischemia, and necrosis of the glans.

Both conditions commonly result from chronic infection from poor local hygiene in uncircumcised males; it can also be due to redundant skin.

86.1 Indications

- Phimosis: signs of acute urinary retention
- Paraphimosis: signs of present or impending *arterial* occlusion

86.2 Contraindications

- Absolute
  - Failure to rule out penile swelling and pain due alternative conditions (e.g., posthitis/balanoposthitis, angioedema, insect bite, constricting band)

86.3 Materials and Medications

- Latex-free gloves (sterile)
- Local anesthetic
  - 2 % lidocaine without epinephrine (preferred)
  - 2 % lidocaine gel or eutectic mixture of local anesthetics (EMLA) cream (2.5 % prilocaine and 2.5 % lidocaine)
- 25- to 27-gauge 1.5-in. needles (2)
- Small plastic syringe, 10 mL (1)
- Bag of ice (1)
- 2-inch elastic pressure dressing (1)
- Sterile gauze (1)

Chen, MD, MSc
Department of Emergency Medicine, North Shore University Hospital, Manhasset, NY, USA
email: chen.justin@gmail.com

M. Waseem, MD (✉)
Department of Emergency Medicine, Lincoln Medical and Mental Health Center, New York, NY, USA
email: waseemm2001@hotmail.com

Springer Science+Business Media New York 2016
Ganti (ed.), *Atlas of Emergency Medicine Procedures*, DOI 10.1007/978-1-4939-2507-0_86

86.4 Procedure: Manual Reduction for Paraphimosis

1. Grasp the swollen foreskin of the penis and apply gentle compression for a few minutes.
2. Grasp the swollen foreskin and elevate upward.
3. Push the glans into the foreskin.
4. Place the patient in the supine position and carefully inspect the penis for constricting bands or foreign bodies (e.g., piercings).
5. Usage of penile block to provide analgesia to the shaft and glans penis depends on urgency, patient age, and cooperativeness (Fig. 86.1).
   (a) Use a 25- to 27-gauge needle to inject lidocaine into the base of the penis, at the junction between the penis and the suprapubic skin, away from the midline to avoid the superficial dorsal vein.
   (b) Inject lidocaine just deep to Buck's fascia (3–5 mm beneath the skin) to form wheals, where a slight "pop" is felt as the needle penetrates the fascial layer.
   (c) Between 1 and 5 mL of local anesthetic should be used, depending on the age of the patient, which can be delivered as follows:
      • Half the volume should be injected at the 10 o'clock position and the remainder at the 2 o'clock position or
      • Full volume of local anesthetic is injected midline through Buck's fascia, directed toward each direction, ensuring negative aspiration of blood.
6. Alternatively, use gauze soaked in topical local anesthetic to cover the penis (2 % lidocaine gel or EMLA cream [2.5 % prilocaine and 2.5 % lidocaine]), which has slower onset.
7. For phimosis
   (a) If acute urinary retention occurs, dilate the foreskin under procedural sedation or penile block to allow Foley catheterization.
8. For paraphimosis
   (a) Once penile analgesia is achieved (typically in 5 min with penile block), relieve tissue edema before attempting reduction by using:
      • Bag of ice (3 min at a time), or
      • Granulated sugar (*contraindicated* in emergent situations owing to time required), or
      • Manual compression (squeezing the glans for 5 min), or
      • Pressure dressing (2-in. elastic bandage over the gland for 5 min)
   (b) Place both thumbs over the glans, with both index fingers and long fingers surrounding the trapped foreskin proximal from the paraphimotic tissue.
   (c) Use the thumbs to push the glans back into the foreskin while pulling the trapped foreskin distally, which may require a few minutes of constant pressure (Fig. 86.2).
   (d) Can also attempt using Babcock (once in each quadrant) or Adson (3 and 9 o'clock positions) forceps to grasp the paraphimotic tissue (Fig. 86.3).
   (e) If ineffective owing to extreme tissue edema, seek emergent urological consultation.
   (f) Follow-up with urologist is always recommended; circumcision may be performed once infection and/or edema have resolved to prevent recurrence (Fig. 86.4).

Fig. 86.1 Penile block to
provide analgesia to the shaft and
glans penis

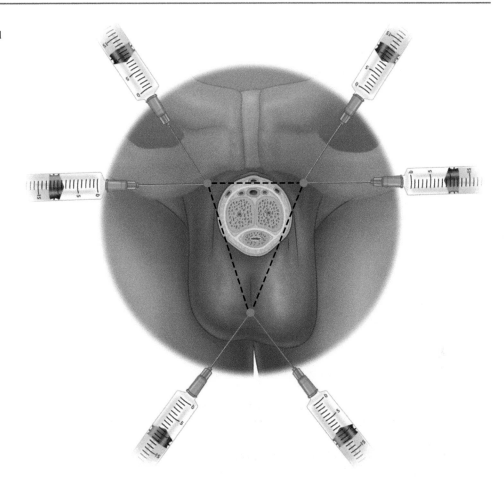

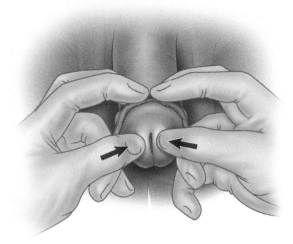

Fig. 86.2 Use the thumbs to push the glans back into the foreskin
while pulling the trapped foreskin distally

a

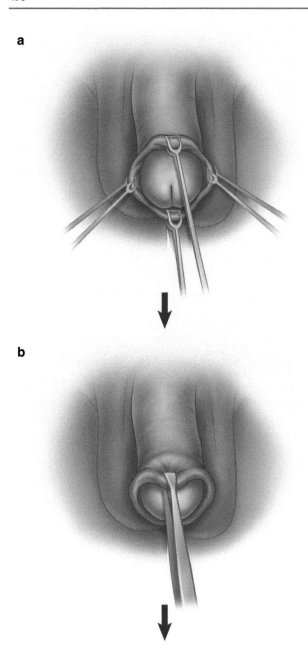

b

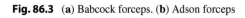

Fig. 86.3 (**a**) Babcock forceps. (**b**) Adson forceps

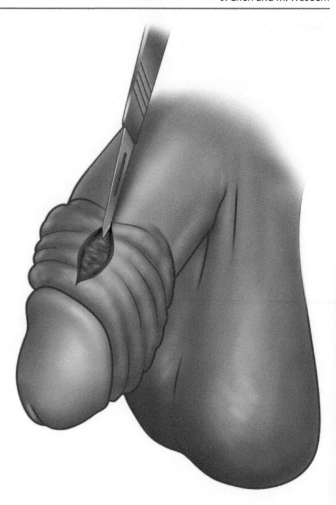

Fig. 86.4 Circumcision may be performed once infection and/or edema have resolved to prevent recurrence

86.5   Complications

- Bleeding/infection of injection site(s).
- Phimosis and scarring due to foreskin manipulation.
- Usage of Adson or Babcock forceps may result in minor bruising and abrasion to the foreskin and glans penis.

86.6   Pearls and Pitfalls

- Pearls
  - Phimosis is a normal occurrence in young males (<5–6 years) and should be treated only in the presence of acute urinary retention.
  - If arterial compromise is imminent in paraphimosis, the emergency physician should attempt reduction if urological consult is unavailable.

- Pitfalls
  - Reduction of phimotic tissue over the coronal sulcus may lead to emergent paraphimosis.

Selected Reading

Doherty GM, editor. Current diagnosis and treatment: surgery. 13th ed. New York: McGraw-Hill Medical; 2010.

King C, Henretig FM, editors. Textbook of pediatric emergency procedures. Philadelphia: Wolters Kluwer Health/Lippincott Williams & Wilkins; 2008.

Knoop KJ, editor. Atlas of emergency medicine. 3rd ed. New York: McGraw-Hill Professional; 2010.

Smith DR, Tanagho EA, McAninch JW, editors. Smith's general urology. New York: Lange Medical Books/McGraw-Hill; 2008.

Manual Testicular Detorsion

87

Brandon R. Allen and L. Connor Nickels

87.1 Indications

- Testicular torsion is a clinical diagnosis (Fig. 87.1).
  - Although no single clinical finding has 100 % sensitivity for the presence of testicular torsion, patients will have one or more of these signs and symptoms: nausea or vomiting, pain for less than 24 h, high position of the testis, and/or abnormal cremasteric reflex [1].
  - If the diagnosis is in question, radionuclide scan or ultrasonography of the testicles may be helpful to assess blood flow and to differentiate torsion from other conditions (Fig. 87.2).

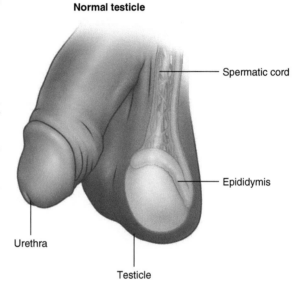

Normal testicle

Spermatic cord

Epididymis

Urethra

Testicle

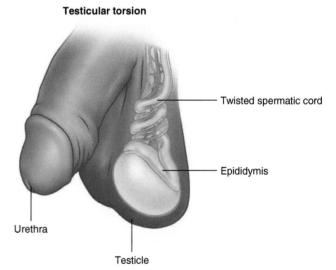

Testicular torsion

Twisted spermatic cord

Epididymis

Urethra

Testicle

Fig. 87.1 Schematic of normal testicle and testicular torsion

.R. Allen, MD • L.C. Nickels, MD, RDMS (✉)
epartment of Emergency Medicine, University of Florida Health
ands Hospital, Gainesville, FL, USA
mail: brandonrallen@ufl.edu; cnickels@ufl.edu

Springer Science+Business Media New York 2016
Ganti (ed.), *Atlas of Emergency Medicine Procedures*, DOI 10.1007/978-1-4939-2507-0_87

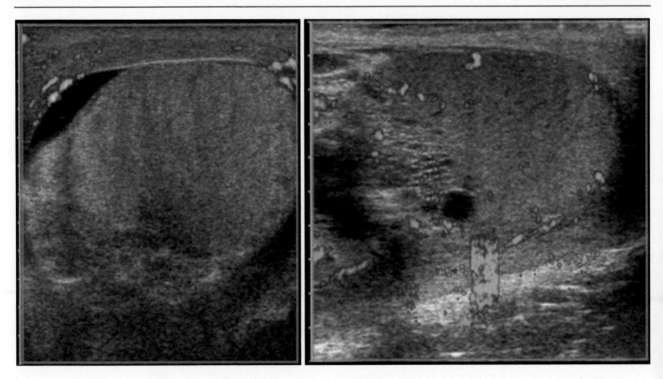

Fig. 87.2 Doppler ultrasound of bilateral testes shows swollen right testis with hypoechoic areas within and reduced arterial signal suggesting testicular torsion with necrosis (*left panel*). This is compared to the left testis which has normal flow (*right panel*) (Reproduced with permission from: Bhagra et al. [4])

87.2   Contraindications

- Do not attempt if the length of symptoms is greater than 24 h.
- Manual detorsion should not delay scrotal exploration and bilateral orchiopexy in the operating room [2].

87.3   Materials and Medications

- Standard precautions barrier protection for the provider
- Local anesthetic (optional to anesthetize the spermatic cord near the external ring)
- Intravenous sedation (optional)

87.4   Procedure

- The physician stands at the patient's feet and rotates the affected testicle away from the midline (as if opening a book) (Fig. 87.3).
  - For detorsion of the left testicle: the physician will place his or her right thumb and index finger on the affected testicle and rotate the testicle 180° from medial to lateral [2].
  - For detorsion of the right testicle: the physician will place his or her left thumb and index finger on the affected testicle and rotate the testicle 180° from medial to lateral.

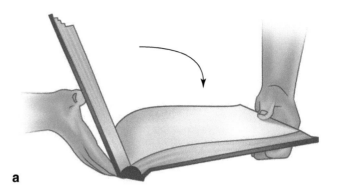

a

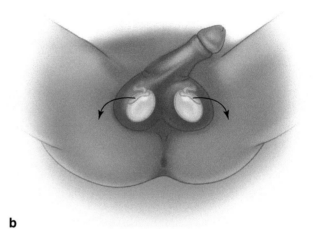

b

Fig. 87.3 (**a**) As if opening a book, rotate the testicle away from the midline. (**b**) Affected testicle should be rotated 180° from medial to lateral

87.5 Pearls and Pitfalls

- Pearls
  - The most common misdiagnosis is epididymitis.
  - Because torsion of greater than 360° degrees is possible, more than one rotation may be needed to fully detorse the affected testis (Fig. 87.4).
  - Only surgical exploration can provide a definitive resolution if testicular torsion is present [2].
- Pitfalls
  - The most common causes of testicular loss after torsion are delay in seeking medical attention (58 %), incorrect initial diagnosis (29 %), and delay in treatment at the referral hospital (13 %) [3]

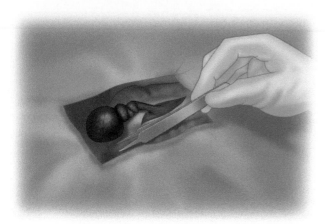

Fig. 87.4 Because torsion of greater than 360° degrees is possible, more than one rotation may be needed to fully detorse the affected testis

References

1. Beni-Israel T, Goldman M, Bar Chaim S, Kozer E. Clinical predictors for testicular torsion as seen in the pediatric ED. Am J Emerg Med. 2010;28:786–9.
2. Ringdahl E, Teague L. Testicular torsion. Am Fam Physician. 2006;74:1739–43.
3. Jones DJ, Macreadie D, Morgans BT. Testicular torsion in the armed services: twelve year review of 179 cases. Br J Surg. 1986;73:624–6.
4. Bhagra A, Suravaram S, Schears RM. Testicular torsion–a common surgical emergency. Int J Emerg Med. 2008;1(2):147.

Local Anesthesia

88

Derek Ailes and Muhammad Waseem

88.1 Indications

- Laceration repair
- Abscess incision and drainage
- Wound exploration
- Vascular access procedures
- Foreign body removal
- Lumbar puncture

88.2 Contraindications

- History of allergy (usually to the ester class [e.g., procaine, tetracaine]), amide class (e.g., lidocaine [Xylocaine], bupivacaine, mepivacaine) may be safely substituted if true allergy to esters and vice versa. One percent diphenhydramine (4 mL normal saline: 1 mL 5 % intravenous [IV] diphenhydramine [Benadryl] mixture) can be used in patients with true allergy.
- Topical preparations on mucous membranes, burns, abraded/denuded skin, or eyes owing to potential toxicity from increased absorption and corneal injury.
- Common teaching is to avoid epinephrine-containing anesthetic solutions in nose, penis, and digits for concern of ischemia owing to end-artery constriction. Recent studies including prospective trials and comprehensive literature reviews, however, do not validate this concern [1, 2].

. Ailes, MD • M. Waseem, MD (✉)
epartment of Emergency Medicine,
incoln Medical and Mental Health Center, New York, NY, USA
mail: derekailes@yahoo.com; waseemm2001@hotmail.com

Springer Science+Business Media New York 2016
Ganti (ed.), *Atlas of Emergency Medicine Procedures*, DOI 10.1007/978-1-4939-2507-0_88

88.3 Materials and Medications (Fig. 88.1)

- 1 % Xylocaine with or without 1:200,000 epinephrine, 0.25 % bupivacaine solution. 8.4 % (1 mL/mL) sodium bicarbonate (optional)

- 18-, 25-, or 27-gauge needles, syringes up to 10 mL
- Sterile and nonsterile gloves, face shield
- Alcohol pads and povidone-iodine swabs

Fig. 88.1 Local anesthesia materials

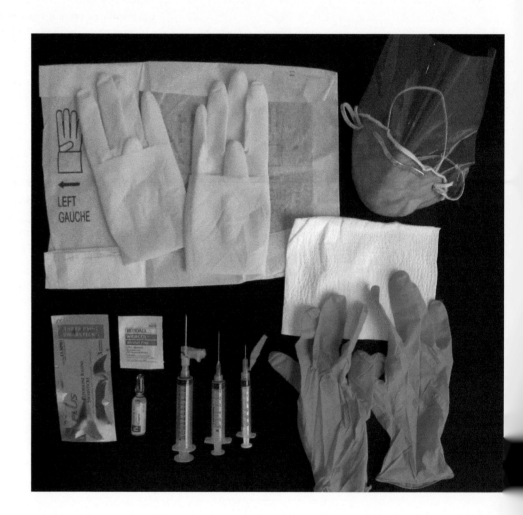

88.4   Procedure

1. Position the patient in a comfortable position (supine, sitting, anticipating vasovagal response).
2. Draw the anesthetic with an 18-gauge needle into a syringe. Be aware of the maximum dose for the particular local anesthetic to avoid systemic toxicity.
3. Take steps to minimize the pain of infiltration (Table 88.1).
4. Prepare the area with povidone-iodine solution; cover surrounding areas with sterile drapes.
5. Inject subcutaneously by direct infiltration with a 25- to 27-gauge needle noting wheal and blanching. If a clean wound, may inject into wound edges. Usually no aspiration is needed because the infiltration is superficial to major blood vessels.
6. For contaminated wounds or abscess incision and drainage, perform field block by inserting the needle into clean intact skin adjacent to the wound and continuing in a circular manner around the wound, injecting into the previously anesthetized area (Fig. 88.2).
7. Wait several minutes for the local anesthetic to provide the maximum effect.
8. Test the area for sharp sensation with a needle tip or other sharp object.

Table 88.1 Common anesthetics and their characteristics

Medication	Time to onset (min)	Length of action	Maximum dose (mg/kg)	Maximum dose with epinephrine (mg/kg)
Marcaine (bupivacaine)	5–10	>3 h, up to 9 h with epinephrine	2.5	2.5–3.5
Xylocaine (lidocaine)	<2	30–75 min (longer with epinephrine)	3	5–7

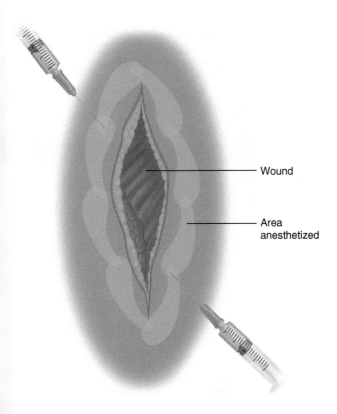

Wound

Area anesthetized

Fig. 88.2 Local infiltration should be performed in a circular fashion with each injection performed over the prior anesthetized area

88.5 Complications

- Systemic toxicity
- Allergic reaction
- Infection
- Digital artery vasospasm from accidental injection of epinephrine (can be reversed with topical nitroglycerine or subcutaneous phentolamine)
- Vasovagal response

88.6 Pearls

- Minimize or reduce the pain of infiltration by use of the following:
  - Warm Xylocaine before infiltration (blanket warmer or water bath) [3].
  - Buffer Xylocaine with 1 mL 8.4 % sodium bicarbonate for every 10 mL of Xylocaine. Buffer bupivacaine with 0.05–0.10 mL sodium bicarbonate for every 10 mL of bupivacaine (greater chance of precipitation).
  - Use a small-gauge needle (e.g., 27 gauge) and inject slowly.
  - Use a small syringe (1–3 mL) to reduce the pressure of injection.
  - Withdraw the needle and, just before exiting the skin, redirect and inject.
  - Inject in a circular manner around the wound with each subsequent injection entering a previously anesthetized area, such that the patient feels only one needle stick (Fig. 88.2).
  - Inject into the subcutaneous plane as opposed to the intradermal plane.
  - Consider using a topical anesthetic before infiltration, especially in pediatrics (lidocaine, epinephrine, tetracaine [LET]).
- Beware of toxicity by not exceeding the maximum dose, especially in large or multiple lacerations. Even at standard doses, toxicity can occur with inadvertent vascular injection, injection into highly vascular areas, or onto mucous membranes [4, 5].

- Convert % mg/mL into mg/kg by moving the decimal one place to the right (e.g., 1 % Xylocaine becomes 10 mg/mL and 0.25 % bupivacaine becomes 2.5 mg/mL).
- Xylocaine can be safely injected up to 3.5 mg/kg every 30 min, up to 300 mg/dose. If the mixture contains epinephrine, 5–7 mg/kg is safe.
- Bupivacaine can be injected at 2.5 mg/kg and 3.5 mg/kg with epinephrine and can be injected every 3 h with daily maximum of 400 mg [5].
- When treating a wound, it is important to first anesthetize so debridement, cleansing, and irrigation can adequately be performed.
- Choose appropriate anesthetics. Xylocaine lasts approximately 75 min, and bupivacaine lasts several hours. Adding epinephrine to either increases vascular constriction, thereby decreasing systemic absorption and significantly increasing the duration of effect.
- Topical anesthetics have a role in pediatric populations and in conjunction with or as an alternate to local infiltrative anesthesia. TAC is a mixture of 0.5 % tetracaine, 0.05 % epinephrine, and 11.8 % cocaine. LET is 4 % lidocaine, 0.1 % epinephrine, and 0.5 % tetracaine. LET has been found to be safer and more cost-effective [6].

References

1. Muck AE, Bebarta VS, Borys DJ, Morgan DL. Six years of epinephrine digital injections: absence of significant local or systemic effects. Ann Emerg Med. 2010;56:270–4.
2. Waterbrook AL, Germann AC, Southall JC. Is epinephrine harmful when used with anesthetics for digital blocks? Ann Emerg Med. 2007;50:472–5.
3. Hogan ME, vanderVaart S, Perampalades K, Machado M, Einarson TR, Teddio A. Systematic review and meta-analysis of the effect of warming local anesthetics on injection pain. Ann Emerg Med. 2011;58:86–98.
4. Reichman EF, Simon RR, editors. Emergency medicine procedures. New York: McGraw-Hill Medical; 2004. p. 937.
5. Marx J, Hockberger R, Walls R, editors. Rosen's emergency medicine: concepts and clinical practice. 7th ed. Philadelphia: Mosby 2010. p. 2425–7.
6. Kravitz ND. The use of compound topical anesthetics. J Am Den Assoc. 2007;138:1333–9.

Regional Anesthesia (Nerve Blocks)

89

Derek Ailes and Muhammad Waseem

89.1 Indications

Repair of wounds where preserving anatomical landmarks or having precise anatomical alignment is important (e.g., vermillion border of lip)

Pain control in dislocation or fracture reductions

Incision and drainage of abscesses

Burn and wound care

Extensive or multiple lacerations (reduces total amount of local anesthetic needed)

Foreign body removal

89.2 Contraindications

- Allergic to local anesthetic (see Chap. 88)
- History of coagulopathy or bleeding disorder
- Injection through infected tissue

D. Ailes, MD • M. Waseem, MD (✉)
Department of Emergency Medicine, Lincoln Medical and Mental Health Center, New York, NY, USA
e-mail: derekailes@yahoo.com; waseemm2001@hotmail.com

© Springer Science+Business Media New York 2016
R. Ganti (ed.), *Atlas of Emergency Medicine Procedures*, DOI 10.1007/978-1-4939-2507-0_89

89.3 **Materials and Medications** (Fig. 89.1)

- Povidone-iodine, alcohol swabs
- Sterile gloves and drapes
- Local anesthetic solution (e.g., lidocaine, Marcaine with or without epinephrine)

- 18-gauge, 20- to 30-gauge needles 2 in. in length
- 22- to 24-gauge spinal needles
- Syringes up to 60 mL

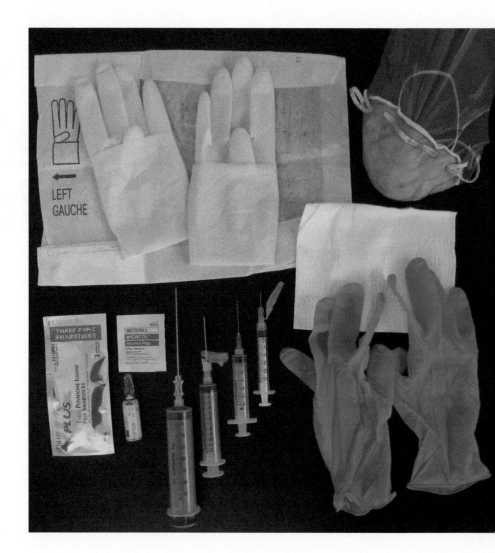

Fig. 89.1 Materials

89.4   Procedure: General Block

1. Obtain consent after explaining the risks of procedure including temporary paresthesias and expected duration of block. Perform neurological examination before procedure, documenting any preexisting deficits.
2. Position the patient comfortably, preferably supine, anticipating vasovagal response.
3. Identify landmarks for the block. Clean area, prepare with povidone-iodine, and surround with sterile drapes.
4. A small skin wheal of local anesthetic may be placed at the site of needle entry before block.
5. Insert the needle into the site while aspirating to ensure it is not in a vessel.
6. If paresthesia is elicited, withdraw the needle slightly allowing paresthesia to improve and inject.
7. Wait 5–15 min for the block to reach full effect.
8. Test for sharp sensation in the anesthetized area and document.

89.5   Complications

- Infection
- Hemorrhage
- Hematoma
- Allergic reaction
- Systemic toxicity (exceeded maximum dose or inadvertent injection into vasculature)
- Paresthesias, pain
- Intraneural injection causing ischemia
- Intra-arterial injection of epinephrine causing vasospasm and tissue ischemia

89.6   Pearls and Pitfalls

- Pearls
  - It is important to aspirate before injecting anesthesia when performing regional anesthesia because, unlike local techniques, the needle is deeper and in proximity to larger vessels.
  - Shooting pain and/or paresthesias occurs when the needle contacts the nerve. When this happens, withdraw the needle 1 mm and wait for the paresthesia to resolve before injecting.
  - Injury can occur to a limb or digit if the patient manipulates it before the anesthesia wears off. The patient should be cautioned not to use the affected area until motor and sensation return. If an extensive block was done, monitor the patient in the emergency department until return of baseline neurological function.
- Pitfalls
  - It is traditionally taught to avoid epinephrine-containing solutions in blocks in end-artery blocks (e.g., digital blocks). However, evidence for any vascular insufficiency and necrosis as a result is lacking in standard commercially available lidocaine with epinephrine preparations. They should, however, be avoided in patients with peripheral artery disease [1, 2].

89.7 Selected Specific Blocks

- Contraindications and materials are the same as general block.

89.7.1 Facial Blocks: Trigeminal Nerve
(Fig. 89.2) [2, 3]

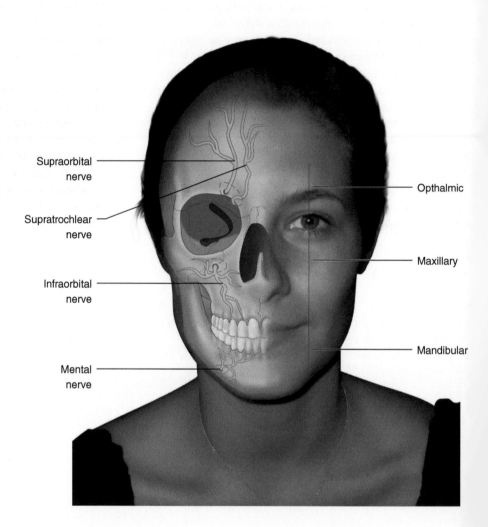

Fig. 89.2 Vertical plane through the midposition of the pupil shows the position of the supraorbital foramen, infraorbital foremen, and mental foramen

89.7.1.1 Supraorbital (Fig. 89.3) and Supratrochlear Nerve Block

- Indications
  - To anesthetize the forehead from the orbital ridge to the vertex of the scalp. The supraorbital nerve emerges from the supraorbital foramen/notch and is a branch of the ophthalmic division of the trigeminal nerve. The supratrochlear nerve also is a branch of the ophthalmic division of the trigeminal nerve and exits through the superior medial aspect of the orbit.
- Procedure
  1. Inject local anesthetic solution over the midline of the forehead at eyebrow level.
  2. Inject a 25- or 27-gauge needle through skin wheal aimed laterally while injecting 3–5 mL local anesthetic subcutaneously. Stop infiltrating when the needle reaches the midline of the orbit.

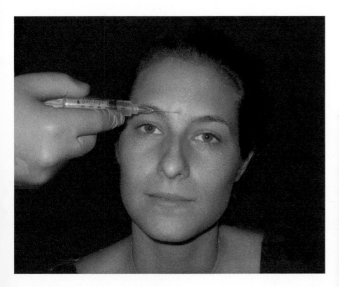

Fig. 89.3 Supraorbital nerve block

89.7.1.2 Infraorbital Nerve Block

- Indications
  - To anesthetize the medial cheek, upper lip, philtrum, skin between the lips and the nose, and nasal ala. The infraorbital nerve emerges from the infraorbital foramen and is a branch of the maxillary division of the trigeminal nerve. Anesthesia to the infraorbital nerve will also provide anesthesia to its terminus, the superior alveolar nerves.
- Procedure: Extraoral Approach (Fig. 89.4)
  1. Palpate the inferior orbital foramen in its midline position. The infraorbital nerve is often tender on palpation as it exits the foramen.
  2. Inject a 25- or 27-gauge needle just above the infraorbital foramen injecting 1–2 mL of local anesthetic.
  3. Take care not to inject into the foramen because there is an increased risk of intraneural injection.
  4. Hold a finger on the inferior orbital rim to avoid ballooning of the lower eyelid with injection.
  5. Intraoral approach is possible and preferred because it is less painful.

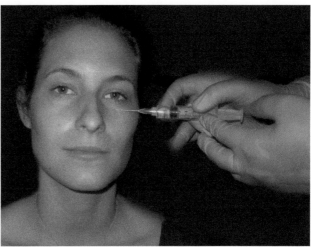

Fig. 89.4 Extraoral approach to the infraorbital nerve block

- Procedure: Intraoral Approach (Fig. 89.5) [3]
  1. Apply topical benzocaine or lidocaine gel to the point of insertion, which is the height of the mucobuccal fold over the first premolar, which is the site of insertion. Wipe off after 1–3 min.
  2. Palpate with the finger of the noninjecting hand over the inferior border of the inferior orbital rim. Retract the lip with the noninjecting hand.
  3. Using a long 25- to 27-gauge needle, with the bevel toward the bone, advance the needle at the insertion site toward the infraorbital foramen. Once the target is reached, aspirate and inject 1 mL of local anesthetic.
  4. Exert pressure on the foramen for 1 min after injection to force the anesthetic through the infraorbital foramen.
  5. If the needle is difficult to advance and the patient experiences pain on insertion, redirect the needle laterally and advance.
  6. If analgesia is attained for the lip but not the eyelid, the analgesia was placed inferior to foramen, and if analgesia is attained for the eyelid but not the lip, placement was superior to the foramen.

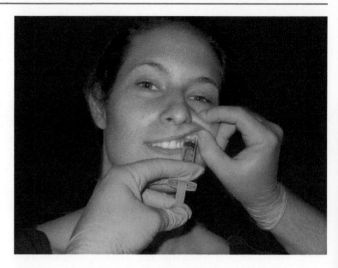

Fig. 89.5 Intraoral approach to the infraorbital nerve block

89.7.1.3 Mental Nerve Block

- Indications
  - To anesthetize the lower lip and chin and is especially useful in laceration repair at those sites. The mental nerve emerges from the mental foramen and is a branch of the mandibular division of the trigeminal nerve. Mental foramen lies in the vertical plane with the midpoint of the pupil and sits in the middle of the body of the mandible.
- Procedure: Extraoral Approach (Fig. 89.6)
  1. Inject local anesthetic solution over the identified location of the mental foramen, creating a skin wheal.
  2. Advance a 25- or 27-gauge needle through the skin wheal until the mandible is contacted, injecting 1–2 mL of local anesthetic.
  3. Intraoral approach is possible and preferred because it is less painful.
- Procedure: Intraoral Approach (Fig. 89.7) [3]
  1. Apply topical benzocaine or lidocaine gel to the point of insertion, which is the mucobuccal fold between the apices of the first and the second premolars. Wipe off after 1–3 min.
  2. Insert a 25- to 27-gauge needle, with the bevel toward the mandible, aimed toward the mental foramen.
  3. After advancing one-third the depth of the mandible and contacting the mandible, inject 1–2 mL of local anesthetic.
  4. By pressing firmly on the mental foramen for 2–3 min after the mental foramen has been blocked, an incisive nerve block is also created. This is useful if anesthesia to the lower anterior teeth is also desired.

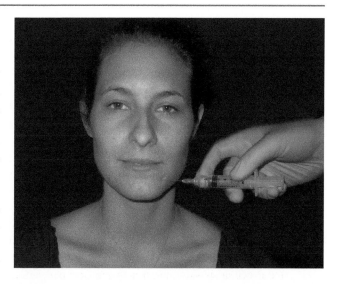

Fig. 89.6 Extraoral approach to the mental nerve block

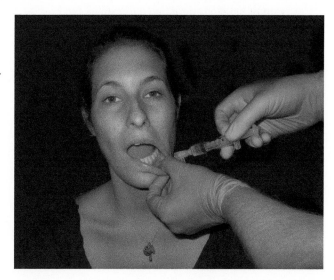

Fig. 89.7 Intraoral approach to the mental nerve block

89.7.2 External Ear Block (Fig. 89.8) [4]

- Indications
  - To anesthetize the entire external ear, excluding the external auditory canal and the concha
  - Especially useful in large lacerations of the ear and surrounding skin, hematoma evacuations, or incision and drainage of abscess.
- Procedure: Auricular Ring Block (Fig. 89.9) [4]
  1. Using a 25- to 27-gauge needle, insert the needle just inferior to the earlobe directing it toward the tragus.
  2. Aspirate and advance the needle superiorly subcutaneously injecting 3–4 mL of local anesthetic (Fig. 89.9, #1).
  3. Withdraw the needle without fully removing it and redirect it posterosuperiorly along the inferior posterior auricular sulcus, aspirating and injecting as before (Fig. 89.9, #2).
  4. Remove the needle and insert it just superior to the point of helix insertion into the scalp.
  5. Advance the needle and aspirate and inject in the direction of the tragus. Inject into the subcutaneous tissue while avoiding the ear cartilage (Fig. 89.9, #3).
  6. Withdraw and redirect the needle posteriorly and inferiorly toward the skin behind the ear, injecting as before (Fig. 89.9,#4).
  7. Beware of inadvertent cannulation of the superficial temporal artery, which crosses the zygomatic arch and crosses medial to the ear. If the artery is violated, it requires 20–30 min application of firm pressure.

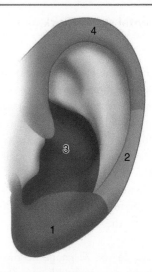

Fig. 89.8 Auricular block anesthetizes four nerves that innervate auricle. *1* Great auricular nerve, *2* lesser occipital nerve, *3* auricu branch of vagus nerve, *4* auriculotemporal nerve

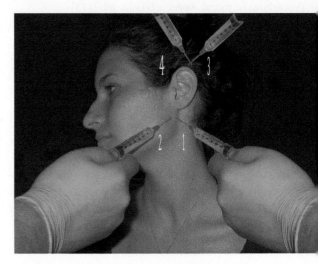

Fig. 89.9 Auricular ring block technique

89.7.3 **Wrist Block** (Fig. 89.10) [3, 5, 6]

- Indications
  - To anesthetize the hand in preparation for laceration repair, fracture or dislocation reduction, or pain relief

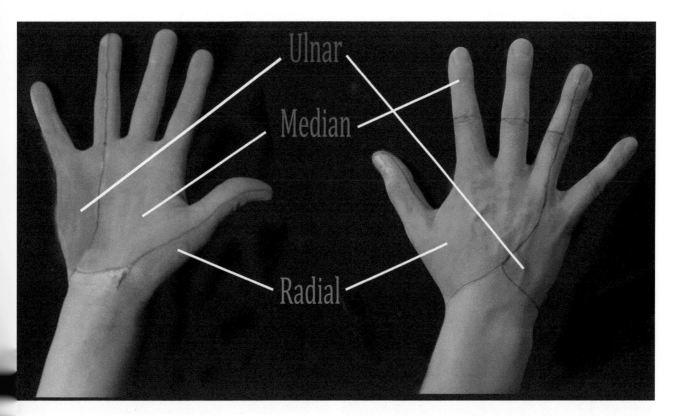

Fig. 89.10 Nerve distribution in the hand

89.7.3.1 Wrist Block: Median Nerve (Fig. 89.11)

- Procedure
  1. Position the patient supine with the palmar surface of the hand face up.
  2. Have the patient make a fist and slightly flex the wrist so that the palmaris longus and flexor carpi radialis tendons become prominent.
  3. Create a skin wheal of local anesthetic between the two tendons between the proximal skin crease and the distal skin crease at the wrist. Alternatively, anesthetic can be injected in line with the ulnar styloid process at the proximal skin crease.
  4. The palmaris longus tendon is absent normally in 10–20 % of the population. In this case, inject over the midpoint of the proximal skin crease at the level of the styloid process.

89.7.3.2 Wrist Block: Radial Nerve (Figs. 89.12 and 89.13) [3, 7]

- Procedure
  1. To block the radial nerve, block multiple peripheral branches on the dorsal and the radial aspects of the lateral wrist.
  2. A field block in and around the anatomical snuffbox may be performed, requiring roughly 5–6 mL of local anesthetic. This anesthetizes the terminal branches of the radius arising from the forearm.
  3. Position the patient's palm face up and inject a skin wheal to the area 1 mm lateral to the radial pulse and in line with the proximal wrist crease. Inject 2 mL of local anesthesia with a 25- to 27-gauge needle. This anesthetizes the terminal trunk of the radial nerve.

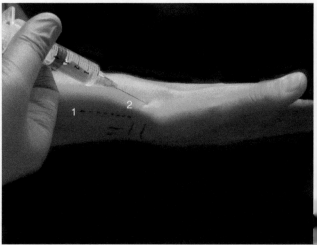

Fig. 89.12 Radial nerve block at the wrist: *1* radial artery, *2* anatomical snuffbox

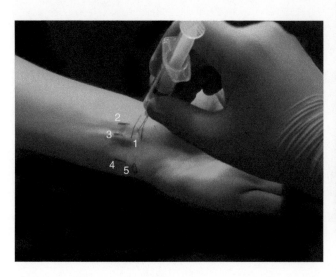

Fig. 89.11 Median nerve block at the wrist: *1* proximal and distal wrist creases radial artery, *2* flexor carpi radialis tendon, *3* palmaris longus tendon, *4* ulnar artery, *5* styloid process

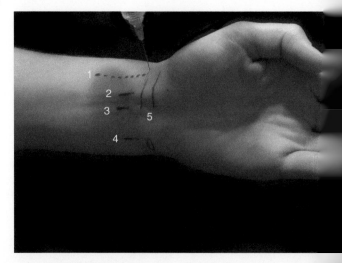

Fig. 89.13 Radial nerve block at the wrist: *1* radial artery, *2* flex carpi radialis tendon, *3* palmaris longus tendon, *4* ulnar artery, *5* pro mal and distal wrist creases

89.7.3.3 Wrist Block: Ulnar Nerve (Fig. 89.14)

- Procedure
  1. Position the patient with the hand face up.
  2. Palpate the styloid process of the ulna and pisiform and find the ulnar artery pulse.
  3. Create a skin wheal of local anesthetic between lateral to the ulnar artery and medial to the flexor carpi ulnaris tendon just proximal to the styloid process. This is at the level of the proximal wrist crease.

Digital Nerve Blocks: Ring, Web Space, and Tendon Sheath (Fig. 89.15) [3, 8, 9]

- Indications
  - To anesthetize the digits in preparation for laceration repair, nail bed repair, joint reduction, or pain relief

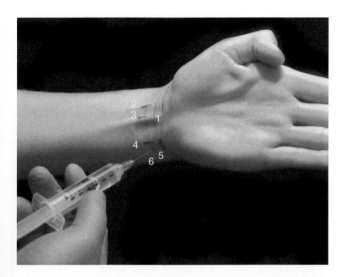

Fig. 89.14 Ulnar nerve block at the wrist: *1* proximal and distal wrist creases, *2* flexor carpi radialis tendon, *3* palmaris longus tendon, *4* ulnar artery, *5* styloid process, *6* flexor carpi ulnaris

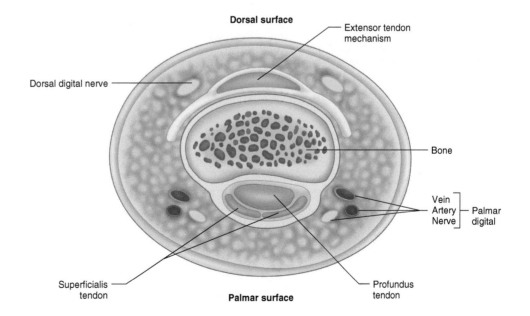

Fig. 89.15 Cross section of finger

89.7.3.4 Ring Block (Fig. 89.16) [3]

- Procedure
  1. Insert a 25-gauge needle on the dorsal surface of the proximal phalanx of the digit to be anesthetized. Inject 1 mL along the dorsal surface and withdraw the needle.
  2. Reinsert the needle again perpendicular to the last injection and running on the lateral surface of the phalanx. Inject 1–1.5 mL of local anesthetic to just past the phalanx base.
  3. Repeat the injection in the same fashion on the medial aspect of the phalanx.
  4. Do not inject more than 5 mL into a digit.
  5. Toe blocks are similar to finger ring blocks, except that the great toe requires plantar surface injection as well, owing to its unique nerve supply.

89.7.3.5 Web Space Digital Block (Fig. 89.17) [9]

- Procedure
  1. Have the patient abduct the fingers.
  2. Palpate the metacarpophalangeal joint and then insert a 25- to 27-gauge needle into the lateral web space subcutaneously, directing it dorsally. Aspirate then inject 1 mL of local anesthetic.
  3. Withdraw the needle but before the exiting skin, redirect toward the palmar aspect until the tip is next to the metacarpophalangeal joint, and inject 1 mL of local anesthetic.
  4. Repeat the procedure on the medial web space of the digit. Each digit blocked requires injection on both the lateral and the medial web spaces.

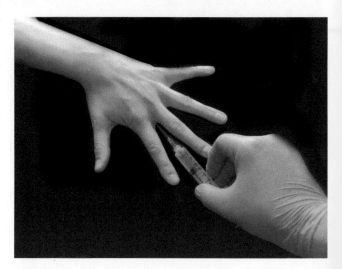

Fig. 89.17 Web space approach to the digital block, requiring injection on the medial and lateral web spaces for a blocked digit

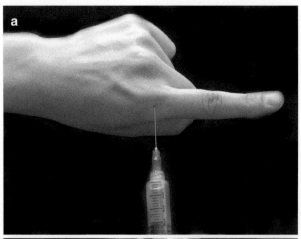

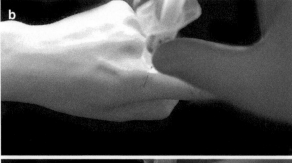

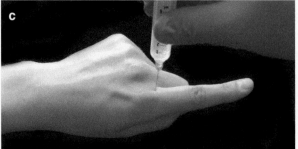

Fig. 89.16 Dorsal surface injection of digital nerve ring block. Digital nerve block is performed by injecting onto the (a) dorsal, (b) lateral, and (c) medial surfaces of the proximal phalanx

89.7.3.6 Intrathecal Digital Block: Flexor Tendon Sheath (Fig. 89.18) [8]

- Procedure
  1. Inject anesthetic directly into the flexor tendon sheath. Palpate on the palmar surface over and proximal to the metacarpophalangeal joint. Gentle flexion of digit may better reveal the sheath. Have the patient abduct the fingers.
  2. Insert a 25-gauge needle at a 45° angle to the skin and along the long axis of the digit directly into the flexor tendon sheath at the level of the distal skin crease.
  3. Inject 2 mL of local anesthetic. The anesthetic should flow freely if it is in the sheath. If it does not, it is likely in the tendon and should be withdrawn slightly.
  4. Contraindications to intrathecal block are local infection and preexisting flexor tendon injury.
  5. Risk of tenosynovitis; sterilize the skin before introducing the needle.
  6. If laceration has involved the tendon, anesthetic may leak from the wound.

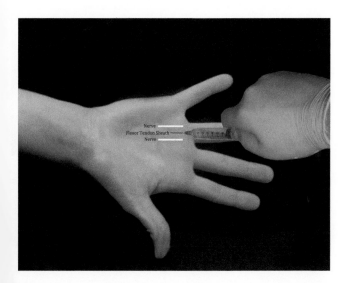

Fig. 89.18 Intrathecal/tendon sheath approach to the digital block

Acknowledgment The authors would like to thank Katy Howard for serving as the subject in many of the photographs in this chapter.

References

1. Muck AE, Bebarta VS, Borys DJ, Morgan DL. Six years of epinephrine digital injections: absence of significant local or systemic effects. Ann Emerg Med. 2010;56:270–4.
2. Waterbrook AL, Germann AC, Southall JC. Is epinephrine harmful when used with anesthetics for digital blocks? Ann Emerg Med. 2007;50:472–5.
3. Reichman EF, Simon RR, editors. Emergency medicine procedures. New York: McGraw-Hill Medical; 2004. p. 961–3.
4. Benko K. Fixing faces painlessly: facial anesthesia in emergency medicine. Available at: Emergency Medicine Practice (ebmedicine.net). 2009;11.
5. Rosh AJ. Ear anesthesia. Medscape reference. Available at: http://emedicine.medscape.com/article/82698-overview#a15.
6. Butterworth JF. Atlas of procedures in anesthesia and critical care. Philadelphia: WB Saunders; 1992. p. 160–4.
7. Brown DL. Atlas of regional anesthesia. Philadelphia: WB Saunders; 1992. p. 52.
8. Morrison WG. Transthecal digital block. Arch Emerg Med. 1993;10:35–8.
9. Mueller J, Davenport M. Digital nerve block (web space and tendon sheath). New York: McGraw-Hill's Access Emergency Medicine. Available at: http://www.accessemergencymedicine.com/videosPDF/DigitalNerveBlock.pdf.

Wound Management and Hemostasis

Rich Teitell and Muhammad Waseem

90.1 Indications for Primary Wound Repair

- Wounds that have been sustained less than 8 h before presentation may be closed primarily.
- If there is suspicion of broken glass or the presence of a foreign body, the patient should receive an x-ray before primary wound repair. Of note, x-ray has poor sensitivity for radiolucent foreign bodies such as wood and plastic.
- Wounds that are free of foreign bodies or show no gross evidence of infection or dead tissue may be closed primarily.

90.2 Contraindications for Primary Wound Repair

- History must address the factors that predispose a wound to greater risks of infection and not implement primary wound closure in such wounds that have had a duration greater than 8–12 h or contamination with saliva, stool, or foreign matter and a wound that has been sustained by blunt or crush mechanism.
- When wounds are highly contaminated with debris or if devitalized tissue is present, the wound should be left open for 3–4 days and then reevaluated.
- After a proper physical examination has been performed that assesses distal pulse and sensory and motor function of the surrounding region and distal extremity, if any of these are compromised, appropriate orthopedic and/or vascular consultation should be sought before wound closure, especially in the setting of a suspicion for open fracture.

Teitell, MD
Department of Emergency Medicine, Waterbury Hospital, Waterbury, CT, USA
email: rjt0013@gmail.com

Waseem, MD (✉)
Department of Emergency Medicine, Lincoln Medical and Mental Health Center, New York, NY, USA
email: waseemm2001@hotmail.com

- Consider delayed closure in wounds over joints.
- Wounds that have a significant loss of skin should be left to heal by secondary intention.

90.3 Procedure for Wound Closure and Hemostasis

1. Wound should be thoroughly prepared with Betadine (10 % povidone with 1 % iodine), which has a rapid onset with greatest antimicrobial effect.
2. Skin surrounding the wound should be covered with sterile drapes (Fig. 90.1) so as to reduce additional contamination within the open wound.
3. The most important determinant for preventing wound infection is adequate high-pressure irrigation.
4. Normal saline is the best solution for irrigation. Use pressures above 7 psi and an 18-gauge needle with a syringe of 30 mL or more; this gauge needle will achieve pressure greater than 7 psi.
5. It has been suggested that tap water irrigation may be just as effective. Because this approach will reduce costs, it can be considered.
6. Sharp debridement should be performed when foreign matter is found in an open wound that does not easily rinse out with saline. In this circumstance, consider wound closure by secondary intention or delayed primary closure.
7. At this point, wounds that do not meet criteria for primary closure must be left open, covered with a sterile dressing, and reevaluated in 3–4 days for consideration of delayed primary closure versus healing by secondary intention.
8. Wounds that do meet criteria as previously discussed for primary closure should be closed with either sutures or staples.
9. Staples are the preferred method of closure of scalp wounds and can be used under low wound tension.

Springer Science+Business Media New York 2016
Ganti (ed.), *Atlas of Emergency Medicine Procedures*, DOI 10.1007/978-1-4939-2507-0_90

10. The angle of the stapler is critical and must be positioned perpendicular to the intended area of delivery. A two-person approach can be utilized for optimal placement of the staple, using forceps to approximate the edges of the tissue.

11. Synthetic or monofilament sutures have a lower rate of infection than braided sutures (for closure techniques with sutures, see Chap. 92).

12. Dermabond should be utilized only for the most superficial linear lacerations and confers the benefit of efficiency of time and less discomfort to the patient. However, it should be mentioned that Dermabond does not offer any statistically significant difference in cosmesis when compared with suturing or other adhesives (see Chap. 93).

13. When a wound presents with deep underlying tissue involvement and direct bleeding is evident, direct pressure may be used to achieve hemostasis within a wound. Surgicel may also be applied with pressure to achieve control of small capillary and venous oozing (Fig. 90.2).

14. When a persistent bleed is visible within a wound that does not respond to direct pressure, a figure-of-eight suture (Fig. 90.3) may be used.

15. If a bleeding vessel is visible within a wound, an alternate method of hemostasis may be achieved by utilizing a hemostat to clamp the vessel and then tying an absorbable suture (Fig. 90.4).

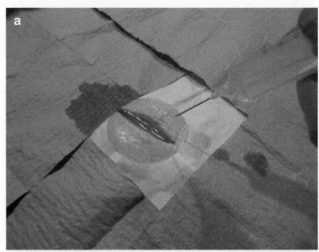
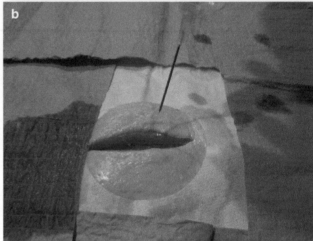

Fig. 90.1 (**a**) High-pressure irrigation using an 18-gauge needle (**b**)

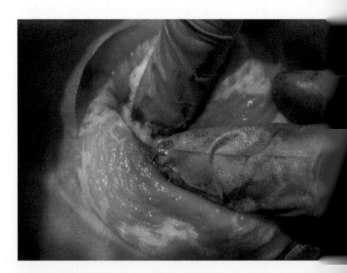

Fig. 90.2 Direct pressure with or without Surgicel may be used achieve hemostasis within a wound and also to achieve control of sm capillary and venous oozing

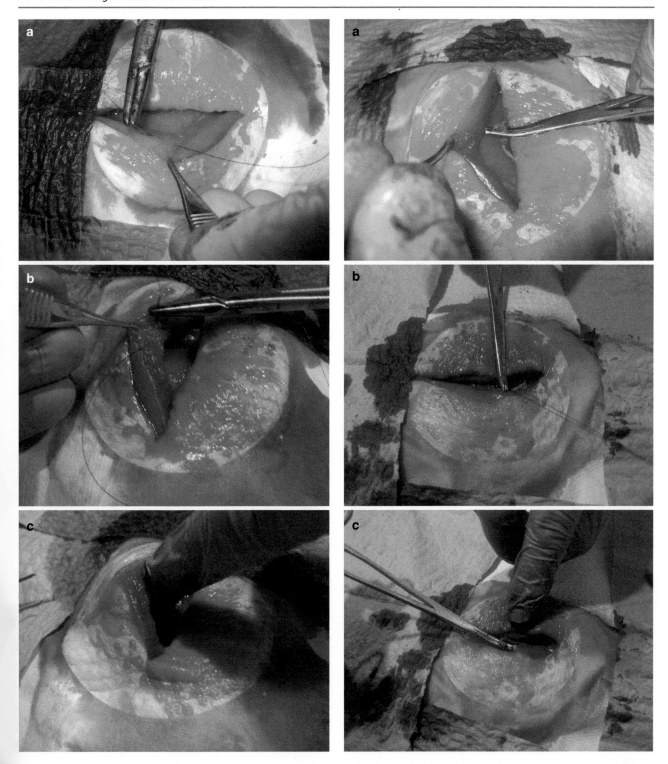

Fig. 90.3 (a) The location of the bleeding vessel in the subcutaneous tissue is identified and an absorbable suture is threaded through the region. (b) In a diagonal direction, a second suture is placed, which when tied will form the shape of an eight. (c) Once tied, the suture forms a figure eight in the tissue and hemostasis is achieved

Fig. 90.4 (a) The culprit vessel is identified and clamped with a hemostat. (b) An absorbable suture is wrapped around the vessel inferior to the hemostat. (c) Once the first tie is placed being driven down with index finger, the hemostat may be removed and the knot can be completed for a total of three or four passes

90.4 Complications

- Hematoma formation
- Infection
- Scar formation

90.5 Pearls and Pitfalls

- Pearls
  - Antibiotic coverage should be employed judiciously depending on the wound and location.
  - Wounds to the face that are not heavily contaminated generally do not require antibiotics because the face and scalp have a significant vascular supply.
  - Patients with diabetes have higher incidences of wound infection, and the physician should consider prophylactic antibiotics in such individuals.
  - Wounds that are clean-contaminated and sutured in the emergency department should have a nonadherent dressing applied for 48 h until epithelialization has occurred. After that, the dressing may be removed, and soap and water gentle washing should commence to keep area clean. Only small amounts of bacitracin should be applied to wound in the interim period before sutures are removed.
- Pitfalls
  - Wounds located on the extremities have greater incidences of infection than those on the trunk or head/face.

Selected Reading

Blankenship RB, Baker T. Imaging modalities in wounds and superficial skin infections. Emerg Med Clin North Am. 2007;25:223–34.

Dimick AR. Delayed wound closure: indications and techniques. Ann Emerg Med. 1988;17:1303–4.

Edlich RF, Rodeheaver GT, Morgan RF, Berman DE, Thacker JG. Principles of emergency wound management. Ann Emerg Med. 1988;17(12):1284–302.

Farion K, Osmond MH, Hartling L, et al. Tissue adhesives for traumatic lacerations in children and adults. Cochrane Database Syst Rev. 2002;(3):CD003326.

Hall S. A review of the effect of tap water versus normal saline on infection rates in acute traumatic wounds. J Wound Care. 2007;16:38–41.

Marx J, Hockberger R, Walls R, editors. Rosen's emergency medicine: concepts and clinical practice. 6th ed. Philadelphia: Mosby-Elsevier; 2006. p. 702–3.

Ritchie AJ, Rocke LG. Staples versus sutures in the closure of scalp wounds: a prospective, double-blind, randomized trial. Injury. 1989;20:217–8.

Singer AJ, Hollander JE, Quinn JV. Evaluation and management of traumatic lacerations. N Engl J Med. 1997;337:1142–8.

Burn Care

Thomas Parry and Jeffrey Pepin

Burns result from exposure to heat, caustic chemicals, electricity, or radiation. Damage to the natural barrier provided by skin results in rapid fluid losses and risk of infection. Permanent scarring is a common long-term complication. They may also be complicated by sensory deficits due to loss of nerve connections and limb loss due to circulatory compromise.

91.1 Burn Description (Fig. 91.1)

- First degree or superficial: burn that remains confined to the epidermis (e.g., sunburn)
- Second degree or partial thickness: burn that extends into the dermis (e.g., blistering scald burns)
- Third degree or full thickness: burn involving the entire depth of the dermis and epidermal appendages

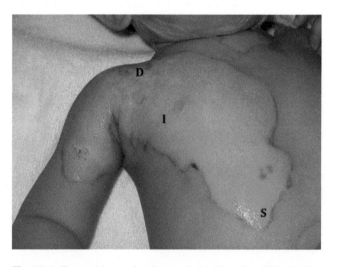

Fig. 91.1 Tea scald over the chest and shoulder of a child showing heterogeneity of burn depth. *D* deep (second or third degree), *I* intermediate (second degree), *S* superficial (first degree) (Reproduced from: Enoch S, Roshan A, Shah M. Emergency and early management of burns and scalds. *BMJ*. 2009;338:b1037, with permission from BMJ Publishing Group Ltd.)

T. Parry, MD (✉)
Department of Emergency Medicine, Lincoln Hospital and Mental Health Center, New York, NY, USA
e-mail: Thomas.parry@nychhc.org

J. Pepin, MD
Department of Emergency Medicine, University of Minnesota Medical Center Fairview, Minneapolis, MN, USA
e-mail: medicone76@hotmail.com

© Springer Science+Business Media New York 2016
L. Ganti (ed.), *Atlas of Emergency Medicine Procedures*, DOI 10.1007/978-1-4939-2507-0_91

91.2 Indications

- Superficial, deep second degree, and third degree.
- First-degree burns generally need only supportive care.

91.3 Materials and Medications

- Appropriate analgesia
- Antibiotic ointment
- Silver sulfadiazine (avoid on face)
- Sulfamylon for ears
- Alternative agents include bacitracin or polymyxin B ointments
- Cleansing solution such as chlorhexidine prep and water
- Basin
- Petroleum gauze
- Several 4×4 gauze pads
- Rolled gauze
- Tape
- Gloves

Airway, breathing, and circulation and cervical spine should be immediately assessed before any burn wound management. It is important to remember that any patient suspected of an inhalation injury or carbon monoxide poisoning should receive 100 % humidified oxygen until carboxyhemoglobin returns to normal. Inhalation injuries may not present themselves until after fluid resuscitation has already been started, so early intubation is recommended in these cases.

91.4 Sizing

Total body surface area (TBSA) of body parts is estimated by multiples of 9 (Rule of Nines)

- Adults
  - Head and neck: 9
  - Arms: 9 each
  - Legs: 18 each
  - Trunk: 18 front and 18 back
  - Perineum and palms: 1
- Infants/children
  - Head and neck: 18
  - Arms: 9 each
  - Legs: 14 each
  - Trunk: 18 front and 18 back

A second way to estimate TBSA in smaller burns is by using the palm surface area: using the patient's palm as a guide, each palmar surface equals 1 %.

A third way to estimate TBSA is via the use of the Lund and Browder chart (Fig. 91.2).

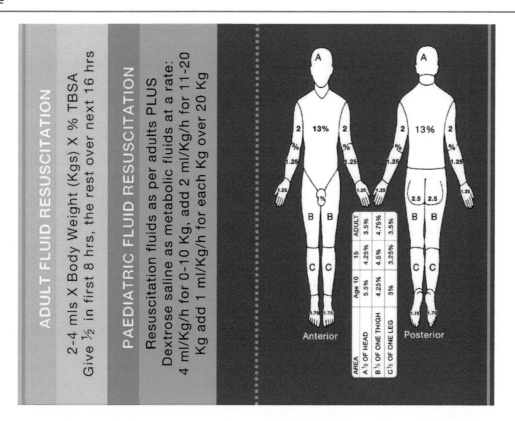

ADULT FLUID RESUSCITATION

2-4 mls X Body Weight (Kgs) X % TBSA
Give ½ in first 8 hrs, the rest over next 16 hrs

PAEDIATRIC FLUID RESUSCITATION

Resuscitation fluids as per adults PLUS
Dextrose saline as metabolic fluids at a rate:
4 ml/Kg/h for 0-10 Kg, add 2 ml/Kg/h for 11-20
Kg add 1 ml/Kg/h for each Kg over 20 Kg

AREA	Age 10	15	ADULT
A ½ OF HEAD	5.5%	4.25%	3.5%
B ½ OF ONE THIGH	4.25%	4.5%	4.75%
C ½ OF ONE LEG	3%	3.25%	3.5%

Anterior   Posterior

Fig. 91.2 Lund Browder chart for estimating total body surface area of burns, with suggested fluid resuscitation guidelines (Reprinted from Malic CC, Karoo RO, Austin O, Phipps A. Resuscitation burn card–a useful tool for burn injury assessment. *Burns*. 2007;33(2)195–9, with permission from Elsevier)

91.5 Fluid Resuscitation

Because fluid resuscitation is absolutely essential in the early aspects of burn care, the Parkland formula has been used to estimate fluid requirements in burn patients. The patient's weight in kilograms is multiplied by the percent body surface area (BSA) involved; this number is multiplied by 4 mL of lactated Ringer's solution. Half of this amount is given during the first 8 h and the remaining amount is given over the next 16 h of resuscitation. The goal is to keep urine output approximately 0.5–1.0 mL/kg/h.

In pediatric cases, the Galveston formula may be used instead: 5000 mL/m^2 BSA burned plus 2000 mL/m^2. TBSA of 5 % dextrose in lactated Ringer's solution intravenously over the first 24 h, half in the first 8 h, and the other half over the next 16 h.

91.6 Procedure

1. Provide appropriate analgesia.
2. Clean the wound with antiseptic solution and water (if it is a dry chemical burn, make sure to brush off as much chemical before using copious amounts of water to clean the wound).
3. Debride any loose skin or foreign debris using a dry 4×4 or rolled gauze.
4. Apply antibiotic ointment or cream to the burn.
5. Apply petroleum gauze in a single layer just over the affected skin.
6. Use loose 4×4 gauzes and "fluff" them to make a thick layer of padding to place over the petroleum gauze.
7. Either wrap the entire area with a rolled gauze or tape a small layer of 4×4 gauze over the "fluffed" layer of 4×4 gauze.

91.7 Complications

- Wound infection
- Nonhealing wound requiring skin graft (deep second-degree and third-degree burns)
- Compartment syndrome (circumferential burns may require escharotomy)
- Rhabdomyolysis

91.8 Pearls and Pitfalls

- Pearls
  - Determination of the depth of burns on initial presentation is difficult (especially when covered with petroleum).

A good rule of thumb is if it blanches and/or hurts, it is a partial thickness burn.
  - First-degree burns are not included in burn size estimations for fluid resuscitation calculation.
  - Burn size determines fluid requirements and transfer decision.
  - Burn of greater than 20 % TBSA should receive intravenous fluids.
  - Patients who have inhalation injury, greater than 10 % TBSA, high-voltage electrical injury, or chemical burns should be referred to burn unit.
  - Fluid resuscitation should be adjusted according to physiological response such as urine output (30–50 mL/h in adults and 1 mL/kg/h in children).
  - Assure tetanus is up to date.
- Pitfalls
  - Keep the patient warm in the first few hours. There is no need to apply ice.
  - All jewelry and rings should be removed.
  - Prophylactic antibiotics are not recommended.
  - Silver sulfadiazine should be avoided in facial burns because of the risk of staining of the skin.

Blister care is a very controversial topic. Current research suggests that it may be beneficial to keep the blister intact unless it appears to be tense or over a joint. Most blisters will rupture in 2–4 days. Ruptured blisters should be debrided with all the extra skin removed. Most burn units will scrub everything off once they receive a patient.

Wounds should be kept clean to prevent an environment that will increase the chances of infection. Wrap in saline-soaked sterile gauze prior to transfer.

Dressing changes should be done daily with all previously applied antibiotic ointment removed before a reapplication of new ointment. It is important to provide analgesic 30 min before a dressing change.

91.9 Admission Criteria

- Partial-thickness burns of noncritical areas not including the eyes, ears, face, hands, feet, or perineum that total BSA of 10–20 % in adults
- Partial-thickness burns of noncritical areas involving 5–10 % of BSA in children younger than 10 years
- Suspicious of non-accidental trauma
- Patients unable to care for wounds in outpatient settings
- Prompt referral to a burn specialist is required in the following cases:
  - Partial-thickness and full-thickness burns greater than 10 % of the TBSA in patients younger than 10 years or older than 50 years of age.
  - Partial-thickness and full-thickness burns greater than 20 % of the TBSA in other age groups.

- Partial-thickness and full-thickness burns involving the face, eyes, ears, hands, feet, genitalia, or perineum or the skin overlying major joints.
- Full-thickness burns greater than 5 % TBSA in any age group.
- Electrical burns, including lightning injury: significant volumes of tissue beneath the surface may be injured and result in acute renal failure and other complications.
- Significant chemical burns.
- Inhalation injury.
- Burn injury in patients with preexisting illness that could complicate management, prolong recovery, or affect mortality.
- Any burn patient in whom concomitant trauma poses an increased risk of morbidity or mortality may be treated initially in a trauma center until stable before transfer to a burn center.

- Children with burns seen in hospitals without qualified personnel or equipment for their care should be transferred to a burn center with these capabilities.
- Burn injury in patients who will require special social and emotional or long-term rehabilitative support, including cases involving suspected child abuse and neglect.

Selected Reading

Bezuhly M, Fish JS. Acute burn care. Plast Reconstr Surg. 2012;130(2):349e–58.

Rex S. Burn injuries. Curr Opin Crit Care. 2012;18(6):671–6.

Wasiak J, Cleland H, Campbell F, Spinks A. Dressings for superficial and partial thickness burns. Cochrane Database Syst Rev. 2013;(3):CD002106.

Wound Closure

92

Oliver Michael Berrett, Jeffrey Joseph Harroch,
Karlene Hosford, and Muhammad Waseem

92.1 Indications

Open wound of skin or mucosal tissues
Purpose
- Preserve function
- Control bleeding
- Promote healing
- Cosmesis

92.2 Contraindications

Wounds caused by animal or human bites
Contaminated, infected, or puncture wounds
Complex wounds (may require operating room)

92.3 Methods

Suture placement
Tissue adhesives
Adhesive tapes
Staples

92.4 Preparation

- Obtain a complete history of injury
  - Mechanism
  - Time since injury
  - Tetanus status
  - Comorbidities
- Examine the extent of the wound, remove any contaminants, debride devitalized tissue, inspect for foreign bodies. Obtain a radiograph if foreign body is suspected.
- Copious irrigation with normal saline.
- Clean around the wound with a povidone-iodine solution.
- Drape the area in sterile manner.
- Inject the anesthetic agent into the wound edges using a 25- or 27-gauge needle. The most common agent is lidocaine 2 % with or without epinephrine 1 % (maximum dose is 3 mg/kg without epinephrine and 5 mg/kg with epinephrine).
- Close the wound using the appropriate technique (see later).
- Dress the wound.
- Update tetanus and diphtheria vaccination if needed.

O.M. Berrett, MD • K. Hosford, MD • M. Waseem, MD (✉)
Department of Emergency Medicine, Lincoln Medical and Mental
Health Center, New York, NY, USA
e-mail: omberrett@gmail.com; krlhos@aol.com;
waseemm2001@hotmail.com

J. Harroch, MD
Department of Emergency Medicine, University of Miami Miller
School of Medicine, University of Miami Hospital,
Miami, FL, USA
e-mail: jharroch@med.miami.edu

© Springer Science+Business Media New York 2016
L. Ganti (ed.), *Atlas of Emergency Medicine Procedures*, DOI 10.1007/978-1-4939-2507-0_92

92.5   Suture Repair

92.5.1 Materials and Medications

- Commercial kits commonly contain all the following except the suture material (Fig. 92.1)
    - Povidone-iodine solution
    - Normal saline for irrigation

- 5- to 12-mL syringe with a 25-gauge needle
- Anesthetic agent
- Needle holder
- Pickups
- Suture scissors
- Suturing material
- Sterile drape or sheet, gloves, gauze

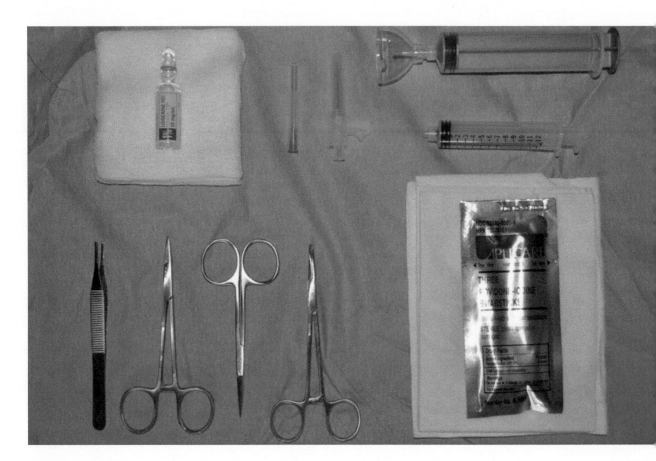

Fig. 92.1 Suture kit

92.5.2 General Guidelines

- Local anesthetic lidocaine 1 % or lidocaine 1 % with epinephrine.
- Minimize direct use of instruments on the tissues.
- Wound edges should be everted to maximize healing and cosmetic effect. This is achieved by inserting the needle at 90° to the skin.
- Sutures should be evenly spaced, placed 1–3 mm apart and 2 mm from the wound edge.
- Optimal tension is achieved by tying the sutures so the edges lightly approximate.

92.5.3 Suture Material

- Nonabsorbable
  - Silk: for specialty use, reactive and weak
  - Nylon (Ethilon), polypropylene (Prolene): good strength, good overall material for cutaneous wounds
  - Polypropylene: good strength, difficult to use
  - Require removal at a specified time

- Absorbable
  - Undergo rapid degradation in tissues, losing their tensile strength within 60 days
  - Indication: buried suture to reduce wound edge tension
  - Vicryl: subcutaneous placement, mucous membranes
  - Chromic: use for intraoral lacerations
  - Removal not required

92.5.4 Suture Size

- 0.0–2.0: thick material for large wounds, trunk
- 0.3–0.4: used on medium-sized wounds, extremities, scalp
- 0.5–0.6: fine sutures, used on facial wounds

92.5.5 Suture Techniques

- Simple interrupted sutures (Fig. 92.2)
  - Most common method
  - Position needle 2 mm from the wound edge at a 90° angle. Enter the needle into the skin and arc through the wound edge and into the opposing edge at the same level, exiting the skin on the opposing side 2 mm from wound edge, tie.
- Deep dermal suture (Fig. 92.3)
  - Also known as buried sutures, used to minimize tension in a wound.
  - Use absorbable suture material.
  - The needle is placed at the base of the wound wall and arched upward, exiting the ipsilateral wall more superficially. The needle is then directed across to the opposing wound wall at the same level and directed downward, exiting deep, tie. Note: The knot will be deep in the wound.
- Simple running suture (Fig. 92.4)
  - This method provides rapid closure of long and relatively linear lacerations.
  - Place the initial suture in the same manner as a simple suture, tie, cut the free strand, and leave the needle attached. Reintroduce the needle into the skin on the opposite side so the suture crosses the wound superficially at a 65° angle. The needle is then inserted perpendicular to the skin, emerging on the opposite side about 3 mm from the wound edge. Repeat without tying until closure is complete, maintaining appropriate tension. When the last stitch is placed, leave a loose loop of suture on one side so that both ends can be tied together.
- Vertical mattress suture (Fig. 92.5)
  - Provides the benefits of both simple and deep techniques. For use on deeper, gaping wounds and wounds over high-tension areas such as joints.
  - Position the needle 1 cm from skin edge, at a 90° angle, drive a deep arc perpendicular through the wound, exiting the skin on the opposing side the same distance from the wound edge. Next, reinsert the needle on the ipsilateral side 2 mm from the edge, emerging on the opposing side and approximate, tie.
- Horizontal mattress suture (Fig. 92.6)
  - For large wounds with tension.
  - Place the initial suture in the same manner as a simple suture, only do not tie. Reposition the needle on the ipsilateral side, horizontally 5 mm to the side of the

exit at the same distance from the wound edge and drive through to the other side, tie. Note: The tie lies parallel to the wound.
- Half-buried horizontal mattress suture (Fig. 92.7)
  - Used on wounds with skin flap.
  - On one side, drive the needle percutaneously, and then pass horizontally through the dermal tissue of the tip of flap, finally passing into the dermis of the opposing edge and exiting the skin, tie.

92.5.6 Recommendations

- Face
  - 5.0–6.0 nylon.
  - Remove after 3–5 days.
- Scalp
  - 2.0–3.0 nylon or staple.
  - Remove at 8–10 days.

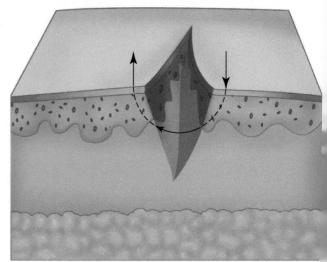

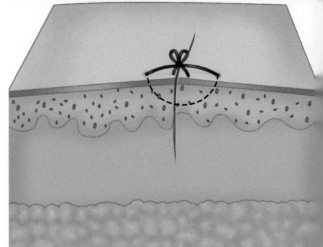

Fig. 92.2 Simple suture

- Hand
  - 4.0–5.0 nylon, consider vertical or horizontal mattress.
  - 5.0–6.0 Monocryl for nail bed.
  - Remove at 10–14 days, use for a longer time if directly over the joint.
- Extremity
  - Nonmobile skin: 3.0–4.0 nylon, remove at 8–10 days
  - Over joint: 3.0–4.0 nylon, remove at 10–14 days
- Trunk
  - Anterior trunk: 3.0–4.0 nylon, remove at 8–10 days.
  - Posterior trunk: 2.0–3.0 nylon, remove at 10–14 days.
  - Consider staples.
- Oral mucosa
  - Thin mucosa: 4.0 Vicryl will absorb; duration, 5–7 days
  - Tongue: 3.0 Vicryl will absorb; duration, 5–7 days

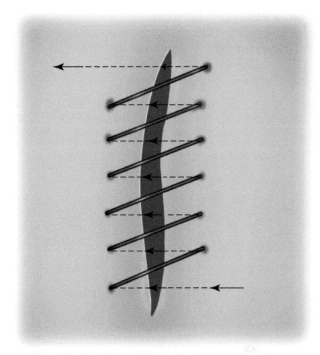

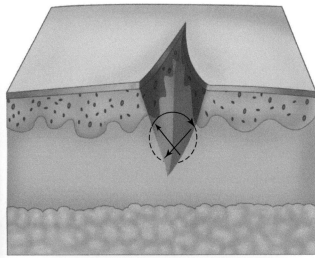

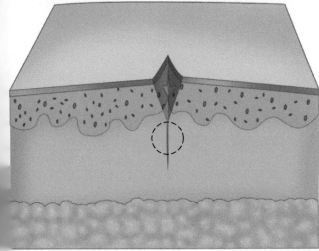

Fig. 92.3 Deep suture

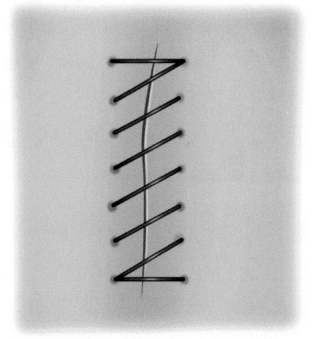

Fig. 92.4 Running suture

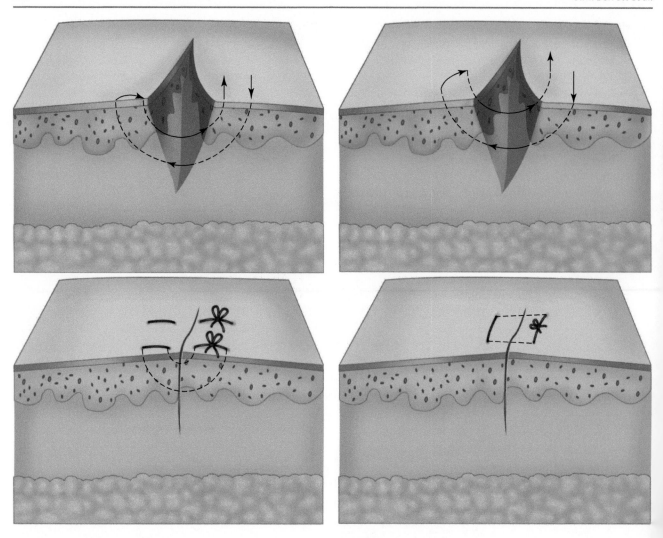

Fig. 92.5 Vertical mattress suture

Fig. 92.6 Horizontal mattress suture

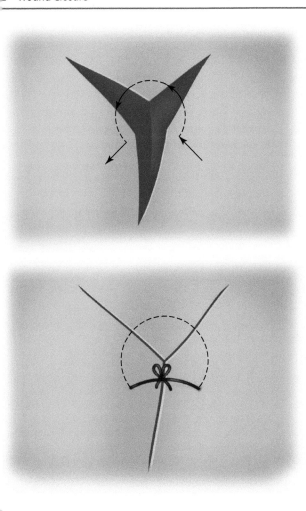

92.6 Alternative Methods of Wound Closure

92.6.1 Cyanoacrylate Tissue Adhesives

See Chap. 93.

92.6.2 Adhesive Tape

- Advantages
  - Rapid and painless application
  - Inexpensive
  - Good cosmetic result
- Disadvantages
  - Minimal strength
- Contraindications
  - Allergy to product
- Precautions
  - For use with wounds under little tension
- Procedure
  - Thoroughly clean the wound as described previously.
  - Approximate the wound edges.
  - Apply adhesive tape directly over the wound with 2–3 mm of space between strips.
  - An adjunct adhesive, such as benzoin, may be used to improve durability.

Fig. 92.7 Half-buried horizontal mattress suture

92.6.3 Staple Closure (Fig. 92.8)

- Advantages
  - Rapid
  - Inexpensive
- Disadvantages
  - Minimal strength
- Contraindications
  - Wounds on face, hands, or feet
- Procedure
  - Thoroughly clean the wound as described previously.
  - Anesthetize the wound edges.
  - Approximate the wound edges (may require an additional set of hands).
  - Apply staples.

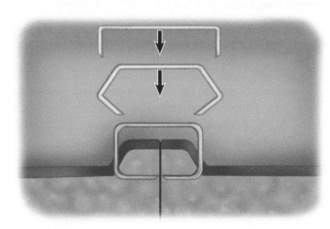

Fig. 92.8 Staple

92.7 Pearls and Pitfalls

- Pearls
  - Sutures should not remain in place longer than the recommended period. If the wound is not completely healed, sutures should be removed and an adhesive tape may be used for edge approximation.
  - Remember to verify tetanus status.
  - Antibiotics should be used judiciously.
- Pitfalls
  - Wound infection.
  - Incomplete healing may lead to wound separation.
  - Tissue reaction to suture or adhesive materials.
  - Allergy to anesthetic agent.

Selected Reading

http://apps.med.buffalo.edu/procedures/repairoflacerations.asp?p=17. Accessed 19 May 2014.

Singer AJ, Hollander JE. Methods for wound closure. In: Ma OJ, Cline DH, Tintinalli JE, Kelen GD, Stapczynski JS, editors. Emergency medicine manual. 6th ed. New York: McGraw Hill; 2003: Chap. 13, Fig. 13–14.

Singer AJ, Hollander JE, editors. Laceration and acute wounds: an evidence-based guide. Philadelphia: FA Davis; 2003. p. 122.

University of Connecticut Health Center, suturing 101. fitsweb.uchc.edu/suturing101. Accessed 19 May 2014.

Zuber TJ. The mattress sutures: vertical, horizontal and corner stitch. Am Fam Physician. 2002;66:2231–6.

Wound Closure with Tissue Adhesive

93

Pratik S. Patel and Latha Ganti

93.1 Indications

- Small superficial skin incisions or laceration repairs which require 5.0 or smaller-diameter sutures.

93.2 Contraindications

- Absolute
  - Large irregular/stellate lacerations
  - Infected/contaminated wounds
  - Animal/human bites
  - Puncture wounds
  - Crush wounds
  - Skin ulcers
  - Mucous membranes and mucocutaneous junctions
  - Axillae and perineum (owing to high moisture)
- Relative
  - Wounds on extremities (unless kept dry)
  - Joints (unless kept immobilized with a splint)

93.3 Materials and Medications

- Dermabond (2-octyl cyanoacrylate)
- Betadine (povidone-iodine) solution
- 0.9 % normal saline solution
- 20-mL sterile syringe
- Sterile gloves
- Dry 4×4 gauze

93.4 Optional Materials

- Topical anesthesia
- 1:1000 epinephrine solution
- Forceps
- Bacitracin ointment or sterile petroleum jelly ointment
- Gown and protective eyeglasses
- Splint

S. Patel, MD
Department of Emergency Medicine, University of Florida Health, Gainesville, FL, USA
email: drpratik@gmail.com

L. Ganti, MD, MS, MBA (✉)
Professor of Emergency Medicine, University of Central Florida, Orlando, FL, USA

Director, SE Specialty Care Centers of Innovation, Orlando Veterans Affairs Medical Center, Orlando, FL, USA
email: lathagantimd@gmail.com

© Springer Science+Business Media New York 2016
L. Ganti (ed.), *Atlas of Emergency Medicine Procedures*, DOI 10.1007/978-1-4939-2507-0_93

93.5 Procedure

1. Have the patient rest comfortably on a chair or bed.
2. Use universal precaution measures: sterile gloves (gown and eye-screen, if necessary for wound irrigation).
3. Wash the wound with 0.9 % normal saline irrigation.
4. Use a topical anesthetic such as LET (lidocaine, epinephrine, tetracaine) or EMLA (eutectic mixture of local anesthetics) cream (lidocaine and prilocaine), or a 1:1000 epinephrine solution soaked into gauze can be used to achieve hemostasis in a bleeding wound.
5. Approximate the edges of the wound with fingers. Toothed forceps or other skin approximation devices may be used as an adjunct. Apply bacitracin ointment or Vaseline to the tips of the forceps and wipe off the excess to prevent sticking of Dermabond glue to the forceps.
6. Crush Dermabond vial between the thumb and the finger while in the inverted position until the adhesive is seen at the applicator tip (Fig. 93.1).
7. Squeeze gently until a drop of adhesive forms at the applicator tip.
8. Gently brush the adhesive at the applicator tip over the approximated wound edges (Fig. 93.2). (Do not force or press the applicator tip over the wound.)
9. Cover the entire wound with single coat of adhesive.
10. Hold the wound edges for 30 s to 1 min until it dries.
11. Apply two or three more coats of adhesive over and around the wound in a circular or oval movement to provide extra strength.
12. Wipe off extra adhesive in the surrounding skin with gauze if needed.
13. Apply a splint (optional) to provide wound stability over the joints.
14. Recommend the patient to keep the wound dry for 4–5 days. Patients may shower but should be instructed to pat dry instead of rubbing a towel over the skin.
15. No topical antibiotic ointment is required before or after application of Dermabond.

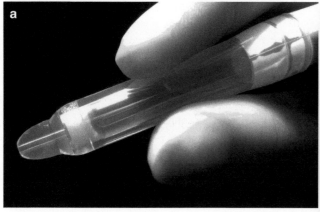
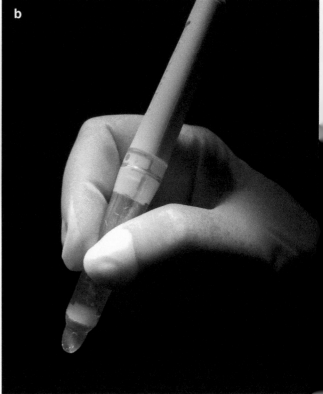

Fig. 93.1 (**a**) Before the tip has been crushed. (**b**) The purple Dermabond is in the tip

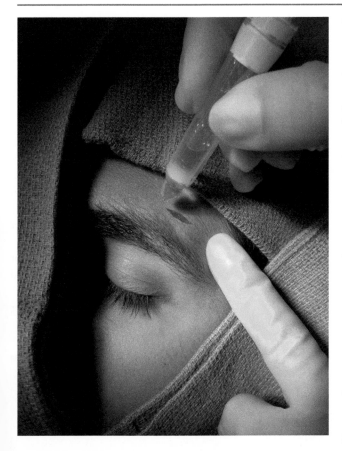

Fig. 93.2 Closing the wound: use tip of Dermabond pen to "paint" over the laceration

93.6   Complications

- Wound dehiscence
- Wound infection

93.7   Pearls and Pitfalls

- Pearls
    - Advantages of tissue adhesives for wound repair compared with sutures include faster repair time, better acceptance by patients (especially children), water-resistant covering, and no need for a second visit to remove sutures (sloughs off in 5–10 days).
- Pitfalls
    - Dermabond is a super adhesive. Take care not to have the glove, finger, drape, gauze, or instrument inadvertently stuck to the wound or the patient by having a bacitracin or petroleum jelly coating around the wound, on gloved fingers, and on forceps as needed.

Selected Reading

Bruns TB, Worthington JM. Using tissue adhesive for wound repair: a practical guide to Dermabond. Am Fam Physician. 2000;61:1383–8.

Farion K, Osmond MH, Hartling L, et al. Tissue adhesives for traumatic lacerations in children and adults. Cochrane Database Syst Rev. 2002;(3):CD003326.

Fishhook Removal

Judith K. Lucas

94.1 Indications

Removal of a fishhook from nonvital structures (Fig. 94.1)

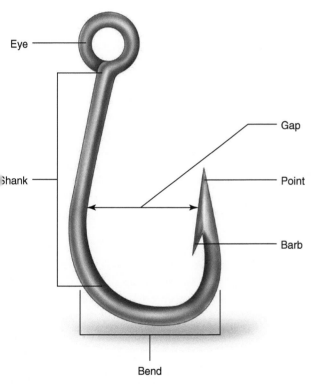

Fig. 94.1 Anatomy of a fishhook

Labels: Eye, Shank, Gap, Point, Barb, Bend

94.2 Contraindications

- Removal of hooks located near/in eyes or eyelids, embedded near or within neurovascular structures, or embedded within vital structures such as peritoneum, testicle, or urethra.
  - Fishhooks in these areas require specialist consultation.

94.3 Materials and Medications

- Antiseptic cleansing solutions
  - Betadine (povidone-iodine)
  - Chloraprep
- Local anesthetic
  - 1 % lidocaine, with or without epinephrine
- Needle drivers or pliers
- 18- or 20-gauge needle
- 3-0 silk suture or umbilical tape
- Wire cutters
- Protective eyewear

K. Lucas, MD
Department of Emergency Medicine,
University of Florida Health Shands Hospital,
Gainesville, FL, USA
e-mail: judithklucas@ufl.edu

Springer Science+Business Media New York 2016
. Ganti (ed.), *Atlas of Emergency Medicine Procedures*, DOI 10.1007/978-1-4939-2507-0_94

94.4 Procedures

- Retrograde technique (Fig. 94.2): simplest, least traumatic, but least successful; good for small to medium hooks, superficially embedded hooks, and hooks with no barbs or a single barb.
  1. Detach extra hooks, line, or foreign materials (e.g., worms, fish, debris).
  2. Cleanse the puncture site and surrounding tissue with antiseptic solution.
  3. Infiltrate the entry site and surrounding area with local anesthetic.
  4. Apply downward pressure on the shank or shaft of the hook, near the eye, thus disengaging the barb from the tissue.
  5. Back the hook out of the skin along the path of entry.
- String and yank technique (Fig. 94.3): Good for small to medium hooks. Often requires no anesthesia. Good for areas of deep soft tissue penetration. Cannot be used on parts of the body that are not fixed, such as earlobes.
  1. Detach extra hooks, line, or foreign materials (e.g., worms, fish, debris).
  2. Cleanse the penetration site and surrounding area with antiseptic wash.
  3. Consider infiltrating the entry site with local anesthetic.
  4. Wrap 3-0 silk suture, fishing line, or umbilical tape several times around the bend of the hook (at the point of greatest curvature).
  5. The loose ends of the string need be held tightly. Sometimes the loose ends can be more firmly held if wrapped around a pencil or tongue depressor.
  6. The skin around the entry site should be well stabilized, while simultaneously depressing the shank, close to the eye of the hook.
  7. While stabilizing the skin and applying downward pressure on the shaft, quickly and firmly yank the string, in a parallel line to the shaft. Be certain downward pressure is applied along the shank.
  8. The hook will "fly" out quickly. Be certain to wear eye protection.
- Needle cover technique (Fig. 94.4): good method to remove large hooks with a single barb, especially if superficially embedded

  1. Detach extra hooks, line, or foreign materials (e. worms, fish, debris).
  2. Cleanse the penetration site and surrounding area w antiseptic wash.
  3. Infiltrate the entry site and surrounding area with lo anesthetic.
  4. Advance an 18-gauge needle along the entrar wound of the hook. Pass the needle parallel to shank. The bevel should be pointed downward, towa the barb and point.
  5. The needle is advanced until it disengages the ba entrapping it within the needle lumen.
  6. The hook and needle are advanced just enough to d engage the barb.
  7. The hook and needle are withdrawn along the track the wound.
- Advance and cut technique (Fig. 94.5). Almost alwa successful but does cause additional tissue trauma.
  1. Detach extra hooks, line, or foreign materials (e. worms, fish, debris).
  2. Cleanse the penetration site and surrounding area w antiseptic wash.
  3. Infiltrate the entry site and surrounding area with lo anesthetic.
  4. If the hook has a single barb:
     - Grip the hook on the shank, near the bend, w either a needle driver or pliers.
     - Push the hook through along its natural trajecto until the point and barb pass completely throu the skin.
     - Clip the point proximal to the barb. Be certain wear eye protection because the point can fly off an unpredictable direction.
     - Withdraw the hook out back along its entry path.
  5. If the hook has multiple barbs (Fig. 94.6):
     - Grip the hook on the shank, near the hook's be with either a needle driver or pliers.
     - Push the hook through along its natural trajecto until the point and barb pass completely throu the skin.
     - Clip the eye of the hook with wire cutters.
     - Grasp the point and withdraw the hook through t skin forward along its natural course.

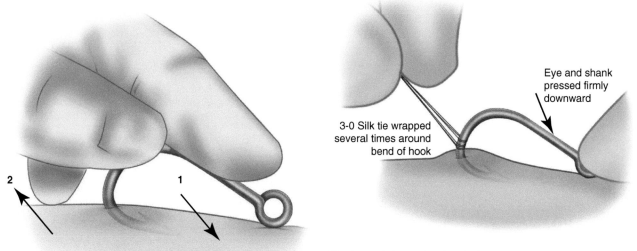

Fig. 94.3 String and yank technique

Eye and shank pressed firmly downward

3-0 Silk tie wrapped several times around bend of hook

Fig. 94.2 Retrograde technique. *1* Push down along whole shank and slightly forward to release the barb. *2* Pull back and out along hook's entry path, applying steady downward pressure

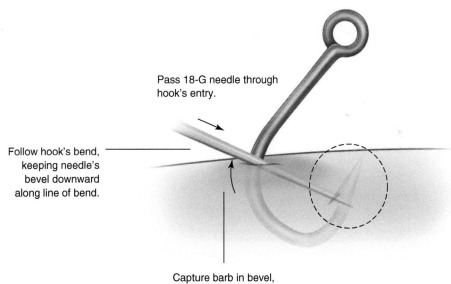

Pass 18-G needle through hook's entry.

Follow hook's bend, keeping needle's bevel downward along line of bend.

Capture barb in bevel, then gently pull needle/hook unit out of skin along path.

Fig. 94.4 Needle technique

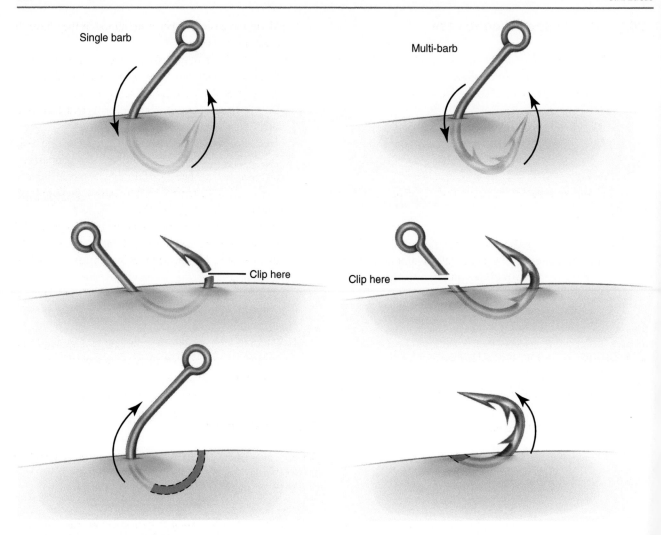

Fig. 94.5 Advance and cut technique

Fig. 94.6 Advance and cut a hook with multiple barbs present

94.5 Postremoval Wound Care

- Immune competent, without peripheral vascular disease:
  1. Explore the wound for possible foreign bodies.
  2. Irrigate or scrub the wound copiously with soapy solution.
  3. Apply antibiotic ointment and sterile dressing.
  4. Tdap (or Dtap) should be given to anyone in whom the last tetanus booster has been longer than 5 years.
  5. Wound check in 24–48 h with care provider.
- Immunocompromised or a patient with peripheral vascular disease:
  1. As previously.
  2. Give strong consideration to treating prophylactically with antibiotics, choosing a fluoroquinolone, third-generation cephalosporin, or aminoglycoside.

94.6 Complications

- Infection
- Retained foreign body
- Injury to neurovascular structures, if method of removal is not carefully selected
- Injury to provider if adequate (eye) protection not used

94.7 Pearls and Pitfalls

- Pearls
  - Begin with either the retrograde method or the string-yank method, because these result in less tissue damage and are the easiest to perform, although they have the lowest rate of success.
  - Eye protection is imperative, especially if utilizing the string-yank method or clipping any portion of the hook (eye or point) because the retraction of the hook, or its parts, is generally at a high velocity and travels an unpredictable path.
  - When trying the advance and cut technique, stop immediately if, when advancing the hook, impasse, or resistance is met because this may indicate bone or neurovascular structures are blocking the natural path of the hook.
  - Fishhooks that embed into or near the eye or lids should be covered with a metal patch or cup and the patient should be sent (immediately) for ophthalmologic consultation.
  - Close follow-up is imperative to watch for signs of infection.
- Pitfalls
  - When utilizing the advance and cut technique, do not cut anything until certain there is another portion of the hook on which to grasp.

Selected Reading

Bothner J. Fish-hook removal techniques. Available at: www.UpToDate.com. Literature review version 19.2, May 2011. Topic last updated: Sep 2010. Accessed 23 June 2014.

Gammons M, Jackson E. Fishhook removal. Am Fam Physician. 2001;63:2231–7.

Wakeman K. Fishhook removal. Available at: www.fishgame.com. Texas Fish and Game, LLC. July 2003. Accessed 23 June 2014.

Tick Removal

David N. Smith and Judith K. Lucas

95.1 Indications

- Tick attachment to the skin

95.2 Contraindications

- None

95.3 Materials and Medications

- Gloves
- Skin disinfectant (commercially available product, such as Chloraprep, isopropyl alcohol, or Betadine [povidone-iodine])
- Fine-toothed forceps

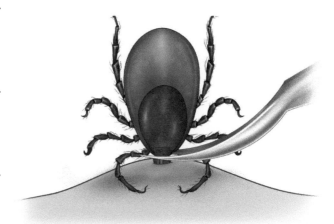

Fig. 95.1 Place the forceps as close to the mouth of the tick as possible, hold firmly, and pull straight up with steady gentle traction

95.4 Procedure

1. Comfortably position the patient with the tick site exposed.
2. Grasp the tick as close to the skin surface as possible (e.g., grasp the mouth parts).
3. Gently pull upward with steady, nontwisting, even traction (Figs. 95.1 and 95.2).
4. After removal, clean the bite area and apply antibiotic ointment.

D.N. Smith, MD
Department of Pediatrics, University of Alabama at Birmingham, Children's of Alabama, Birmingham, AL, USA
e-mail: dsmith@peds.uab.edu

J.K. Lucas, MD (✉)
Department of Emergency Medicine,
University of Florida Health Shands Hospital,
Gainesville, FL, USA
e-mail: judithklucas@ufl.edu

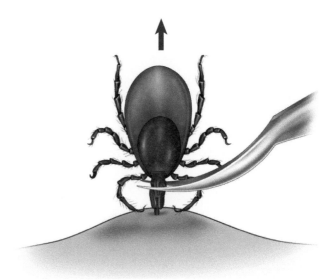

Fig. 95.2 Steady upward traction

© Springer Science+Business Media New York 2016
R. Ganti (ed.), *Atlas of Emergency Medicine Procedures*, DOI 10.1007/978-1-4939-2507-0_95

95.5 Complications

- Multiple diseases including:
  - Lyme disease
  - Human granulocytic and monocytic ehrlichiosis
  - Babesiosis
  - Relapsing fever
  - Rocky Mountain spotted fever
  - Colorado tick fever
  - Tularemia
  - Q fever
  - Tick paralysis
- Secondary infection (methicillin-resistant *Staphylococcus aureus* [MRSA] and group A streptococcus).
- Scratching can lead to lichenification.
- Rare cases of alopecia when tick located in the scalp.

95.6 Pearls and Pitfalls

- Pearls
  - Do not twist or jerk the tick out (may cause breakage of mouth parts; they may remain in the skin).
  - Do not squeeze the body of the tick.
  - Do not use a hot match, gasoline, or other noxious stimulus for removal (causes irritation of tick and release of internal contents).
  - Lyme disease transmission increases significantly after 24–48 h of attachment, so early removal is the key.
  - Patients should be monitored for up to 30 days for signs of tick-borne diseases, including erythema migrans (bull's-eye rash) indicating Lyme disease (Fig. 95.3).
  - Prophylactic antibiotic treatment, a single dose of doxycycline, is used only in patients with an identified *Ixodes scapularis* tick that has been attached for longer than 36 h and if treatment can start within 72 h of tick removal.
    - Serological testing for Lyme disease is not indicated for a reported tick bite.
- Pitfalls
  - Use of lidocaine subcutaneously can irritate the tick and cause it to regurgitate its stomach contents, increasing the risk of disease transfer.

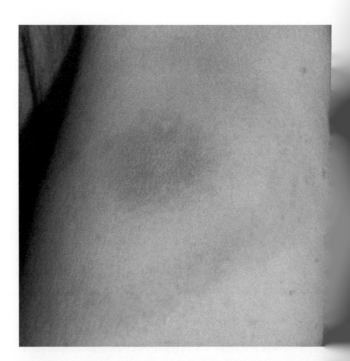

Fig. 95.3 Erythema migrans (the bull's-eye rash), the rash typical associated with Lyme disease. Often the rash is so pale as to go unnoticed

Selected Reading

Centers for Disease Control and Prevention. Tick removal. In: Ticks. 2014. http://www.cdc.gov/ticks/removing_a_tick.html. Accessed 23 Feb 2014.

Needham GR. Evaluation of five popular methods for tick removal. Pediatrics. 1985;75:997–1002.

Sexton DJ. Evaluation of a tick bite for possible Lyme disease. Up To Date; 2010. http://uptodate.com.

Sloan S. Background. In Tick removal. 2014. http://emedicine.medscape.com/article/1413603-overview. Accessed 23 Feb 2014.

Subungal Hematoma Drainage

96

Pratik S. Patel and Latha Ganti

96.1 Causes

- Crushing injury to the finger or toe
- Ill-fitted shoes/inadequate space for toes

96.2 Indications

- Pain that is not tolerable with nail edges intact

96.3 Contraindications

- Relative
  - Disrupted nail edges
  - Tolerable pain that can be managed conservatively
  - Skin infections around toe/finger
  - Bleeding disorder

96.4 Materials and Medications

- 18-gauge needle
- Betadine (povidone-iodine) solution
- Gloves
- Topical antibiotic

96.4.1 Optional materials

- Electrocautery tool
- Paper clip or sewing needle and sterilizing flame
- Finger splint
- Lidocaine (1 or 2 % with epinephrine)

P.S. Patel, MD
Department of Emergency Medicine, University of Florida Health, Gainesville, FL, USA
e-mail: drpratik@gmail.com

L. Ganti, MD, MS, MBA (✉)
Professor of Emergency Medicine, University of Central Florida, Orlando, FL, USA

Director, SE Specialty Care Centers of Innovation, Orlando Veterans Affairs Medical Center, Orlando, FL, USA
e-mail: lathagantimd@gmail.com

© Springer Science+Business Media New York 2016
L. Ganti (ed.), *Atlas of Emergency Medicine Procedures*, DOI 10.1007/978-1-4939-2507-0_96

96.5 Procedure

1. Have the patient rest the affected finger comfortably on a flat surface.
2. Use universal precaution measures: gloves, gown, and eye screen.
3. Sterile skin preparation with Betadine.
4. Optional (for complicated subungal hematoma): use 1 or 2 % lidocaine with epinephrine for providing local digital block.
5. Using the thumb and index finger gently twist the 18-gauge needle with light pressure over the base of the nailbed or in the center of the hematoma until no resistance is felt. Do not apply any further pressure in order to avoid nailbed damage. Nail penetration is confirmed by return of dark blood from the hole. This procedure is known as trephination (Figs. 96.1 and 96.2).
6. Apply light pressure around the tip of the finger and hematoma to facilitate drainage. In case of continuous bleeding elevate the digit and apply firm and continuous pressure over the nail with a gauze piece.
7. Apply topical antibiotic ointment (e.g., bacitracin) over the puncture hole.
8. Apply a gauze dressing or a bandage over the wound site/fingernail.
9. Apply a finger splint (optional) to provide additional comfort.
10. Recommend the patient to keep the finger or toe dry (avoid soaking) and elevated for 1–2 days.

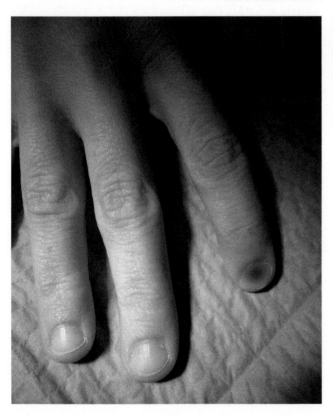

Fig. 96.1 Subungal hematoma of right index finger

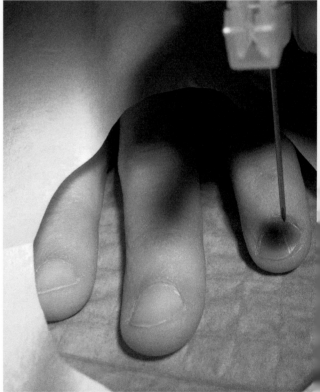

Fig. 96.2 Positioning of needle to perform subungal hematom drainage

96.6 Complications (Rare)

- Infection
- Injury to nail bed or underlying bone if too much pressure is applied with puncture
- Onycholysis when there is incomplete drainage in rare cases

96.7 Pearls and Pitfalls

- Pearls
  - Multiple holes may be necessary for appropriate drainage of the hematoma.
  - When using electrocautery for hole puncture, execute high caution with acrylic nails because they are flammable.
  - When using a paper clip or regular needle, make sure to sterilize the tip over a flame.
  - Take a radiograph of the finger whenever necessary to rule out phalangeal fracture.
  - Check for avulsion of the extensor tendon.
  - Inform the patient that the existing nail may fall off and will regenerate in few months if the nailbed is intact.
  - Systemic or oral antibiotics are not recommended.
- Pitfalls
  - Development of a dark color change over the nailbed without any history of trauma should raise suspicion of a tumor and should be evaluated accordingly.
  - Do not remove the nail to evaluate injury to nailbed.

Selected Reading

Brown RE. Acute nail bed injuries. Hand Clin. 2002;18:561–75.

Dean B, Becker G, Little C. The management of the acute traumatic subungual haematoma: a systematic review. Hand Surg. 2012;17:151–4.

Incision and Drainage of Abscess

Nicholas D. Caputo, Karlene Hosford,
and Muhammad Waseem

97.1 Indications

- Abscess greater than 5 mm in diameter and in accessible areas (e.g., axilla, extremities, trunk)

97.2 Contraindications

- Absolute
  - Absence of fluctuation
  - Large, deep, and complicated (multiloculated) abscesses
  - Location
    - Perianal
    - Mastoid
- Relative
  - Location
    - Face (e.g., nose, nasolabial fold)
    - Palms

- Coagulopathy
- Recurrent pilonidal cysts (may mandate operative excision)
- Area of cosmetic importance where aspiration may be preferred

97.3 Materials and Medications

- Incision and drainage tray (Fig. 97.1)
  - Drape
  - Betadine (povidone-iodine) swabs
  - 1 % lidocaine
  - 18- and 27-gauge needles
  - 12-mL syringes, gauze pads
  - #11 scalpel, mosquito clamps (hemostat)
  - Iodoform packing of appropriate size
- Ultrasound machine (Fig. 97.2)

.D. Caputo, MD, MSc
.mergency Department Critical Care, Lincoln Medical and Mental
.ealth Center, New York, NY, USA
.mail: Ncaputo.md@gmail.com

. Hosford, MD • M. Waseem, MD (✉)
.epartment of Emergency Medicine, Lincoln Medical and Mental
.ealth Center, New York, NY, USA
.mail: krlhos@aol.com; waseemm2001@hotmail.com

.Springer Science+Business Media New York 2016
.Ganti (ed.), *Atlas of Emergency Medicine Procedures*, DOI 10.1007/978-1-4939-2507-0_97

Fig. 97.1 Supplies necessary for incision and drainage

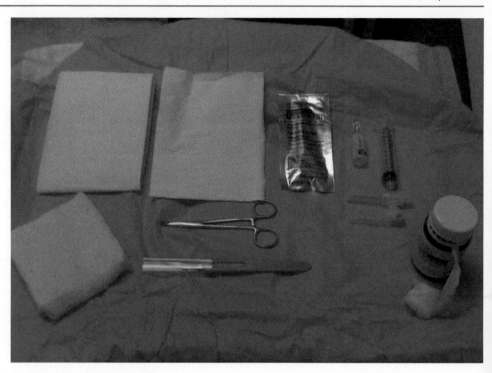

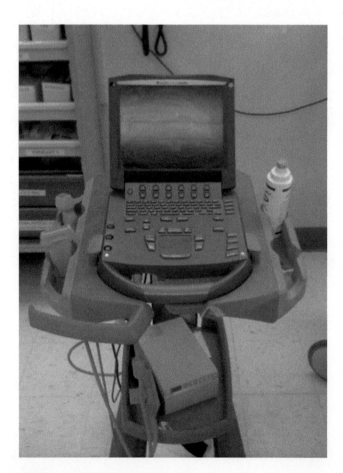

Fig. 97.2 Bedside SonoSite ultrasound

97.4   Procedure

1. Ultrasound (optional) may be helpful when abscess is suspected in the absence of fluctuation. Using the vascular probe (7 mHz), confirm the clinical suspicion of abscess and check the depth and width of the abscess (Fig. 97.3).
2. Sterile skin preparation with Betadine swab and sterile drape.
3. Anesthetize the appropriate area subcutaneously with 5 mL of 1 % lidocaine by inserting the 27-gauge needle at an acute angle into the intradermal space (Fig. 97.4a, b).
4. Using a #11 blade, make an approximately 1- to 2-cm skin incision over the desired area parallel to the Langer lines. The incision must approach into the abscess cavity (Fig. 97.4c).
   - Some physicians still advocate the technique of making a cruciate incision. This may leave a larger scar and should be discussed with patient before doing so because of cosmetic consequences.

5. Allow for spontaneous drainage. After resolution of drainage, you may express more pus with gentle downward pressure.
6. Using the hemostat, enter the incision to break any suspected loculations. This should be done with the clamps closed and curved part down. The clamps should then be opened and removed slowly (Fig. 97.4d).
7. After clearing the remaining loculations, the wound should be packed.
   - Evidence suggests that packing the abscesses does not prevent recurrence; however, this is still practiced. If packing the wound, follow the next step.
8. Take the iodoform packing with the hemostat, and place the packing into the incision site until no further packing will fit.
9. Cut the packing leaving a tail out of the incision site (Fig. 97.4e).
10. Apply dressing with 4×4 gauze and adhesive tape (2 in.).

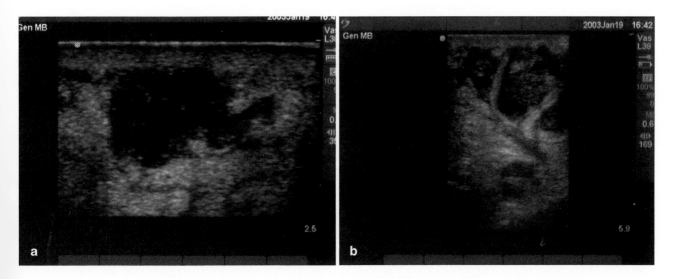

Fig. 97.3 (**a**) Example of an abscess as viewed on bedside ultrasound. (**b**) A multiloculated abscess

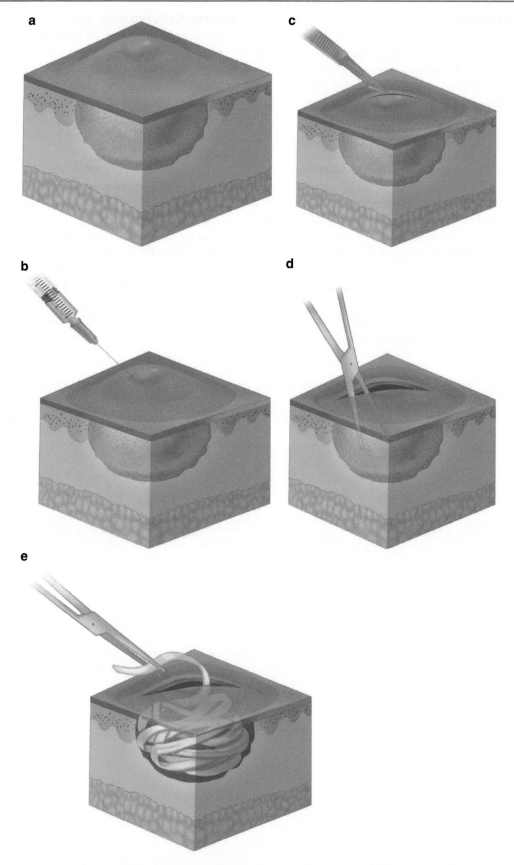

Fig. 97.4 (**a**) Abscess with overlying erythema. (**b**) Lidocaine injection in the superficial layer. (**c**) Linear incision with #11 blade. (**d**) Expression of purulent material and breaking of loculations with clamps. (**e**) Optional placement of packing

97.5   Complications

- Recurrence of abscess
- Progression of cellulitis
- Neurovascular injury to adjacent structures

97.6   Pearls

Antibiotic coverage is a controversial topic. Methicillin-resistant *Staphylococcus aureus* (MRSA) is a concern not only in the immunocompromised and diabetic patients. *S. aureus* has been detected in up to 51 % of patients with abscesses. Of these isolates, approximately 75 % were MRSA. Bactrim (trimethoprim/sulfamethoxazole) should be utilized for all prophylactic measures.

Selected Reading

Barnes SM, Milsom PL. Abscess: an open and shut case. Arch Emerg Med. 1988;5:200–5.

Burney RE. Incision and drainage procedures: soft tissue abscesses in the emergency service. Emerg Med Clin North Am. 1986;4:527–42.

Duong M, Markwell S, Peter J, Barenkamp S. Randomized, controlled trial of antibiotics in the management of community-acquired skin abscesses in the pediatric patient. Ann Emerg Med. 2010;55:401–7.

Fitch MT, Manthey DE, McGinnis HD, Nicks BA, Pariyadath M. Abscess incision and drainage. N Engl J Med. 2007;357:e20.

Frazee BW, Lynn J, Charlebois ED, Lambert L, Lowery D, Perdreau-Remington F. High prevalence of methicillin-resistant *Staphylococcus aureus* in emergency department skin and soft tissue infections. Ann Emerg Med. 2005;45:311–20.

Hankin A, Everett WW. Are antibiotics necessary after incision and drainage of a cutaneous abscess? Ann Emerg Med. 2007;50:49–51.

O'Malley GF, Dominici P, Giraldo P, et al. Routine packing of simple cutaneous abscesses is painful and probably unnecessary. Acad Emerg Med. 2009;16:470–3.

Splinting

98

Christopher H. Stahmer and Muhammad Waseem

98.1 Indications

- Need for immobilization for fracture, dislocation, or soft tissue injury
- Suspicion for occult injury of an extremity
- Immobilization for pain management

98.2 Contraindications

- Absolute
  - Open fracture (requires operative intervention)
- Relative
  - Infection
  - Compartment syndrome

98.3 Materials and Medications (Fig. 98.1)

- Plaster of Paris
- Fast drying: 5–8 min to set
- Extra fast drying: 2–4 min to set
  - Variety of widths depending upon splint of choice:
  - Splints may take up to 2 days to dry and achieve maximum strength.
- Prefabricated splinting materials
  - Plaster OCL® (Orthopedic Casting Laboratories)
    - 10–20 sheets of plaster with padding and cover
    - Faster setup time but less customizable

- Fiberglass splints
  - Cure rapidly
  - Less messy
  - Less moldable
  - Stronger and lighter
- Stockinette.
  - Protects the skin.
  - Variety of sizes available.
- Soft wrap (Webril™).
  - Provides padding.
  - Five to six layers depending on anticipated swelling.
    - Too much padding reduces the stability of the splint.
  - Use extra padding over bony prominences.
  - Pad between digits for splinting of digits.
  - Avoid wrinkles, which generate pressure points.
  - Do not wrap circumferentially.
    - Increased risk of ischemia.
- Ace wraps.
  - Variety of sizes depending.
    - Larger widths over legs.
    - Narrow widths around fingers and joints.
      - Avoid bunching by using narrow widths at joints.
- Water
  - Warm water and splint sets more quickly but increases the risk of burns.
    - Splint drying is an exothermic or heat-releasing reaction.
  - Hot water leaves less time to mold the splint.

C.H. Stahmer, MD • M. Waseem, MD (✉)
Department of Emergency Medicine, Lincoln Medical and Mental Health Center, New York, NY, USA
e-mail: stahmer@gmail.com; waseemm2001@hotmail.com

© Springer Science+Business Media New York 2016
R. Ganti (ed.), *Atlas of Emergency Medicine Procedures*, DOI 10.1007/978-1-4939-2507-0_98

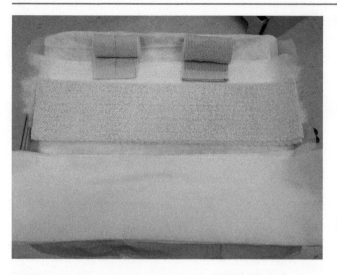

Fig. 98.1 Posterior splint materials: plaster of Paris, Ace wraps, soft roll. Note there are two layers of soft wrap: the inner layer to face the patient (eight layers) and the outer layer to pad the exterior (two layers)

98.4 Procedure

1. Completely expose and examine the afflicted body part for tissue, vascular, or neurological injury.
   - Address respective injuries before proceeding.
2. Lay out all splinting materials before initiating procedure.
   - Layer plaster of Paris.
     - Upper extremity: 8–10 layers.
     - Lower extremity: 12–15 layers.
     - Up to 20 for a large person.
     - More layers of plaster of Paris increase the risk of burn and the weight of the splint.
3. Administer appropriate anesthesia.
   - Conscious sedation
   - Hematoma block
   - Intra-articular injection
   - Intravenous pain medication
   - Oral pain medication
4. Hang fractures as indicated for improved success of reduction to relax muscles before reduction attempt.
5. Reduce afflicted extremity.
6. While maintaining reduction, apply respective splint.
7. Apply in the following order for plaster of Paris splint.
   - Stockinette (not necessary).
   - Soft wrap.
   - Select appropriate layers of plaster of Paris.
   - Prepare plaster of Paris to create splint:
     - Layer plaster with no overlap.
     - Submerge completely into water.
     - Crumple into ball without letting go of the ends of the splint.
     - Release the lower end of the splint while holding the top tightly together.
     - Run fingers in a "squeegee" manner from top to bottom to smooth the splint (Fig. 98.2).
       - This also removes excess water.
       - Repeat until the splint is smooth and free of dripping water.
     - Apply soft wrap layers to the splint.
       - Apply thicker layer to the patient's body.
       - Apply two or three layers of soft wrap to the exterior of plaster of Paris for padding and to facilitate drying.
     - Apply Ace wrap to hold the splint and assist in contouring the splint to the patient's extremity (Fig. 98.3).
       - Applying the Ace wrap too tightly may cause ischemia. Observe the patient after splinting for 30 min for tingling, burning, pain, or discomfort.
     - Mold the splint without making indentations with the fingertips (Fig. 98.4).
       - An indentation may cause a pressure point which may result in an ulcer.

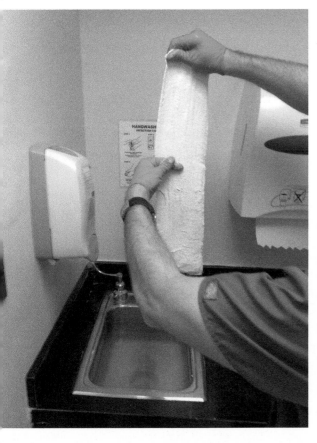

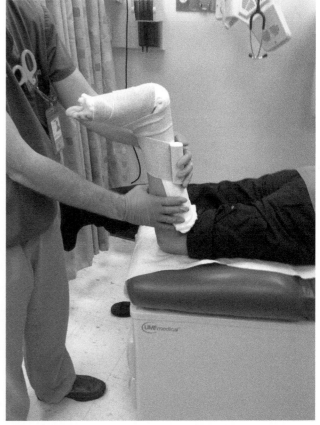

Fig. 98.2 Hold the top of the saturated plaster securely with one hand while removing excess water with the other hand

Fig. 98.3 Apply Ace wrap to hold the splint and assist in contouring the splint to the patient's extremity

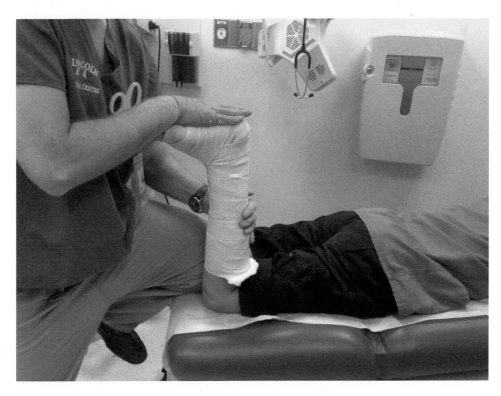

Fig. 98.4 Hold the splint in a neutral anatomical position while taking care not to make indentations with the fingertips

– Allow the splint to cure while the practitioner maintains the appropriate position. This will take approximately 5 min depending upon water temperature and splint thickness.

98.5 Complications

- Ischemia may result in compartment syndrome.
  - Advise the patient to unwrap the splint for the following indications.
    - Increasing pain.
    - Discoloration of fingers, toes, or the splinted extremity.
    - Loss of sensation of splinted extremity.
- Burns
  - Plaster drying releases heat.
  - Increased risk with limited layers of padding.
  - If pain is troubling the patient, remove the splint and add more padding.

- Pressure sores
  - Apply ample padding.
  - Smooth all wrinkles.
  - Instruct the patient to return for increased discomfort.
- Infection
  - Clean and débride all devitalized tissue before application.
  - Requires close follow-up to reevaluate wounds.

Selected Reading

Fitch MT, Nicks BA, Pariyadath M, McGinnis HD, Manthey DE. Basic splinting techniques. N Engl J Med. 2008;359:e32.

Marx JA, Hockberger R, Walls R, editors. Rosen's emergency medicine: concepts and clinical practice. 7th ed. Philadelphia: Mosby; 2010.

Simon R, Sherman S, Koenigsknecht S. Emergency orthopedics—the extremities. New York: McGraw-Hill; 2007.

Ulnar Gutter Splint

99

Jeffrey Kile, Katrina John, and Amish Aghera

99.1 Indications

- Fractures and soft tissue injuries of the ring or little finger
- Fractures of the neck, shaft, or base of the fourth or fifth metacarpal

99.2 Contraindications

- Relative
  - Evidence of compartment syndrome or any neurovascular compromise

99.3 Materials (Fig. 99.1)

- Splint roll (plaster of Paris, prefabricated foamcore, or fiberglass)
- Stockinette
- Cotton padding, such as simple cotton sheet wadding or a newer alternative such as Webril (Curity), Specialist (Johnson & Johnson), and so on
- Elastic bandages, such as Ace (3M) or similar
- Shears
- Adhesive tape
- Gloves

Kile, MBBS, PhD, MPH (✉) • K. John, MBBS
Department of Emergency Medicine, Eisenhower Medical Center,
Rancho Mirage, CA, USA
email: jeffrey.kile@gmail.com; trenjohn@me.com

Aghera, MD
Department of Emergency Medicine, Maimonides Medical Center,
New York, NY, USA
email: aaghera@maimonidesmed.org

Springer Science+Business Media New York 2016
Ganti (ed.), *Atlas of Emergency Medicine Procedures*, DOI 10.1007/978-1-4939-2507-0_99

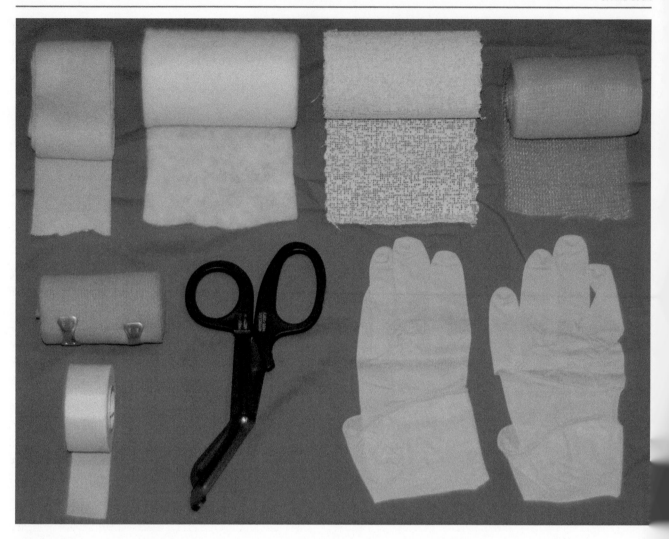

Fig. 99.1 Materials and medications

99.4 Procedure

1. Select the appropriate diameter stockinette according to the size of the forearm.
   - Generally, 3-in. diameter stockinette is used for the ulnar gutter splint.
2. Cut the stockinette to a length approximately 20 cm longer than the total length of the desired splint.
3. Apply the stockinette to the injured limb so that the stockinette extends approximately 10 cm beyond the region to be splinted proximally and distally.
4. Cut the distal aspect of the stockinette to free the thumb and also the index and middle finger (Fig. 99.2).
5. Insert cotton padding cut to the appropriate size between the ring and the little fingers to prevent skin degradation (Fig. 99.3).
6. Wrap cotton padding circumferentially around the entire region to be splinted, with each turn overlapping the previous turn by approximately 25 % of its width.
   - Generally, 3-in.-wide padding is used for the ulnar gutter splint.
   - Apply padding to an approximate thickness of 1 cm, with extra padding placed over the bony prominences of the wrist and carpometacarpal joints.
   - Extend the padding at least an inch beyond the desired splint length so that it may later be folded back over the jagged ends of the plaster or fiberglass splint roll (Fig. 99.4).
7. Unwrap and prepare an appropriate length splint.
   - The width of splinting material used should be approximately one-half the circumference of the extremity measured at the wrist, such that it is wide enough to extend approximately halfway around the distal forearm once applied.
   - Layer the splint eight sheets thick if using plaster roll and six sheets thick if using fiberglass roll.
   - It is best to begin with a generous length of splinting material because both plaster and fiberglass splint rolls shrink slightly once moistened. If the wet splint turns out too long, the ends can be either folded back or cut with shears before hardening.

8. Apply the dry splinting material to the ulnar aspect of the extremity from the midforearm to just beyond the distal interphalangeal joint of the little finger and cut the splint to approximately 20 cm longer than the desired length.
9. Submerge the dry splint in water until bubbling stops.
10. Remove the splint from water, place on a hard flat surface, and smooth out the excess water to ensure no wrinkles are present.
11. Apply to the splint to the limb over the cotton padding.
    - If the splint is too long at this stage, the ends may be folded back or cut with shears to the proper length.
12 Once positioned properly, fold the side of the splint up around the ulnar aspect of the forearm and hand to form a gutter (Fig. 99.5).
13. Fold the underlying cotton padding and stockinette back over the ends of the splint, which both protects the skin and holds the splint in place.
14. Secure the loose end(s) of the elastic bandage with adhesive tape.
    - Avoid using the metal clips often packaged with elastic bandages because these can become displaced and embed in the skin.
15. Manipulate the forearm and hand into the "neutral" position: (1) the wrist in slight extension (10–20°), (2) the metacarpophalangeal joints in 50° of flexion, and (3) the proximal and distal interphalangeal joints of the ring and little finger in slight flexion (10–15°) (Fig. 99.6).
    - When splinting a boxer's (i.e., metacarpal neck) fracture, the metacarpophalangeal joint should be flexed to 90°.
16. Mold the splint to the contour of the extremity (Fig. 99.7).
    - Use only the palms of the hands when molding because the fingertips may cause indentations, resulting in excessive skin pressure.
17. Wrap the extremity with an elastic bandage in a distal-to-proximal direction to secure the splint in place (Fig. 99.8).
18. Ensure the extremity is neurovascularly intact.
19. Instruct the patient to loosen the elastic bandage if it feels too tight.

Fig. 99.2 Stockinette applied to the forearm and hand

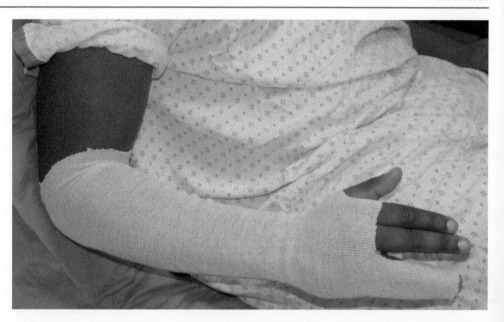

Fig. 99.3 Cotton padding applied to the ring and little fingers

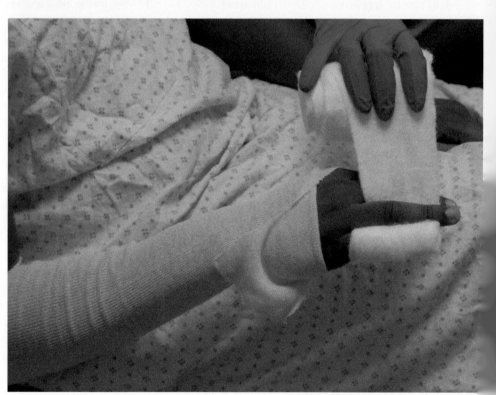

Fig. 99.4 Cotton padding applied to the forearm and hand

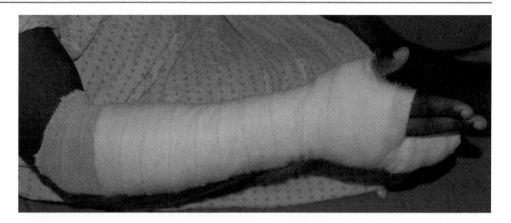

Fig. 99.5 Splint folded around the ulnar aspect of the forearm and hand

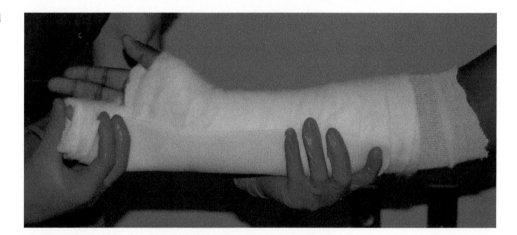

Fig. 99.6 Forearm and hand in the neutral position (without splint)

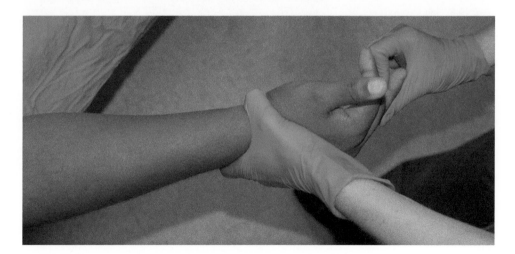

Fig. 99.7 Splint molded to maintain the forearm and hand in the neutral position

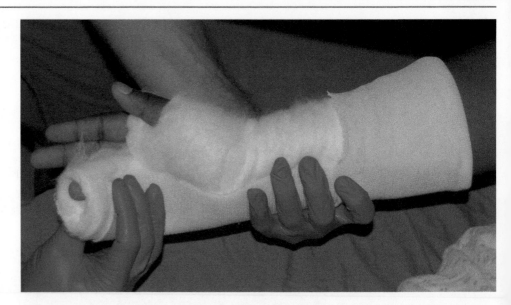

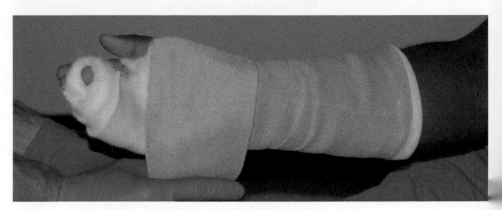

Fig. 99.8 Splint secured in place with an elastic bandage

99.5   Complications

- Neurovascular or other soft tissue compromise (if the splint/bandage is too tight)
- Soft tissue degradation (if the splint is left in place too long)

99.6   Pearls and Pitfalls

- Pearls
  - Simple plaster of Paris splints are inexpensive and allow a thoroughly customizable fit but can be damaged by water and require more time to set and more clean up than prefabricated foamcore or fiberglass splint rolls.
  - Simple fiberglass splints set quickly, are not damaged by water, are stronger and lighter than simple plaster and prefabricated splints, and offer a fully customized fit, but are not applied as quickly as prefabricated splints.
  - Prefabricated fiberglass splints are quickly applied, require virtually no clean up, and are not damaged by water, but are relatively expensive and provide a somewhat less customizable fit than simple splint rolls.
  - Stockinette protects the skin and, when folded back over the ends of the plaster or fiberglass splint roll, holds the wet splint in place before the elastic bandage is placed, and provides a padded rim with a professional appearance.
- Pitfalls
  - Avoid wrinkling the cotton padding applied between the stockinette and the splinting material because, once under the pressure of the elastic bandage, wrinkles can cause unnecessary skin pressure.
  - Avoid using more or fewer layers of splinting material than recommended. Additional layers can result in excessive heat during the setting process and a splint that is too heavy, whereas insufficient layers can result in a splint that is too weak.

Selected Reading

Harrison BP, Hilliard MW. Emergency department evaluation and treatment of hand injuries. Emerg Med Clin North Am. 1999;17: 793–822.

Henry MH. Fractures of the proximal phalanx and metacarpals in the hand: preferred methods of stabilization. J Am Acad Orthop Surg. 2008;16:586–95.

Margic K. External fixation of closed metacarpal and phalangeal fractures of digits. A prospective study of one hundred consecutive patients. J Hand Surg Br. 2006;31:30–40.

McMahon PJ, Woods DA, Burge PD. Initial treatment of closed metacarpal fractures. A controlled comparison of compression glove and splintage. J Hand Surg Br. 1994;19:597–600.

Viegas SF, Tencer A, Woodard P, Williams CR. Functional bracing of fractures of the second through fifth metacarpals. J Hand Surg Am. 1987;12:139–43.

Shoulder Dislocation Reduction Techniques

100

Katrina Skoog Nguyen, L. Connor Nickels, and Rohit Pravin Patel

00.1 Indications

Subjective history of new-onset dislocation or recurrent dislocations combined with clinical assessment consistent with shoulder dislocation

- Anterior dislocations (96 %)
  - Typical mechanism of injury being indirect, with combination of abduction, extension, and external rotation. Rarely, the etiology is a direct blow to the posterior shoulder.
  - Prominent acromion with a palpable drop off below the acromion and subclavicular region fullness is consistent with anterior shoulder dislocation.
- Posterior dislocations (4 %)
  - Mechanism of injury is indirect with a combination of internal rotation, adduction, and flexion. Precipitating events include seizure, electrical shock, and falls.

- More subtle presentation. Patient will maintain arm locked in internal rotation and adduction; he or she cannot externally rotate. Shoulder is flattened anteriorly and rounded posteriorly.
- Ultrasound can be used to prevent missed or delayed diagnosis (Figs. 100.1 and 100.2 show probe positioning and a diagram of abnormal ultrasound anatomy).
- Inferior dislocations (luxation erecta)
  - Arm will be held fixed in overhead position.
- Radiographs reveal shoulder dislocation.
- Ultrasound can be used to identify the nature of the dislocation (anterior or posterior) and can be determined by the position of the humeral head relative to the transducer and glenoid. Although at this point, it should not replace radiographs owing to missed fractures. Advantages may include less radiation (decreased need for postreduction x-rays) and re-sedation if reduction is not complete.

, Skoog Nguyen, DO
orthwest Community Hospital, Arlington Heights, IL, USA
mail: katrinaskoog@hotmail.com

C. Nickels, MD, RDMS (⊠) • R.P. Patel, MD
epartment of Emergency Medicine, University of Florida Health
ands Hospital, Gainesville, FL, USA
mail: cnickels@ufl.edu; rohitpatel@ufl.edu

Springer Science+Business Media New York 2016
Ganti (ed.), *Atlas of Emergency Medicine Procedures*, DOI 10.1007/978-1-4939-2507-0_100

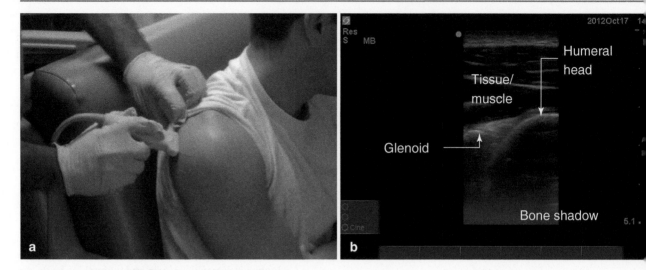

Fig. 100.1 (**a**, **b**) Ultrasound image of normal shoulder anatomy. "Dot fits the Dot" means when looking at the ultrasound machine from the sonographer's standpoint, the side of the probe marker corresponds to the side the marker is on the screen. This ensures when doing procedures, the direction of needle correction is the same as the orientation the probe (Images courtesy of Dr. Rohit Patel)

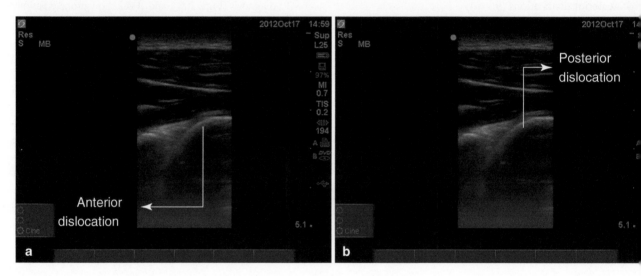

Fig. 100.2 Anterior (**a**) and posterior (**b**) dislocations (Images courtesy of Dr. Rohit Patel)

100.2 Contraindications

- Associated fracture
  - This warrants orthopedic evaluation.
- Associated neurovascular deficit
  - May attempt reduction once but avoid multiple attempts.

100.3 Materials and Medications

- 1 % lidocaine, with syringe and needle and povidone-iodine prep if administering local anesthesia
- Moderate sedation medications if administering moderate sedation
- Bed sheet for traction-countertraction method
- Dangling weight for Stimson maneuver

100.4 Procedure

- Physical examination
  - Compare affected with unaffected shoulder.
  - Perform a complete neurovascular examination: test axillary, radial, ulnar, and median nerves for sensory deficit and motor function.
- Radiographs
  - Always obtain before attempting reduction for assessment of possible fracture and type and position of dislocation.
  - Obtain three views: anteroposterior, scapular Y, and axillary lateral views.
  - Anterior dislocations: humeral head appears anterior to the glenoid fossa on lateral or Y views.

- Posterior dislocations: on anteroposterior view (vacant glenoid sign, 6-mm sign, lightbulb sign; on lateral or Y view: humeral head appears posterior to glenoid fossa).
- Pain management and sedation
  - Decide whether to use intra-articular lidocaine versus procedural sedation and analgesia.
  - For intra-articular lidocaine
    - Use 10–20 mL of 1 % lidocaine.
    - Attach a 1.5-in., 20-gauge needle.
    - Prepare the shoulder with povidone-iodine.
    - Insert the needle lateral to the acromion process and 2 cm inferiorly into the sulcus.
    - After withdrawing to ensure that the needle is not in a vessel, inject 10–20 mL lidocaine into the joint.
- Reduction techniques: it is important for the emergency department physician to be familiar with several different techniques. The following techniques are presented:

100.4.1 Stimson Maneuver (Fig. 100.3)

1. Patient is placed prone with 2.5–5 kg of weight hanging from the wrist.
2. Reduction may be facilitated by traction and external rotation of the arm.
3. A success rate of 96 % has been reported using the combined prone position, hanging weights, intravenous drug therapy, and scapular manipulation.

- Advantage: can be performed by one person only.
- Disadvantages: requires time to gather materials; the danger involved in the patient falling off the stretcher, requiring staff to monitor the patient.

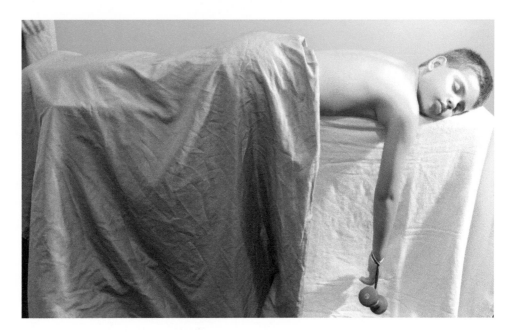

ig. 100.3 Stimson maneuver

100.4.2 Scapular Manipulation Technique (Fig. 100.4)

1. Place the patient in the prone position with the affected arm hanging downward.
2. Apply traction down on the arm.
3. Locate the inferior tip of the scapula. Simultaneously push the inferior tip of the scapula medially toward the spine and use the other hand push the superior scapula laterally.

- Advantages: high success rate, greater than 90 %; very safe to perform.
- Disadvantages: it requires the patient to assume the prone position; may require another person to perform traction.

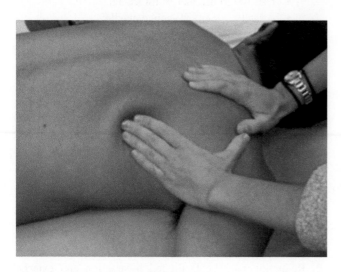

Fig. 100.4 Scapular manipulation method

100.4.3 External Rotation Method
(Fig. 100.5)

1. Place the patient in the supine position with the affected arm adducted directly next to the patient's side with the elbow flexed to 90°.
2. The operator uses one hand to direct downward traction on the affected arm while maintaining it next to the patient's side.

3. The operator uses the other hand to hold the patient's wrist and guide the arm into slow external rotation.
4. Reduction usually takes place between 70° and 110° of external rotation.

• Advantages: requires no strength by operator; well tolerated by patients.
• Disadvantage: patient may have persistent dislocation during procedure, requiring operator to make adjustments.

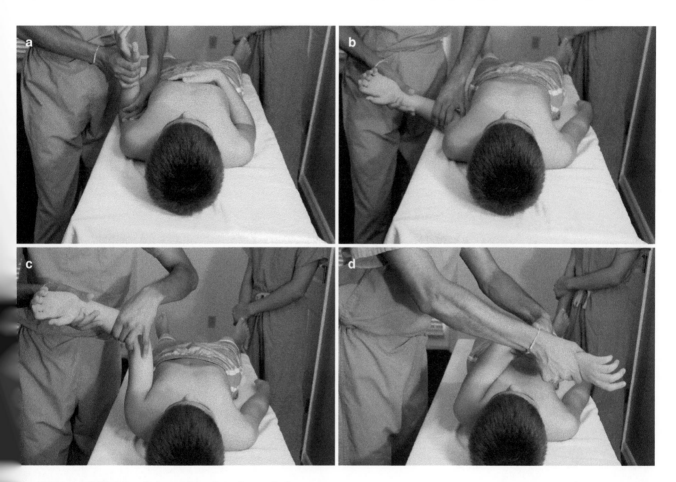

Fig. 100.5 (a–d) Kocher technique: external rotation method

100.4.4 Milch Technique (Fig. 100.6)

1. Technique looks as though one is reaching up to grab an apple from a tree.
2. Abduct the injured arm up to the overhead position.
3. Once in the overhead position, apply gentle vertical traction with external rotation.
4. An adjustment may need to be made if the reduction does not occur easily; push the humeral head upward into the glenoid fossa.

- Advantages: lack of complications; patient tolerance
- Disadvantage: variable success rate reported: 70–90 %

100.4.5 Spaso Technique (Fig. 100.7)

1. Place the patient in the supine position.
2. Operator grasps the affected arm at the wrist and lifts the straight arm directly upward while applying longitudinal traction.
3. Apply external rotation.

- Advantages: single operator, high level of success
- Disadvantage: may require more time to allow the shoulder muscles to relax

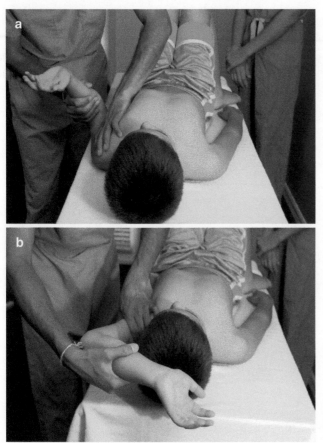

Fig. 100.6 (**a, b**) Milch technique

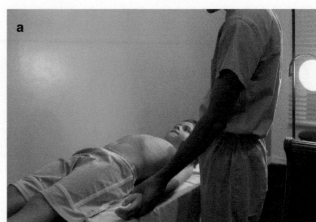

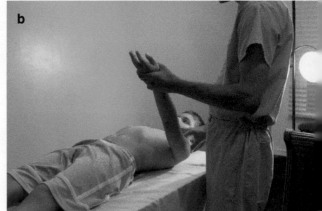

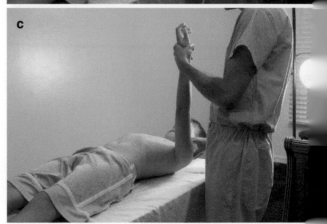

Fig. 100.7 (**a–c**) Spaso technique (Photographs courtesy of Dr. Pra... S. Patel)

100.4.6 Traction-Countertraction Technique (Fig. 100.8)

1. With the patient is sitting up, have an assistant wrap a sheet around the upper chest and under the axilla of the affected shoulder. Have the assistant wrap the sheet behind her or his back. Now have the patient lay supine.
2. Wrap another sheet around the flexed elbow of the affected arm and behind the operator's back.
3. Both the operator and the assistant lean back, applying gentle traction.

- Advantage: many older physicians are familiar with this method and, therefore, have a high degree of success.
- Disadvantages: requires two people; may cause skin tears on elderly patients.

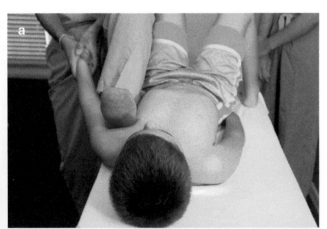

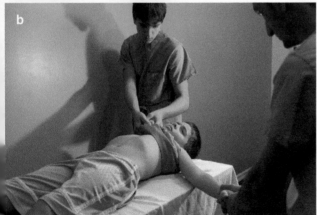

Fig. 100.8 (**a, b**) Hippocrates method/traction-countertraction method

100.4.7 Posterior Shoulder Dislocation Reduction

1. Give adequate premedication.
2. Place the patient supine and apply lateral traction on the proximal humerus.
3. Have an assistant apply anterior pressure to the posteriorly located humeral head.

- Advantage: logical methods for reduction
- Disadvantages: require sufficient premedication because often posterior dislocations present late; may require open reduction

100.4.8 Postreduction

- Obtain postreduction x-rays. There is some literature on using ultrasound to confirm adequate reduction, which allows repetitive assessments throughout procedure, as well as reduce radiation (see Fig. 100.2 for ultrasound of anterior and posterior dislocations).
- Do a postreduction neurovascular examination.
- Sling and swath or shoulder immobilizer for 2–3 weeks.
- Orthopedic follow-up in 1 week.

100.5 Complications

- Fractures
- Adhesive capsulitis, or frozen shoulder; especially a concern in the elderly with prolonged immobilization in sling
- Brachial plexus injury, especially of the axillary nerve
- Vascular laceration, most commonly of the axillary artery
- Rotator cuff tears

100.6 Pearls

- It is imperative to document the pre- and postreduction neurovascular status in the medical record.
- If unsure whether the reduction was successful, attempt to place the palm of the injured extremity on the contralateral shoulder. This is a good sign the reduction was successful.

Acknowledgment The authors would like to thank Karthik Stead for serving as the subject in many of the photographs in this chapter.

Selected Reading

Beck S, Chilstrom M. Point-of-care ultrasound diagnosis and treatment of posterior shoulder dislocation. Am J Emerg Med. 2013;31:449. e3–5.

Blakeley CJ, Spencer O, Newman-Saunders T, Hashemi K. A novel use of portable ultrasound in the management of shoulder dislocation. Emerg Med J. 2009;26:662–3.

Dala-Ali B, Penna M, McConnell J, Vanhegan I, Cobiella C. Management of acute anterior shoulder dislocation. Br J Sports Med. 2014;48(16):1209–15.

Simão MN, Noqueira-Barbosa MH, Muqlia VF, Barbieri CH. Anterior shoulder instability: correlation between magnetic resonance arthrography, ultrasound arthrography, and intraoperative findings. Ultrasound Med Biol. 2012;38:551–60.

Yuen CK, Chung TS, Mok KL, Kan PG, Wong YT. Dynamic ultrasonographic sign for posterior shoulder dislocation. Emerg Radiol. 2011;18:47–51.

Elbow Dislocation Reduction

Katrina John, Jeffrey Kile, and Amish Aghera

101.1 Indications

- Any dislocation of the elbow joint. Direction of the dislocation (i.e., anterior, posterior, lateral and divergent radius, and ulnar dislocations) is determined by the position of the ulna relative to the joint space (Fig. 101.1).

Fig. 101.1 Anatomical depiction

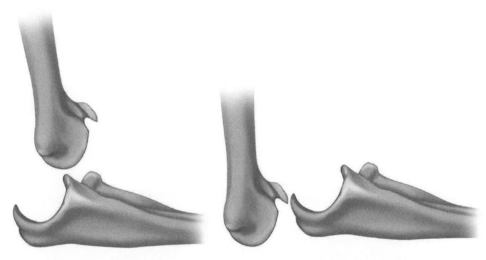

Posterior dislocation   **Anterior dislocation**

101.2 Contraindications

- Relative
  - Compound fracture dislocation

K. John, MBBS • J. Kile, MBBS, PhD, MPH (✉)
Department of Emergency Medicine, Eisenhower Medical Center,
Rancho Mirage, CA, USA
e-mail: trenjohn@me.com; jeffrey.kile@gmail.com

A. Aghera, MD
Department of Emergency Medicine, Maimonides Medical Center,
New York, NY, USA
e-mail: aaghera@maimonidesmed.org

© Springer Science+Business Media New York 2016
. Ganti (ed.), *Atlas of Emergency Medicine Procedures*, DOI 10.1007/978-1-4939-2507-0_101

101.3 Materials and Medications

- Parenteral sedation and analgesia medications
- Local anesthetic for local and intra-articular anesthesia
- Splinting material
- Stockinette
- Padding
- Elastic bandage
- Tape
- Sling

101.4 Procedure for Posterior Dislocations

1. Obtain a true lateral and anteroposterior radiographs of the affected elbow.
2. Ensure adequate sedation and analgesia.
3. Consider intra-articular analgesia.
4. Check the neurovascular status of affected extremity.
5. Follow a selected method for reduction as detailed later.
6. Following successful reduction gently flex the elbow to ensure full range of motion.
7. Place a long-arm posterior splint with the elbow in at least 90° flexion and secure the arm in a regular sling.
8. Check neurovascular status.
9. Obtain a postreduction radiograph of the elbow.

101.4.1 Method A (Fig. 101.2)

1. Position the patient on a stretcher in the supine position.
2. Apply steady traction at the supinated distal forearm keeping the elbow slightly flexed, while an assistant applies countertraction to the midhumerus with both hands.

101.4.2 Method B (Fig. 101.3)

1. Position the patient on a stretcher in the supine position.
2. Extend the affected extremity over the edge of the stretcher.
3. Apply traction to the supinated forearm slightly flexed at the elbow, while an assistant holds the distal humerus with both hands and uses thumbs to apply pressure to the olecranon as if pushing it away from the humerus.

101.4.3 Method C (Fig. 101.4)

1. Position the patient on a stretcher in the prone position.
2. Hang the affected extremity over the side of the stretcher toward the floor.
3. Apply downward traction to the pronated distal forearm and with the other hand just above the patient's antecubital fossa lift the humerus toward you.

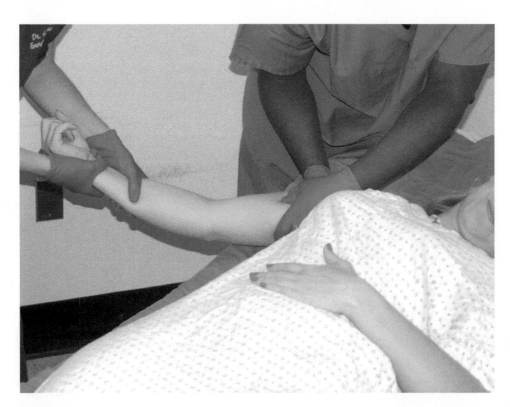

Fig. 101.2 Posterior method A

101.3 Posterior method B

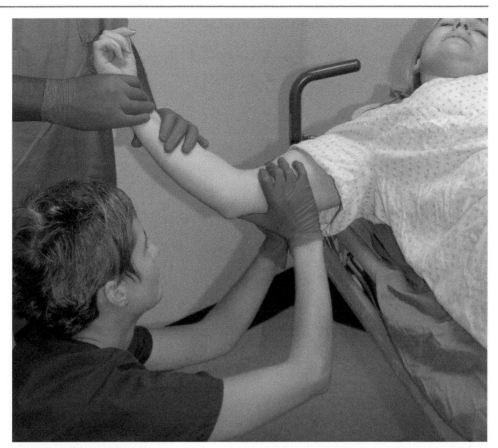

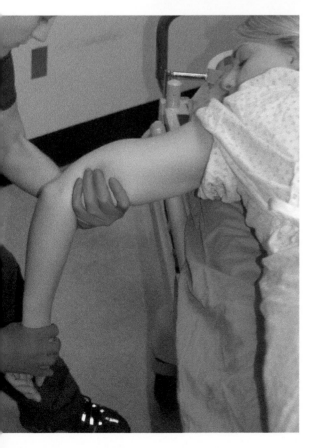

101.4 Posterior method C

101.5 Procedure for Anterior Dislocations
(Fig. 101.5)

1. Follow pre- and postprocedure steps as documented for the posterior dislocation.
2. Position the patient on a stretcher in the supine position.

3. With one hand, apply traction to the supinated distal forearm with the elbow extended, while an assistant applies countertraction with both hands around the distal humerus.
4. With the other hand apply downward and backward pressure over the proximal forearm just below the antecubital fossa.

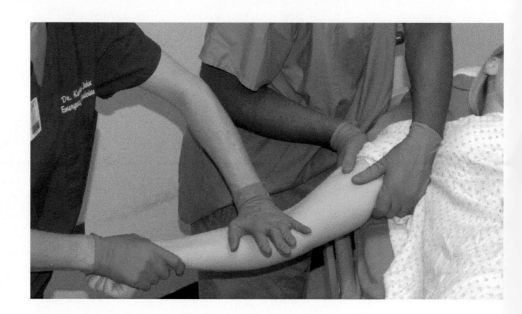

Fig. 101.5 Anterior elbow

101.6 Procedure for Radial Head Subluxations (See Also Chap. 127)

1. This procedure can normally be performed without any sedation or parenteral analgesia.
2. Position the patient, most commonly a child aged 1–3 years, facing forward on the caretaker's lap.
3. Hold the flexed elbow of the affected extremity placing your thumb firmly over the radial head.
4. With the other hand, take the child's hand and wrist, and in one continuous movement, hyperpronate and flex the forearm (Figs. 101.6 and 101.7).

5. Another method is to supinate and flex the forearm instead of hyperpronating it (Fig. 101.8).
6. Leave the room, encourage the caretaker to engage the child with distracting activities and reexamine the child in 10–20 min, at which stage, if reduction was successful, the child should be using the extremity normally again.
7. No postreduction radiograph or immobilization is required.

Fig. 101.6 Subluxation hyperpronated

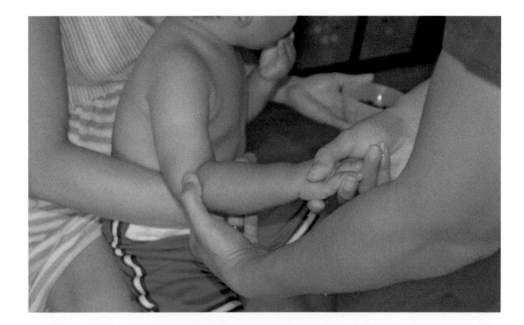

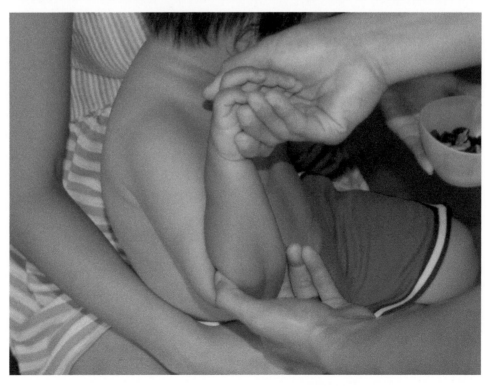

Fig. 101.7 Subluxation hyperpronated and flexed

Fig. 101.8 Subluxation
supinated

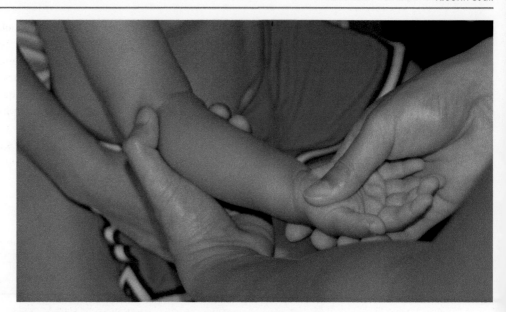

101.7 Complications

- Concomitant fractures
- Vascular injury, most commonly to the brachial artery
- Median nerve injury/entrapment
- Recurrent dislocation—rare

101.8 Pearls and Pitfalls

- Pearls
  - A true lateral radiograph is necessary to accurately detect and identify elbow fractures, dislocations, and soft tissue abnormalities (i.e., the fat pad sign). It is obtained with the patient's elbow in 90° flexion, in neutral rotation with the thumb pointing up and the arm and forearm resting on the radiograph cassette and the beam nearly perpendicular to the cassette. On a true lateral, the "hourglass" or "figure-of-eight" formation at the distal humerus should be clearly visible, and the rings of the capitellum and trochlea should be concentric.
  - During nursemaid elbow reduction, provide age appropriate distractions to divert the child's attention and minimize resistance.
- Pitfalls
  - On the pre- and postreduction radiographs, search for commonly associated fractures of the distal humerus, radial head, and coronoid process.

- Inability to range the elbow after apparent reduction indicates possible trapped fracture fragments and the need for operative intervention.
- Vascular or open injuries are common with anterior dislocations, and early orthopedic consultation is advised.
- Ninety percent of simple elbow dislocations are posterior, and this injury is rarely associated with vascular injury. However, it does occur, and vascular evaluation after every reduction is good clinical practice.

Selected Reading

Jain K, Shashi Kumar Y, Mruthyunjaya, Ravishankar R, Nair AV. Posterior dislocation of elbow with brachial artery injury. J Emerg Trauma Shock. 2010;3:308.

Kuhn MA, Ross G. Acute elbow dislocations. Orthop Clin North Am. 2008;39:155–61.

McDonald J, Witelaw C, Goldsmith LJ. Radial head subluxation. Comparing two methods of reduction. Acad Emerg Med. 1999;6:715.

Sheps DM, Hildebrand KA, Boorman RS. Simple dislocations of the elbow: evaluation and treatment. Hand Clin. 2004;20:389–404.

Villarin Jr LA, Belk KE, Freid R. Emergency department evaluation and treatment of elbow and forearm injuries. Emerg Med Clin North Am. 1999;17:843–58.

Distal Interphalangeal Joint Reduction

102

Justin Chen and Muhammad Waseem

stal interphalangeal (DIP) joint dislocation is rare. It occurs
.en an axial force is applied to the distal phalanx (Fig. 102.1).

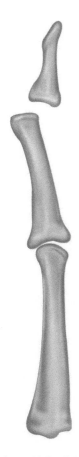

102.1 Distal interphalangeal joint dislocation

102.1 Indications

- DIP joint reduction is performed to alleviate functional and anatomical derangements resulting from DIP joint dislocation, commonly dorsal, from axial compression.

102.2 Contraindications

- Absolute
  - Absence of radiographic confirmation (anteroposterior, true lateral, and oblique) of simple DIP joint dislocation, especially in pediatric cases
- Relative
  - Open joint dislocation, associated fracture, or entrapped volar plate
  - Digital neurovascular compromise

102.3 Materials and Medications

- Latex-free gloves
- Local anesthetic: 2 % lidocaine without epinephrine, 1.5 % mepivacaine, 0.5 % ropivacaine, or 0.5 % bupivacaine
- 25-gauge × 1.5-in. needle (can substitute with 27 or 30 gauge)
- Small plastic syringe, 10 mL
- Padded, malleable, aluminum digital splint

'hen, MD, MSc
)artment of Emergency Medicine, North Shore University
spital, Manhasset, NY, USA
ail: chen.justin@gmail.com

Waseem, MD (✉)
)artment of Emergency Medicine, Lincoln Medical and Mental
lth Center, New York, NY, USA
ail: waseemm2001@hotmail.com

pringer Science+Business Media New York 2016
;anti (ed.), *Atlas of Emergency Medicine Procedures*, DOI 10.1007/978-1-4939-2507-0_102

102.4 Procedure

1. Place the patient in the seated position with the arms at rest on a bedside table or supported by an assistant.
2. Pronate the patient's hand, remove rings if present, and rest on a flat surface.
3. Insert a 25-gauge needle at the dorsolateral aspect of the base of the finger to form a wheal to reduce patient discomfort.
4. Advance the needle and direct anteriorly toward the phalangeal base.
5. Inject 0.5–1 mL of local anesthetic as the needle is withdrawn 1–2 mm from the point of bone contact.
6. Inject an additional 1 mL of local anesthetic continuously as the needle is withdrawn.
7. The injection should never render the tissue tense nor be circumferential.
8. Hyperextend the DIP joint while applying longitudinal traction, followed by immediate joint flexion at the base of the distal phalanx.
9. Place finger(s) in an aluminum digital dorsal splint in slight flexion for 2 weeks (Fig. 102.2).
10. Postreduction radiograph is recommended for confirmation.

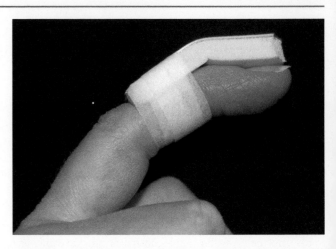

Fig. 102.2 Padded aluminum splint applied to block the DIP joint in flexion but allow further flexion, which encourages active flexion of that joint when the PIP joint flexes (Reproduced with permission from: HandLab Clinical Pearls Feb 2011, No 12. www.handlab.com)

102.5 Complications

- Irreducible dislocations
- Stiffness
- Recurrent dislocation
- Extensor lag in joints with residual subluxation
- Associated with dorsal joint prominences, swan-neck/boutonnière deformity, and degenerative arthritis

102.6 Pearls and Pitfalls

- Pearls
  - Lidocaine without epinephrine is preferred owing to the risk of vasoconstriction of the digital vessels with epinephrine.
  - Regardless of the mechanism of trauma, all joints (DIP, proximal interphalangeal, metacarpophalangeal) should be assessed for instability.

- Joint dislocations involving volar plate entrapment may require surgical repair (open reduction internal fixation) for successful reduction.
- Pitfalls
  - Irreducible DIP joint dislocations may be due to entrapment of an avulsion fracture, the profundus tendon, or the volar plate.

Selected Reading

Calfee RP, Sommerkamp TG. Fracture-dislocation about the finger joints [review]. J Hand Surg Am. 2009;34:1140–7.

Knoop KJ. Atlas of emergency medicine. 3rd ed. New York: McGraw-Hill Professional; 2010.

Simon RR, Sherman SC, Sharieff GQ. Emergency orthopedics. 6th ed. New York: McGraw-Hill Medical; 2011.

Stone CK, Humphries RL. Current diagnosis & treatment emergency medicine. 6th ed. New York: McGraw-Hill; 2008.

Tintinalli JE, Stapczynski JS, Ma OJ, Cline D, Cydulka R, Meckler G, editors. Tintinalli's emergency medicine: a comprehensive study guide. 7th ed. New York: McGraw-Hill; 2012.

Hip Dislocation Reduction

Katrina John, Jeffrey Kile, and Amish Aghera

103.1 Indications

Displacement of the femoral head in relation to the acetabulum without concomitant femoral neck, head, or acetabulum fractures:

- Posterior hip dislocations make up 80–90 % of cases.
- Anterior hip dislocations make up 10–15 % of cases. These are classified into obturator, pubic, iliac, central, or inferior types. Central dislocations are associated with comminuted acetabulum fractures, and inferior dislocations are a rare occurrence normally occurring in children younger than 7 years of age.
- Prosthetic hip dislocations

103.2 Contraindications

- Absolute
  - Femoral neck fracture: attempted reduction may increase the displacement of the fracture and increase the probability of avascular necrosis.
- Relative
  - Fractures in other parts of the affected lower extremity: these may limit the pressure that can be applied necessary for traction during reduction.

103.3 Materials and Medications

- Parenteral sedation and analgesia medications
- Sheet or belt to fix the pelvis to the stretcher
- Knee immobilizer
- Abduction pillow

103.4 Procedure

1. Check the neurovascular status of the affected extremity.
2. Obtain anteroposterior (AP) views of the pelvis and lateral views of the hip.
3. Ensure adequate parenteral sedation and analgesia.
4. Decide upon a technique, as detailed later, and position the patient accordingly.
5. Once the hip has been successfully reduced, test the joint for stability by moving it gently thought its range of motion.
6. Place a knee immobilizer and an abduction pillow between the knees.
7. Check the neurovascular status.
8. Obtain repeat AP films of the pelvis.

K. John, MBBS • J. Kile, MBBS, PhD, MPH (✉)
Department of Emergency Medicine, Eisenhower Medical Center,
Rancho Mirage, CA, USA
e-mail: trenjohn@me.com; jeffrey.kile@gmail.com

A. Aghera, MD
Department of Emergency Medicine, Maimonides Medical Center,
New York, NY, USA
e-mail: aaghera@maimonidesmed.org

© Springer Science+Business Media New York 2016
S. Ganti (ed.), *Atlas of Emergency Medicine Procedures*, DOI 10.1007/978-1-4939-2507-0_103

103.4.1 Stimson Maneuver

1. Place the patient prone on the stretcher with the affected extremity hanging over the edge and the hip flexed to 90°.
2. Flex the knee and the foot to 90°.
3. Apply downward pressure to the area just distal to the popliteal fossa with a hand (Fig. 103.1) or knee (Fig. 103.2) while using the opposite hand to internally and externally rotate the hip at the ankle.
4. Have an assistant simultaneously manipulate the displaced femoral head into position with both hands, applying downward pressure over the affected buttock (Fig. 103.3).

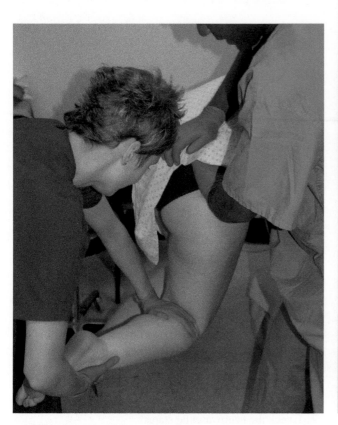

Fig. 103.1 Stimson maneuver with hand

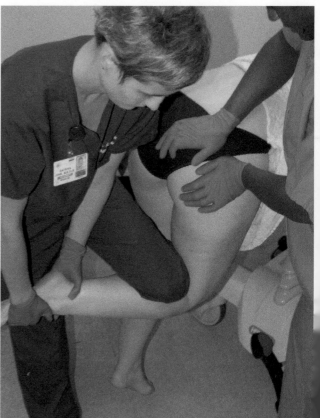

Fig. 103.2 Stimson maneuver with knee

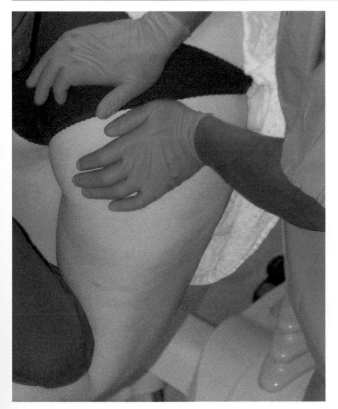

Fig. 103.3 Manipulation of the femoral head

103.4.2 Allis Maneuver

1. Position the patient supine on the stretcher.
2. The operator should stand on the stretcher to achieve maximum leverage or have the patient on a backboard on the ground.
3. Have an assistant apply downward pressure to both iliac crests.
4. Apply constant, gentle upward traction in line with the deformity while maneuvering the hip to 90° flexion and through internal and external rotation (Fig. 103.4).
5. Have a second assistant provide lateral traction to the midthigh.
6. Once the femoral head has cleared the outer lip of the acetabulum, continue traction while keeping the hip in external rotation and gently abducting and extending the hip (Fig. 103.5).

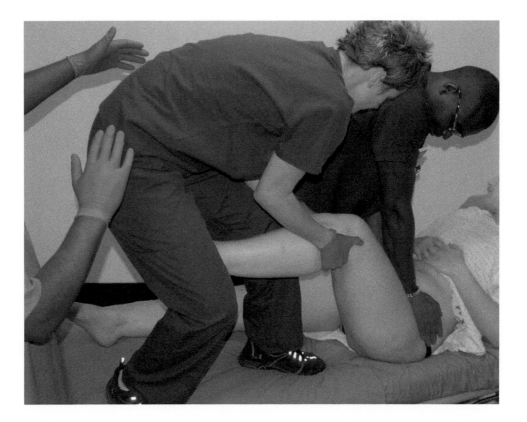

Fig. 103.4 Allis flexion

Fig. 103.5 Allis extension

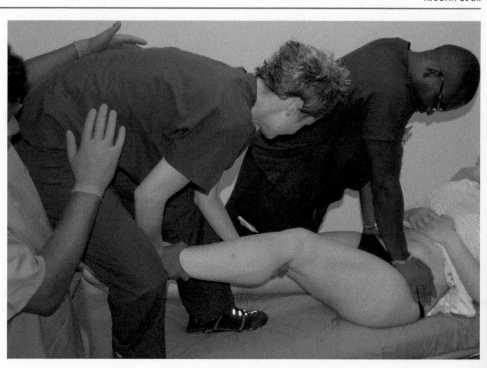

103.4.3 Whistler Technique

1. Position the patient supine on the stretcher with the knee and hip flexed to 45°.
2. Have an assistant stabilize the pelvis with downward pressure on both iliac crests.
3. Stand on the side of the affected extremity and place one arm under the knee, resting the hand on the flexed knee of the unaffected extremity.
4. Secure the ankle of the affected extremity with the other hand and elevate the shoulder of the opposite arm, providing upward traction at the distal thigh and a strong fulcrum to reduce the dislocation (Fig. 103.6).
5. Internal and external rotation can be achieved with the opposite hand at the ipsilateral ankle.

103.4.4 Captain Morgan Technique

1. Position the patient supine on the stretcher with the knee and hip flexed to 90°.
2. Stabilize and fix the pelvis with a sheet tied securely over the pelvis and under the stretcher.
3. Standing on the side of the affected extremity, the operator's foot should be resting perpendicular on the stretcher with the knee placed under the patient's knee.
4. With the opposite hand, apply downward pressure to the ankle and provide a sustained upward force to the patient's thigh by elevation of the knee through plantar flexion of the toes and upward pressure of the other hand placed behind the patient's knee.
5. Internal and external rotation can be applied simultaneously if necessary by gently twisting the ankle (Fig. 103.7).

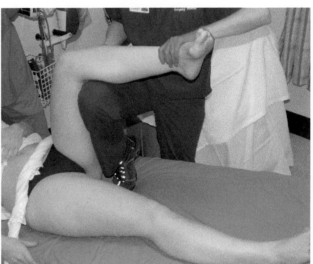

Fig. 103.7 Captain Morgan technique

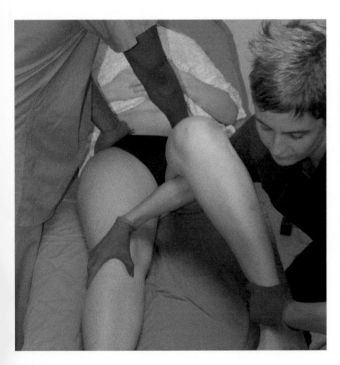

Fig. 103.6 Whistler technique

103.5 Complications

- Sciatic nerve injury
- Avascular necrosis of the femoral head due to delay in adequate reduction
- Inability to perform reduction due to occult fractures and fracture fragments, incarceration of the joint capsule, or associated tendons
- Unstable or irreducible dislocations
- Traumatic arthritis and joint instability

103.6 Pearls and Pitfalls

- Pearls
  - On AP radiograph, posterior dislocations can be more easily detected by the presence of a smaller femoral head compared with the unaffected side and poor visualization of the lesser trochanter.
  - On AP radiographs, anterior dislocations can be detected by a larger femoral head and a clear lesser trochanter seen in profile alongside the femoral shaft.
  - Pay close attention to the femoral vessels and the sciatic nerve. Injury to the sciatic nerve most commonly affects the common peroneal branch, therefore causing weakness in great toe extension and foot dorsiflexion. Sensation may also be reduced over the dorsum of the foot.
  - Check the femoral head is intact and clearly in the acetabulum and for intact Shenton lines, symmetrical intra-articular spaces, and clear outlines of the lesser trochanters.
  - For any of the techniques requiring stabilization of the pelvis, an alternative is to fix it to the stretcher using a sheet or belt.
  - To overcome the powerful muscles that oppose successful reduction, it is important to provide adequate muscle relaxation and steady, prolonged traction.
  - An assistant should stand on the floor behind to support the operator if standing on a stretcher.

- Pitfalls
  - Owing to the force necessary to dislocate a native hip, this injury should serve as a red flag to the physician to consider other potentially life- or limb-threatening occult injuries.
  - Hip dislocation is a true orthopedic emergency and must be treated without delay. Delay in reduction, especially greater than 6 h, results in increased incidence of avascular necrosis of the femoral head and sciatic nerve injury.
  - Review imaging carefully because associated fractures of the femoral head, neck, and acetabulum are often present.
  - It is recommended that anterior dislocations be reduced by orthopedic surgeons under general anesthetic in the operating room. These are often more complicated and difficult to reduce, and failure at closed reduction in the operating room can be followed by an open procedure.
  - Multiple attempts at reduction should not be performed in the emergency department because these are unlikely to be successful and will only delay definitive management and lead to an increased risk of complications.

Selected Reading

Hendey GW, Avila A. The captain Morgan technique for the reduction of the dislocated hip. Ann Emerg Med. 2011;58:536–40.

Newton EJ, Love J. Emergency department management of selected orthopedic injuries. Emerg Med Clin North Am. 2007; 25:763–93.

Nordt WE. Maneuvers for reducing dislocated hips. Clin Orthop Relat Res. 1999;360:160–4.

Rupp JD, Schneider LW. Injuries to the hip joint in frontal motor vehicle crashes: biomechanical and real-world perspectives. Orthop Clin North Am. 2004;35:493–504.

Walden PD, Hamer JR. Whistler technique used to reduce traumatic dislocation of the hip in the emergency department setting. J Emerg Med. 1999;17:441–4.

Knee Dislocation Reduction

104

Katrina John, Jeffrey Kile, and Amish Aghera

104.1 Indications

- Dislocation of the knee/fibular head/patella

104.2 Contraindications

- Absolute
  - None
- Relative
  - Immediate availability of orthopedic consultation

104.3 Materials and Medications

- Parenteral sedation and analgesia medications
- Knee immobilizer or splinting materials

104.4 Procedure

104.4.1 Knee (Femur/Tibia) Dislocation Reduction

1. Assess neurovascular function.
2. Pretreat the patient with sedation or analgesia as appropriate.
3. Position the patient supine with the affected leg fully extended.
4. Instruct an assistant to stand near the patient's hip and, facing the patient's affected knee, grasp the distal femur firmly with both hands to fix it in place.

5. Stand near the patient's foot and, facing the patient's affected knee, grasp the distal tibia and apply straight traction in a distal direction.
   - Longitudinal traction-countertraction alone, as described previously, will usually reduce the dislocation. If reduction does not occur, proceed with the following steps.
6. While applying straight traction in a distal direction to the tibia with the dominant hand, with the nondominant hand:
   (a) Anterior dislocation: push the proximal tibia in a posterior direction (Fig. 104.1)
   (b) Posterior dislocation: lift the proximal tibia in an anterior direction (Fig. 104.2)
   (c) Lateral dislocation: push the proximal tibia in a medial direction (Fig. 104.3)
   (d) Medial dislocation: push the proximal tibia in a lateral direction (Fig. 104.4)
   (e) Rotary dislocation: rotate the proximal tibia into proper linear alignment with the femoral condyles (Fig. 104.5)
   - Reduction may be facilitated by the use of two assistants rather than just one. The second assistant grasps the distal tibia and applies straight traction in a distal direction, freeing the operator to manipulate the proximal tibia as described previously using both hands.
7. After reduction, reassess neurovascular function and, if available, obtain angiography.
8. Immobilize the knee in 15° of flexion in a knee immobilizer or long-leg posterior splint.

K. John, MBBS • J. Kile, MBBS, PhD, MPH (✉)
Department of Emergency Medicine, Eisenhower Medical Center, Rancho Mirage, CA, USA
e-mail: trenjohn@me.com; jeffrey.kile@gmail.com

A. Aghera, MD
Department of Emergency Medicine, Maimonides Medical Center, New York, NY, USA
e-mail: aaghera@maimonidesmed.org

© Springer Science+Business Media New York 2016
. Ganti (ed.), *Atlas of Emergency Medicine Procedures*, DOI 10.1007/978-1-4939-2507-0_104

Fig. 104.1 Anterior dislocation of the knee: the proximal tibia is pushed in a posterior direction. The *arrows* indicate the direction in which force should be applied by the operator during reduction of dislocation

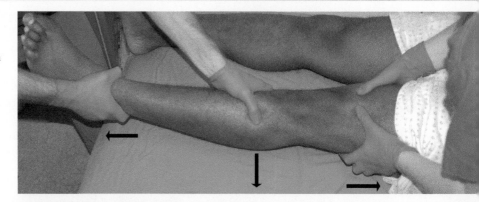

Fig. 104.2 Posterior dislocation of the knee: the proximal tibia is pushed in an anterior direction. The *arrows* indicate the direction in which force should be applied by the operator during reduction of dislocation

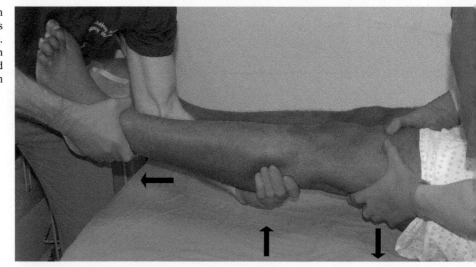

Fig. 104.3 Lateral dislocation of the knee: the proximal tibia is pushed in a medial direction. The *arrows* indicate the direction in which force should be applied by the operator during reduction of dislocation

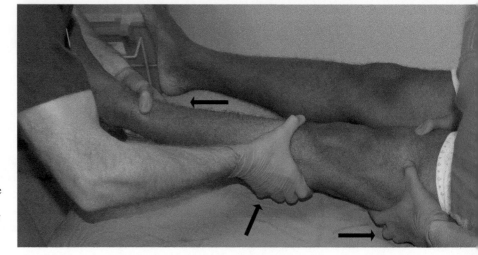

Fig. 104.4 Medial dislocation
of the knee: the proximal tibia is
pushed in a lateral direction. The
arrows indicate the direction in
which force should be applied by
the operator during reduvction of
dislocation

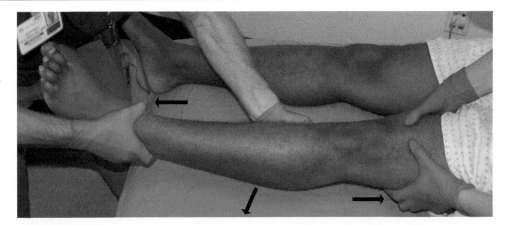

Fig. 104.5 Rotary dislocation of
the knee: the proximal tibia is
rotated into proper alignment
with the femoral condyles. The
arrows indicate the direction in
which force should be applied by
the operator during reduction of
dislocation

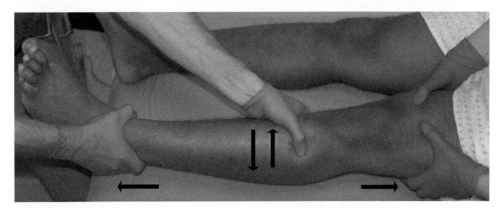

104.4.2 Fibular Head Dislocation Reduction

1. Assess neurovascular function.
2. Pretreat the patient with sedation or analgesia as appropriate.
3. Position the patient supine.
4. Flex the knee to 90° to relax the biceps femoris tendon.
5. Instruct an assistant to stand near the patient's hip and, facing the patient's affected knee, grasp the distal femur firmly with both hands to fix it in place.
6. Stand near the patient's foot and, facing the patient's affected knee, grasp the distal tibia and apply straight traction in a distal direction with the dominant hand and with the nondominant hand.
   (a) Anterior dislocation: push the fibular head in a posterior direction (Fig. 104.6)
   (b) Posterior dislocation: push the fibular head in an anterior direction (Fig. 104.7)
      - Reduction may be facilitated by the use of two assistants rather than just one. If a second assistant is available, instruct the second assistant to stand near the patient's foot and, facing the patient's affected knee, grasp the distal tibia and apply straight traction in a distal direction. This enables the operator to grasp and move the proximal fibula as described previously using both hands.
   - Reduction is often signified by a palpable and audible click as the fibula snaps back into position.
7. After reduction, reassess neurovascular function and, if available, obtain angiography.
   - After reduction, patients should receive orthopedic referral, avoid weight-bearing for the first 2 weeks, and then gradually increase weight-bearing over the next 6 weeks.
   - Typically, immobilization is not required following reduction of an i.solated fibular head dislocation.

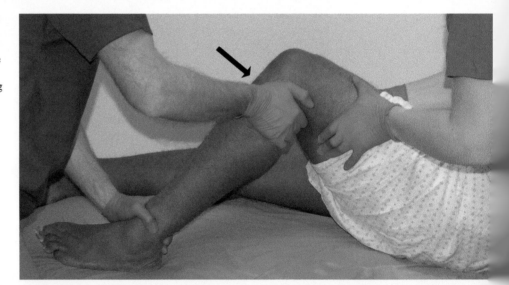

Fig. 104.6 Anterior dislocation of the fibular head: the fibular head is pushed in a posterior direction. The *arrow* indicate the direction in which force should be applied by the operator during reduction of dislocation

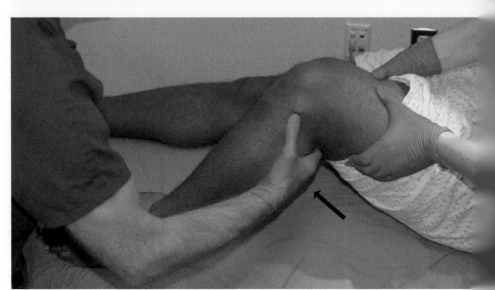

Fig. 104.7 Posterior dislocation of the fibular head: the fibular head is pushed in an anterior direction. The *arrow* indicate the direction in which force should be applied by the operator during reduction of dislocation

104.4.3 Lateral Patellar Dislocation Reduction

1. Pretreat the patient with sedation or analgesia as appropriate.
2. Stand at the side of the affected knee and, facing the knee, grasp the distal tibia and slowly extend the knee with one hand, and with the other hand simultaneously apply gentle pressure to the patella in a medial direction.

- The lateral edge of the patella may be lifted slightly to facilitate its travel over the femoral condyle during reduction (Fig. 104.8).
- After reduction, the knee should be immobilized in full extension in a knee immobilizer or long-leg posterior splint, and the patient should receive orthopedic referral, avoid weight-bearing for the first 2 weeks, and then gradually increase weight-bearing over the next 6 weeks.

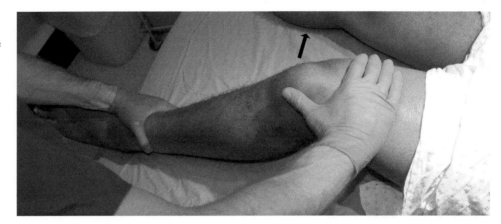

Fig. 104.8 Lateral dislocation of the patella: the patella is pushed in a medial direction. The *arrow* indicate the direction in which force should be applied by the operator during reduction of dislocation

104.5 Complications

104.5.1 Knee (Femur/Tibia) Dislocations

- Distal ischemia (even requiring amputation)
- Degenerative arthritis
- Joint instability due to ligamentous injury

104.5.2 Fibular Head Dislocations

- Peroneal nerve injury
- Fibular head instability/subluxation
- Degenerative arthritis

104.5.3 Patellar Dislocations

- Failure of reduction
- Degenerative arthritis
- Recurrent dislocation/subluxation

104.6 Pearls and Pitfalls

104.6.1 Knee (Femur/Tibia) Dislocations

- Pearls
  - Dislocations of the knee are described in terms of the tibia's position in relation to the femur.
  - All knee dislocations require orthopedic evaluation at the earliest possible opportunity.
  - Owing to the frequency of associated popliteal artery and peroneal nerve injury, a neurovascular examination should be performed before and after any attempts at reduction or manipulation of the knee.
  - Dislocations of the knee should be reduced as soon as possible, particularly if distal neurovascular compromise exists.
  - Operative ligamentous repair is often required approximately 2 weeks postreduction (once acute swelling has resolved) to achieve the maximum functional recovery.
- Pitfalls
  - If the knee hyperextends more than 30° when the horizontal leg is lifted by the foot, the knee is considered severely unstable. This is likely due to a previous dislocation, and thus, the knee should be evaluated for the neurovascular complications of dislocation.

- Because the joint capsule is commonly disrupted during knee dislocation, synovial fluid may diffuse into the surrounding tissue, such that an effusion is not always present.
- A posterolateral dislocation may be irreducible because the medial femoral condyle traps the medial capsule within the joint.

104.6.2 Fibular Head Dislocations

- Pearls
  - Fibular head dislocations are usually anterolateral, but these do not result in neurovascular compromise.
  - A knee joint effusion is usually not seen in a fibular head dislocation because the tibiofibular ligaments are contained within a separate synovium.
  - Anterior dislocations typically result from a fall on the flexed, adducted leg, often combined with ankle inversion.
  - Flexion of the knee relaxes the fibular collateral ligament, reducing the stability of the tibiofibular joint.
  - Superior dislocation is accompanied by interosseus membrane damage and proximal displacement of the lateral malleolus.
- Pitfalls
  - Posterior fibular head dislocations usually result from direct trauma to the flexed knee and may be accompanied by peroneal nerve injury.

104.6.3 Patellar Dislocations

- Pearls
  - Patellar dislocation occurs most frequently among adolescents.
  - Patellar dislocation typically occurs in the setting of external rotation combined with a strong valgus force and quadriceps contraction.
  - Patellar dislocations are described in terms of the patellar relationship to the normal knee joint.
  - The most common patellar dislocations are lateral.
  - If a spontaneous reduction has occurred, a knee effusion and tenderness along the medial aspect of the patella are likely to be present on examination, and the patellar apprehension test will be positive.
  - To perform the patellar apprehension test, flex the knee 30° and push the patella laterally. If the patient senses impending redislocation, the test is considered positive

- Isolated lateral patellar dislocations do not usually require hospitalization, but orthopedic follow-up is recommended owing to the likelihood of persistent instability.
- Intracondylar and superior dislocations require surgical reduction.
- Patients with an isolated patellar dislocation typically present with the knee in 20–30° of flexion and the patella displaced laterally.
- Pitfalls
  - Dislocations tend to be recurrent, particularly in patients with patellofemoral anatomical abnormalities.

Selected Reading

Martinez D, Sweatman K, Thompson EC. Popliteal artery injury associated with knee dislocations. Am Surg. 2001;67:165–7.

Peskun CJ, Levy BA, Fanelli GC, et al. Diagnosis and management of knee dislocations. Phys Sportsmed. 2010;38:101–11.

Rihn JA, Groff YJ, Harner CD, Cha PS. The acutely dislocated knee: evaluation and management. J Am Acad Orthop Surg. 2004;12:334–46.

Roberts DM, Stallard TC. Emergency department evaluation and treatment of knee and leg injuries. Emerg Med Clin North Am. 2000;18:67–84. v–vi.

Wascher DC, Dvirnak PC, DeCoster TA. Knee dislocation: initial assessment and implications for treatment. J Orthop Trauma. 1997;11:525–9.

Ankle Dislocation Reduction

Katrina John, Jeffrey Kile, and Amish Aghera

105.1 Indications

- Dislocation of the ankle joint. This is defined by the articulation of the talus with the mortise that is formed by the distal tibia and fibula. Dislocations can be posterior, anterior, superior, or lateral and are classified by the position of the talus in relation to the tibial mortise.

105.2 Contraindications

- Relative
  - Open dislocations where there is no evidence of acute neurovascular compromise are better managed definitively in the operating room to avoid further contamination.

105.3 Materials and Medications

Parenteral sedation and analgesia medications
Local anesthetic for local and intra-articular anesthesia
Splinting material

- Stockinette
- Padding
- Elastic bandage
- Tape
- Sheet

105.4 Procedure

1. Check the neurovascular status of the affected foot and ankle.
2. If there is no evidence of critical neurovascular compromise, obtain a lateral and an anteroposterior radiograph of the affected ankle.
3. Ensure adequate parenteral sedation and analgesia to maximize success and limit pain and suffering.
4. Position the patient on a stretcher with the knee flexed at 90° over a folded pillow or rolled-up sheet or with the lower leg and knee hanging over the edge of the stretcher.

John, MBBS • J. Kile, MBBS, PhD, MPH (✉)
Department of Emergency Medicine, Eisenhower Medical Center,
Rancho Mirage, CA, USA
email: trenjohn@me.com; jeffrey.kile@gmail.com

Aghera, MD
Department of Emergency Medicine, Maimonides Medical Center,
New York, NY, USA
email: aaghera@maimonidesmed.org

Springer Science+Business Media New York 2016
Ganti (ed.), *Atlas of Emergency Medicine Procedures*, DOI 10.1007/978-1-4939-2507-0_105

105.4.1 Posterior Dislocations

1. Hold the heel in one hand and pull with longitudinal traction.
2. With the other hand, hold the top of the foot and gently plantarflex it downward, while an assistant provides countertraction at the back of the midcalf (Fig. 105.1).
3. Continue longitudinal traction at the heel and countertraction at the calf.
4. Dorsiflex the foot while another assistant applies downward pressure to the distal anterior leg (Fig. 105.2).
5. Examine foot for restoration of normal anatomy and for any new lacerations or defects to the skin.
6. Recheck neurovascular integrity.
7. Place the leg in a sugar-tong splint with the foot at 90°.
8. Recheck neurovascular integrity.

Fig. 105.1 Plantarflexion with longitudinal heel traction

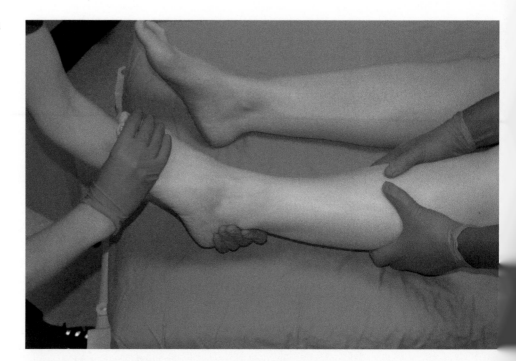

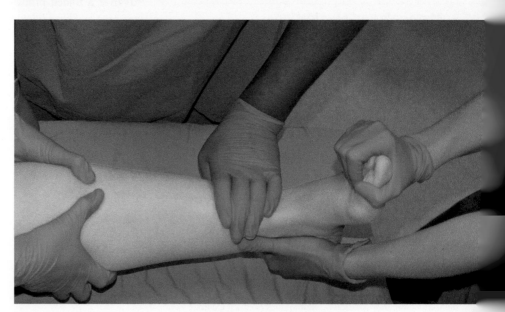

Fig. 105.2 Dorsiflexion with longitudinal heel traction

105.4.2 Anterior Dislocations

1. Hold the heel in one hand and pull with longitudinal traction.
2. With the other hand, hold the top of the foot and dorsiflex, while an assistant provides countertraction at the back of the midcalf (Fig. 105.3).
3. Continue longitudinal traction at the heel and countertraction at the calf.

4. Keeping the foot at 90° to the leg, hold the foot firmly and push the foot downward toward the floor while another assistant applies upward pressure to the distal posterior leg (Fig. 105.4).
5. Examine the foot for restoration of normal anatomy and for any new lacerations or defects to the skin.
6. Recheck neurovascular integrity.
7. Place the leg in a sugar-tong splint with the foot at 90°.
8. Recheck neurovascular integrity.

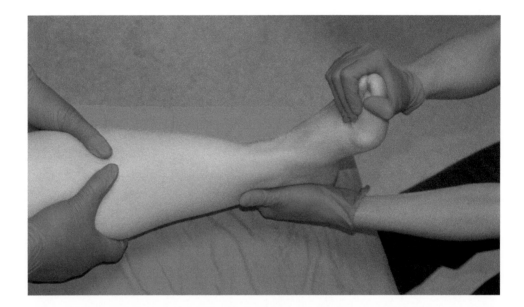

Fig. 105.3 Dorsiflexion with longitudinal heel traction

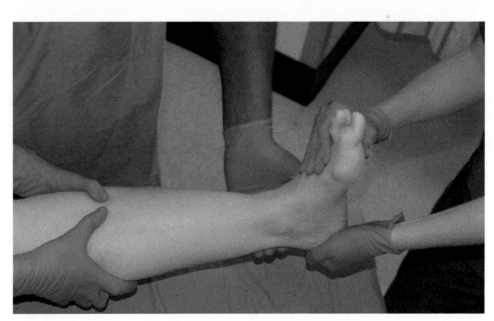

Fig. 105.4 Downward movement of foot (toward the floor) with longitudinal heel traction

105.5 Complications

- Compound fractures
- Neurovascular injury
- Skin and soft tissue damage
- Compartment syndrome

105.6 Pearls and Pitfalls

- Pearls
  - The ankle rarely dislocates without associated fractures.
- Pitfalls
  - Ankle dislocation is an orthopedic emergency, and reduction should not be delayed by imaging if there is evidence of neurovascular impairment. Complications that are exacerbated by delay in management include concomitant fractures, gross deformity of the ankle, severe stretching and tenting of the skin with resultant skin blisters, skin necrosis, and possible conversion to a compound fracture.
  - Be sure to check the radiograph carefully for commonly associated fractures notably of the malleoli.

Selected Reading

Collins DN, Temple SD. Open joint injuries: classification and treatment. Clin Orthop. 1989;243:48.

Hamilton WC. Injuries of the ankle and foot. Emerg Med Clin North Am. 1984;2:361.

Kelly PJ, Peterson FP. Compound dislocations of the ankle without fractures. Am J Surg. 1986;103:170.

Simon RR, Sherman SC, Koenigsknecht SJ, editors. Emergency orthopedics—the extremities. 5th ed. New York: McGraw-Hill; 2007. p. 264.

Wedmore IS, Charette J. Emergency department evaluation and treatment of ankle and foot injuries. Emerg Med Clin North Am. 2000;18:85.

Arthrocentesis

Shalu S. Patel and Bobby K. Desai

106.1 Indications

- Diagnosis of septic joint
- Diagnosis of traumatic effusion
- Diagnosis of inflammatory effusion
- Diagnosis of crystal-induced arthritis
- Therapeutic relief of pain from effusion

106.2 Contraindications

- Severe coagulopathy
- Skin infection over the needle insertion site
- Joint prosthesis
- Patients with bacteremia or sepsis (except to diagnose a septic joint)

106.3 Materials and Medications

- Betadine (povidone-iodine) or other skin antiseptic
- Sterile gloves
- Sterile towels
- Lidocaine 1 % or 2 % (5 mL) or other anesthetic of choice
- 18- to 22-gauge needle, 25-gauge needle
- Syringes (5 mL, 5–50 mL)
- Sterile gauze (4×4)
- Band-aid

106.4 Procedure

1. Informed consent may be required.
2. Position the patient appropriately. The joint should be placed in slight flexion.
3. Palpate the joint and identify anatomical landmarks.
   (a) For knee arthrocentesis, the needle should be inserted at the midpoint of either the medial or the lateral side of the patella (Fig. 106.1).
   (b) For acromioclavicular (AC) joint arthrocentesis, the needle should be inserted at the superior surface of the AC joint (Fig. 106.2).
   (c) For glenohumeral joint arthrocentesis, there are two approaches.
      (i) In the anterior approach, the needle is inserted into the groove lateral to the coracoid process (Fig. 106.3).
      (ii) In the posterior approach (preferred), the needle is inserted below the posterior border of the acromion process and lateral to the border of the scapula (Fig. 106.4).
4. Prepare the skin and drape in a sterile fashion.
5. Using lidocaine (drawn up in 5-mL syringe), anesthetize the skin with the 25-gauge needle.
6. Secure the 18- to 22-gauge needle on the 5- to 50-mL syringe (depending on the size of the joint) and insert it into the skin.
7. Advance the needle slowly into the joint space while aspirating until joint fluid can easily be withdrawn. While inserting the needle into the joint space, avoid scraping the needle against the bone.

S.S. Patel, MD
Department of Emergency Medicine, Florida Hospital Tampa, Florida Hospital Carrollwood, Tampa, FL, USA

B.K. Desai, MD (✉)
Department of Emergency Medicine, University of Florida Health Shands Hospita, Gainesville, FL, USA
e-mail: bdesai@ufl.edu

© Springer Science+Business Media New York 2016
. Ganti (ed.), *Atlas of Emergency Medicine Procedures*, DOI 10.1007/978-1-4939-2507-0_106

8. If fluid cannot be aspirated easily, the catheter can be repositioned further in the joint space or turned by 45° sequentially as needed.
9. Once the joint fluid is aspirated, pull out the needle and hold pressure with gauze. Bleeding should be minimal.

10. Place a band-aid or other dressing over the site.
11. Send the synovial fluid to the laboratory. Generally, laboratory analyses may include crystals, protein, glucose, cell count and differential, culture and sensitivity, and Gram stain.

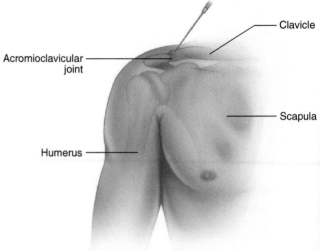

Fig. 106.2 Acromioclavicular joint arthrocentesis

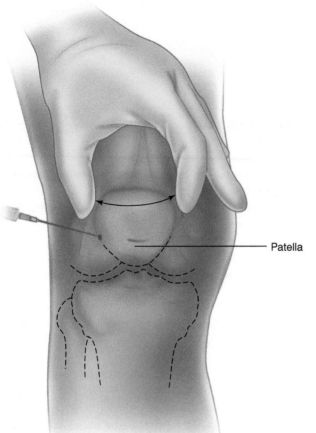

Fig. 106.1 Knee arthrocentesis

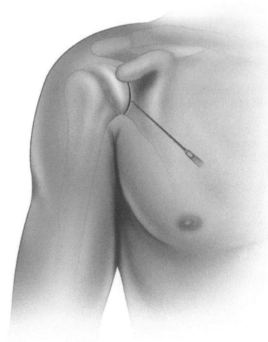

Fig. 106.3 Glenohumeral joint arthrocentesis: anterior approach

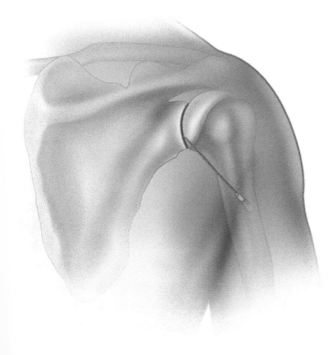

Fig. 106.4 Glenohumeral joint arthrocentesis: posterior approach

106.5 Complications

- Introduction of infection
- Bleeding

106.6 Pearls and Pitfalls

- The preferred site of entry is over the extensor surface of the joint. This will reduce the risk of damage to tendons, ligaments, and blood vessels.
- When assessing synovial fluid, the Rule of Twos may be used to differentiate among normal, inflammatory, and septic fluid. Normal synovial fluid has less than 200 white blood cells (WBCs)/mm^3. Noninflammatory synovial fluid has 200–2000 WBCs/mm^3. Inflammatory synovial fluid has greater than 2000 WBCs/mm^3 (but <50,000 WBCs/mm^3). Septic synovial fluid has greater than 75,000 WBCs/mm^3.
- Only septic synovial fluid will have a positive Gram stain and culture.

Selected Reading

Biundo JJ, Roberts N, Deodhar A. Regional musculoskeletal complaints. In: Stone JH, editor. A clinician's pearls and myths in rheumatology. New York: Springer Science; 2009. p. 433–4.

Parrillo SJ, Fisher J. Arthrocentesis. In: Roberts JR, Hedges J, editors. Clinical procedures in emergency medicine. 4th ed. Philadelphia: Saunders; 2004. p. 1042–57.

Self WH, Wang EE, Vozenilek JA, del Castillo J, Pettineo C, Benedict L. Dynamic emergency medicine. Arthrocentesis. Acad Emerg Med. 2008;15:298.

Thomsen TW, Shen S, Shaffer RW, Setnik GS. Arthrocentesis of the knee. N Engl J Med. 2006;354:e19.

Intra-articular Injection

Bharat Kothakota and Muhammad Waseem

107.1 Indications

- Aspiration of fluid (arthrocentesis)
  - For diagnosis: to rule out infection
  - To relieve pressure from large, painful joint effusion
- Injection of joints with inflammatory arthritis
  - Tendinitis
  - Bursitis
  - Rheumatoid arthritis (RA)
- Injection of joints with osteoarthritis (OA)
  - Injection of large weight-bearing joints
  - Injection of small joints of hands
- Intra-articular anesthetic
  - Shoulder reduction
  - Ankle impingement syndrome

107.2 Contraindications

- Cellulitis
- Bacteremia
- Fracture

107.3 Materials and Medications

- Glucocorticoid
  - Duration of effect inversely proportional to solubility
    - Less soluble → longer acting
  - Choice of steroid is the personal preference of the physician
  - Methylprednisone (Depo-Medrol) and triamcinolone acetonide (Kenalog)
    - Less likely to induce postinjection flare
  - Kenalog and triamcinolone hexacetonide (Aristospan)
    - Longest-acting agents
- Local anesthetic
  - 1 % Lidocaine
- Needle
  - 18- to 22-gauge used for knee, ankle, hip, elbow, and shoulder
  - 25-gauge or smaller used for smaller joints (interphalangeal)
- Syringe

B. Kothakota, MD • M. Waseem, MD (✉)
Department of Emergency Medicine, Lincoln Medical and Mental Health Center, New York, NY, USA
e-mail: bharatkothakota@yahoo.com; waseemm2001@hotmail.com

© Springer Science+Business Media New York 2016
Ganti (ed.), *Atlas of Emergency Medicine Procedures*, DOI 10.1007/978-1-4939-2507-0_107

107.4 Procedure

1. Selecting an injection approach.
   - Knee
     – Lateral approach: 1 cm inferior to the patella laterally (Fig. 107.1)
     – Medial approach: 1 cm inferior to the patella medially (Fig. 107.2)
   - Ankle
     – Lateral approach: just inferior to the lateral malleolus (Fig. 107.3)
     – Medial approach
       - Plantar flex the foot.
       - Angle the needle cephalad to pass between the medial malleolus and the tibialis anterior tendon (Fig. 107.4).
   - Shoulder
     – Posterior approach
       - Insert the needle 1 cm inferior and 1 cm medial to the posterolateral corner of the acromion.
       - Direct the needle anterior and medial toward the coracoid process (Fig. 107.5).
2. Skin preparation.
   - Make three separate concentric outward spirals with iodine disinfectant
   - Scrub with cyclohexidine preparation
3. Mark the injection site by impressing the skin with a hard object.
   - Sterile end of needle sheath
   - Ball point pen with tip retracted
4. Local anesthesia.
   - 1 % Lidocaine injected into the skin and subcutaneous tissue
   - Short burst of ethyl chloride spray before iodine preparation
   - Mixing lidocaine with glucocorticoid preparation
5. Always aspirate joint fluid before injecting the corticosteroids.
   - Use a 1.5-inch 18-gauge needle for aspiration.
   - Confirm that the needle is in the joint space.
   - Reduced effusion size before injection can improve outcomes.
   - Compress the opposite side of the joint to aid in aspiration (Fig. 107.6).
6. After aspirating, change the syringe.
   - Use a sterile hemostat or hand to stabilize the needle within the joint space (Fig. 107.7).
   - Avoid injecting corticosteroids if the aspirate appears purulent.
7. Injection of medication.
   - Can use the same needle used for aspiration.
   - Insert needle 0.75–1.25 inch in depth for injection.
8. Remove the needle, wipe the iodine solution clean, and apply the bandage.
9. Postinjection care.
   - First 48 h: bedrest versus minimize walking
   - Next 2–3 weeks: crutches or cane

Fig. 107.1 Knee arthrocentesis, lateral approach

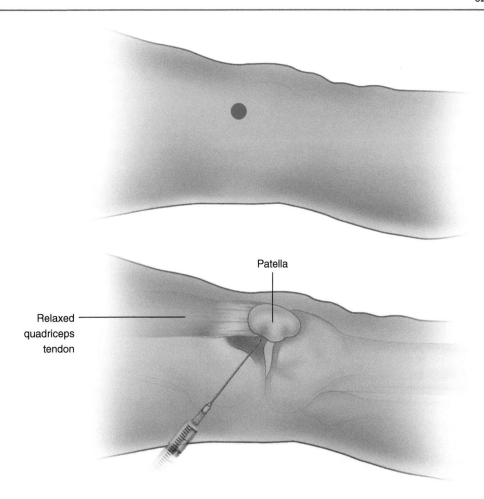

Patella

Relaxed quadriceps tendon

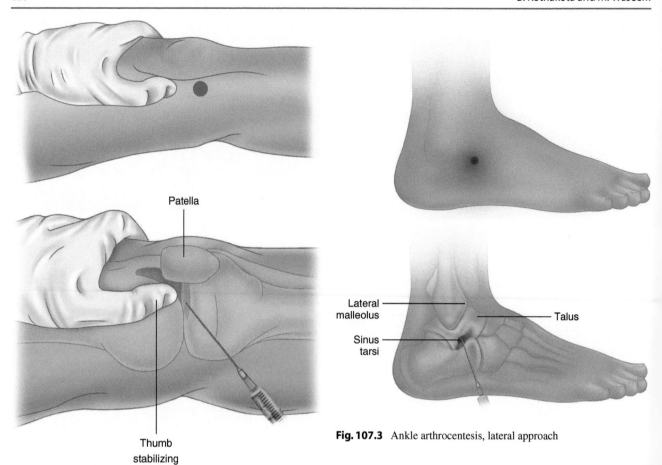

Fig. 107.2　Knee arthrocentesis, medial approach

Fig. 107.3　Ankle arthrocentesis, lateral approach

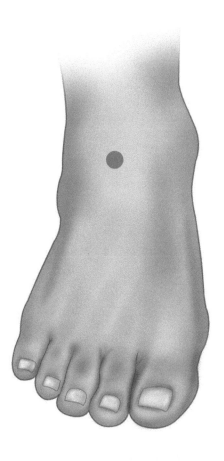

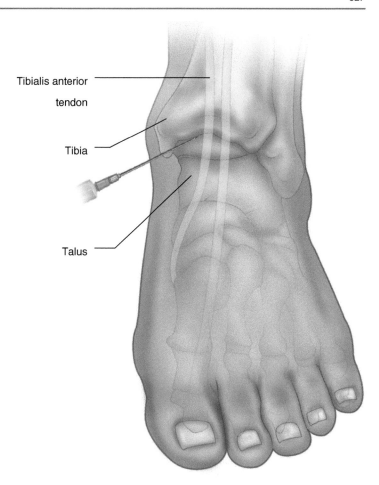

Fig. 107.4   Ankle arthrocentesis, medial approach

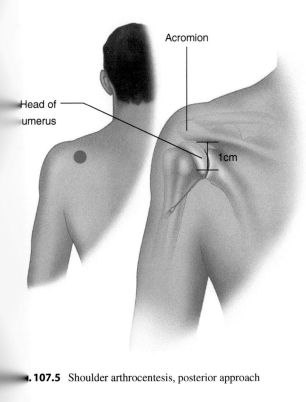

107.5   Shoulder arthrocentesis, posterior approach

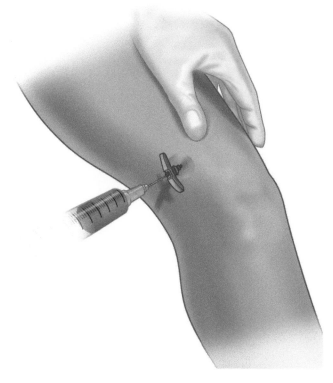

Fig. 107.6   Compress opposite side of joint to aid in aspiration

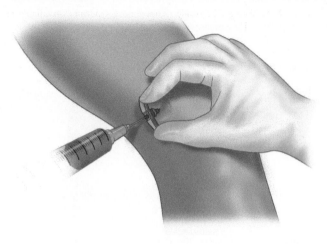

Fig. 107.7 Use hemostat or hand to stabilize needle within joint space

107.5 Complications

- Local postinjection flare
  - Irritation of the synovium by steroid microcrystals
  - Can be confused for infection
  - Occurs and resolves within 48 h after injection
  - Treat with ice and appropriate analgesics.
- Iatrogenic joint infection
  - Suspect if it begins later than, or lasts longer than, flare
  - Increasing pattern of pain
  - Fever, malaise, redness, or drainage around injection site
  - *Staphylococcus aureus* most common
- Subcutaneous atrophy and depigmentation
  - Leakage of corticosteroids into soft tissues
- Aspiration of blood
  - Indicative of trauma or bleeding disorder (hemophilia)
- Systemic absorption
  - Water-soluble preparations
  - Dose dependent
  - Injection into multiple joints
  - Transient hyperglycemia in diabetic patients
  - Avascular necrosis of the femoral head

107.6 Pearls

- Mixing lidocaine with glucocorticoids
  - Reduces pain caused by injection of steroids into joint space
  - Less likely to cause soft tissue atrophy and tendon rupture
  - Immediate relief from anesthetic indicates proper injection
- Limiting intra-articular glucocorticoid injections per joint
  - OA
    - Four injections per lifetime of the joint
    - Injections reduce the rate of accelerated degeneration in joints
  - RA
    - Limit of one injection per month
    - No evidence of glucocorticoid-induced cartilage loss

Selected Reading

Aponte EM, Schraga ED. Joint reduction, shoulder dislocation, anterior. Available at: http://emedicine.medscape.com/article/109130-overview#a08.

Cianflocco AJ. Intra-articular injections of the knee: a step-by-step guide. J Fam Pract. 2011;60(Suppl):S48–9. Available at: http://www.jfponline.com/pages.asp?id=10062.

Lavelle W, Lavelle ED, Lavelle L. Intra-articular injections. Anesthesiol Clin. 2007;25:835–62.

Molis MA, Young CC. Ankle impingement syndrome. Available at: http://emedicine.medscape.com/article/85311-overview.

Neustadt DH. Intra-articular injections for osteoarthritis of the knee. Cleve Clin J Med. 2006;73:897–911.

Roberts WN. Intraarticular and soft tissue injections: what agents(s) to inject and how frequently? Available at: www.uptodate.com.

Roberts WN. Joint aspiration or injection in adults: techniques and indications. Available at: www.uptodate.com.

Sugar-Tong Splint

108

Katrina John, Jeffrey Kile, and Amish Aghera

108.1 Indications

- Fractures to the wrist or forearm
- To prevent motion at the wrist and elbow
- To prevent supination and pronation

108.2 Contraindications

- Relative
  - Evidence of compartment syndrome or any neurovascular compromise

108.3 Materials (Fig. 108.1)

- Stockinette
- Padding
- Splint material: fiberglass/plaster of Paris or prefabricated splint rolls, 2, 3, 4 inches depending on age and body habitus
- Trauma shears/scissors
- Elastic bandage
- Tape
- Container with water
- Gloves, eyemask, sheet
- Sling

K. John, MBBS • J. Kile, MBBS, PhD, MPH (✉)
Department of Emergency Medicine, Eisenhower Medical Center,
Rancho Mirage, CA, USA
e-mail: trenjohn@me.com; jeffrey.kile@gmail.com

A. Aghera, MD
Department of Emergency Medicine, Maimonides Medical Center,
New York, NY, USA
e-mail: aaghera@maimonidesmed.org

© Springer Science+Business Media New York 2016
L. Ganti (ed.), *Atlas of Emergency Medicine Procedures*, DOI 10.1007/978-1-4939-2507-0_108

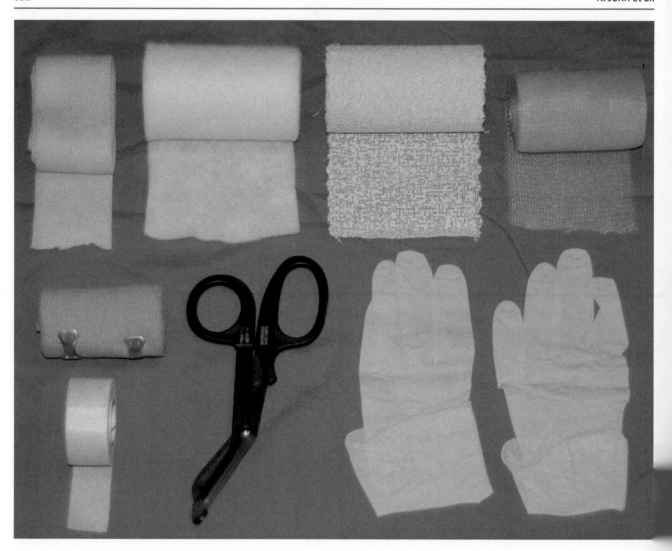

Fig. 108.1 Equipment

108.4 Procedure

1. Ensure the skin of the affected extremity is clean, dry, and intact.
2. Cover the patient with a sheet or gown to protect the patient's clothing and the surrounding area.
3. Position the patient's arm abducted at 90° at the shoulder and internally rotated with the elbow flexed at 90° (Fig. 108.2).
4. Measure the splinting material by running a single layer from the metacarpal heads of the dorsum of the hand along the extensor surface of the forearm over the elbow and humeral condyles and back down the flexor surface of the forearm to the palmar aspect of the hand to the metacarpal heads.
5. If using non-prefabricated splint rolls, lay the measured piece of splinting material out on a flat surface and multiply the layers to the same length, 6–8 layers for fiberglass and 10–12 layers for plaster.
6. Measure the stockinette from the finger tips to the midhumerus and cut a hole for the thumb.
7. Place the stockinette on the arm (Fig. 108.3).
8. Use a 3- to 4-inch padding roll to apply several layers of circumferential padding extending from the metacarpal heads to the midhumerus below the level of the stockinette (Fig. 108.4).
9. Wet the already prepared and measured splinting material and remove the excess water.
10. Ensure the forearm is in the aforementioned position, and apply the splinting material from the metacarpal heads of the dorsum of the hand along the extensor surface of the forearm over the elbow and humeral condyles and back down the flexor surface of the forearm to the palmar aspect of the hand to the metacarpal heads (Fig. 108.5).
11. Fold each end of the stockinette down over the padding and splinting material.
12. An extra layer of padding can be added at this stage.
13. Secure the entire splint with two elastic bandages/ace wrap and apply tape to ensure the bandages stay in place (Fig. 108.6).
14. Place the arm in a sling.

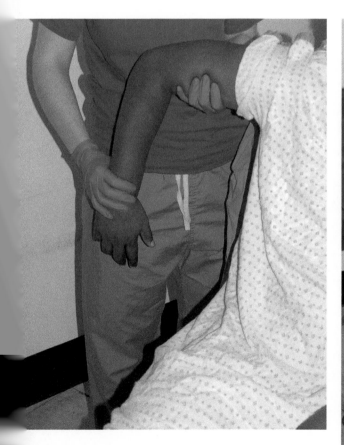

Fig. 108.2 Arm positioning

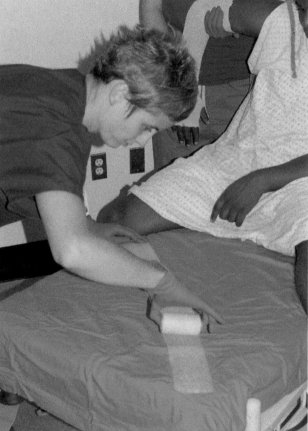

Fig. 108.3 Fiberglass being measured and stockinette on patient

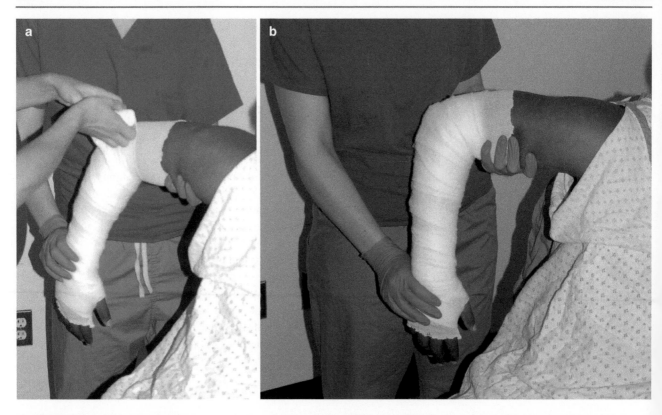

Fig. 108.4 (**a**) Application of padding over the stockinette (partial), (**b**) Application of padding over the stockinette (complete)

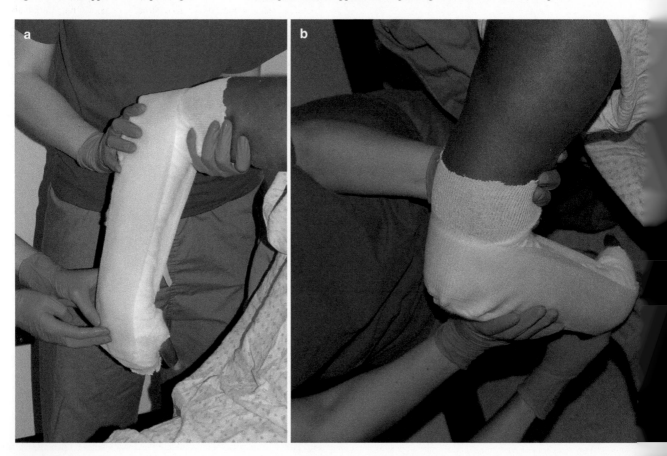

Fig. 108.5 (**a**) Application of splinting material over padding (anteromedial view), (**b**) Application of splinting material over padding (anterolateral view)

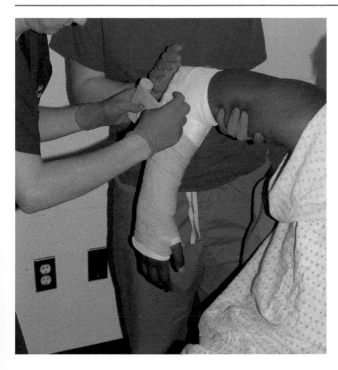

Fig. 108.6 Application of elastic bandage over splinting material

108.5 Complications

- Compartment syndrome

108.6 Pearls and Pitfalls

- Pearls
  - This procedure is best done with an assistant to hold the extremity in the desired position and to prevent the splint slipping as it is secured.
  - Having the patient in the illustrated position enables the practitioner to use gravity to hold the splint in the correct position while securing it; especially helpful if an assistant is not available.
- Pitfalls
  - If the splint is too short, it fails to immobilize the wrist.
  - If the splint is too long, it will cause reduced motion and stiffness at the metacarpophalangeal joints and swelling of the fingers due to immobility.

Selected Reading

Bong MR, Egol KA, Leibman M, Koval KJ. A comparison of immediate postreduction splinting constructs for controlling initial displacement of fractures of the distal radius: a prospective randomized study of long-arm versus short-arm splinting. J Hand Surg Am. 2006;31:766–70.

Denes AE, Goding R, Tamborlane J, Schwartz E. Maintenance of reduction of pediatric distal radius fractures with a sugar-tong splint. Am J Orthop (Belle Mead NJ). 2007;36:68–70.

Gartland JJ. The sugar tong splint. Am J Orthop. 1963;5:131.

McGeorge DD, Stilwell JH. The sugar tong splint: a reliable method of arm splintage in the child. J Hand Surg Br. 1989;14:357.

Simon RR, Koenigsknecht SJ, editors. Emergency orthopedics—the extremities. 3rd ed. New York: McGraw Hill; 1995.

Fetal Heart Rate Monitoring

Nathaniel Lisenbee and Joseph A. Tyndall

109.1 Indications

- Fetal heart rate (FHR) monitoring is important because it provides basic patterns that can be correlated to the acid–base status, circulatory volume, and oxygenation status of the fetus through brainstem detection and subsequent cardiac response. It has numerous indications during the antepartum and intrapartum stages [1].
- Antepartum indications include:
  - Nonstress test (consists of monitoring FHR in conjunction with fetal movements)
  - Contraction stress test (consists of monitoring FHR during contractions, which are induced pharmacologically)
  - Biophysical profile (BPP; consists of a nonstress test with an additional ultrasound)
- Intrapartum indications include monitoring FHR during:
  - Uterine contractions
  - Pain medications/anesthetic administration to the mother during labor
  - Procedures performed during labor
  - Second stage of labor
  - High-risk pregnancies, which can be defined by a number of conditions including [2, 3]:
    - Maternal diabetes, asthma, preeclampsia/eclampsia
    - Multiple gestations
    - Intrauterine growth restriction
    - Premature rupture of membranes
    - Lack of prenatal care

Lisenbee, MD
S. Air Force Medical Center Keesler,
loxi, MI, USA
mail: nate4085@ufl.edu

A. Tyndall, MD, MPH (✉)
partment of Emergency Medicine, University of Florida Health,
inesville, FL, USA
mail: tyndall@ufl.edu

109.2 Contraindications

- Contraindications for internal FHR monitoring
  - Presence of placenta previa
  - Lack of ability to identify the portion of the fetal body where device application is being considered
  - Active herpes, active hepatitis, or human immunodeficiency virus (HIV) in the mother
- Contraindications for external FHR monitoring
  - None

109.3 Methods

- Two methods for FHR monitoring:
  - Auscultation monitoring
    - Defined as auscultating FHR every 15 min in the first stage of labor and auscultating every 5 min in the second stage
    - Does not provide strips with information on FHR variability or the shape of FHR accelerations and decelerations
- Electronic FHR monitoring
  - Allows for real-time continuous monitoring of FHR activity
  - Provides strips with information on FHR variability or the shape of FHR accelerations and decelerations
  - Can be performed by Doppler ultrasound or internal fetal electrocardiography (ECG)

When comparing the two methods for electronic FHR monitoring, both are equally as reliable in most settings. Thus, external monitoring is the preferred method because it is noninvasive. However, in instances in which external monitoring becomes difficult owing to poor quality or technical difficulties, invasive monitoring is indicated.

pringer Science+Business Media New York 2016

Ganti (ed.), *Atlas of Emergency Medicine Procedures*, DOI 10.1007/978-1-4939-2507-0_109

109.4 Equipment and Procedures

Multiple methods exist for electronic FHR monitoring [4]. The most commonly used are external monitoring by Doppler ultrasound and internal monitoring by fetal ECG.

109.4.1 Doppler Ultrasound is a Noninvasive Method to Monitor FHR (Fig. 109.1)

- Equipment
  - Electronic FHR monitor
  - Contraction monitor sensor with belt
  - FHR sensor with belt (consists of ultrasound transducer and ultrasound sensor)
  - Ultrasound coupling gel
- Procedure
  1. Place the patient in a supine position.
  2. Palpate the fetal anatomy through the maternal abdomen to find the approximate location of the fetal heart.
  3. Place ultrasound coupling gel on the maternal abdomen at the sight of suspected fetal cardiac activity.
  4. Place the transducer probe on gel and locate the fetal heart tones.
  5. Once the fetal heart tones are located, secure the FHR sensor to the maternal abdomen with the attached belt.
  6. Place the contraction monitor sensor near the fundus in order to monitor uterine contractions.
  7. Attach the FHR sensor and contraction monitor to the electronic FHR monitor to obtain printouts of FHR and uterine contractions.

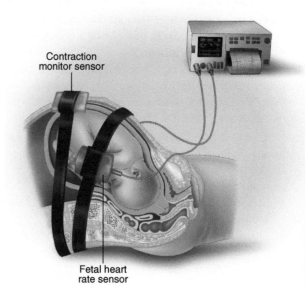

Fig. 109.1 External fetal heart rate monitoring

09.4.2 Internal Fetal ECG is an Invasive Method to Monitor FHR and is Used Only in the Intrapartum Period
(Fig. 109.2)

Equipment
- Fetal scalp monitoring electrode
- Leg plate electrode
- Sterile vaginal lubricant
- Electronic FHR monitor

Procedure (Fig. 109.3)
1. Place the patient in a dorsal lithotomy position.
2. Sterilize the perineal area.
3. Perform a bimanual vaginal examination to identify the presenting fetal head. (Note: rupture of membranes must occur before scalp electrode placement.)
4. Place the spiral electrode guide tube on the fetal scalp and advance the electrode until it contacts the scalp.
5. Rotate the drive tube clockwise approximately one rotation while maintaining pressure on the guide tube and drive tube.
6. Release the electrode locking device by pressing together the arms on the drive tube grip.
7. Carefully slide the drive and guide tubes off the electrode wires while holding the locking device open.
8. Attach the leg plate to the inner thigh of the mother as a means to eliminate electrical interference.
9. Attach the spiral electrode wires to the color-coded leg plate, which is then connected to the electronic fetal monitor.

10. Do not forget to sterilize the area of electrode placement after delivery is completed and the scalp electrode is removed.

When comparing the two methods, both are equally reliable in most settings. Thus, external monitoring is the preferred method because it is noninvasive. However, in instances in which external monitoring becomes difficult owing to poor quality or technical difficulties, invasive monitoring is indicated.

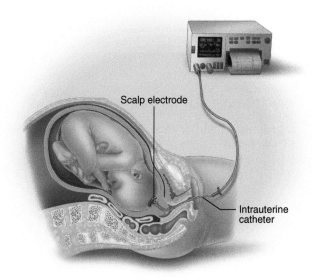

Scalp electrode

Intrauterine catheter

Fig. 109.2 Internal fetal heart rate monitoring

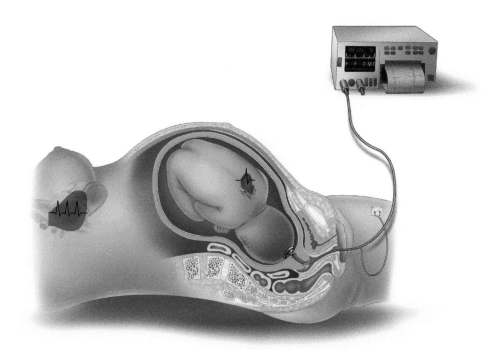

g. 109.3 Internal fetal heart
e monitoring

109.5 Complications

- Complications of external FHR monitoring
  - Confusing maternal aortic pulsations with FHR
  - Inability to locate FHR
- Complications of internal FHR monitoring
  - Fetal or maternal hemorrhage, fetal infection (usually scalp abscess at the site of insertion)
  - Uterine perforation
  - Subsequent fetal infection due to the invasive nature of the procedure

References

1. Hobel CJ. Intrapartum clinical assessment of fetal distress. Am J Obstet Gynecol. 1971;110:336–42.
2. Byrd JE. Intrapartum electronic fetal heart rate monitoring (EFM) and amnioinfusion. In: Advanced life support in obstetrics course syllabus. Kansas City: American Academy of Family Physicians; 1996. p. 97–106.
3. Queenan JT, Hobbins JC, Spong CY. Protocols for high-risk pregnancies. New York: Wiley; 2010. Retrieved 16 Jan 2012, from http://lib.myilibrary.com?ID=268955.
4. External and internal heart rate monitoring of the fetus. New Haven: Yale Medical Group; 2012. Retrieved from http://www.yalemedicalgroup.org/stw/.

Selected Reading

Alfirevic Z, Devane D, Gyte GM. Continuous cardiotocography (CTG) as a form of electronic fetal monitoring (EFM) for fetal assessment during labour. Cochrane Database Syst Rev. 2006;(3):CD006066.

American College of Obstetricians and Gynecologists. Fetal heart rate patterns: monitoring, interpretation, and management, ACOG technical bulletin, vol. 207. Washington, DC: ACOG; 1995.

Cunningham FG, Leveno KJ, Bloom SL, Hauth JC, Rouse DJ, Spong CY. Chapter 18: Intrapartum assessment. In: Williams obstetrics. 23rd ed. New York: McGraw Hill; 2010.

Freeman RK. Problems with intrapartum fetal heart rate monitoring interpretation and patient management. Obstet Gynecol. 2002;100:813.

Gomella LG, Haist SA. Chapter 13: Bedside procedures. In: Clinician's pocket reference. 11th ed. Columbus: McGraw-Hill; 2007.

Sweha A, Hacker TW, Nuovo J. Interpretation of the electronic fetal heart rate during labor. Am Fam Physician. 1999;59:2487–500.

Ultrasonography for Ectopic Pregnancy

L. Connor Nickels

An ectopic pregnancy is a pregnancy occurring outside of the uterine cavity (fundus) (Fig. 110.1).

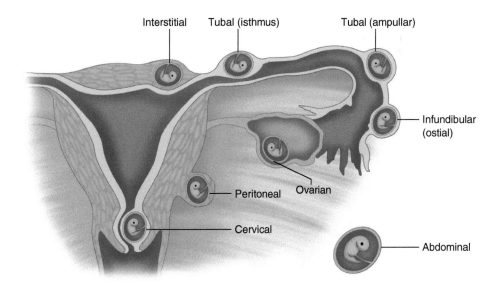

Interstitial   Tubal (isthmus)   Tubal (ampullar)

Infundibular (ostial)

Peritoneal   Ovarian

Cervical

Abdominal

Fig. 110.1 Ectopic pregnancy diagram: pregnancy occurring outside of the uterine cavity

L.C. Nickels, MD, RDMS
Department of Emergency Medicine,
University of Florida Health Shands Hospital,
Gainesville, FL, USA
e-mail: cnickels@ufl.edu

Springer Science+Business Media New York 2016
Ganti (ed.), *Atlas of Emergency Medicine Procedures*, DOI 10.1007/978-1-4939-2507-0_110

110.1 Indications

- Patient in the first trimester of pregnancy with any combination of the following:
  - Vaginal bleeding.
  - Acute pelvic pain.
  - Hypotension or shock.
  - Dizziness or syncope.
  - Positive pregnancy test.
  - Adnexal mass.
  - Cervical tenderness.
  - Abnormal rise in the serum human chorionic gonadotropin (hCG).
  - No specific sign or symptom is absolute; therefore, the index of suspicion must be high.
- Risk factors for ectopic pregnancy
  - Pelvic inflammatory disease (PID)
  - Previous or current intrauterine device
  - Infertility treatment
  - Previous tubal surgery
  - Tubal ligation
  - Advanced maternal age
  - Previous ectopic pregnancy
- Usually a sonographic diagnosis
- Sonographic signs of an ectopic can include any of the following:
  - Gestational sac seen in one of the following:
    - Adnexa with any of the following:
      - Yolk sac (Figs. 110.2 and 110.3)
      - Fetal pole with or without cardiac activity
      - Both of these
    - Low position in the cervix (cervical ectopic)
    - Seemingly in the uterus, but off to one side and with minimal surrounding myometrium (interstitial ectopic)
    - Within the peritoneal cavity, outside of the tubes (abdominal ectopic)

- Pseudogestational sac seen in the uterus
  - Uterine enlargement or decidual reaction (single outline only) in the endometrium without a gestational sac
- Other unidentifiable adnexa mass
- Free fluid in the pelvis or other gravity-dependent area (i.e., Morison's pouch in the right upper quadrant in a supine or reverse Trendelenburg patient) (Fig. 110.4)
  - Small free fluid: tracks less than one third of the posterior cul-de-sac
  - Moderate free fluid: tracks less than two third of the posterior cul-de-sac
  - Large free fluid: tracks greater than two third of the posterior cul-de-sac
  - Right upper quadrant free fluid: 100 % predictability for ectopic
- Empty uterus with serum hCG >1000 mIU/mL
- Patient in the first trimester of pregnancy with a serum hCG at or above the discriminatory zone (i.e., 1000 mIU/mL) without a sonographically normal gestational sac visualized within the uterus has an ectopic pregnancy until proven otherwise and should have an obstetrics consult in the emergency department.
  - Discriminatory zone may differ depending on the reference, but typically serum hCG between 1000 and 2000 mIU/mL.
  - For this chapter, we have used serum hCG greater than 1000 mIU/mL [1].
- Yolk sac should be first sign of definitive intrauterine pregnancy for emergency physicians because the decidual reaction and gestational sac are not 100 % accurate.
- May be treated surgically or medically depending on findings.
  - Decision to be made by obstetrics consultant

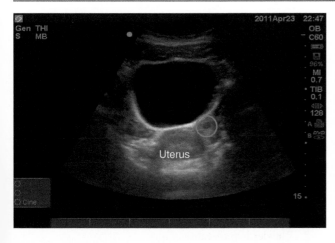

Fig. 110.2 Transabdominal transverse image of the uterus shows an ectopic pregnancy in the left adnexa (red circle) with the yolk sac present (Photo courtesy of L. Connor Nickels, MD, RDMS)

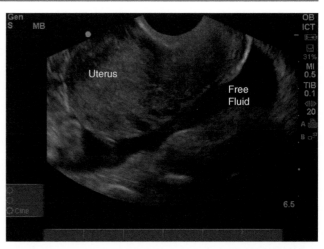

Fig. 110.4 Transvaginal sagittal image of an empty uterus and large free fluid in the posterior cul-de-sac in a patient with a presumed ectopic pregnancy (Photo courtesy of L. Connor Nickels, MD, RDMS)

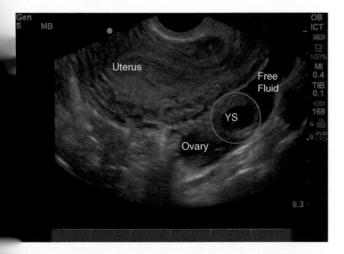

Fig. 110.3 Transvaginal sagittal image of an empty uterus with an ectopic pregnancy (in red circle) noted just posterior in the adnexa, adjacent to the ovary. The gestational sac contains a yolk sac and there is free fluid surrounding the ectopic, concerning for rupture (Photo courtesy of L. Connor Nickels, MD, RDMS). YS–yolk sac

110.2 Contraindications

- Treating ectopic pregnancy medically when there is a fetal pole with fetal cardiac activity present
- Failing to consult obstetrics/gynecology when the patient has a serum hCG above the discriminatory zone and no sonographic findings to diagnose intrauterine pregnancy

110.3 Materials and Medications

- Ultrasound machine
- Probes: transabdominal and transvaginal
- Gel
- Skilled ultrasound operator
- Endocavitary probe covers
- Pelvic setup (speculum and cultures)
- Cardiac monitor, two large-bore intravenous needles
- Laboratory work: serum quantitative hCG, hemoglobin, group and Rh, type and screen
  - May add additional laboratory tests depending on the stability and symptoms of the patient

110.4 Procedure

- Ultrasound machine in obstetrics preset
- Transabdominal
  1. Place the patient in the supine position.
  2. Ideally, the bladder will be full for a good acoustic window.
  3. Using a curvilinear probe, 3.5–5.0 MHz.
  4. Begin scanning the patient in a sagittal position to identify the uterus as it lies in position with the bladder. Scan through the uterus completely in this plane, looking for signs of intrauterine pregnancy.
  5. Imaging in the transverse plane should be done in the same fashion.
  6. Any signs of an intrauterine pregnancy should be clearly identified and measured.
     - Gestational sac diameter
     - Yolk sac diameter
     - Fetal pole with crown rump diameter
       - If present, fetal cardiac activity should be recorded by using M mode to obtain a tracing and measure the fetal heart rate.
  7. Although sometimes limited transabdominally, an attempt to identify the adnexa should be performed in both planes bilaterally.
  8. Any abnormalities identified should be noted.
     - Free fluid surrounding the uterus (anterior or posterior cul-de-sac) or ovaries

- On pelvic imaging or FAST examination
- Intrauterine contents not consistent with an intrauterine pregnancy and/or not clearly, centrally visualized within the fundus of the uterus
- Masses or contained fluid collections outside the uterus
- Yolk sac or fetal pole with or without fetal cardiac activity seen outside the uterus
  9. Transvaginal scanning should be performed if a definitive intrauterine pregnancy is not identified on transabdominal imaging.
- Transvaginal
  1. Place the patient in the lithotomy position.
  2. Bladder is preferably empty.
  3. Use a transvaginal probe, 5–7.5 MHz.
  4. Repeat same steps as transabdominal imaging previously.
- The procedure is the same for all pelvic ultrasounds including transabdominal and transvaginal imaging because this should be performed in a systematic fashion so as to not miss pertinent findings. Therefore, the findings may change, but the examination remains the same.
- Yolk sac should be first sign of definitive intrauterine pregnancy for emergency physicians because the decidual reaction and gestational sac are not 100 % accurate.

110.5 Complications

- Bleeding: internal and/or external
- Maternal death if ectopic ruptures
  - Nine percent of pregnancy-related deaths
  - Leading cause of maternal death in the first trimester
- Sterility if tube(s) are damaged or surgically removed

110.6 Pearls and Pitfalls

- Pearls
  - Following the algorithm despite the patient being asymptomatic can help avoid missed ectopic pregnancies.
  - Cervical ectopic pregnancy can be difficult to distinguish from a spontaneous abortion. If the patient aborting, the ultrasound findings should change quickly and the patient should have vaginal bleeding
  - Double decidual reaction versus pseudogestational sac can be a very subtle distinction and should not be made by emergency physicians; hence, the statement made earlier, requiring a yolk sac as the earliest definitive sign of an intrauterine pregnancy.

- Fibroids, bicornuate uterus, and eccentrically located normal pregnancy can all appear similar to a cornual pregnancy.
- The majority of times when the patient is pregnant, has an empty uterus on sonographic imaging, and has vaginal bleeding, the final diagnosis is still unknown because it could still be an early normal pregnancy or an ectopic pregnancy.
- Pitfalls
  - Failing to obtain a pregnancy test in all reproductive-age women who have not undergone a hysterectomy
  - Failing to identify subtle signs of ectopic pregnancies

Reference

1. Ma OJ, Mateer JR, Blaivas M, editors. Emergency ultrasound. 2nd ed. New York: McGraw-Hill Professional; 2007.

Selected Reading

Gabbe SG, Niebyl JR, Galan HL, et al., editors. Obstetrics: normal and problem pregnancies. 5th ed. Philadelphia: Churchill Livingstone; 2007.

Marx J, Hockberger R, Walls R, editors. Rosen's emergency medicine: concepts and clinical practice. 7th ed. Philadelphia: Mosby; 2010.

Sanders RC, Winter T, editors. Clinical sonography: a practical guide. 4th ed. Philadelphia: Lippincott Williams & Wilkins; 2007.

Stead LG, Behera SR. Ectopic pregnancy. J Emerg Med. 2007;32(2):205–6.

Ultrasonography for Hydatidiform Mole

111

L. Connor Nickels

Definition: molar pregnancy = hydatidiform mole = anomalous growth of trophoblastic tissue
- Complete: 46,XX or 46,XY
  - Completely paternal in origin
  - Contains no fetal tissue
  - Most recognizable by clinical symptoms
- Incomplete (partial mole): 69,XXX or 69,XXY
  - Maternal and paternal in origin
  - Contains fetal tissue
  - More subtle clinical presentation

111.1 Indications

- Clinical presentation of any combination of the following:
  - Vaginal bleeding
  - With or without vomiting, persistent hyperemesis gravidarum
  - High blood pressure
  - Uterine size large for dates
- Serum human chorionic gonadotropin (hCG) very elevated (more than would be consistent for dates)
  - Usually greater than 100,000 mIU/mL

111.2 Contraindications

- Conservative management

L.C. Nickels, MD, RDMS
Department of Emergency Medicine,
University of Florida Health Shands Hospital,
Gainesville, FL, USA
e-mail: cnickels@ufl.edu

111.3 Materials and Medications

- Ultrasound machine
- Probes: curvilinear (abdominal) and endocavitary (transvaginal)
- Gel
- Skilled ultrasound operator
- Endocavitary probe covers
- Pelvic setup (speculum and cultures)
- Lab work: serum quantitative hCG, hemoglobin, group and Rh
  - May add additional laboratory tests depending on the stability and symptoms of the patient

111.4 Procedure

- Ultrasound machine in obstetrics preset
- Transabdominal imaging
  1. Place the patient in the supine position.
  2. Ideally the bladder will be full for a good acoustic window.
  3. Using a curvilinear probe, 3.5–5.0 MHz, begin scanning the patient in a sagittal position to identify the uterus as it lies in position with the bladder. Scan through the uterus completely in this plane, looking for signs of intrauterine pregnancy.
  4. Rotate the probe to a transverse position (counterclockwise), with the probe indicator toward the patient's right. Scan through the uterus completely in this plane, looking for signs of intrauterine pregnancy.
  5. Any signs of an intrauterine pregnancy should be clearly identified and measured.
  6. Sonographic findings of a molar pregnancy include:
     - Uterus filled with heterogeneous material.
       - Echogenic material interspersed with anechoic areas known as the "snowstorm" is the most common appearance of a mole (Fig. 111.1).

© Springer Science+Business Media New York 2016
Ganti (ed.), *Atlas of Emergency Medicine Procedures*, DOI 10.1007/978-1-4939-2507-0_111

- Can be confused with missed abortion or fibroid, underscoring the importance of the serum hCG because this will be markedly elevated, which would make the alternative diagnoses less likely.
- Theca lutein cysts are present in the adnexa.
  - Multiple cysts that occur with trophoblastic disease, multiple pregnancies (e.g., twins, triplets, quadruplets), and induced ovulation.
7. Although sometimes limited transabdominally, an attempt to identify the adnexa should be performed in both planes bilaterally.
8. Any abnormalities should be noted.
9. Transvaginal scanning should be performed if a definitive intrauterine pregnancy is not identified on transabdominal imaging.
- Transvaginal imaging
  1. Place the patient in the lithotomy position.
  2. Bladder is preferably empty.
  3. Use an endocavitary probe, 5–7.5 MHz.
  4. Repeat the same steps as for transabdominal imaging previously discussed (#2).
  5. After scanning through the uterus in sagittal and transverse planes, the adnexa should be scanned in the same format bilaterally, looking for any abnormalities, as mentioned previously.
  6. Again, any abnormalities should be noted:
     - Free fluid surrounding the uterus (anterior or posterior cul-de-sac) and/or ovaries
     - Masses or contained fluid collections outside the uterus
     - Yolk sac or fetal pole with or without fetal cardiac activity seen outside the uterus

- The procedure is the same for all pelvic ultrasounds, transabdominal and transvaginal imaging, because this should be performed in a systematic fashion so as to not miss pertinent findings. Therefore, the findings may change, but the examination remains the same.
- Yolk sac should be the first sign of definitive intrauterine pregnancy for emergency physicians because the decidual reaction and gestational sac are not 100 % accurate.

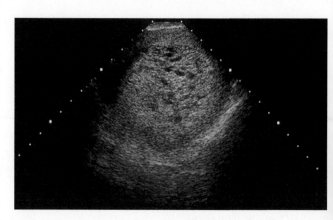

Fig. 111.1 Uterus with "cluster of grapes" represents a molar pregnancy (With kind permission from Springer Science+Business Media: Swisher E, Greer B, Montz FJ, Stenchever M. Chapter 14. In: *Atlas of Clinical Gynecology*. Vol. 4. 2002)

111.5 Complications

- Multiple complications can occur and include the following:
  - Invasive mole: when a hydatidiform mole recurs after a dilation and curettage and, subsequently, invades the muscle of the uterus.
    - Molar tissue is extremely vascular and necessitates an ultrasound with color flow to visualize any residual invasive tissue.
  - Choriocarcinoma: molar tissue develops into an aggressive malignancy, metastasizing early throughout the body.
    - In this scenario, the tumor takes on a very cystic appearance with an echogenic rim. When this is seen, one should attempt to view the liver as well for heterogeneous appearance consistent with metastasis or consider other imaging tests (more comprehensive ultrasound, computed tomography, or magnetic resonance imaging) as indicated to further assess concerns for malignancy.
    - Extremely sensitive to chemotherapy, but most favorable results are seen when diagnosed and treated early.

111.6 Pearls and Pitfalls

- Pearls
  - An obstetrics consult must be obtained in the emergency department when this diagnosis is made.
    - Patient must have a dilation and curettage to evacuate the mole.
  - Serum hCG must be followed to less than detectable levels because they have a high rate of recurrence (invasive mole) and potential for malignancy (choriocarcinoma).
  - May occur with intrauterine or ectopic pregnancies or after spontaneous abortions or full-term pregnancies
  - Qualitative and quantitative β-hCG results may be falsely negative in the setting of a molar pregnancy secondary to the "high-dose hook effect" found in sandwich immunoassays in which there is an overabundance of antigen. This error can be corrected by diluting the urine or serum sample and repeating the test.
- Pitfalls
  - Many pitfalls with potentially life-threatening consequences surround this diagnosis. Meticulous observation of the entire picture, including clinical presentation, laboratory results, and ultrasound findings, will help to avoid these outcomes.

Selected Reading

Gabbe SG, Niebyl JR, Galan HL, et al., editors. Obstetrics: normal and problem pregnancies. 5th ed. New York: Churchill Livingstone; 2007.

Hunter CL, Ladde J. Molar pregnancy with false negative â-hCG urine in the emergency department. West J Emerg Med. 2011;12:213–5.

Lentz GM, Lobo RA, Gershenson DM, et al., editors. Comprehensive gynecology. 6th ed. Philadelphia: Mosby; 2012.

Ma OJ, Mateer JR, Blaivas M. Emergency ultrasound. 2nd ed. New York: McGraw Hill Professional; 2008.

Sanders RC, Winter T, editors. Clinical sonography: a practical guide. 4th ed. Philadelphia: Lippincott Williams & Wilkins; 2007.

Ultrasonography for Blighted Ovum (Anembryonic Gestation)

112

Katrina Skoog Nguyen and L. Connor Nickels

112.1 Indications

- A blighted ovum or anembryonic gestation is a pregnancy in which the embryo never develops in the gestational sac (Fig. 112.1).
- Presents as first-trimester vaginal bleeding and/or pelvic pain or cramping
- Criteria for defining an anembryonic pregnancy:
  - Based, in part, on mean gestational diameter (MGD), which is an average of three orthogonal measurements of the gestational sac
    - MGD greater than or equal to 25mm with no embryo
    - 5 MHz or less
      - MGD greater than or equal to 20 mm without a yolk sac
  - May have abnormally low sac position

- References differ in their measurements depending on the approach, transabdominal versus transvaginal, and the frequency of the probe (e.g., 5 MHz vs. 6.5 MHz or greater).

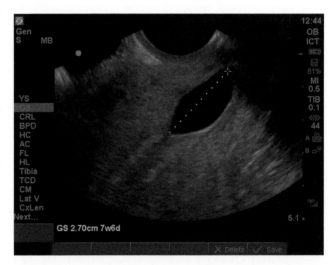

Fig. 112.1 Low-lying empty gestational sac consistent with blighted ovum (Photo courtesy of L. Connor Nickels, MD, RDMS)

K.S. Nguyen, DO • L.C. Nickels, MD, RDMS (✉)
Department of Emergency Medicine,
University of Florida Health Shands Hospital,
Gainesville, FL, USA
e-mail: katrinaskoog@hotmail.com; cnickels@ufl.edu

Springer Science+Business Media New York 2016
Ganti (ed.), *Atlas of Emergency Medicine Procedures*, DOI 10.1007/978-1-4939-2507-0_112

112.2 Contraindications

- Misinterpreting images as blighted ovum when any of the following could potentially be present:
    - Early intrauterine pregnancy
    - Pseudogestational sac
    - Molar pregnancy
- Discussions with the patient should always involve an obstetrics consult or referral for definitive decisions and treatment.

112.3 Materials and Medications

- Ultrasound machine
- Probes: transabdominal and transvaginal
- Ultrasound gel
- Endocavitary probe covers
- Skilled ultrasound operator
- Laboratory tests: serum quantitative human chorionic gonadotropin (hCG), hemoglobin, group, and Rh
    - May add additional laboratory tests depending on the stability and symptoms of the patient

112.4 Procedure

- Ultrasound machine in obstetrics preset
- Transabdominal
    1. Place the patient in the supine position.
    2. Ideally the bladder will be full for a good acoustic window.
    3. Use a curvilinear probe, 3.5–5.0 MHz.
    4. Begin scanning the patient in a sagittal position to identify the uterus as it lies in position with the bladder. Scan through the uterus completely in this plane, looking for signs of intrauterine pregnancy.
    5. Imaging in the transverse plane should be done in the same fashion.
    6. Any signs of an intrauterine pregnancy should be clearly identified and measured.
        - In this case, gestational sac and any other intrauterine contents
    7. Although sometimes limited transabdominally, an attempt to identify the adnexa should be performed in both planes bilaterally.
    8. Any abnormalities should be noted.
        - Free fluid surrounding the uterus (anterior or posterior cul-de-sac) or ovaries
        - Masses or contained fluid collections outside the uterus
        - Yolk sac or fetal pole with or without fetal cardiac activity seen outside the uterus

9. Transvaginal scanning should be performed if a definitive intrauterine pregnancy is not identified on transabdominal imaging.
- Transvaginal
    1. Place the patient in the lithotomy position.
    2. Bladder is preferably empty.
    3. Use a transvaginal probe, 5–7.5 MHz.
    4. Repeat the same steps as for transabdominal imaging previously discussed (#2).
- The procedure is the same for all pelvic ultrasounds including transabdominal and transvaginal imaging because this should be performed in a systematic fashion so as to not miss pertinent findings. Therefore, the findings may change, but the examination remains the same.
- Yolk sac should be first sign of definitive intrauterine pregnancy for emergency physicians because the decidual reaction and gestational sac are not 100 % accurate.

112.5 Complications

- Bleeding
- Retained products of conception

112.6 Pearls and Pitfalls

- Pearls
    - See "Contraindications." If following an algorithm, a blighted ovum would fall into indeterminate category and obstetrics consult is recommended in the emergency department.
- Pitfalls
    - It is imperative to inform all pregnant patients that obstetrical ultrasonography performed by emergency physicians is limited and not used to detect fetal health and/or anatomy.

Selected Reading

Cosby K, Kendall J, editors. Practical guide to emergency ultrasoun Philadelphia: Lippincott Williams & Wilkins; 2006.

Doubilet PM, Benson CB, Bourne T, Blaivas M. Diagnostic criteria f nonviable pregnancy early in the first trimester. N Engl J Me 2013;369(15):1443–51.

Ma OJ, Mateer JR, Blaivas M, editors. Emergency ultrasound. 2nd e New York: McGraw Hill Professional; 2007.

Morin L, Van den Hof MC. Ultrasound evaluation of first trimes pregnancy complications. J Obstet Gynaecol Ca 2005;161:581–5.

Sanders RC, Winter T, editors. Clinical sonography: a practical gui 4th ed. Philadelphia: Lippincott Williams & Wilkins; 2007.

Shah K, Mason C, editors. Essential emergency procedur Philadelphia: Lippincott Williams & Wilkins; 2008.

Ultrasonography for Threatened, Incomplete, or Compete Abortion

113

L. Connor Nickels and Giuliano De Portu

Key Points

Threatened abortion: closed os, no passage of products of conception (POC).

Inevitable abortion: open os, no POC.

Incomplete abortion: open os, passage of POC.

Complete abortion: closed os, empty uterus (all POC passed).

Missed abortion: fetus has died and the uterus has failed to enlarge any further.

113.1 Indications

- Vaginal bleeding in the setting of early intrauterine pregnancy

113.2 Contraindications

- There are no contraindications to ultrasonography.

113.3 Materials and Medications

- Ultrasound machine
- Probes: curvilinear (transabdominal) and endocavitary (transvaginal)
- Gel
- Endocavitary probe covers
- Towels
- Skilled ultrasound operator
- Pelvic setup (speculum and cultures)
- Cardiac monitor and intravenous access if bleeding is significant
- Laboratory tests: serum human chorionic gonadotropin (hCG), hemoglobin, group and Rh, type, and screen

L.C. Nickels, MD, RDMS (✉) • G. De Portu, MD
Department of Emergency Medicine, University of Florida Health
Shands Hospital, Gainesville, FL, USA
e-mail: cnickels@ufl.edu; gdeportu@ufl.edu

113.4 Procedure

The procedure is the same for all pelvic ultrasounds including transabdominal and transvaginal imaging because this should be performed in a systematic fashion so as to not miss pertinent findings. Therefore, the findings may change, but the examination remains the same.

1. Place the patient in the supine position.
2. Ultrasound machine in obstetrics preset with abdominal probe and gel.
3. Begin scanning the patient in a transabdominal sagittal plane to identify the uterus as it lies in position with the bladder. Scan through the uterus completely in this plane looking for signs of intrauterine pregnancy (gestational sac, yolk sac, fetal pole, fetal cardiac activity).
   - For our purposes as emergency physicians, a yolk sac (at the least) must be seen within the uterus to definitively report an intrauterine pregnancy (Fig. 113.1). The decidual reaction and/or presence of gestational sac is not 100 % accurate.
4. Transabdominal imaging in the transverse plane should be done in the same fashion.
5. If an intrauterine pregnancy is clearly identified on transabdominal scanning, appropriate measurements can be taken to estimate dates:
   - Gestational sac diameter.
   - Yolk sac diameter or crown rump length (CRL).
   - If present, fetal cardiac activity should be recorded by using M mode to obtain a tracing and measure the fetal heart rate (Fig. 113.2).
6. For a complete examination, the adnexa should be scanned in an attempt to identify the ovaries bilaterally.
7. Any abnormalities identified should be noted:
   - Free fluid surrounding the uterus (anterior or posterior cul-de-sac) or ovaries
     - On pelvic imaging or focused assessment with sonography in trauma (FAST) examination

Ganti (ed.), *Atlas of Emergency Medicine Procedures*, DOI 10.1007/978-1-4939-2507-0_113

- Intrauterine contents not consistent with an intrauterine pregnancy and/or not clearly, centrally visualized within the fundus of the uterus
- Any masses or contained fluid collections noted outside the uterus
- Yolk sac or fetal pole with or without fetal cardiac activity seen outside the uterus

8. Transvaginal scanning with the endocavitary probe should be performed if a definitive intrauterine pregnancy is not identified on transabdominal imaging.
9. Transvaginal imaging is performed in the sagittal and transverse planes to identify an intrauterine pregnancy, with bladder preferably empty.

10. Measurements should be taken of any intrauterine findings.
    - Same as #5.
    - CRL >7 mm on transvaginal ultrasound should have fetal cardiac activity.
11. Each adnexa should be scanned in the sagittal and transverse planes.
12. Any abnormalities identified should be noted.
    - Same as #7.
13. The uterus will be empty in the case of a complete abortion (Figs. 113.3 and 113.4).

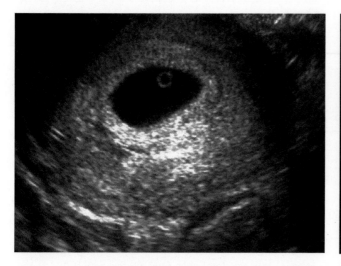

Fig. 113.1 Yolk sac present within the gestational sac with double decidual reaction (With kind permission from Springer Science+Business Media: Buja LM, Chandrasekhar C. Chapter 7: pathology of the breast and female genital tract. In: Krueger GRF, Buja LM, eds. *Atlas of Anatomic Pathology with Imaging*. 2013)

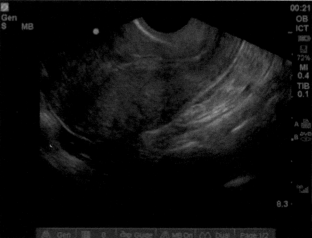

Fig. 113.3 Transvaginal sagittal image of an empty uterus (Photo courtesy of L. Connor Nickels, MD, RDMS)

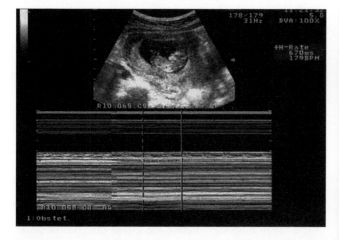

Fig. 113.2 Fetal cardiac activity recorded using M mode to obtain a tracing and measure the fetal heart rate (With kind permission from Springer Science+Business Media: Hanprasertpong T, Phupong V. First trimester embryonic/fetal heart rate in normal pregnant women. *Archives of Gynecology and Obstetrics*. 2006;274(5))

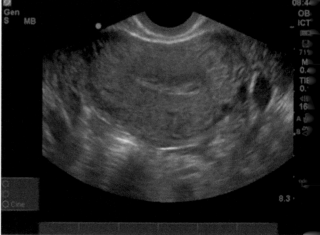

Fig. 113.4 Transvaginal transverse image of an empty uterus (Photo courtesy of L. Connor Nickels, MD, RDMS)

113.5 Complications

- Vaginal bleeding
- Miscarriage
- Rh isoimmunization

113.6 Pearls and Pitfalls

- Pearls
  - Threatened abortion:
    - Threatened abortion is not visible sonographically. It is the presumed diagnosis when a patient presents with vaginal bleeding in the first 20 weeks of pregnancy, an intrauterine pregnancy is found with dates corresponding to the patient's dates, and the cervix is closed.
    - Fetal cardiac activity suggests a better prognosis than those without.
    - Fetal heart rate less than 120 bpm suggests impending fetal death (only 6 % survival).
  - Completed abortion:
    - There are only three scenarios in which this diagnosis can confidently be made in the emergency department:
      1. Intact gestation is passed and identified in the emergency room.
      2. Ultrasound shows an empty uterus in the setting of a prior known intrauterine pregnancy.
         - Small internal echoes within the uterus may represent blood rather than retained products of conception, but this determination should be made in consultation with obstetrics.
      3. Negative pregnancy test result in the setting of a prior known intrauterine pregnancy.
    - In all other cases, the quantitative β-hCG must be followed until it is less than 2 mIU/mL.
- Pitfalls
  - Treating threatened abortion as fetal demise or abortion – many of these pregnancies actually go on to completion with a normal fetus.
  - If there is any concern for alternative diagnoses in any of the abortion types (i.e., ectopic gestation), obstetrics consult should be obtained.
  - Failing to order a quantitative serum hCG to rule out other possibilities (e.g., molar pregnancy) and to ensure that it is trending downward (if others to compare).
  - Failing to establish follow-up for an incomplete abortion to ensure appropriate management. The patient may eventually require a dilation and curettage if products do not pass naturally.

Selected Reading

Doubilet PM, Benson CB, Bourne T, Blaivas M. Diagnostic criteria for nonviable pregnancy early in the first trimester. N Engl J Med. 2013;369(15):1443–51.

Gabbe SG, Niebyl JR, Galan HL, et al., editors. Obstetrics: normal and problem pregnancies. 5th ed. Orlando: Churchill Livingstone; 2007.

Ma OJ, Mateer JR, Blaivas M, editors. Emergency ultrasound. 2nd ed. New York: McGraw-Hill Professional; 2007.

Marx J, Hockberger R, Walls R, editors. Rosen's emergency medicine. 7th ed. Philadelphia: Mosby; 2010.

Sanders RC, Winter T, editors. Clinical sonography: a practical guide. 4th ed. Philadelphia: Lippincott Williams & Wilkins; 2007.

Ultrasonography for Placenta Previa

114

L. Connor Nickels and Giuliano De Portu

Placenta previa is a condition in which the placenta covers the internal cervical os. It is the leading cause of antepartum hemorrhage. There are four grades of the condition:

- Complete: Placenta completely covers the internal os.
- Partial: Placenta partially covers the internal os.

- Marginal : Lower margin of placenta reaches the internal os but does not cover it (within 3 cm).
- Low lying: Lower margin of placenta is located in the lower uterine segment but does not reach the internal os (Fig. 114.1).

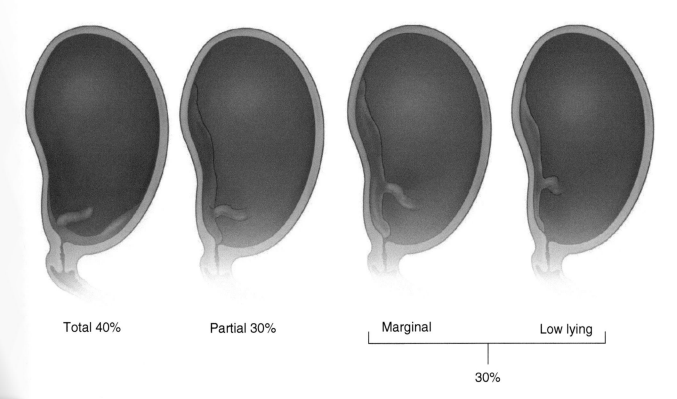

Total 40%   Partial 30%   Marginal   Low lying

30%

Fig. 114.1 Varying degrees of placenta previa

.C. Nickels, MD, RDMS (✉) • G. De Portu, MD
Department of Emergency Medicine, University of Florida Health
Shands Hospital, Gainesville, FL, USA
e-mail: cnickels@ufl.edu; gdeportu@ufl.edu

Springer Science+Business Media New York 2016
Ganti (ed.), *Atlas of Emergency Medicine Procedures*, DOI 10.1007/978-1-4939-2507-0_114

114.1 Indications

- A patient in the second half of pregnancy who presents to the emergency room with bright red, painless vaginal bleeding OR premature labor should be evaluated for this condition.

114.2 Contraindications

- Absolute:
  - There are no absolute contraindications to transabdominal ultrasonography.
- Relative:
  - Transvaginal ultrasound should be carried out with caution, so as to avoid hemorrhage.

114.3 Materials and Medications

- Ultrasound machine
- Probes: curvilinear or phased array, endocavitary
- Sterile gel
- Endocavitary probe covers
- Towels
- Sterile speculum (see previously)
- Cardiac monitor, two large-bore intravenous needles, laboratory tests

114.4 Procedure

1. Place the patient in the supine position.
2. Ultrasound machine with abdominal probe and gel.
3. Begin scanning the patient in a transabdominal sagittal position (Fig. 114.2) to determine the placental position and whether it is lying in the lower uterine segment.
4. The patient should then be scanned in a transverse fashion to further evaluate the exact position of the placenta.
5. If the placenta appears to lie in the lower uterine segment, the patient should be scanned in the oblique plane as well.
6. The bladder should initially be full for best visualization. However, if the placenta appears to reside low or lie over the internal os, the scanning should be repeated after the patient has voided.
   - An overdistended bladder may create the appearance of a placenta previa. The anterior wall of the uterus is compressed against the posterior wall by the distended bladder, shortening the distance between the placenta and the internal os (Fig. 114.3).
7. The following ultrasonographic findings exclude placenta previa [1]:
   - Direct apposition of the presenting part of the fetus and the cervix without space for interposed tissue
   - Presence of amniotic fluid between the presenting part of the fetus and the cervix, without the presence of placental tissue
   - Distance of greater than 2 cm between the inferior aspect of the placenta
   - Indirect visualization of the internal cervical os
8. If placenta previa cannot be ruled out with transabdominal ultrasound, the patient should then be scanned transvaginally with the endocavitary probe because this is more sensitive for diagnosing placenta previa.
9. A sterile speculum examination should be performed before transvaginal scanning to assess the cervix and ensure there are no presenting parts or bulging membranes. Transvaginal imaging is contraindicated if the patient has ruptured or bulging membranes.
10. The probes should be swapped out and a sterile cover placed on the endocavitary probe with gel inside the cover and sterile gel on the outside of the cover.
11. The endocavitary probe should be inserted into the vaginal canal, ensuring that caution is taken to stay off the cervix and distal to it, keeping the cervix in view on the screen.
12. The patient should be scanned in both the sagittal and the transverse planes to assess the inferior margin of the placenta.

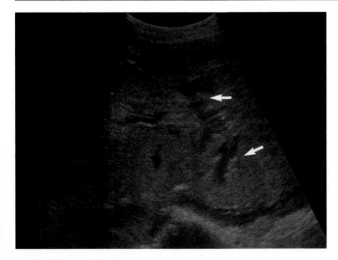

Fig. 114.2 Transabdominal ultrasound of placenta previa. Note loss of the decidual interface between the placenta and the myometrium on the lower part of the uterus and multiple intraplacental lacunae (*arrows*) (Reproduced with permission from *J Korean Med Sci*. 2010; 25(4):651–5)

13. If the inferior margin appears to be located near the internal os, then the distance should be measured.
    - Steps 8 through 13 should only be performed by the emergency physician if he or she feels confident in this ultrasound skill and there is no obstetrics available. If obstetrics is available, these steps should be performed in conjunction with them or by them to ensure the best outcome for the patient.

Fig. 114.3 (**a**) Overdistended bladder creating the appearance of placenta previa, (**b**) empty bladder showing the more accurate position of the placenta

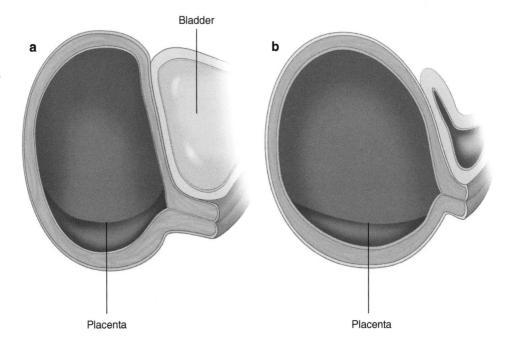

114.5 Complications

- Bleeding:
  - May range from self-limited to life-threatening hemorrhage
- Maternal and/or fetal distress or death

114.6 Pearls and Pitfalls

- Pearls
  - Risk factors include:
    - Multiparity
    - Multiple pregnancy
    - Advanced maternal age
    - Previous placenta previa
    - Cigarette smoking
    - Cocaine abuse
    - Hypertension
    - Previous cesarean delivery/uterine surgeries
  - Myometrium contraction: can mimic placenta previa by temporarily displacing the placenta in the lower uterine segment.
  - If ultrasound capabilities are not available, but the patient is in the second half of pregnancy and having vaginal bleeding, do not perform a digital cervical examination.
- Pitfalls
  - Digital examination should be avoided because this may precipitate life-threatening hemorrhage and/or death.

- Always consult obstetrics as soon as possible if this is suspected or known and the patient is symptomatic. Not consulting obstetrics could be detrimental to the mother and fetus.
- Gentle sterile speculum examination should be done only if an obstetrician is not available. This is to ensure the bleeding is coming from the cervix. If placenta previa is suspected or known and obstetrics are available, then abdominal ultrasound evaluation alone should be sufficient for the examination of the patient.

Reference

1. American College of Radiology. Role of imaging in second and third trimester bleeding. In: ACR Appropriateness Criteri. Reston: American College of Radiology; 2001.

Selected Reading

Gabbe SG, Niebyl JR, Galan HL, et al., editors. Obstetrics: normal and problem pregnancies. 5th ed. Orlando: Churchill Livingstone; 2007.

Ma OJ, Mateer J, Blaivas M, editors. Emergency ultrasound. 2nd ed. New York: McGraw Hill Professional; 2007.

Marx J, Hockberger R, Walls R, editors. Rosen's emergency medicine: concepts and clinical practice. 7th ed. Philadelphia: Mosby; 2010.

Sanders RC, Winter T, editors. Clinical sonography: a practical guide. 4th ed. Philadelphia: Lippincott Williams & Wilkins; 2007.

Vaginal Delivery

Umarfarook Javed Mirza, Christopher Shields, and Muhammad Waseem

115.1 Indications

- Inevitable delivery of the fetus (cervix fully dilated at 10 cm and fully effaced 1 mm with crowning of the head)

115.2 Contraindications

- Absolute:
  - Indications for emergent cesarean section (C-section)
  - Prolapsed cord
  - Prior C-section with classic vertical incision
  - Placenta previa – complete/partial
  - Breech presentation – footling
- Relative:
  - Placenta previa – marginal/low lying
  - Breech presentation – complete/incomplete/frank

115.3 Materials and Medications (Fig. 115.1)

- 4 Crile clamps or Kelly clamps
- 1 Mayo scissor curved and 1 Mayo scissor straight
- 2 sponge forceps
- 2 towel clamps
- 1 Mayo-Hegar needle holder
- 1 mouse-tooth forceps
- Suction bulb
- Betadine (povidone-iodine)
- Umbilical cord clamp (Fig. 115.2)
- Incubator warmer (Fig. 115.3)
- Most importantly, help.

J. Mirza, DO
Department of Emergency Medicine,
Baylor University Medical Center, Dallas, TX, USA
email: Umarfarook.Mirza@gmail.com

Shields, MD • M. Waseem, MD (✉)
Department of Emergency Medicine,
Lincoln Medical and Mental Health Center, New York, NY, USA
email: cpatrickshields@hotmail.com; waseemm2001@hotmail.com

© Springer Science+Business Media New York 2016
Ganti (ed.), *Atlas of Emergency Medicine Procedures*, DOI 10.1007/978-1-4939-2507-0_115

Fig. 115.1 Equipment: delivery set

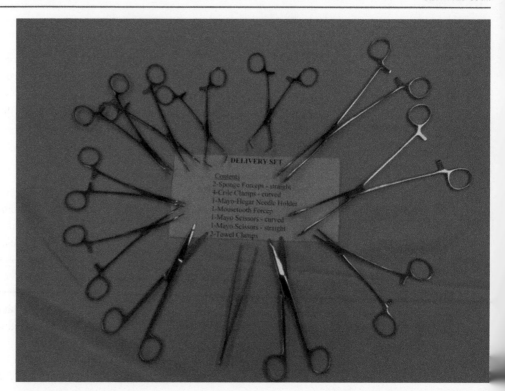

Fig. 115.2 Equipment: umbilical clamp

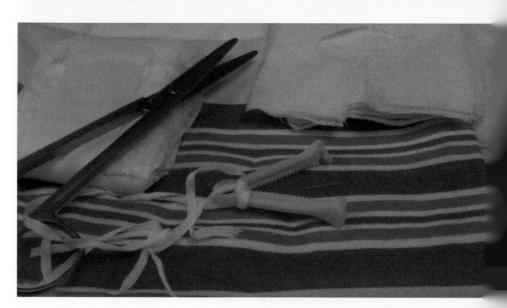

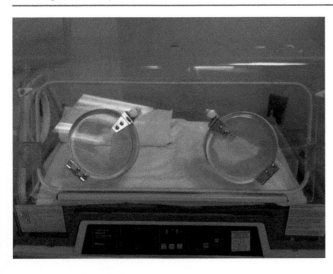

Fig. 115.3 Equipment: incubator warmer

115.4 Procedure

1. Determine the fetal presentation (breech or cephalic) with Leopold's maneuvers or bedside ultrasound.
2. If breech, follow the breech pathway.
3. Perform a vaginal examination.
4. Check for cord prolapse.
5. Check effacement.
6. Check dilation.
7. Prepare the site.
8. Position the mother in the extreme lithotomy position.
9. Deliver the head in a controlled manner.
10. Check to see if the cord is wrapped around the neck. If present, follow cord presentation pathway.
11. Deliver the anterior shoulder with downward traction of the head.
12. Check for shoulder dystocia. If present, follow the McRobert-Rubin maneuvers (see Chap. 116).
13. Deliver the posterior shoulder by gently pulling the trunk upward.
14. Suction the airway.
15. Clamp the cord 5 cm from the umbilicus in two places and cut.
16. Obtain Apgar score of the baby. Initiate resuscitation if required.
17. Keep the baby warm in the incubator.
18. Clamp the cord again closer to the vaginal opening.
19. Use this clamp to help deliver the placenta. Use gentle controlled traction on the clamp with one hand while placing the other hand suprapubically to push the uterus upward.
20. If the placenta does not deliver easily, stop and wait a few minutes to allow it to come away from the uterine wall naturally and then try again.
21. Placenta must be fully intact. If not, check for retained intrauterine placental products, and manually remove them; retained placenta may cause postpartum hemorrhage.
    - Massage the fundus externally to prevent uterine atony, but only after all products have been removed.
22. Repair any vaginal or cervical lacerations.

115.5 Complications

- Postpartum hemorrhage due to uterine atony or retained products
- Uterine inversion
- Rectal or urethral injuries
- Shoulder dystocia
- Meconium aspiration

115.6 Pearls and Pitfalls

- Pearls
  - Postpartum hemorrhage has a high incidence during the first hour postpartum.
  - Be aware of possible second delivery.
  - Oxytocin or Methergine (methylergonovine maleate) may be used after delivery of the placenta; both help increase uterine contractions and decrease postpartum hemorrhage.

- Pitfalls
  - Rushing delivery of the head/shoulders can lead to trauma to the mother/baby.
  - Rushing delivery of the placenta, when the placenta is not ready to detach, may cause placental or cord tearing or uterine inversion. Remember: it may take up to 20 min for the placenta to detach from the uterus.

Selected Reading

Desai S, Henderson SO, Mallon WK. Labor and delivery and their complications. In: Marx J, Hockberger R, Walls R, editors. Rosen's emergency medicine: concepts and clinical practice. 7th ed. Philadelphia: Mosby; 2010.

Liao JB, Buhimschi CS, Norwitz ER. Normal labor: mechanism and duration. Obstet Gynecol Clin North Am. 2005;32:145–64.

Norwitz ER, Robinson JN, Repke JT. Labor and delivery. In: Gabbe SG, Niebyl JR, Simpson JL, editors. Obstetrics: normal and problem pregnancies. 4th ed. Philadelphia: Saunders; 2001. p. 353–94.

Shoulder Dystocia Management

Irina Fox Brennan and Joseph A. Tyndall

116.1 Indications

- Retracting fetal head ("turtle sign")
- Failure of anterior shoulder delivery following gentle downward traction
- Difficult face-chin delivery
- Failure of shoulders to descend

116.2 Contraindications

- Mother with diabetes and fetus larger than 4500 g
- Mother without diabetes and fetus larger than 5000 g
- History of shoulder dystocia with prior birth

- Factors that signal the need for cesarean section:
    - Complete/partial placenta previa
    - Cord prolapse
    - Brow/face presentation
    - Non-reassuring fetal heart rate
    - Extensive uterine surgery and previous classic uterine incision

116.3 Materials and Medications

- No specialized materials/equipment required.
- Team coordination is of utmost importance.

.F. Brennan, MD • J.A. Tyndall, MD, MPH (✉)
Department of Emergency Medicine, University of Florida Health, Gainesville, FL, USA
-mail: ibrennan@ufl.edu; tyndall@ufl.edu

Springer Science+Business Media New York 2016
. Ganti (ed.), *Atlas of Emergency Medicine Procedures*, DOI 10.1007/978-1-4939-2507-0_116

116.4 Procedure

1. *Accurate documentation*: Designate a team member to document the progress of labor, the position and rotation of the infant's head, the time of delivery for the head and body, the presence of episiotomy, anesthesia requirements, the duration of shoulder dystocia, whether the shoulder is anterior or posterior at the time of delivery, the onset/duration/results of maneuver(s) performed, and Apgar scores.

   The HELPERR mnemonic is commonly employed:

2. *Help recruitment*: Involve anesthesiology, pediatric resuscitation, and obstetric/gynecology colleagues either as part of advance preparations or via activation of protocol during labor.

3. *Episiotomy consideration*: Not required but might be of benefit if more space is needed for rotation maneuvers.
   - Episiotomy alone will not release the impacted shoulder.

4. *Legs positioned for the McRoberts maneuver*: Position the woman's thighs onto her abdomen by abducting and flexing her hips. Have two assistants help her, one on either side. This increases the functional size of the bony pelvis by rotating the pubic symphysis toward the mother's head, hence aiding delivery (Fig. 116.1).

Fig. 116.1 McRoberts maneuver: hyperflexion of the maternal thighs against the abdomen

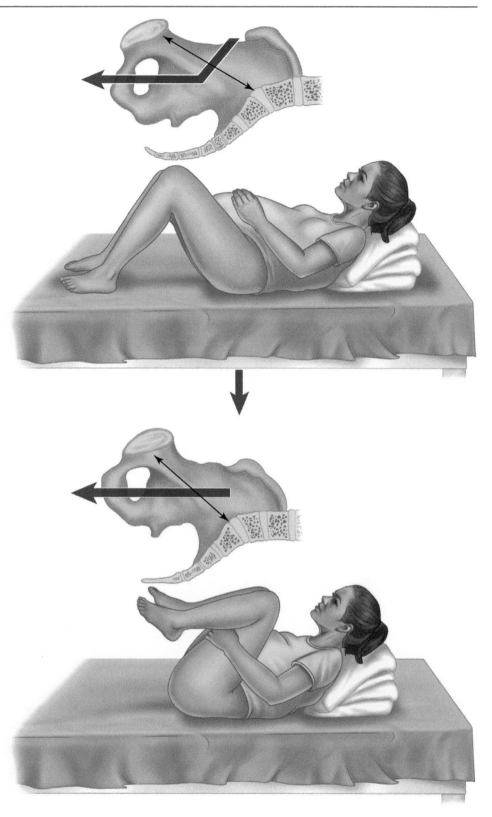

5. *Pressure suprapubically (Rubin I maneuver)*: While continuing downward traction, have a colleague place his or her hand suprapubically on the fetal anterior shoulder and apply pressure down and laterally on its posterior aspect in 30-second increments. This allows the fetal shoulders to enter the pelvis in an oblique fashion (pelvic inlet is widest in the transverse plane) (Fig. 116.2).

6. *Enter maneuver (internal rotation)*: Rotate the anterior shoulder into the oblique plane and under the maternal symphysis.
   - It may be necessary to push the fetus slightly up into the pelvis in order to successfully perform this maneuver.
     - (a) *Rubin II maneuver*: Insert one hand vaginally behind the fetal anterior shoulder and rotate the shoulder toward the chest. This will reduce the diameter of the fetal shoulder girdle and facilitate delivery (Fig. 116.3).
     - (b) *The Woods corkscrew maneuver*: Place one hand at the front of posterior shoulder and push upward gently. This can be combined with the Rubin II maneuver (Fig. 116.4).

   - (c) *The reverse Woods corkscrew maneuver*: Place one hand behind the fetal posterior shoulder and rotate in the direction opposite to that of the Woods corkscrew maneuver to adduct the shoulder.

7. *Remove the posterior arm*: Flex the fetal elbow and deliver the forearm in a sweeping motion over the fetal anterior chest wall. This allows the fetus to drop into the sacral hollow, freeing the anterior shoulder impaction.
   - Avoid grasping and pulling on the fetal arm directly because it may fracture the fetal humerus.

8. *Roll the patient (Gaskin maneuver)*: Position the patient on all fours (this acts as an upside-down McRoberts maneuver). Continue gentle traction. The turning itself, as well as gravity, will often dislodge the impacted shoulder.

   Last-resort maneuvers:

9. *Deliberate fracture of the fetal clavicle*: Apply direct pressure upward in the middle of the clavicle to reduce the shoulder-to-shoulder distance.

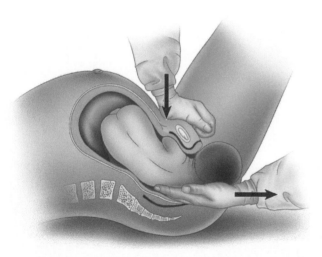

Fig. 116.2 Ruben I maneuver: suprapubic pressure is directed at the anterior shoulder

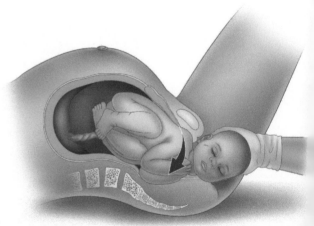

Fig. 116.3 Ruben II maneuver: pressure is applied to the most acce sible part of the fetal shoulder and rotated toward the chest

Fig. 116.4 The Woods corkscrew maneuver: pressure is applied to the clavicle of the posterior arm, enabling rotation and dislodgement of the anterior shoulder

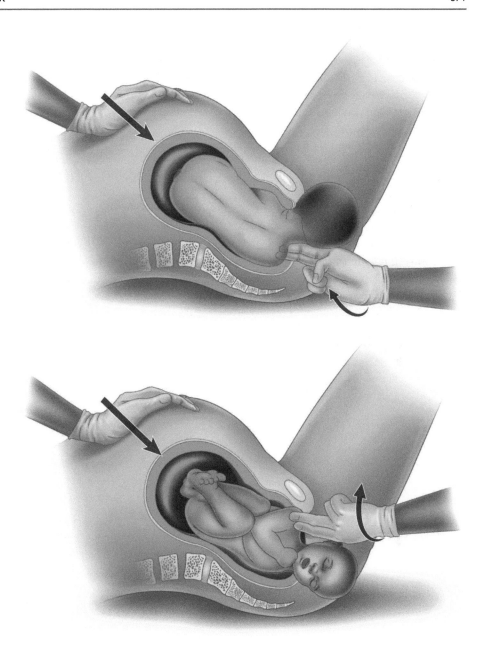

10. *Zavanelli maneuver*: Rotate the fetal head into the direct occiput anterior position, flex, and push back into the birth canal. Continue holding upward pressure until cesarean delivery. Ensure the operating and anesthesiology teams are present (Fig. 116.5).
    • Do not perform this maneuver if the nuchal cord has been clamped or cut.
11. *Symphysiotomy*: Place the patient in the exaggerated lithotomy position, insert a transurethral catheter, displace the urethra laterally, and separate the cephalad portion of fibrous cartilage of the symphysis pubis under local anesthesia with either a scalpel blade or Kelly clamp.
    • This technique is associated with significant maternal morbidity, including bladder neck injury and infection. It is truly the last resort and should be used only when all other methods have failed and cesarean delivery is unavailable.

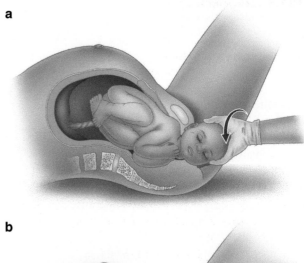

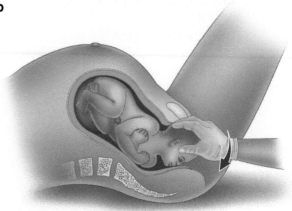

Fig. 116.5 Zavanelli maneuver: the fetal head is rotated into the direct occiput anterior position, flexed, and pushed back into the birth canal. (**a**) Rotation of the head to the occiput anterior position. (**b**) Replace head with constant firm pressure on occiput with palm of hand flexing head

116.5 Complications

- Maternal:
  - Postpartum hemorrhage
  - Fourth-degree laceration/soft tissue damage to cervix and vagina
  - Uterine rupture
  - Bladder atony
  - Symphyseal separation with or without femoral neuropathy (transient)
  - Sacroiliac dislocation
- Fetal:
  - Brachial plexus palsies (Erb, Klumpke): most resolve within 6–12 months; permanent injury occurs in less than 10 % of patients
  - Clavicular and/or humeral fractures
  - Ischemia/hypoxia/asphyxia due to umbilical cord compression with or without neurological damage
  - Significant fetal acidosis, with pH drop of 0.04 U/min between delivery of the head and trunk
  - Death

116.6 Pearls and Pitfalls

- Pearls
  - Many cases of shoulder dystocia and birth trauma are encountered in the absence of risk factors and in non-macrosomic infants. Shoulder dystocia is largely neither predictable nor preventable.
  - Presence of risk factors for shoulder dystocia should prompt advance preparation in anticipation of a difficult delivery. Risk factors include maternal diabetes, obesity, multiparity, advanced maternal age, prolonged pregnancy, macrosomia (fetal weight >4,500–5,000 g), male fetal gender, and prior birth complicated by shoulder dystocia.

- Pitfalls
  - Do not cut and clamp the nuchal cord if at all possible in order to avoid fetal hypoxia and hypotension should shoulder dystocia arise.
  - Labor induction or prophylactic cesarean delivery of macrosomic fetuses has not decreased rates of shoulder dystocia.
  - Avoid fundal pressure in shoulder dystocia because it has been shown to increase the risk of permanent neurological damage and uterine rupture.

Selected Reading

Acker DB. A shoulder dystocia intervention form. Obstet Gynecol. 1991;78:150–1.

Athukorala C, Middleton P, Crowther CA. Intrapartum interventions for preventing shoulder dystocia. Cochrane Database Syst Rev. 2006;4:CD005543.

Baxley EG, Gobbo RW. Shoulder dystocia. Am Fam Physician. 2004;69:1707–14.

Chauhan SP, Gherman R, Hendrix NW, Bingham JM, Hayes E. Shoulder dystocia: comparison of the ACOG practice bulletin with another national guideline. Am J Perinatol. 2010;27:129–36.

Gherman RB, Chauhan S, Ouzounian JG, Lerner H, Gonik B, Goodwin TM. Shoulder dystocia: the unpreventable obstetric emergency with empiric management guidelines. Am J Obstet Gynecol. 2006;195:657–72.

Gottlieb AG, Galan HL. Shoulder dystocia: an update. Obstet Gynecol Clin North Am. 2007;34:501–31.

Hoffman MK, Bailit JL, Branch DW, et al. Consortium on safe labor. A comparison of obstetric maneuvers for the acute management of shoulder dystocia. Obstet Gynecol. 2011;117:1272–8.

Patterson DA, Winslow M, Matus CD. Spontaneous vaginal delivery. Am Fam Physician. 2008;78:336–41.

Sokol RJ, Blackwell SC, American College of Obstetricians and Gynecologists. Committee on Practice Bulletins–Gynecology. ACOG practice bulletin no. 40: shoulder dystocia. November 2002 (replaces practice pattern no. 7, October 1997). Int J Gynaecol Obstet. 2003;80:87–92.

Breech Delivery in the Emergency Department

Kristin Stegeman, Sapnalaxmi Amin, Anton A. Wray, and Joseph A. Tyndall

Breech presentation: the buttocks enter the pelvis before the head (Fig. 117.1)

- Frank (extended):
  - Hips flexed and knees extended, buttocks presenting
  - Most common

- Incomplete/complete (flexed):
  - One or both hips and knees flexed, buttocks presenting
- Footling:
  - One or both hips and knees extended, foot presenting

The emergent delivery of a breech baby is one of the most challenging situations for an emergency physician.

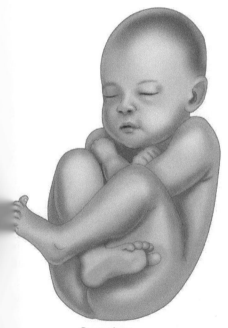
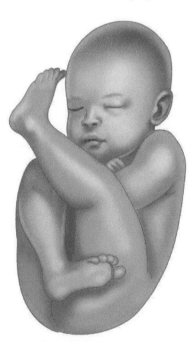
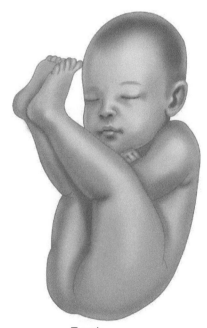

Complete breech	Incomplete breech	Frank breech

Fig. 117.1 Variations of the breech presentation

Stegeman, MD • A.A. Wray, MD (✉)
Department of Emergency Medicine, The Brooklyn Hospital
Center, New York, NY, USA
e-mail: kristin.stegeman@gmail.com; anw9071@nyp.org

Amin, MD
Department of Family Medicine/Urgent Care,
side Urgent Care Center, Clearwater, FL, USA
e-mail: sapna_amin59@yahoo.com

J.A. Tyndall, MD, MPH
Department of Emergency Medicine, University of Florida Health,
Gainesville, FL, USA
e-mail: tyndall@ufl.edu

Springer Science+Business Media New York 2016
Ganti (ed.), *Atlas of Emergency Medicine Procedures*, DOI 10.1007/978-1-4939-2507-0_117

117.1 Indications

- Inevitable delivery of fetus with complete or frank breech presentation
- Absence of vertex presentation

117.2 Contraindications

- Footling presentation (increased risk of cord prolapse and entrapment of the after-coming head).
- There is adequate time to transfer the mother safely to labor and delivery in the knee/chest position (administer subcutaneous terbutaline before transfer).

117.3 Materials and Medications

- Supplemental oxygen for mother
- Ultrasound machine
- Piper forceps
- Sterile towels/gloves
- Betadine (povidone-iodine) or another antiseptic preparing solution
- Sterile lubricant (Surgilube)
- Instruments to cut the umbilical cord/perform episiotomy/resuscitate baby (Kelly clamps/scissors/#10 scalpel/bulb suction)
- Available emergency department staff
- Pediatric, obstetrics, and anesthesia practitioners

117.4 Procedure

1. Assess the health of the mother and the baby (vitals/physical examination/history).
2. Listen to the fetal heart with stethoscope or Doppler ultrasound.
   - Should be 120–160 beats/min.
3. Identify the type of presentation by bedside ultrasound or by digital exam.
4. Perform a sterile digital examination to confirm the position of the baby and the stage of labor.
   - Membranes should not be artificially ruptured. The amniotic sac will help to dilate the cervix, lubricate the canal, and protect the umbilical cord from compression.
5. If footling presentation: await OB/general surgery for emergency C-section.
6. If frank/complete/incomplete: instruct the patient to push when the cervix is completely dilated.
7. When the breech has descended to the perineum, consider performing an episiotomy if more space is needed. Cleanse the perineum with antiseptic and sterile lubricant beforehand.
8. Allow the baby to extrude to the umbilicus with maternal efforts alone. Do not exert traction before this time.
9. If frank: deliver the posterior leg by gently guiding the sacrum anteriorly, grasping the thigh and flexing the leg at the knee.
10. Deliver the anterior leg in a similar manner while guiding the sacrum posteriorly.
11. If incomplete: deliver the extended leg as #8 or #9 as appropriate.
12. Delivery continues as it would for a complete presentation.
13. Wrap the legs/buttocks in a clean towel to decrease trauma (create grip).
14. Grasp the upper legs with the index fingers holding the anterior iliac crests. Place the thumbs on the sacrum (Fig. 117.2).
15. Apply gentle traction as the mother pushes until the scapulae and axillae are visible.
16. If there is difficulty delivering the shoulders, deliver the posterior shoulder by rotating the trunk 90° and applying gentle downward traction to rotate the shoulder anteriorly.
17. Rotate the baby 180° so as to deliver the anterior arm a similar manner.
18. If the arms do not spontaneously deliver, a finger can hooked over the shoulders to bring the arm down while rotating the trunk as above (Fig. 117.3).
19. Use the McRoberts position to increase the diameter the pelvis (Fig. 117.4).

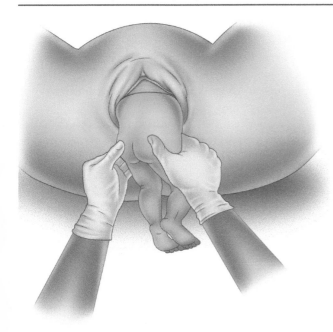

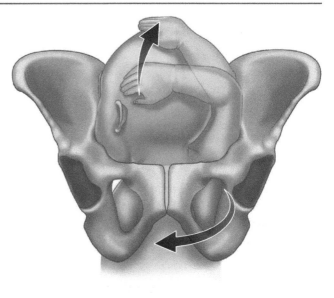

Fig. 117.3 Rotation toward maternal symphysis pubis to avoid nuchal arm

Fig. 117.2 Correct placement of hands on sacrum

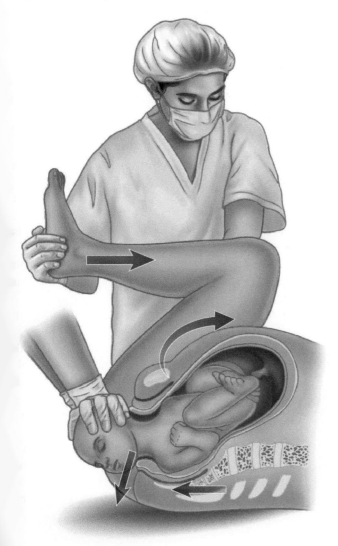

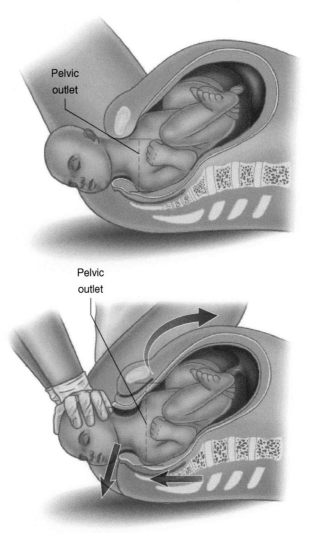

Pelvic outlet

Pelvic outlet

g. 117.4 The McRoberts maneuver in vertex (head-first) presentation

20. Maintain the baby in the same plane as the vagina (support the body with the forearm) and place the second and fourth fingers over the maxilla of the baby. Place the middle finger in the mouth or on the chin and the other hand on the upper back/occiput (Fig. 117.5).
    • Avoid extreme elevation of the fetus to prevent hyperextension and cervical spine injury. Piper forceps may also be used to promote flexion.
21. Deliver the head in the flexed position.
    • If the baby descends with the neck and abdomen facing anteriorly: Grasp the shoulders posteriorly with two fingers of one hand while the other hand flexes the abdomen and the baby's feet are brought upward (Fig. 117.6).
    • If the baby's neck remains extended: Leave the baby hanging (weight = traction). When the hairline appears under the symphysis, grab the baby by the feet and elevate upward (Fig. 117.7).
22. Clamp and cut the umbilical cord (collect arterial and venous samples for pH).
23. Suction the baby's mouth and nose, and resuscitate as indicated.
24. Deliver the maternal placenta.
25. Repair tears or episiotomy made during delivery.

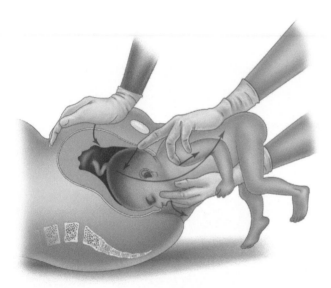

Fig. 117.5 Delivery of head in flexed position

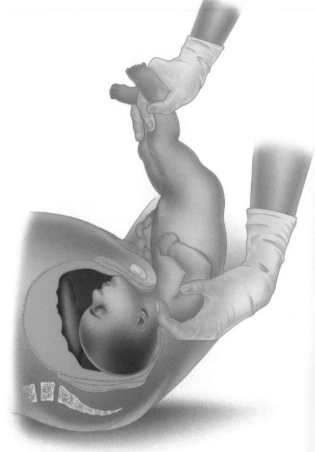

Fig. 117.6 Correct hand placement if abdomen facing anterior

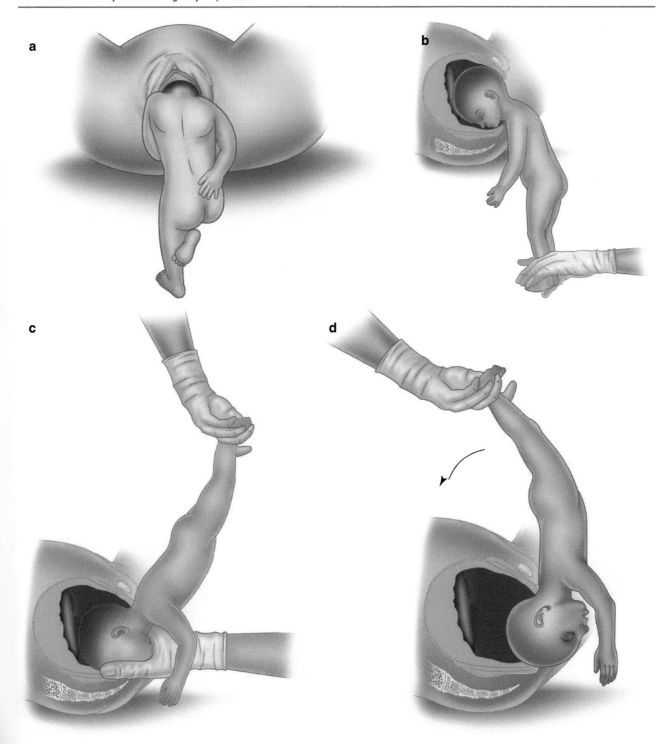

Fig. 117.7 The Burns-Marshall maneuver. (**a**) Allow baby to hang until you can see the hair at the nape of his neck; (**b**) swing the baby's head clear of the birth canal; (**c**) left hand guards and slips the perineum over fetal mouth; suction baby's air passage to clear mucus; (**d**) hold baby's feet

117.5 Complications

- Umbilical cord prolapse
- Brachial plexus injury (from the nuchal arm)
- Fetal head entrapment
- Cervical spine injury (from hyperextension of the neck)
- Birth asphyxia

117.6 Pearls and Pitfalls

- Pearls
  - Allow the uterine contractions to help deliver the baby.
- Pitfalls
  - Do not rush the delivery or use too much force. This can increase the risk of trauma to the baby and mother.
  - Beware of nuchal arm. To avoid brachial plexus injury: Rotate the face of baby toward the maternal symphysis pubis. This will reduce the tension keeping the arm around the back of the fetal head (Fig. 117.3).

Selected Reading

Auerbach PS. Gynecologic and obstetric emergencies. In: Wilderness medicine. 6th ed. Philadelphia: Elsevier; 2012.

Buckley RG, Knoop KJ. Gynecologic and obstetric conditions. In: Knoop KJ, Stack LB, Storrow AB, Thurman RJ, editors. The atlas of emergency medicine. 3rd ed. New York: McGraw Hill; 2010.

Cunningham FG, Leveno KJ, Bloom SL, Hauth JC, Rouse DJ, Spong CY. Breech presentation and delivery. In: Williams obstetrics. 23rd ed. New York: McGraw Hill; 2010.

Kish K, Collea JV. Chapter 21. Malpresentation & cord prolapse. In: DeCherney AH, Nathan L, editors. Current diagnosis & treatment: obstetrics & gynecology. 10th ed. New York: McGraw Hill; 2007.

Kotaska A, Menticoglou S, Gagnon R. Vaginal delivery of breech presentation. Int J Gynecol Obstet. 2009;107:169–76.

Probst BD. Emergency childbirth. In: Roberts JR, Hedges JR, editors. Clinical procedures in emergency medicine. 5th ed. Philadelphia: Elsevier; 2010.

Management of Primary Postpartum Hemorrhage

Megan Kwasniak, Anton A. Wray, and Joseph A. Tyndall

Postpartum hemorrhage (PPH) is defined as $\geq$500 ml blood loss within 24 h of vaginal delivery or 1000 ml loss within 24 h of cesarean section. It is the leading cause of maternal mortality worldwide.

118.1 Indications

- Excessive vaginal bleeding with or without pain and/or hemodynamic instability within 24 h of delivery

118.2 Contraindications

There are no absolute contraindications to the management of PPH.

18.3 Materials and Medications

Sterile technique
Good lighting
Sponge forceps
Gauze
Towels

Kwasniak, MD
nergency Department, The Brooklyn Hospital Center,
w York, NY, USA
nail: megan.kwasniak@gmail.com

A. Wray, MD (✉)
partment of Emergency Medicine, The Brooklyn Hospital
nter, New York, NY, USA
ail: anw9071@nyp.org

Tyndall, MD, MPH
partment of Emergency Medicine, University of Florida Health,
nesville, FL, USA
ail: tyndall@ufl.edu

- IV fluids
- Type and screen/crossmatch of blood
- Absorbable suture with curved needle
- Needle holder
- Tooth forceps

118.4 Procedure

- Standard resuscitation measures: Place IV, O_2, monitor.
- Assessment and treatment should occur simultaneously.
- All techniques should be performed under strict sterile conditions.

118.4.1 Uterine Exam

1. Assess by placing the hand on the uterine fundus and checking its size and firmness.
2. High, soft, or boggy uterus implicates retained placenta or uterine atony. Start external fundal massage.
3. Non-palpable uterus implicates uterine inversion.

118.4.2 Vaginal Exam

1. Keeping one hand on the abdomen, gently examine the vaginal canal using the other sterilely gloved hand.
2. Gently scoop out any clots/retained placenta that are easily removable.
3. Look for traumatic sources of bleeding from the perineum, vaginal walls, and cervical lacerations.
4. Gauze-wrapped ring forceps can be used to assist direct visualization and clearing of clots.

pringer Science+Business Media New York 2016
anti (ed.), *Atlas of Emergency Medicine Procedures*, DOI 10.1007/978-1-4939-2507-0_118

118.4.3   If Uterine Atony Suspected

1. Continue external fundal massage with the abdominal hand. Make a fist with the vaginal hand and start bimanual massage. Raise the uterus from the pelvis and pivot it anteriorly, compressing it between the external hand and the internal fist. This maneuver will result in expression of any clots present and decrease uterine bleeding via direct compression (Fig. 118.1).
2. Administer oxytocin (20–40 units in 1 L of normal saline or lactated Ringer's solution intravenously [IV]; alternatively give 10 units intramyometrially with a spinal needle).
3. Methylergonovine may also be used at this time if oxytocin fails to reduce uterine bleeding (100 or 125 mcg IV or intramyometrially; alternatively 200 or 250 mcg may be given intramuscularly).
4. Continue massage until bleeding slows and the uterus becomes more firm. This can take 15–30 mins.

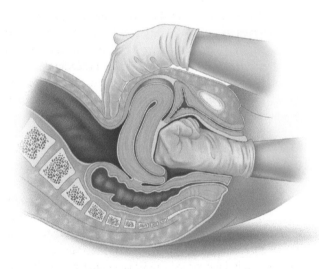

Fig. 118.1 Intrauterine massage for uterine atony

118.4.4   If Retained Placenta Suspected

1. Manual removal of the placenta or any of its retained tissue should be facilitated with sedation or additional analgesia.
2. Keeping the thumb and fingers together in a teardrop shape and using sterile technique as described previously, insert the hand through the vaginal canal and the cervix into the lower uterine segment.
3. Keep the other hand on the lower abdomen to continue gentle yet firm upward pressure and massage.
4. Find the placental edge within the uterus, grasp it gently, detach it from the uterine wall, and withdraw the hand from the patient.
5. Repeat the maneuver as necessary; remove any additional clots from the uterus and continue bimanual massage until it becomes firm and bleeding decreases.
6. If the entire placenta has been removed this way, an assistant should be available to inspect it for completeness and any torn vessels.
7. If the bleeding is particularly severe and placenta accreta is strongly suspected, pack the uterus with gauze and prepare the patient for urgent surgical intervention.

118.4.5   If Uterine Inversion Suspected

1. Using sterile technique, insert a fist through the vaginal canal and push the inverted fundus back through the cervical canal with pressure directed toward the umbilicus.
2. If the uterus has contracted, tocolytics such as IV magnesium sulfate or terbutaline can be used to aid myometrial relaxation. Alternatively, provided the patient is not overly hypotensive, nitroglycerin 50–100 mcg IV may be administered to relax the myometrium and facilitate return to normal uterine position.
3. If manual replacement is ineffective, hydrostatic reduction may be attempted. Warm fluids are run into the upper vagina under high pressure while occluding the introitus

18.4.6 Trauma: Genital and Perineal Lacerations

For significant cervical lacerations: use absorbable sutures with a continuous interlocking stitch technique to close (Fig. 118.2).

For vaginal wound repair: place the initial and final stitch above the apices of the lacerations and grab a good amount of tissue with the needle. Small bites can lead to ongoing bleeding and hematoma formation.

Observe the repaired lacerations for any additional bleeding after the torn edges have been sutured.

- Apply additional pressure to any site that continues to ooze blood; gauze-wrapped ring forceps may be used for this purpose if necessary.

If none of the above causes are apparent, consider underlying coagulopathies and treat appropriately. This may require administration of fresh-frozen plasma, platelets, or clotting factors as indicated.

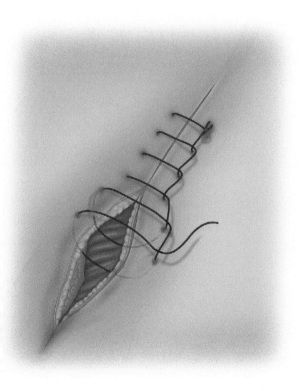

Fig. 118.2 Continuous interlocking stitch: perineal lacerations repair

118.5 Complications

- Uterine perforation and scarring
- Urinary and genital tract trauma and injury
- Genitourinary and genitointestinal fistula
- Pelvic hematoma
- Genital vascular injury
- Infection and sepsis
- Disseminated intravascular coagulation (DIC)
- Maternal death

118.6 Pearls and Pitfalls

- Pearls
  - Causes of PPH can be divided into the "5 Ts":
    - Tone: uterine atony, occurring within the first 4 h after delivery.
    - Tissue: retention of the placenta, especially placenta accreta and its fragments, more common at extreme preterm deliveries.
    - Trauma: injury to the uterus, cervix, and perineal structures after delivery of a large fetus, use of forceps and/or vacuum, frequent vaginal manipulation during delivery, and episiotomy procedures.
    - Thrombosis: intrinsic or acquired coagulation disorders, including idiopathic thrombocytic purpura (ITP); hemolysis, elevated liver enzymes, and low platelets (HELLP) syndrome; and disseminated intravascular coagulation (DIC), as well as preexisting conditions such as von Willebrand disease.
    - Traction: inversion of the uterus during placental delivery secondary to excessive traction on the umbilical cord. The uterine fundus can be within the endometrial cavity, in the cervical canal, or outside the external os and within the vaginal canal.
  - The administration of broad-spectrum antibiotics should be strongly considered following any manual removal, exploration, or instrumentation of the uterus and the genital tract.
  - Bedside ultrasonography can be very helpful for identifying uterine abnormalities, retained placental tissue, free fluid in the pelvis, and/or intrauterine hematoma.
  - Risk factors for PPH include prolonged active phase of labor, previous PPH, multiple pregnancy, and history of a bleeding disorder.
- Pitfalls
  - Failure to recognize and treat PPH early increases morbidity and mortality.
  - Underestimating the potential blood loss of PPH. The gravid uterus at term has a blood flow of 600 ml/min (non-gravid: 60 ml/h).

Selected Reading

Anderson J, Duncan E. Prevention and management of postpartum hemorrhage. Am Fam Physician. 2007;75:875–82.

Druelinger L. Postpartum emergencies. Emerg Med Clin North Am. 1994;12:219–37.

Leduc D, Senikas V, Lalonde AB, et al. Active management of the third stage of labour: prevention and treatment of postpartum hemorrhage. J Obstet Gynaecol Can. 2009;31:980–93.

Miller S, Lester F, Hensleigh P. Prevention and treatment of postpartum hemorrhage: new advances for low-resource settings. J Midwifery Womens Health. 2004;49:283–92.

Sheiner E, Sarid L, Levy A, Seidman DS, Hallak M. Obstetric risk tors and outcome of pregnancies complicated with early postpar hemorrhage: a population-based study. J Matern Fetal Neor Med. 2005;18:149–54.

Tessier V, Pierre F. Risk factors of postpartum hemorrhage during l and clinical and pharmacological prevention. J Gynecol Obstet Reprod (Paris). 2004;33(8 suppl):4S29–56.

World Health Organization. World health report 2005: make e mother and child count. Available at: http://www.who.int/whr/2 whr2005_en.pdf.

Perimortem Cesarean Section

119

Jordana J. Haber, Elaine B. Josephson,
and Muhammad Waseem

119.1 Indications

- Maternal arrest with a viable fetus (gestation >24 weeks)

119.2 Contraindications

- Stable mother
- Fetus less than 24 weeks' gestation
- Extreme fetal prematurity
- Maternal hypoxia longer than 15 min

119.3 Materials and Medications

- Cesarean section instrument tray if available
  - #10 or #11 scalpel blade, scissors, bladder retractor, 2 large retractors, gauze sponges, hemostats, suction, forceps, and straight and curved clamps
- Skin antiseptic preparing solution, such as Betadine (povidone-iodine)
- Silk suture with needle driver or skin stapler
- Sterile drapes
- Sterile gloves
- Obstetrical pack (See Chap. 115)
  - Bulb syringe and umbilical cord clamp
- Clean blanket or towels for delivery
- Neonatal resuscitation equipment

Owing to the rarity of this procedure in the emergency department, it is unlikely to have a prepared cesarean section tray available. In this case, a thorocotomy or thorocostomy tray combined with an obstetrical pack would contain all the supplies needed. At a minimum, a scalpel and an obstetrical pack are necessary.

J.J. Haber, MD
Department of Emergency Medicine, Maimonides Medical Center, New York, NY, USA
e-mail: Jordana.haber@gmail.com

E.B. Josephson, MD
Department of Emergency Medicine, Lincoln Medical and Mental Health Center, Weill Cornell Medical College of Cornell University, Bronx, New York, NY, USA
e-mail: elaine.Josephson@nychhc.org

M. Waseem, MD (✉)
Department of Emergency Medicine, Lincoln Medical and Mental Health Center, New York, NY, USA
e-mail: waseemm2001@hotmail.com

Springer Science+Business Media New York 2016
Ganti (ed.), *Atlas of Emergency Medicine Procedures*, DOI 10.1007/978-1-4939-2507-0_119

119.4 Procedure

1. Prepare skin with antiseptic solution and a sterile drape.
2. Insert a Foley catheter to empty the bladder.
3. Continue cardiopulmonary resuscitation until delivery.
4. Obtain emergent obstetrician and neonatologist consult if available, but do not delay procedure.
5. Using a #10 or #11 blade, make a vertical midline incision beginning 4–5 cm below the xiphoid process and extend the incision to the pubic symphysis (Fig. 119.1).
6. Incise through the subcutaneous fat no further than the rectus sheath.
7. Lift the rectus sheath with a toothed forceps and make an incision with scissors to expose the uterus (Fig. 119.2).
8. With forceps and scissors, lift and incise the peritoneal membrane in the midline.
9. Identify and lift the bowel and cover it with saline-soaked gauze.
10. Retract the rectus sheath and bladder with a bladder retractor or, if not available, use saline-soaked gauze or a towel.
11. Create a 2- to 4-cm midline vertical opening in the uterus.
12. Place a finger in the opening directed caudally to protect the fetus while making a superior incision through the uterine wall. Once complete, repeat this step in the inferior direction.
13. Use a clamp to rupture the amniotic membranes. Immediately deliver the fetus and clamp the umbilical cord.
14. Expulse the head by placing a hand between the pubic symphysis landmark and the fetal occiput. Then, gently flex the fetus while simultaneously moving the head superiorly and anteriorly until delivery (Fig. 119.3).
15. Suction the mouth and nose with a bulb syringe immediately.
16. Deliver the shoulders, followed by the torso and extremities. Secure the umbilical cord with a hemostat or umbilical cord clamp 10 cm distal to the fetus and a second clamp 2 cm distal to this clamp. With scissors, incise the umbilical cord between the two clamps.
17. Immediately begin resuscitation of the infant (Fig. 119.4).
18. If the patient is still alive or regains vital signs, prepare to deliver the placenta. Begin with an oxytocin infusion at 20 U in 1 L at 10 mL/h. Apply cautious traction to the umbilical cord until the placenta separates from the uterus (Fig. 119.5).
19. Following delivery, the uterus should be closed using two layers with either 2-0 or 1-0 suture. In the case of maternal death, skin staples or a running stitch is an acceptable method of skin closure.

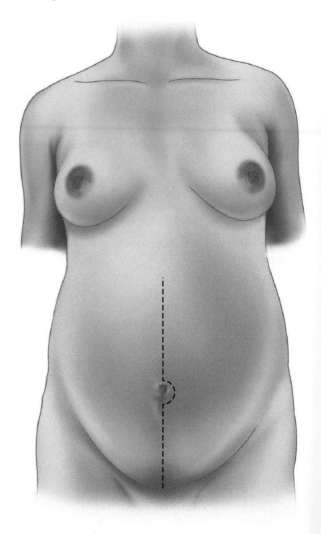

Fig. 119.1 Vertical incision

Fig. 119.2 Exposing rectus sheath

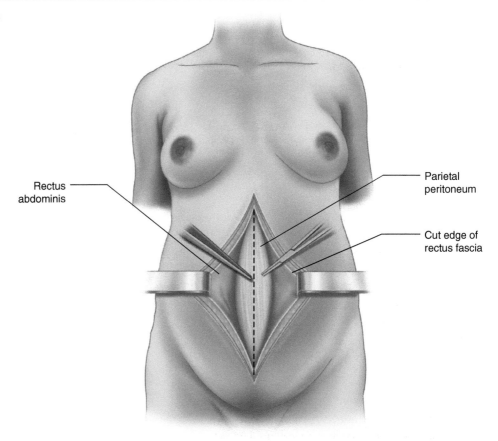

Rectus
abdominis

Parietal
peritoneum

Cut edge of
rectus fascia

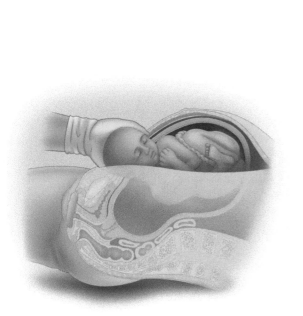

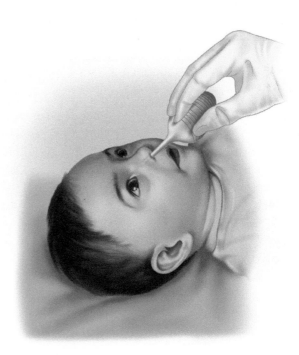

119.3 Delivery of the fetus

Fig. 119.4 Suctioning newborn as part of resuscitation

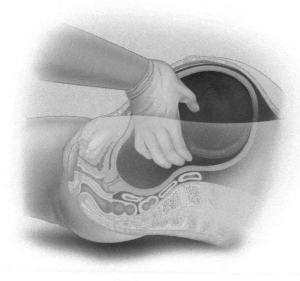

Fig. 119.5 Delivery of the placenta

119.5 Complications

- Maternal sepsis
- Maternal visceral injury
- Maternal hemorrhage
- Maternal death
- Fetal injuries and laceration
- Fetal sepsis

119.6 Pearls and Pitfalls

- Pearls
  - Perimortem cesarean section, although rarely performed, should be considered in any maternal arrest when the fetus is greater than 24 weeks' gestation.
  - In addition to saving the life of the fetus, this procedure may aid in resuscitation of the mother. Emptying of the uterus may improve thoracic compliance and, therefore, improve maternal ventilation.
- Pitfalls
  - The decision to perform an emergency cesarean section must be made early. There is a higher chance of survival if performed no more than 5 min after the onset of maternal cardiac arrest.

Selected Reading

Doan-Wiggins L. Emergency childbirth. In: Roberts JR, Hedges JR, editors. Clinical procedures in emergency medicine. 4th ed. Philadelphia: Saunders; 2004. p. 1117–43.

Flippin A, Hendricks S. Perimortem cesarean section. In: Reichman EF, Simon RS, editors. Emergency medicine procedures. New York: McGraw Hill Medical; 2004. p. 1070–8.

Gianopoulos JG. Emergency complications of labor and delivery. Emerg Med Clin North Am. 1994;12:201–17.

Jeejeebhoy FM, Zelop CM, Windrim R, Carvalho JC, Dorian P, Morrison LJ. Management of cardiac arrest in pregnancy: a systematic review. Resuscitation. 2011;82:801–19.

Whitten M, Irvine LM. Postmortem and perimortem caesarean section: what are the indications? J R Soc Med. 2000;93:6–9.

Peripheral Venous Catheterization

David N. Smith and Judith K. Lucas

120.1 Indications (See Also Chap. 2)

- Fluid resuscitation
- Medication administration
- Blood draws

120.2 Contraindications

- Relative
  - Avoid catheterizing areas of trauma in which extravasation of fluid is possible (e.g., burns, open wounds, or severe edema in tissue).
  - Avoid catheterizing in an area of local infection for risk of inoculating the circulation with bacteria (e.g., cellulitis).
- Absolute
  - None

120.3 Materials and Medications

- Gloves
- Skin disinfectant (isopropyl alcohol, chlorhexidine, or Betadine [povidone-iodine])
- Appropriate-sized catheter (18- to 24-gauge [IV]) (Fig. 120.1)
  - Large child: 18 to 20 gauge
  - Infant or small child: 22 to 24 gauge
- Tourniquet
- Sterile 2×2 gauze
- Appropriate-sized Tegaderm transparent dressing
- Adhesive tape
- IV bag with solution set (tubing flushed and ready) or saline lock
- Sharps container

D.N. Smith, MD
Department of Pediatrics, University of Alabama at Birmingham,
Children's of Alabama, Birmingham, AL, USA
e-mail: dsmith@peds.uab.edu

J.K. Lucas, MD (✉)
Department of Emergency Medicine,
University of Florida Health Shands Hospital,
Gainesville, FL, USA
e-mail: judithklucas@ufl.edu

© Springer Science+Business Media New York 2016
S. Ganti (ed.), *Atlas of Emergency Medicine Procedures*, DOI 10.1007/978-1-4939-2507-0_120

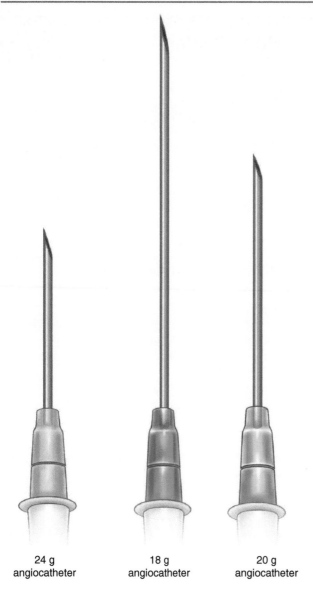

24 g
angiocatheter

18 g
angiocatheter

20 g
angiocatheter

Fig. 120.1 24-Gauge angiocatheter (*yellow*), 18-gauge angiocatheter (*red*), 20-gauge angiocatheter (*blue*)

120.4 Procedure

1. Comfortably position the patient with the site exposed.
2. Assemble the equipment and don a pair of (nonlatex) examination gloves.
3. Apply the tourniquet to the extremity above the site to be catheterized (Fig. 120.2).
4. Visualize and palpate the vein.
5. Cleanse the site with a disinfectant swab using an expanding circular motion.
6. Prepare and inspect the catheter and flush the tubing; be certain that the stylet and catheter separate easily, then fit again into the notch, aligning the bevel with the hub.
7. Stabilize the vein and apply countertension to the skin, being careful not to touch the cleansed area.
8. Insert the stylet through the skin and then reduce the angle while advancing through the vein (Fig. 120.3).
9. Observe for "flashback" as blood slowly fills the flashback chamber.
10. Advance the needle approximately 1–2 mm further into the vein, depending on the gauge and age of the patient, to ensure that the catheter is within the vein.
11. Slowly advance the catheter into the vein while keeping tension on the vein and skin (Fig. 120.4).
12. While advancing the catheter, be certain to hold the stylet portion with the thumb and forefinger, so as to avoid advancing the needle portion into and through the opposite side of the vessel, thus "blowing" the vein.
13. When the catheter is advanced about halfway, slowly withdraw and remove the stylet while simultaneously continuing to advance the catheter to its hub.
14. Attach a 3-mL non-Luer-Lok syringe to the hub.
15. Remove the tourniquet.
16. Gently attempt to aspirate blood. The blood should be free flowing.
17. Secure the catheter by either placing a transparent occlusive dressing (e.g., Tegaderm) over the lower half of the catheter hub or taping over the catheter hub in a cruciat

fashion, taking care not to cover the IV tubing connection (Fig. 120.5).

18. Remove the cover from the end of the IV tubing and insert the IV tubing into the hub of the catheter (the tubing must have been flushed with IV solution before connecting with the catheter hub: the unit from the solution bag/bottle through the catheter must be air free).

19. Open up the IV roller clamp and observe for drips forming in the drip chamber.

20. Place a piece of tape over the catheter hub then make a small (kink-free) loop in the IV tubing and place a second piece of tape over the first piece to secure the loop (Fig. 120.6).

21. Place a third piece of tape over the IV tubing above the site.

22. Ensure that the IV is properly secured and infusing properly.

23. Ensure that all "sharps" are placed in the sharps container.

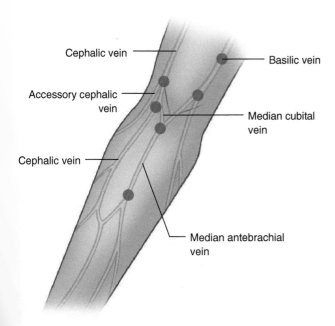

Fig. 120.2 Anatomy of the volar surface antecubital fossa and forearm

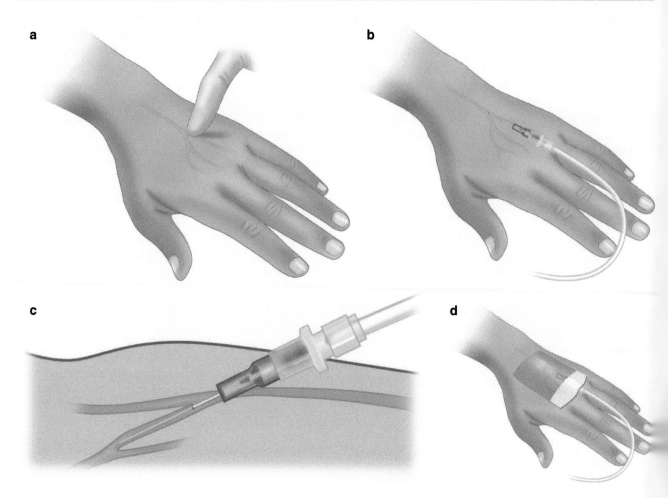

Fig. 120.3 (**a**–**d**) After applying the tourniquet, palpate a vein, as straight as possible, and ideally without many "knots" (i.e., valves)

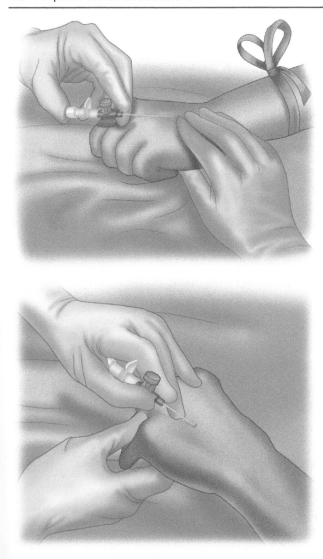

Fig. 120.4 With the tourniquet "up," and the vein distended, apply traction to the skin, pierce the skin, and pass the catheter tip (into the vein) until blood return is noted in the catheter hub

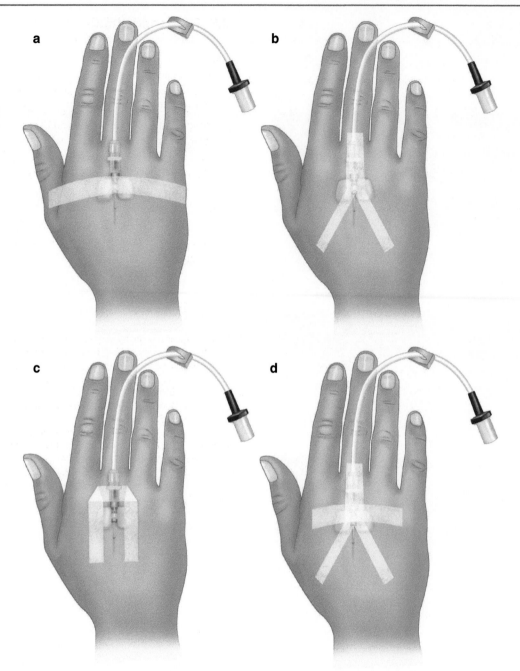

Fig. 120.5 (**a–d**) Securing the intravenous line utilizing the cruciate taping style

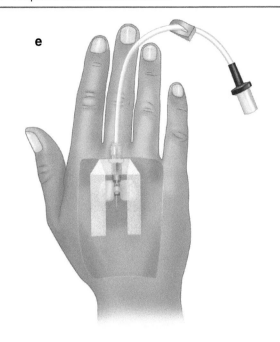

e

Fig. 120.5 (continued)

120.5 Pearls and Pitfalls

- Pearls
    - Start catheter attempts distal in the extremities and move proximally with each subsequent attempt.
    - The use of ultrasound or a light source in infants can aid in location of the vessel and placement of the line.
    - In an emergent situation, in which fluids or medications are needed quickly, intraosseous access (see Chap. 122) can be obtained if venous catheterization fails.
- Pitfalls
    - The use of lidocaine subcutaneously can improve patient comfort, but it does disrupt anatomical landmarks.

Selected Reading

Bailey P. Vascular (venous) access for pediatric resuscitation and other pediatric emergencies. UpToDate. http://www.uptodate.com/contents/vascular-venous-access-for-pediatric-resuscitation-and-other-pediatric-emergencies. Accessed 23 June 2014.

Department of Emergency Medicine, University of Ottawa. Peripheral intravenous access. 2003. http://www.med.uottawa.ca/procedures/iv/. Accessed 23 June 2014.

Kost S. Ultrasound-guided vascular (venous) access. UpToDate. http://www.uptodate.com/contents/principles-of-ultrasound-guided-venous-access. Accessed 23 June 2014.

Nursing Resource Administration. Medical procedure: insertion of peripheral IV line. http://nursing-resource.com/iv-insertion/. Accessed 23 June 2014.

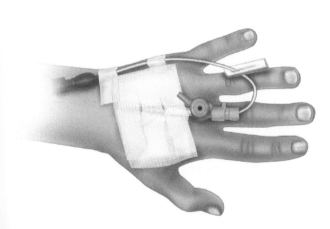

Fig. 120.6 Commercially available hub stabilizer, minimizing the need for excessive tape

Umbilical Venous Catheters (Insertion and Removal)

121

Judith K. Lucas

121.1 Indications

- Temporary vascular access for infants up to roughly 10 days of life (between 7 and 14 days) with shock or cardiopulmonary failure
- Emergency vascular access in this age group, when peripheral intravenous (IV) access cannot be rapidly obtained
- Preferred vascular access in infants less than 1000 g

121.2 Contraindications

Omphalitis
Omphalocele
Necrotizing enterocolitis
Peritonitis

121.3 Materials and Medications

- Anesthetic: not necessary; procedure is painless
- Soft ties to restrain infant's extremities
- Sterile gloves/gowns
- Antiseptic solution
- Sterile towels/drapes
- 3.5- (infants <1500 g) or 5-French (>1500 g) umbilical venous catheter
- 5-French feeding tube
- Three-way stopcock
- 10-mL syringe with heparinized saline flush (1 U/mL)
- Umbilical tape or 3-0 silk on a cutting needle
- Non-toothed forceps
- Small hemostats (2)
- #11 scalpel and blade
- Scissors
- Graph depicting length of catheter insertion, if placing umbilical venous catheter (UVC) above the diaphragm in either very small infants or infants for whom measurement of central venous pressure (CVP) is indicated (Fig. 121.1)

. Lucas, MD
partment of Emergency Medicine,
versity of Florida Health Shands Hospital,
nesville, FL, USA
ail: judithklucas@ufl.edu

pringer Science+Business Media New York 2016
anti (ed.), *Atlas of Emergency Medicine Procedures*, DOI 10.1007/978-1-4939-2507-0_121

Fig. 121.1 (**a**) Instrumentation suggested for umbilical venous catheter placement.
(**b**) Umbilical venous catheters (in an emergency, 5 F feeding tube is an acceptable alternative)

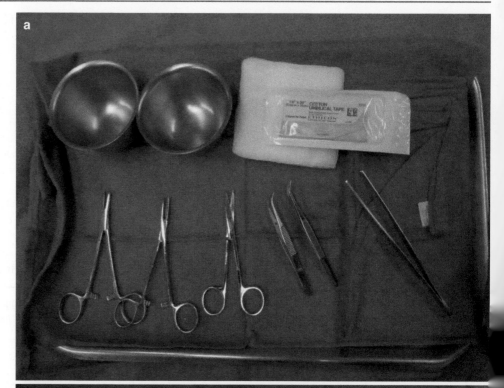

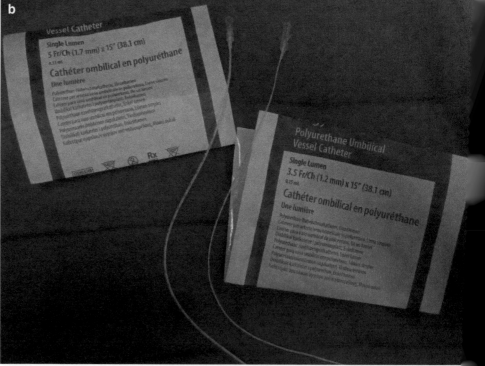

121.4 Procedure (Insertion)

1. Place the infant under a radiant warmer.
2. Using soft ties, restrain the infant's extremities.
3. Scrub the umbilicus and surrounding abdomen with antiseptic solution.
4. Drape the umbilicus and area in sterile manner (leave the infant's head exposed).
5. Tie a loose loop with the umbilical tape around the base of the cord OR run the 3-0 silk through the skin *of the cord* in a purse-string fashion.
   - This will be used later to anchor the line after placement and to provide hemostasis should the line accidentally be pulled out and bleeding ensue.
6. Using the scalpel blade, cut the umbilical cord horizontally approximately 2 cm above the junction between the cord and the skin.
7. Identify the umbilical vessels
   - The vein is thinner walled, larger in diameter, and somewhat floppy appearing, relative to the umbilical arteries, and typically located at the 12 o'clock position.
   - The arteries are smaller, thick walled, and paired (a single umbilical artery often signifies the presence of a congenital malformation/syndrome) and located at the 4 and 8 o'clock positions (Fig. 121.2).

8. Place the stopcock on the receiving end of the umbilical catheter or the 5-French feeding tube and flush with heparinized saline solution, and then close the stopcock.
   - It is imperative that there is no air in the catheter.
9. Introduce a closed smooth-surfaced forceps into the lumen of the umbilical vein and allow the forceps to separate, allowing the vein to dilate (Fig. 121.3).
10. Insert the catheter (or feeding tube) into the lumen and gently advance, directing the catheter toward the right shoulder (Fig. 121.4).
11. Advance the catheter only until good blood flow is noted and then another 1 to 2 cm (this should be a total of only 4–5 cm in a term infant).
    - *Do not force the advancement.*
    - At this level the tip of the catheter should still be inferior to the liver (Fig. 121.5).
12. Tighten the umbilical tie or the purse-string suture.
13. Secure the catheter with a tape bridge (Figs. 121.6, 121.7, and 121.8).
14. Although if placed only up to point of blood return, the catheter tip should be below the liver; it is best to get an abdominal x-ray to confirm; many solutions are caustic to the liver and can result in complications.

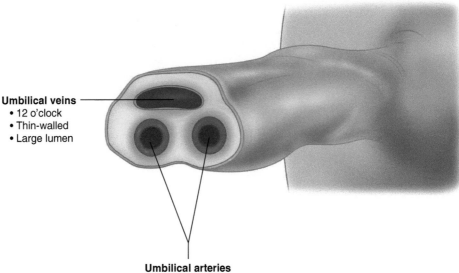

Umbilical stump

Umbilical veins
- 12 o'clock
- Thin-walled
- Large lumen

Umbilical arteries
- Usually paired
- Thick-walled
- Small lumen

Fig. 121.2 Anatomy of the umbilical cord when cut transversely approximately 2 cm from abdominal wall

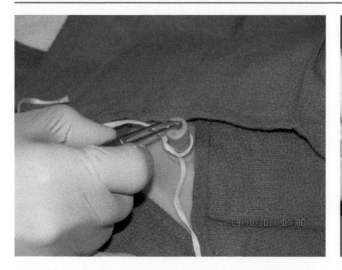

Fig. 121.3 Sterilely draped umbilicus, with umbilical tape loosely tied at base of umbilical cord. This tie will be cinched and secured once the catheter is placed, but meanwhile, can assist with homeostasis should the catheter be inadvertently dislodged during placement. Gently dilate the umbilical vein with a smooth toothed forceps. Insert the distal most couple of mm of a closed forceps into umbilical vein and relax, so the forceps tips smoothly separate

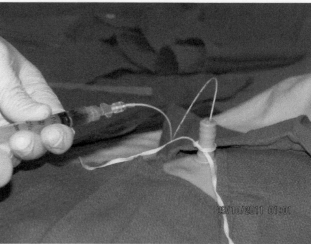

Fig. 121.5 Once there is easy blood return, pass the catheter an additional 1–2 cm. The catheter should still be inferior to the liver at this point

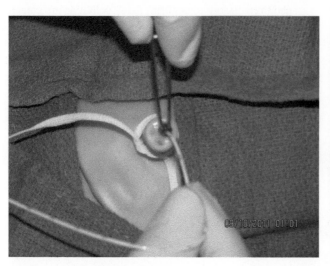

Fig. 121.4 Gently pass the umbilical venous catheter (or 5 F feeding tube) until there is easy blood return

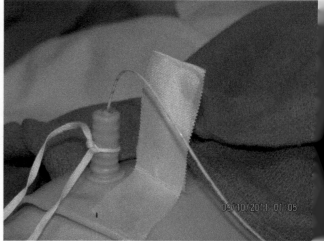

Fig. 121.6 Creating an umbilical catheter tape bridge: the uprights

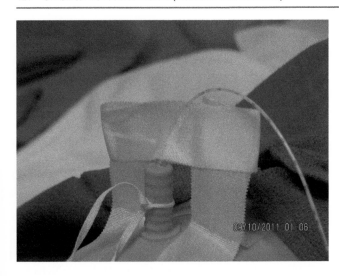

Fig. 121.7 Umbilical tape catheter bridge: the "cross bar" secures the catheter without applying tape to the umbilical stump

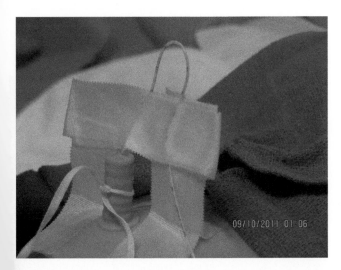

Fig. 121.8 Fold the catheter over to create a "U." Be careful not to kink the catheter, and secure with a second taped cross bar to lend additional security to the catheter and prevent displacement

121.5 Procedure (Removal)

1. The UVC should be removed as soon as adequate peripheral venous access is obtained (unless in an infant estimated to weigh <1000 g).
2. Turn infusions off.
3. Be certain the stopcock is closed to the infant.
4. It is imperative that there be no air in the catheter before withdrawal (if air is present and infant takes inspiration, the negative pressure generated can pull significant amount of air into the central vasculature).
5. Remove the securing tape from the infant.
6. Withdraw the catheter gradually as a single maneuver.

121.6 Complications

- Infection
- Bleeding due to disconnection of tubing (*always use Luer-Lok connections*) or perforation of vessels
- Arterial injury by accidental perforation
- Hepatic injury and necrosis if the catheter sits within a portal vein
- Thrombosis
- Air embolus
- Dysrhythmia or pericardial tamponade or perforation if catheter is advanced too far

121.7 Pearls and Pitfalls

- Pearls
  - The umbilical vein is 2–3 cm long before it widens into the umbilical recess, just before intersecting with the left portal vein and the ductus venosus.
  - Be certain to include the length of the umbilical stump in any calculations for placement.
  - If using the calculating graph, measure from the right shoulder to the umbilicus (Fig. 121.9).
- If choosing the above-diaphragm site for placement, corkscrewing the catheter clockwise while passing the catheter will encourage it to pass through the ductus venosus.
  - A kidney, ureter, and bladder study is mandatory in high UVC placement.
- Pitfalls

- When preparing with Betadine (povidone-iodine), be certain to wipe away and remove any pooled Betadine along the infant's side because this will cool the infant initially; as the Betadine is warmed, it becomes highly irritating to newborn skin.

Selected Reading

Sudbury, Jones, Bartlett. Emergency vascular access. In: APLS: the pediatric emergency medicine resource. 5th ed., p. 741.

Magnan JP. Umbilical Vein Catheterization. http://emedicine. medscape.com/article/80469-overview.

Schlesinger AE, Braverman RM, DiPietre MA. Neonates and umbilical venous catheters: normal appearance, anomalous positions, complications, and potential aid to diagnosis. Presented at the 2001 annual meeting of the American Roentgen Ray Society, Seattle, Apr 2001.

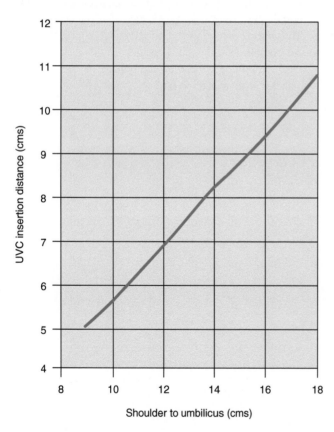

Fig. 121.9 Graph for estimation of insertion distance of the catheter; be certain to add the length (cm) of the umbilical stump to the insertion distance

Intraosseous Access

Judith K. Lucas

122.1 Indications

- During cardiac arrest: Failure to attain vascular access after three peripheral intravenous attempts or 90 s, whichever comes first
- Inability to gain vascular access in pediatric patients presenting in shock due to hemorrhage (trauma), sepsis, profound dehydration, or cardiac failure

122.2 Contraindications

Absolute
- Fracture of the long bone considered for intraosseous (IO) access

Relative
- Previous IO access attempt in the same long bone
- Cellulitis over the insertion site
- Inferior vena cava injury (circulatory access proximal to the injury site is preferred).
- Osteogenesis imperfecta

122.3 Materials and Medications

- Preparation materials, such as an antiseptic solution and sterile drapes, IF the patient's stability offers the time.
- Lidocaine without epinephrine: If it becomes necessary to place an IO in a conscious patient, use lidocaine to anesthetize the skin to the bony cortex; then once accessed, infiltrate 2–3 mL into the marrow to alleviate some of the pain of medications infusing through the marrow.
- IO needle (a few examples shown) (Figs. 122.1, 122.2, and 122.3).

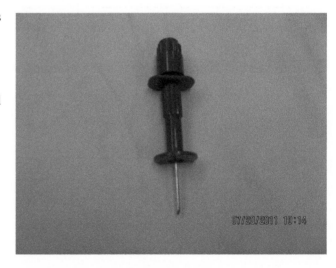

Fig. 122.1 Jamshidi disposable sternal/iliac aspiration needle (Jamshidi, Cardinal Health Dublin, OH)

. Lucas, MD
partment of Emergency Medicine,
versity of Florida Health Shands Hospital,
nesville, FL, USA
ail: judithklucas@ufl.edu

pringer Science+Business Media New York 2016

anti (ed.), *Atlas of Emergency Medicine Procedures*, DOI 10.1007/978-1-4939-2507-0_122

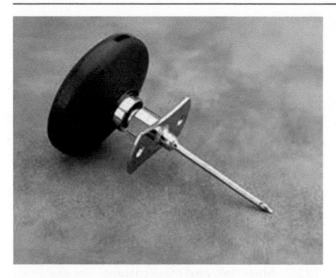

Fig. 122.2 Cook intraosseous needle (Cook Critical Care, Bloomington, IN)

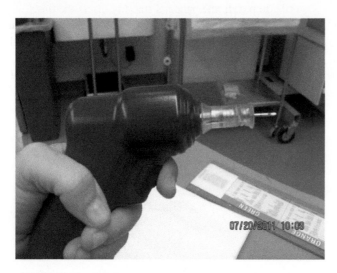

Fig. 122.3 EZ-IO (Vida-Care, San Antonio, TX)

122.4 Procedure

- Most common site: proximal tibia
  1. Patient should be supine, with the intended leg slightly externally rotated and flexed at the hip. Flex the knee about 90°.
  2. Place a towel underneath the knee and the proximal lower leg.
  3. Palpate the tibial tuberosity. Then move fingers 2 cm distal to the tuberosity (1–2 fingerbreadths) and 2 cm medial. This area is consistently flat and is distal to the growth plate (Figs. 122.4 and 122.5).
  4. If the patient is stable, create a sterile field focused on the insertion site.
  5. Insertion site should be cleaned with an antiseptic solution.
  6. Pass the needle through the skin and subcutaneous tissue to the cortex.
  7. Once bone is reached, stabilize the IO with the thumb and first fingers adjacent to where the needle penetrates the skin.
  8. Apply steady and firm pressure downward and with a twisting motion (back and forth) with the palm on the end of the device. Although inserting the needle perpendicularly to the bone is totally acceptable, ideally angling the needle caudally slightly (~15°) will avoid the growth plate (Fig. 122.6).
  9. As the cortex is fully penetrated indicating entrance into the marrow space, one *may* feel an ease in resistance. Do not advance the needle further. The needle should be able to stand up without support.
  10. Remove the inner trocar (Fig. 122.7).
  11. Attempt to aspirate marrow/blood. Not being able to do so DOES NOT mean inadequate or inaccurate placement. Instead, if marrow cannot be aspirated affix a 10-mL syringe with normal saline and attempt to infiltrate. Resistance to flow should be minimal and one should not appreciate either extravasation around the insertion site, coolness, or tissue expansion posterior to the site (indicating the fluid is passing through the IO).

12. Once placement is confirmed, connect an intravenous line, using a three-way stop-cock.
13. Secure the needle with tape and gauze (Fig. 122.8).

- Alternative sites
  - Distal tibia
    - The landmarks are the medial aspect of the tibia (the flat portion), 2 fingerbreadths proximal to the medial malleolus.
    - Again, externally rotate and abduct the hips, with the knee flexed about 60° (as with the proximal tibia).
    - Angle the needle toward the knee (cephalad) about 10–15° to avoid the distal tibia growth plate.
    - The remainder of the IO insertion is identical to the procedure for proximal tibia placement.
  - Distal femur
    - Slightly flex and externally rotate the hip.
    - Flex the knee enough that the quadriceps muscle group is relaxed.
    - The landmarks for the distal femur are the anterior thigh, midline, about 3 fingerbreadths proximal to the medial and lateral condyles.
    - The IO is inserted perpendicular to the bone (because there is no growth plate in the distal femur other than the condyles).
    - The remainder of the procedure is identical to the procedure for placement in the proximal tibia.

  - Proximal humerus (Fig. 122.9)
    - The patient should be supine, with the shoulder, upper arm, and elbow as close to the body as possible, yet still on the bed. The elbow should be flexed at 90°, with the forearm and palm resting on the patient's abdomen.
    - The provider slides his or her thumb up the anterior shaft of the humerus toward the shoulder until the greater humerus tubercle is palpated, which identifies the surgical neck of the humerus.
    - The insertion site is perpendicular to the humerus, approximately 1–2 fingerbreadths proximal to the tubercle.
    - The remainder of the insertion is identical to that for the proximal tibia.
  - Sternum (not usually recommended for small children).
    - Requires a special IO needle and system.
    - Method of placement is specific to the insertion system chosen.
    - Manubrium is the desired site (as opposed to the body of the sternum, which would interfere with cardiopulmonary resuscitation).
    - Risks specific to sternal placement include pneumothorax, mediastinitis, and great vessel injury.

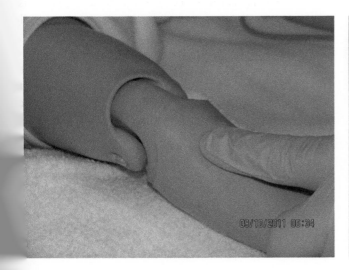

Fig. 122.4 Step 1. Identify the tibial tuberosity

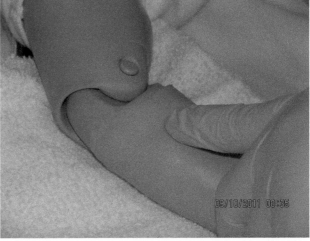

Fig. 122.5 Step 2. One to 2 fingerbreadths below the tuberosity and medially, to the flat aspect of the proximal tibia

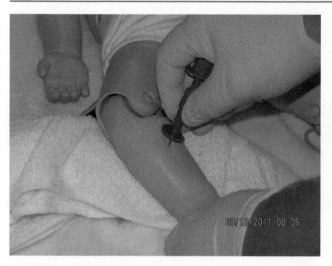

Fig. 122.6 Step 3. Angle the device slightly caudal to avoid growth plate

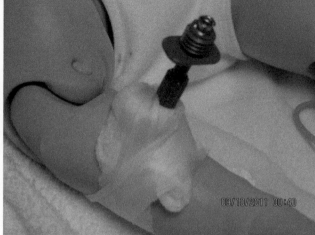

Fig. 122.8 Step 5. Stabilize the intraosseous cannula

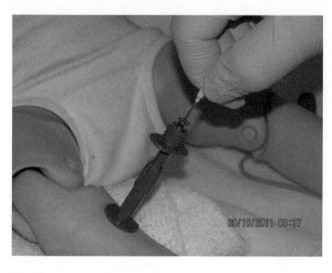

Fig. 122.7 Step 4. Uncap the top of the device and remove the trocar

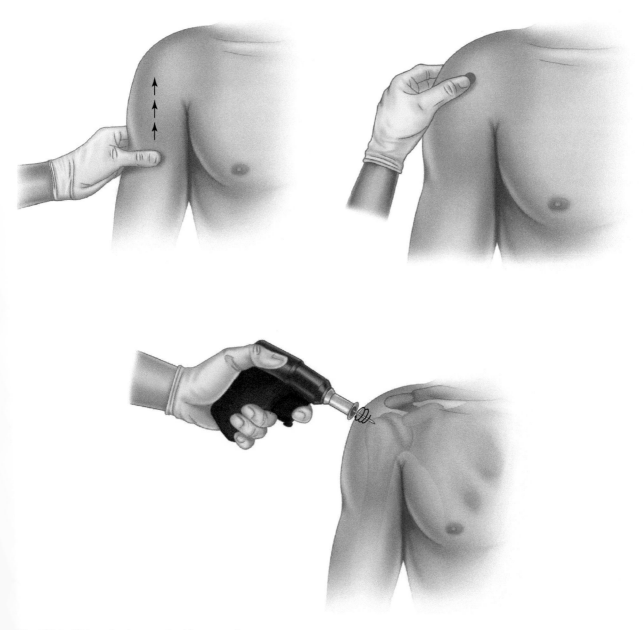

Fig. 122.9 IO insertion into proximal humerus site

122.5 Complications

- Extravasation of fluid.
  - Occurs as a result of a misplaced IO, either not completely in the marrow space anteriorly or through the cortex posteriorly.
  - Tissue necrosis.
- Compartment syndrome if extravasation is not recognized.
- Fracture and growth plate injury.
- Infection and osteomyelitis are rare complications if sterile technique is used.
- Fat embolism, considered rare and only in adult patients.

122.6 Pearls and Pitfalls

- Be certain to avoid placing a hand beneath the IO site during placement in order to prevent possible IO penetration into the provider's tissue.
- Do not rely on the sensation of a "pop" to determine appropriate penetration into the cortex, especially in infants.

- Likewise, one may not be able to aspirate bone marrow or blood, even with an appropriately placed IO. DO NOT pull out the IO if marrow cannot be aspirated. Rather, gently but firmly infiltrate 10 mL normal saline.
- Blood gases, body chemistries, and blood typing can be obtained from IO samples, but the sample CANNOT be used for hematocrit determination.

Selected Reading

Bohn D. Intraosseous vascular access: from archives to the ABC. Crit Care Med. 1999;27:1053.

DeCaen AR, Reis A, Bhutta A. Vascular access and drug therapy in pediatric resuscitation. Pediatr Clin North Am. 2008;55:909–27.

Deitch K. Intraosseous infusion. In: Roberts JR, Hedges JR, editors. Clinical procedures in emergency medicine. 5th ed. Philadelphia: Saunders; 2009. Chap. 25.

EMS World. Intraosseous infusion: not just for kids anymore. Posted Jan. 12, 2011. Updated from Mar 2005. EMSWorld.com. Cygnus Business Media Site.

Halm B, Yamamoto LG. Comparing ease of intraosseous needle placement: Jamshidi versus Cook. Am J Emerg Med. 1998;16:420.

Lumbar Puncture in Pediatrics

Maritza A. Plaza-Verduin and Judith K. Lucas

123.1 Indications

- Evaluation of cerebrospinal fluid (CSF) for infection or malignancy
- Measurement of opening pressure
- Treatment of pseudotumor cerebri
- Diagnosis of central nervous system (CNS) metastases
- Instillation of intrathecal chemotherapy
- Injection of radiopaque dye for spinal cord imaging

123.2 Contraindications

Increased intracranial pressure
Bleeding diathesis (platelet count <50,000)
Overlying skin infection near the area of puncture site
Spinal cord trauma or spinal cord compression
Signs of progressive cerebral herniation
Condition of the patient (e.g., unstable airway, potentially dangerous breathing problem, severe circulatory instability) that could cause an abrupt decompensation
Known spinal cord deformity

123.3 Materials and Medications

- Lumbar puncture (LP) tray (Fig. 123.1)
  - Sterile drapes
  - Betadine (povidone-iodine) swabs or tray to pour Betadine
  - Sterile sponges for preparing the puncture site
  - Sterile 3-mL syringe with needle for lidocaine injection
  - Sterile collecting tubes (4)
  - Sterile spinal needle with stylet (size depending on age of patient)
    - Premature infant: 22 gauge or smaller, 1.5 inch
    - Neonate to 2 years: 22 gauge, 1.5 inch
    - 2–12 years: 22 gauge, 2.5 inch
    - Older than 12 years: 20 or 22 gauge, 3.5 inch
  - Pressure manometer column with a three-way stopcock
- Betadine solution
- Sterile gloves
- Mask
- Lidocaine (1–2 % without epinephrine)
- 4 % Lidocaine cream (LMX-4) or lidocaine and prilocaine mixture (EMLA [eutectic mixture of local anesthetics])

A. Plaza-Verduin, MD
liatric Division, Department of Emergency Medicine, Arnold
mer Hospital for Children, Orlando, FL, USA
ail: mari.plazav@gmail.com

. Lucas, MD (⊠)
artment of Emergency Medicine,
versity of Florida Health Shands Hospital,
nesville, FL, USA
ail: judithklucas@ufl.edu

pringer Science+Business Media New York 2016
anti (ed.), *Atlas of Emergency Medicine Procedures*, DOI 10.1007/978-1-4939-2507-0_123

Fig. 123.1 Lumbar puncture
(LP) tray

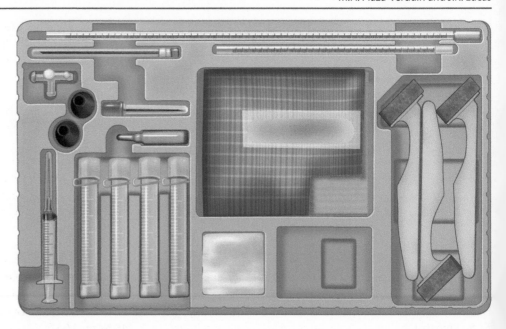

23.4 Procedure

. Position the child (Figs. 123.2 and 123.3).
  (a) Can be positioned in either the sitting or the lateral recumbent position with the hips, knees, and neck flexed.
  (b) For small infants or any patient with any degree of cardiorespiratory compromise, keep close monitoring of heart rate, respirations, and oxygen saturation while in the flexed position.

. Palpate the top of the iliac crest and draw an imaginary line connecting the two across the back, which should cross the midline just above the fourth lumbar spine (Fig. 123.4).

. Palpate L3–4 or L4–5 space along this line.

. Place EMLA or LMX-4 on the area at this time and allow some time for anesthesia to occur (can take up to 30 min to be effective).

. Prepare the skin in sterile fashion with Betadine solution using enlarging circles that begin at the puncture site.

. Drape the patient with sterile towels, exposing the puncture site.
  (a) If an infant, do so conservatively to be able to monitor the infant during the procedure.

. Locate the intervertebral space (L3–4 or L4–5) once again.
  (a) Make a small mark on the chosen intervertebral space with a fingernail depression or the plastic cap of the spinal needle.

. If desired, or if anesthetic cream was not previously used or more is needed, apply a small wheal of lidocaine at the desired puncture site using a 25-gauge needle.

. Insert the spinal needle in the intervertebral space.
  (a) Puncture the skin in the midline just caudal to the palpated spinous process.
  (b) Bevel should be positioned so that the dura mater is pierced parallel to its fibers (which will reduce the likelihood of CSF leakage).
    (i) If in the lateral recumbent position, the bevel of the needle should be positioned horizontally.
    (ii) If in the sitting position, the bevel of the needle should be positioned vertically.
    (iii) Angle the needle slightly cephalad toward the umbilicus and parallel to the bed if the patient is in the lateral recumbent position or slightly caudal (perpendicular to the skin) if the patient is in the sitting position.

. Advance the needle several millimeters at a time and withdraw the stylet frequently to check for CSF flow.
  (a) Advance the needle until a loss of resistance is felt or approximately 1–2 cm.
    (i) In the infants, whose dura are not so thick and a "pop" or give may be unnoticeable, after passing between the spiny processes and approximately 2 cm through the skin, remove the stylet frequently to check for CSF return. This will allow you to avoid passing through the subarachnoid space.
    (ii) After the change in resistance occurs, if resistance is met again, pull back gently on the needle to reposition in the subarachnoid space and remove the stylet to check for CSF fluid.

11. Once CSF is free flowing, attach a pressure manometer to the needle hub via the three-way stopcock (Fig. 123.5).
  (a) Make sure to hold the spinal needle with one hand in place while attaching the manometer to prevent movement of the needle.
  (b) Measure the CSF pressure once the CSF reaches the highest level in the manometer column.
  (c) CSF pressures will be best obtained in the lateral recumbent position with the neck and legs extended.
  (d) Normal CSF pressure is 5–20-cm H_2O with the neck and legs extended, 10–28-cm H_2O with the neck and legs flexed.
  (e) Have an assistant hold the top of the pressure manometer while the spinal needle is supported at the connection of the manometer and stopcock.

12. Remove the manometer and collect the CSF into sterile tubes.
  (a) Make sure to keep the needle in place when removing the manometer.
  (b) Continue to drain fluid into the collecting tubes, approximately 1 mL per tube.
  (c) The tubes should be labeled for specific studies, depending on the order of collection.
    (i) First tube for gram stain and culture.
    (ii) Second tube for quantitative glucose and protein.
    (iii) Third or fourth tube for cell count and differential.
    (iv) Leftover tube for any additional studies that may be needed.
    (v) When the LP is to assess for possible subarachnoid blood, the first and fourth tubes are sent for cell count.

13. Replace the stylet and remove the spinal needle.

14. Cleanse the puncture area to avoid staining with the Betadine solution.

15. Apply a sterile dressing to the puncture site.

16. Patients 4 years and older should remain in the supine position, with the head elevated no more than the height of a pillow (for comfort), for at least an hour to avoid spinal tap headaches.

17. Likewise, after the LP, giving a fluid bolus of normal saline (10–20 mL/kg in children; 1 L in non-volume-sensitive adults) will also assist with avoidance of spinal tap headaches.

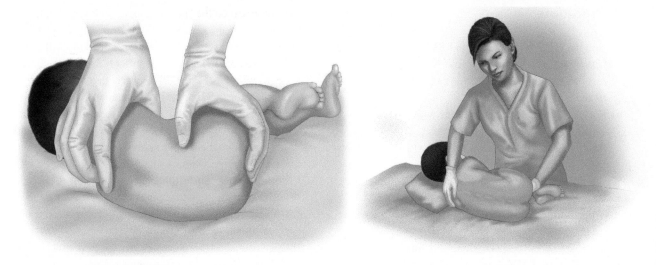

Fig. 123.2 Curling up for an LP

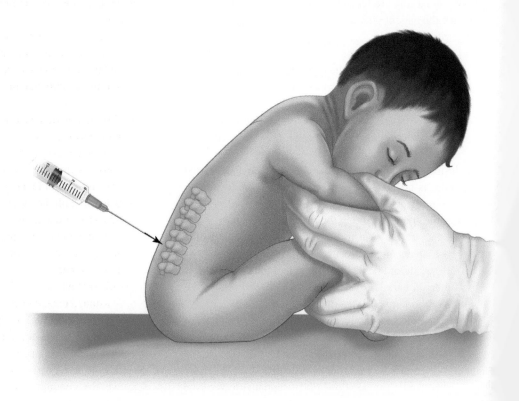

Fig. 123.3 Having the LP

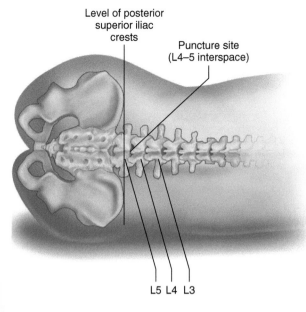

Fig. 123.4 Anatomy of the lumbar spine showing the sites for dural puncture

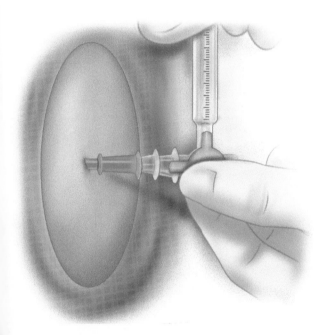

Fig. 123.5 Pressure manometer attached to the needle hub via the three-way stopcock

123.5 Complications

- Minor
  - Localized back pain
  - Transient paresthesia during procedure
  - Post-LP headache
- Major
  - Severe back pain associated with neurological signs (may be subdural or epidural spinal hematoma)
  - LP-induced meningitis
  - Cerebral herniation
  - Acquired epidermoid tumor
  - Damage to adjacent structures (disk herniation, retroperitoneal abscess, spinal cord hematoma)

123.6 Pearls and Pitfalls

- Pearls
  - Success of the LP depends on the positioning of the patient.
    - Goal of positioning is to stretch the ligamentum flavum and increase the interlaminar spaces.
    - In the recumbent position, the shoulder and hips should be perpendicular to the bed, keeping the spinal cord straight, with no rotation.
    - Sitting position is useful with older, cooperative patients or with very young infants who are unlikely to struggle and may have increased respiratory distress in the lateral recumbent position.
  - Administration of an anxiolytic (e.g., midazolam) can be used to facilitate the procedure in an older child. In some cases, procedural sedation may be required.
  - Placing the tip of the thumb on the spinous process just above the space being entered can ensure good alignment of the needle.
  - In older patients a "pop" may often be felt as a change in resistance occurs once the dura is penetrated; however, in infants and neonates, that "pop" may be exceedingly subtle or not palpable.
  - If no CSF returns, attempt the following options:
    - Ensure the needle is in the appropriate position, withdrawing the needle slowly if necessary.
    - Rotate the needle 90°.
    - If an infant, have the assistant massage the anterior fontanel to help facilitate CSF flow.
    - If the procedure continues without CSF, withdraw the needle to just under the skin and redirect it.
    - If the procedure continues without CSF, withdraw the needle and insert a new needle with stylet at an alternate site.

- If these steps do not yield CSF, the infant may be dehydrated, not allowing for adequate CSF flow.
  - Give the patient a bolus and reattempt later.
  - Attempt putting the infant in a sitting position to increase flow.
- Pitfalls
  - Traumatic LP
    - Bloody CSF fluid, which usually clears as the CSF drains if the needle is in the correct space.
    - Occurs with improper technique (inserting the needle too far to one side into an epidural venous plexus or through the subarachnoid space into or adjacent to the vertebral body).
    - Can occur with proper technique as well.
    - If fluid does not clear and clots form in the tubes, LP should be reattempted at a different site.
  - Failed LP attempts despite proper procedure and positioning
    - Ultrasound can be used to visualize the area and determine the reason for failure or the likelihood of success with future attempts.

Selected Reading

Coley BD, Shiels WE, Hogan MJ. Diagnostic and interventional ultrasonography in neonatal and infant lumbar puncture. Pediatr Radiol. 2001;31:399–402.

Cronan KM, Wiley JF. Lumbar puncture. In: King C, Henretig FM, editors. Textbook of pediatric emergency procedures. 2nd ed. New York: Lippincott Williams & Wilkins; 2008.

Ebinger F, Kosel C, Pietz J, Rating D. Headache and backache after lumbar puncture in children and adolescents: a prospective study. Pediatrics. 2004;113:1588–92.

Friedman AG, Mulhern RK, Fairclough D, et al. Midazolam premedication for pediatric bone marrow aspiration and lumbar puncture. Med Pediatr Oncol. 1991;19:499–504.

Partin WR. Emergency procedures. In: Stone CK, Humphries RL, editors. Current diagnosis & treatment: emergency medicine. 6th ed. New York: McGraw-Hill; 2007.

Suprapubic Bladder Aspiration

Maritza A. Plaza-Verduin and Judith K. Lucas

124.1 Indications

- Collection of sterile urine for urinalysis and culture (avoiding urethral contamination)
- Collection of sterile urine in a child with gastroenteritis and frequent diarrheal stools
- Female child with labial adhesions or male child with minimally retractable foreskin
- Urinary retention

124.2 Contraindications

Empty or nonpalpable bladder
Urination within 1 h before the procedure
Anatomical abnormalities of the gut or genitourinary tract
Bleeding diathesis
Intestinal obstruction

- Overlying cellulitis on abdominal wall
- Lower abdominal scars or wounds

124.3 Materials and Medications

- Sterile gloves
- Lidocaine (1–2 %) with syringe and needle
- EMLA (eutectic mixture of local anesthetics) cream
- Betadine (povidone-iodine) solution
- Sterile syringe, 5–20 mL
- Sterile needle 22 or 23 gauge, 1.5 inch
- Sterile specimen container
- Sterile towels
- Sterile gauze
- Sterile dressing
- Adhesive bandage

A. Plaza-Verduin, MD
Pediatric Division, Department of Emergency Medicine,
Arnold Palmer Hospital for Children, Orlando, FL, USA
e-mail: mari.plazav@gmail.com

J. Lucas, MD (✉)
Department of Emergency Medicine,
University of Florida Health Shands Hospital,
Gainesville, FL, USA
e-mail: judithklucas@ufl.edu

© Springer Science+Business Media New York 2016
E. Ganti (ed.), *Atlas of Emergency Medicine Procedures*, DOI 10.1007/978-1-4939-2507-0_124

124.4 Procedure

1. Place the infant in the supine, frog-leg position (Fig. 124.1).
2. Localize the bladder.
3. Palpate the midline between the umbilicus and the pubis symphysis to feel for bladder fullness.
   - Use a portable ultrasound device to localize the bladder and allow for approximation of bladder size (see later).
4. Localize the symphysis pubis and the imaginary line midline from the umbilicus to the pubic symphysis (Fig. 124.2).
5. Sterilize the area from the umbilicus to the urethra.
6. Drape the area with sterile towels, keeping the puncture site area exposed.
7. Area of insertion should be midline 1–2 cm above the symphysis pubis on the abdominal wall.
   - The suprapubic crease can usually be used as a guideline to the puncture site.
8. Place a small wheal of anesthetic at the intended puncture site or can apply EMLA cream.
   - For use of EMLA cream, place before sterilization and allow some time for anesthesia to occur.
9. Occlude the urethral opening to avoid spontaneous loss of urine specimen.
   - In males, apply gentle pressure to the base of the penis against the pubic symphysis.
   - In females, directly apply pressure to the urethral meatus.
10. Puncture the skin with the needle (attached to the syringe).
    - Puncture at a 10–20° angle to the perpendicular, aiming slightly cephalad (Fig. 124.3).
11. Apply negative pressure to the syringe as the needle is advanced until urine enters the syringe; do not advance more than 1 inch.
    - If unsuccessful, draw back the needle until it rests in the subcutaneous fat and redirect 10° in either direction.
    - Do not attempt more than three times.
12. Cleanse the area of antiseptic solution and apply an adhesive dressing.

a

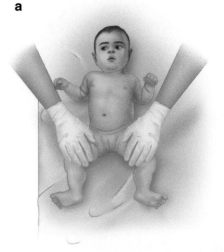

b

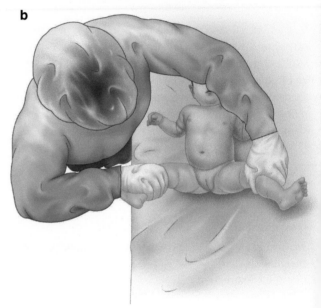

Fig. 124.1 Frog-leg position

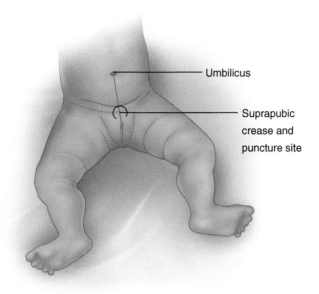

Fig. 124.2 Landmarks

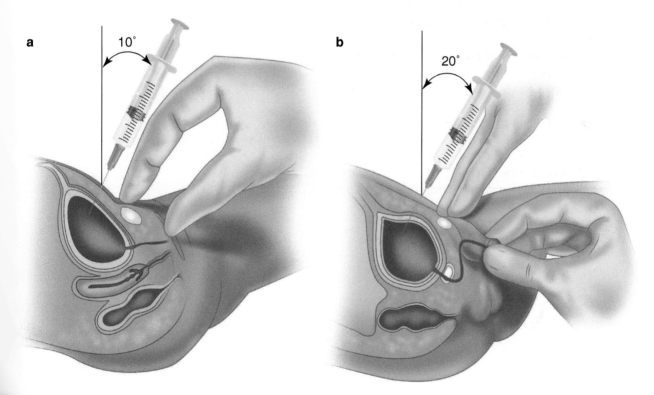

Fig. 124.3 Insert the needle 10–20° perpendicular to the skin

124.5 Complications

- Peritoneal perforation with or without bowel perforation
- Infection
- Hematuria
- Inability to aspirate urine

124.6 Pearls and Pitfalls

- If no fluid is obtained:
  - Hydrate the child and reattempt in 1 h.
- Ultrasound can be used to identify bladder size or for ultrasound-guided aspiration:
  - Use a portable ultrasound device with a standoff 7.5-MHz sector probe to allow for superficial scanning and measurement of the diameter of the bladder.
  - Bladder diameter measurement:
    1. Apply approximately 5 mL of ultrasound transmission gel to the infant's suprapubic region.
    2. Apply pressure to the ureteral meatus as previously described.
    3. Gently apply the probe to the suprapubic region in the midline and scan the area in transverse plane, with the probe directed caudad or cephalad as needed to maximize bladder image.
       - Bladder will appear anechoic below the brighter reflections of the rectus muscle and bladder wall.
    4. When maximum bladder size obtained, freeze the image.
       - Measure the anteroposterior and transverse internal bladder diameters.
       - Goal measurement is 2 cm or more of each diameter. If either diameter is less than 2 cm, the bladder is considered to be empty.

- Ultrasound-guided bladder aspiration:
  1. After preparing the sterile field, place a sterile sheath over the ultrasound probe and proximal cable.
     (a) Gel should be placed within the sheath to eliminate the air interface between the probe and the sheath.
  2. Apply gel to the abdomen above the symphysis pubis.
  3. Locate the bladder and measure the maximum diameter as described previously.
  4. Insert the needle midline at the location where the bladder wall is closest to the probe.
  5. Continue steps for aspiration as described previously.

Selected Reading

Kozer E, Rosenbloom E, Goldman D, et al. Pain in infants who are younger than 2 months during suprapubic aspiration and transurethral bladder catheterization: a randomized, controlled study. Pediatrics. 2006;118:e51–6.

Leong Y, Tang KW. Bladder aspiration for diagnosis of urinary tract infection in infants and young children. J Singapore Paediatr Soc. 1976;18:43–7.

Loiselle JM. Ultrasound-assisted suprapubic bladder aspiration. In: King C, Henretig FM, editors. Textbook of pediatric emergency procedures. 2nd ed. New York: Lippincott Williams & Wilkins; 2008.

Pollack CV, Pollack ES, Andrew ME. Suprapubic bladder aspiration versus urethral catheterization in ill infants: success, efficiency and complication rates. Ann Emerg Med. 1994;23:225–30.

Polnay L, Fraser AM, Lewis JM. Complication of suprapubic bladder aspiration. Arch Dis Child. 1975;50:80–1.

Removal of Hair/Thread Tourniquet

Judith K. Lucas

125.1 Indications

Consider the diagnosis when presented with an append-age that has a well-demarcated, circumferential, painful, edematous distal segment, adjacent to a nonedematous, nonerythematous proximal portion (Fig. 125.1).

Removal is imperative in all cases of tourniquet syndrome and should be undertaken without delay.

Method of removal is determined by degree of constriction.

- Unwrapping: in situations with minimal or no edema and the ability to visualize the offending hair or thread
- Blunt probe, cutting: mild to moderate edema
- Incision: severe swelling or inability to visualize the constricting band; epithelialization
- Depilatory: for areas with mild to moderate edema, but without epithelialization

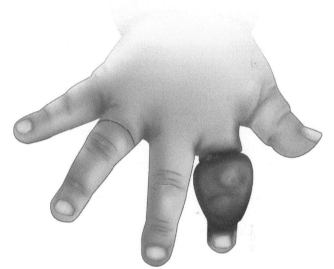

Fig. 125.1 Hair tourniquet

K. Lucas, MD
epartment of Emergency Medicine,
niversity of Florida Health Shands Hospital,
inesville, FL, USA
nail: judithklucas@ufl.edu

Springer Science+Business Media New York 2016
Ganti (ed.), *Atlas of Emergency Medicine Procedures*, DOI 10.1007/978-1-4939-2507-0_125

125.2 Contraindications

- Absolute
  - There are no absolute contraindications; the tourniquet must be removed.
- Relative
  - Based more on the specific approach (e.g., avoid incising the skin of a patient with hemophilia; avoid depilatory creams in a patient with known allergies to such)

125.3 Materials and Medications

- Unraveling technique
  - Fine-tipped, non-rat-tooth forceps or small fine hemostats
- Blunt probe and tourniquet cutting
  - Antiseptic solution of choice
  - Lidocaine 1 % without epinephrine for local or regional anesthesia
  - Scalpel blade #11 or Iris scissors
  - Blunt probe or metal earwax curette
- Incision technique
  - Antiseptic solution of choice
  - Lidocaine 1 % without epinephrine for local or regional anesthesia
  - Scalpel blade #11
  - Fine-tipped, non-rat-tooth forceps or small, fine hemostats
- Depilatory technique
  - Commercial depilatory cream

125.4 Procedures

- Unraveling method (Fig. 125.2)
  1. Place the appendage in an orientation that maximizes exposure.
  2. Apply skin traction such that as much of the tourniquet and base of the constriction can be seen.
  3. Look closely to identify a free end of the hair or thread. If no free end is visible, identify an area of bunching or a knot. Break the knot from the strand and grasp the end with the forceps or hemostat.
  4. Slowly and gently pull and unwind the hair.
  5. This may take several attempts because the hair strand or thread may break repeatedly during removal. Sometimes more than one hair strand may be involved.
- Blunt probe and cutting method (Figs. 125.3 and 125.4)
  1. Apply gentle traction to the skin to maximally expose the involved area and to make the base of the wedge caused by the tourniquet as shallow as possible.
  2. Gently impose a blunt probe or a metal ear curette between the skin and the tourniquet, starting proximally to the band and sliding distally beneath the constriction.
  3. Cut the tourniquet by sliding the scalpel blade along the edge of the probe, placing the blunt edge of the scalpel against the skin and slicing the constricting material in a movement away from the skin, in order to avoid inadvertently cutting the skin.
  4. Once an end of the tourniquet has been created, the remainder of the offending strap can be removed via unraveling.

- Incision technique for digits (Fig. 125.5)
  1. Perform a digital nerve block to anesthetize the extremity proximal to the constriction.
  2. Sterilize the involved area with antiseptic solution of choice and drape in typical protocol to allow as sterile a procedure as is possible outside a surgical suite.
  3. Incise the skin across the demarcation indicating the presence of the tourniquet at the 3 o'clock or 9 o'clock position or the midline dorsal area (12 o'clock), passing the scalpel blade proximally to distally and down to the bone (Fig. 125.6). Incision at these locations will avoid the laterally located neurovascular bundles of the digits.
- Incision technique for severe penile tourniquet
  1. Begin with a dorsal nerve block (Fig. 125.7).
  2. Sterilize the involved area with antiseptic solution of choice and drape in typical protocol to allow as sterile a procedure as is possible outside a surgical suite.
  3. A longitudinal incision is made at either the 4 o'clock or the 8 o'clock position, in order to avoid the penile neurovascular structures located dorsally.

  4. The incision should be made perpendicular to the tourniquet, but shallowly, in order to avoid penetration through the deep fascia. It will be necessary to repeat the incision, staying within the original incision, gently but repeatedly in order to cut through the whole tourniquet. In this way the constriction is relieved, but the integrity of the corpus cavernosum and the corpus spongiosum is maintained (Fig. 125.8).
  5. Once the layers of the tourniquet have been interrupted, grasp an end of the hair/thread and remove the remainder of the tourniquet utilizing the unraveling method.
- Depilatory method
  1. Depilatories work only on hair and will not work on threads.
  2. Apply the depilatory cream directly to the hair tourniquet with a saturated cotton swab, so as to avoid applying this potential irritant to surrounding tissue.
  3. Wait the recommended amount of time, as dictated by whatever brand of depilatory is used.
  4. After the appropriate time has elapsed, wash off the cream thoroughly with soap and water.

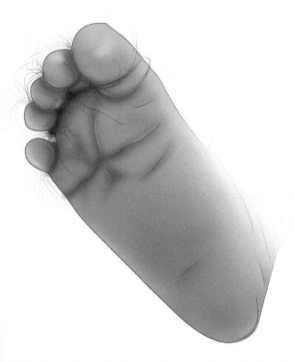

125.2 A good example for use of the unraveling technique. The ~ma is minimal and the hair is easily identifiable

Fig. 125.3 Blunt and cut method.
Notice the cutting edge of the
scalpel blade is away from the skin
as it is placed adjacent to the probe
and slips beneath the tourniquet

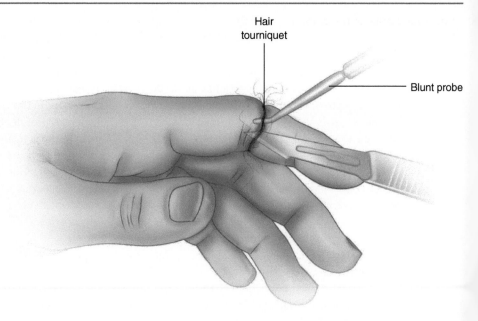

Hair
tourniquet

Blunt probe

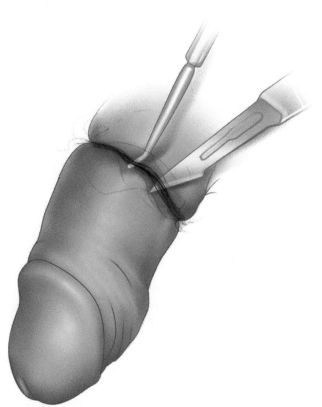

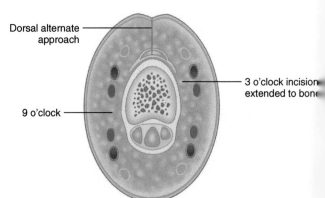

Dorsal alternate
approach

9 o'clock

3 o'clock incision
extended to bone

Fig. 125.5 Incision technique for digits

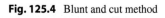

Fig. 125.4 Blunt and cut method

Fig. 125.6 Incision at 12 o'clock preferred

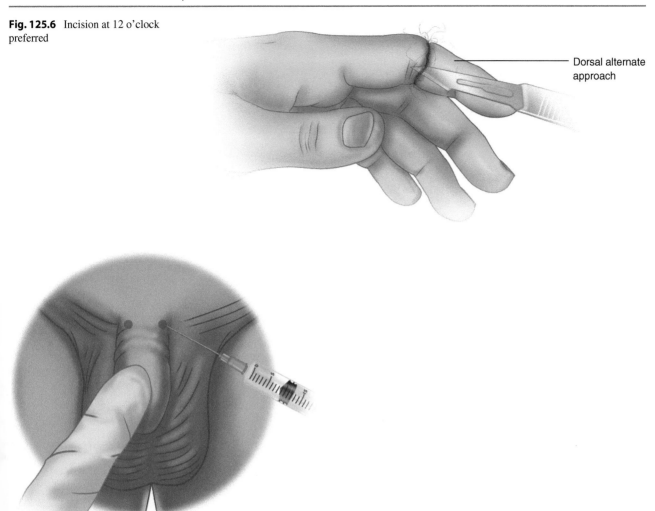

Dorsal alternate approach

Fig. 125.7 Dorsal nerve block

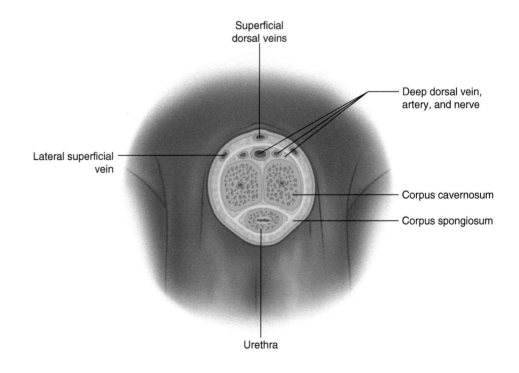

Superficial dorsal veins

Deep dorsal vein, artery, and nerve

Lateral superficial vein

Corpus cavernosum

Corpus spongiosum

Urethra

g. 125.8 Penile tourniquet hematic

125.5 Complications

- Necrosis of tissue distal to the tourniquet
- Neurovascular damage secondary to prolonged ischemia
- The incision technique can cut into the tendon insertions or neurovascular bundles of the digits or into the corpus callosum of the penis. Be certain to ascertain function after incision.
- Infection, especially after incision.

125.6 Pearls and Pitfalls

- Pearls
  - All tourniquets must come off.
  - The easiest way to get to the bottom of the tourniquet, regardless of method used, is to identify the knot or bunched area if possible.
  - When using the incision technique, keep the incision in the longitudinal plane of the appendage and perpendicular to the tourniquet.
  - Do not use depilatories on open wounds.
  - 24-h follow-up is mandatory, although if the tourniquet has been present for an extended period of time, it may actually take several days for return of color and blood flow.

- Be certain to document neurovascular status before and after tourniquet removal.
- Consider surgical consult in cases of severe tissue edema or distorted anatomy.
- Tourniquets have been described in the child abuse literature. Consider that possibility in the preverbal child.
- Pitfalls
  - The depilatories will not work on nonorganic tourniquets.

Selected Reading

Bothner J. Hair entrapment removal techniques. UpToDate. Accessed 30 Nov 2010.

Cardriche, D. Hair tourniquet removal. Medscape reference: drugs, diseases, and procedures. Available at: http://emedicine.medscape.com/article/1348969-overview. Accessed 17 May 2009.

Klusmann A. Tourniquet syndrome—accident or abuse? Eur J Pediatr. 2004;163:495–8.

Lundquist ST, Stack LB. Genitourinary emergencies: diseases of the foreskin, penis, and urethra. Emerg Med Clin North Am. 2001;19:529–46.

Peleg D, Steiner A. The Gomco circumcision: common problems and solutions. Am Fam Physician. 1998;58:891–8.

Use of the Broselow Tape

Judith K. Lucas

126.1 Indications

- To determine the equipment size and the medication doses during a pediatric resuscitation, without having to take the time to perform calculations

126.2 Contraindications

- Premature infant or newborn whose heel, while the infant is fully extended, does not fall at least into the white area (corresponding to 3, 4, and 5 kg).
- The length of the child exceeds the distal end of the green area (36 kg).

126.3 Materials

- Broselow Pediatric Emergency Tape (Armstrong Medical Industries, Wilshire, IL) (Figs. 126.1 and 126.2)

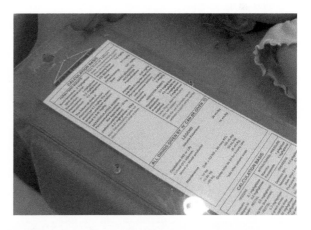

Fig. 126.1 Broselow tape, proximal end (at patient's head)

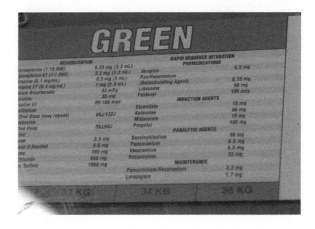

Fig. 126.2 Broselow tape, distal end (the tape will accommodate a 36-kg child, at most)

.K. Lucas, MD
Department of Emergency Medicine,
University of Florida Health Shands Hospital,
Gainesville, FL, USA
e-mail: judithklucas@ufl.edu

Springer Science+Business Media New York 2016
Ganti (ed.), *Atlas of Emergency Medicine Procedures*, DOI 10.1007/978-1-4939-2507-0_126

126.4 Procedure (Figs. 126.3, 126.4, and 126.5)

- Place the infant or child on the bed in the supine position.
- Extend the Broselow Pediatric Emergency Tape next to the patient, placing the red line at the top of the patient's head.
- With the patient fully extended, especially through the hips and knees, align the bottom of the heel, while the ankle is flexed and toes upward, with the color on the tape adjacent to the heel.

- The color on the tape corresponds to the patient's weight.
- The side of the tape with weights noted along the bottom has medication doses for resuscitation, rapid-sequence intubation (RSI), and paralytics (Fig. 126.6).
- The top half of the other side of the tape has the appropriate dosing for managing seizures, overdoses, elevating intracranial pressure, and fluids. The bottom half of this side has the appropriate equipment sizes, such as endotracheal tubes, nasogastric tubes, chest tubes, and other equipment, that correspond to the patient's weight (Fig. 126.7).

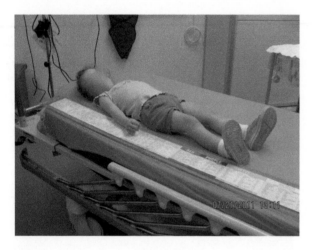

Fig. 126.3 Placement of the child on the tape

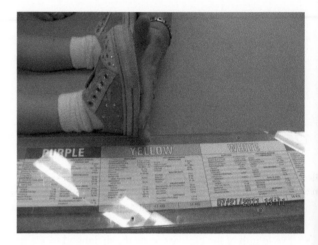

Fig. 126.5 Placement of the child on the tape

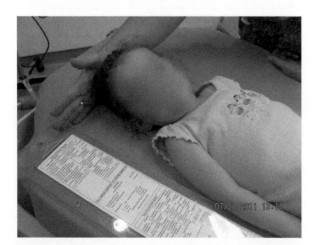

Fig. 126.4 Placement of the child on the tape

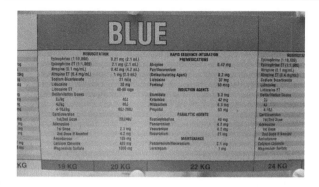

Fig. 126.6 Front of tape. Weight groupings are noted at the bottom. This is the side with resuscitation and RSI medications

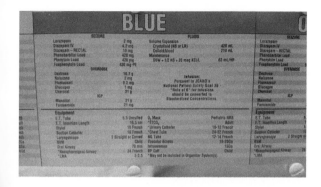

Fig. 126.7 Reverse side of tape. This side has medications for critical interventions aside from the primary survey, as well as equipment sizes

126.5 Pearls and Pitfalls

- Pearls
    - Be certain that the top of the head is at the red line and that the patient's body is fully extended. Infants tend to lay flexed at the hips and knees.
    - Determining the appropriate color code depends on noting the bottom of the heel while the ankle is flexed and the toes are pointing upward.
- Pitfalls
    - Beware of the child who is unusually heavy compared with other children of the same height.

Selected Reading

Luten R. Error and time delay in pediatric trauma resuscitation: addressing the problem with color-coded resuscitation aids. Surg Clin North Am. 2002;82:303–14, vi.

Luten R, Broselow J. Standardization of product concentration in emergency dosing: a response to Fineberg and Arendt. Ann Emerg Med. 2008;52:477–8.

Rosenberg M, Greenberger S, Rawal A, Latimer-Pierson J, Thundiyil J. Comparison of Broselow tape measurements versus estimations of pediatric weights. Am J Emerg Med. 2011;29:482–8.

Nursemaid's Elbow

Judith K. Lucas

127.1 Definition

- An injury commonly seen in children between 6 months and late preteens, although generally seen between 1 and 3 years
- A subluxation of the radial head, usually resulting from sudden, longitudinal traction on an extended arm with the wrist pronated
- Often occurs when a parent/caregiver is holding the child by the hand while walking and suddenly pulls the child away from a dangerous situation (Fig. 127.1)

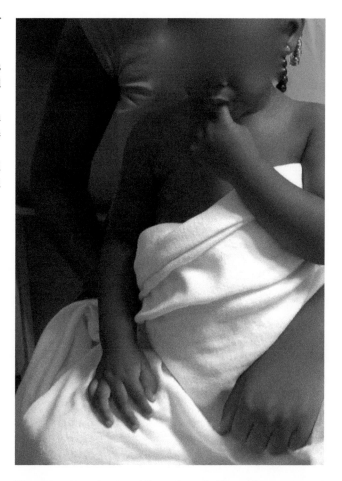

Fig. 127.1 Note that the toddler prefers to hold her right arm pronated and somewhat flexed at the elbow. When asked where it hurts, she may as often point to her wrist as to her elbow. There will be no soft tissue swelling anywhere along the upper extremity

K. Lucas, MD
Department of Emergency Medicine,
University of Florida Health Shands Hospital,
Gainesville, FL, USA
email: judithklucas@ufl.edu

Springer Science+Business Media New York 2016
Ganti (ed.), *Atlas of Emergency Medicine Procedures*, DOI 10.1007/978-1-4939-2507-0_127

127.2 Clinical Diagnosis

- History of pulling-type injury.
- Child presents with arm held slightly flexed at elbow and pronated.
- Patient may point to elbow or wrist as source of pain, but both areas are without any swelling and are nontender on palpation.
- Elbow can be flexed and extended, but the forearm cannot be supinated.
- Radiography is not helpful.

127.3 Indications

- Clinical presence of subluxed radial head

127.4 Contraindications

- Absolute
  - Radiographic evidence of elbow or forearm fracture
  - Swelling or pain about the elbow, forearm, or wrist
- Relative
  - Unknown history or witnessing of pulling-type injury

127.5 Materials and Medications

- None

127.6 Procedure

127.6.1 Method A: Superpronation (preferred method) (Fig. 127.2)

1. Explain to the caretaker that the reduction will cause the child *very brief* discomfort.
2. Seat the child on the lap of a parent/caregiver or an assistant, facing the operator and holding the child in such a way as to hold the child's humerus against her or his side.
3. The person performing the procedure holds the elbow at approximately 90° and grasps the elbow, with the physician's thumb over the region of the radial head (this is done in order to be able to palpate the reduction "clunk" or "click").
4. The physician then holds the patient's wrist firmly and rapidly hyperpronates the forearm. A palpable or audible "click" signifies successful reduction but may not be appreciable.
5. The child may cry for a few minutes after reduction; however, the provider should leave the bedside for 5–10 min and instruct the parents to allow the child to simply play, without focusing on the affected arm.
6. After approximately 10 min, return to the bedside and reevaluate the child, who should have full use of her or his arm by then.

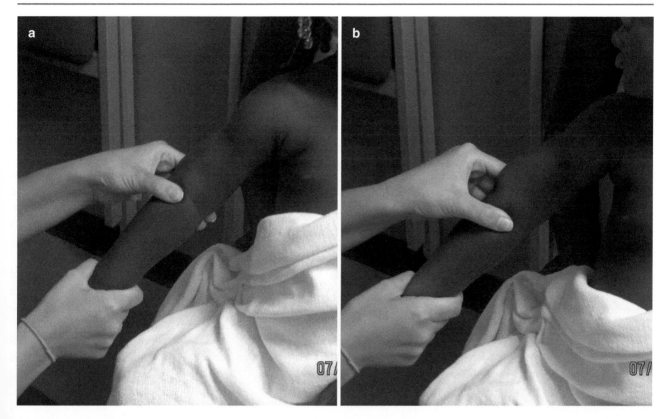

Fig. 127.2 Pronation: (**a**) The examiner's left hand holds the patient's radial head and medial condyle to better appreciate palpable reduction of the subluxation, (**b**) The examiner's right hand gently, but firmly, hyperpronates the patient's forearm from the level of the wrist. Within this maneuver, the examiner should feel or sense a "pop"

127.6.2   Method B: Supination
(Fig. 127.3)

1. Follow the first three steps in Method A.
2. While holding the patient's wrist firmly, the operator steadily supinates the patient's forearm completely,

followed by flexing the elbow, bringing the patient's wrist up to the shoulder.
3. Return to the fifth and sixth steps in Method A.

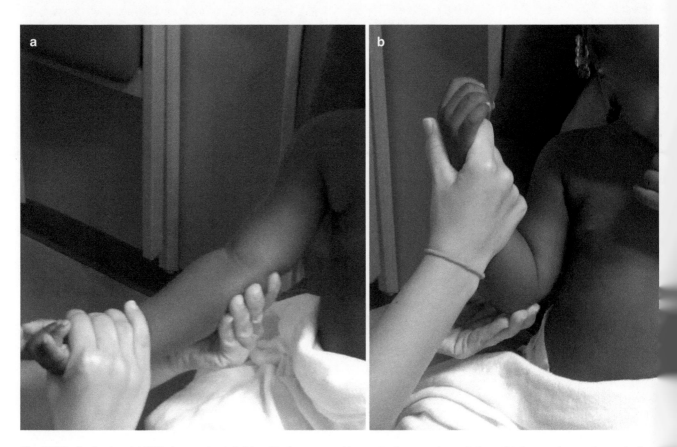

Fig. 127.3 Supination: (**a**) With the examiner's left hand in the same position as for the pronation technique, (**b**) the examiner supinates the forearm, from the level of the wrist, and fully flexes at the elbow. In either of these two maneuvers, the examiner should feel or sense a "pop"

127.7 Evaluation After Procedure

- If the child has complete use of the arm, no further intervention is required.
- If the child is still unable to supinate the forearm after 20–30 min, consider a repeat attempt at reduction.
- If there is still no return to full function after 30 min and/or repeated attempts at reduction, X-rays should be considered.
- In a child who still refuses to use the arm and X-rays are negative, the child should be reevaluated in 24 h.

127.8 Pearls and Pitfalls

- Pearls
  - Once reduced, there is rarely the need for analgesic medications. However, should the need arise, stay with ibuprofen because it is a proven anti-inflammatory.
  - If not seeing improvement within 15 min of reduction, consider this to be a fracture and obtain appropriate views of the elbow and forearm.

- Pitfalls
  - The longer the radial head has been subluxed, the longer it will take the child to return to full use.

Selected Reading

Krul M, van der Wouden JC, Koes BW, Schellevis FG, van Suijlekom-Smit LW. Nursemaid's elbow: its diagnostic clues and preferred means of reduction. J Fam Pract. 2010;59:e5–7.

Krul M, van der Wouden JC, van Suijledom-Smit LW, Koes BW. Manipulative interventions for reducing pulled elbow in young children. Cochrane Database Syst Rev. 2009;4:CD007759. doi: 10.1002/14651858.CD007759.pub2.

Macias CG, Bothner J, Wiebe R. A comparison of supination/flexion to hyperpronation in the reduction of radial head subluxations. Pediatrics. 1998;102:e10–8.

Quan L, Marcuse EK. The epidemiology and treatment of radial head subluxation. Am J Dis Child. 1985;139:1194–7.

Switzer JA, Ellis T, Swiontkowski MF. Wilderness orthopaedics. In: Auerbach PS, editor. Wilderness medicine. 5th ed. Philadelphia: Elsevier; 2007. p. 573.

Index

Springer Science+Business Media New York 2016
Ganti (ed.), *Atlas of Emergency Medicine Procedures*, DOI 10.1007/978-1-4939-2507-0